Coding for Pediatrics 2026

A Manual for Pediatric Documentation and Payment

31ST EDITION

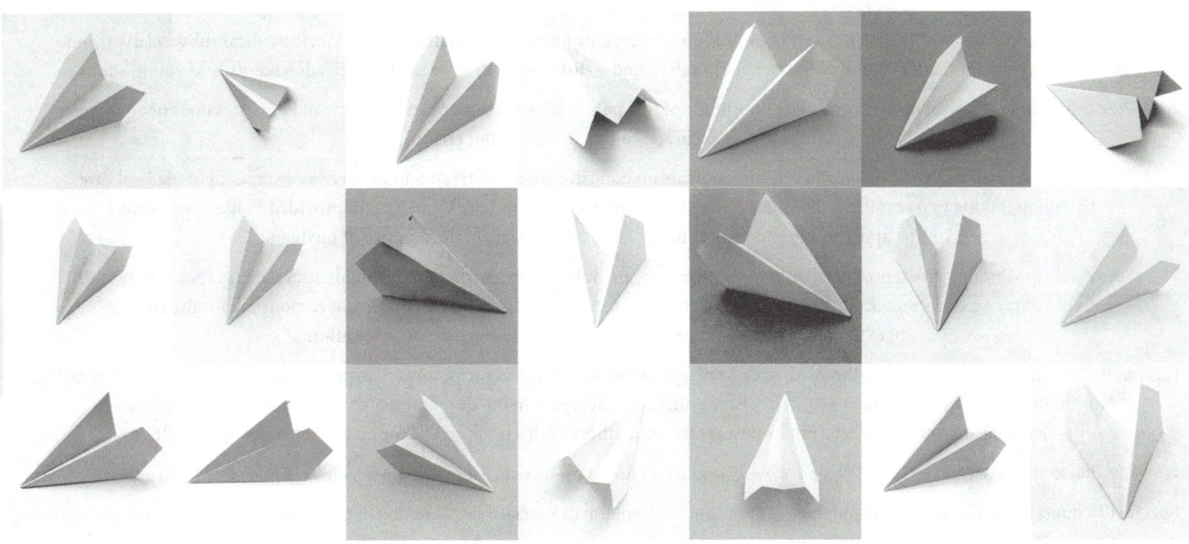

For Use With AMA *CPT® 2026* and *ICD-10-CM*

Author

Committee on Coding and Nomenclature
American Academy of Pediatrics

Editors

Editor in Chief
Linda D. Parsi, MD, MBA, CPEDC, FAAP

Associate Editors
Kathryn B. Lalor, MD, FAAP
Sheri L. Nemerofsky, MD, FAAP

American Academy of Pediatrics
DEDICATED TO THE HEALTH OF ALL CHILDREN®

American Academy of Pediatrics Publishing Staff
Mark Grimes, *Vice President, Publishing*
Laura Underhile, *Senior Editor, Professional/Clinical Publishing*
Grace Klooster, *Editor, Professional/Clinical Publishing*
Jason Crase, *Senior Manager, Production and Editorial Services*
Leesa Levin-Doroba, *Production Manager, Practice Management*
Amanda Helmholz, *Medical Copy Editor*
Peg Mulcahy, *Manager, Art Direction and Production*
Soraya Alem, *Manager, Digital Publishing*
Mary Louise Carr, MBA, *Marketing Manager, Professional Resources*

Published by the American Academy of Pediatrics
345 Park Blvd
Itasca, IL 60143
630/626-6000
www.aap.org

The American Academy of Pediatrics is an organization of 67,000 primary care pediatricians, pediatric medical subspecialists, and pediatric surgical specialists dedicated to the health, safety, and well-being of all infants, children, adolescents, and young adults.

While every effort has been made to ensure the accuracy of this publication, the American Academy of Pediatrics does not guarantee that it is accurate, complete, or without error.

The recommendations in this publication do not indicate an exclusive course of treatment or serve as a standard of medical care. Variations, taking into account individual circumstances, may be appropriate. Vignettes are provided to illustrate correct coding applications and are not intended to offer advice on the practice of medicine.

Any websites, brand names, products, or manufacturers are mentioned for informational and identification purposes only and do not imply an endorsement by the American Academy of Pediatrics (AAP). The AAP is not responsible for the content of external resources. Information was current at the time of publication.

This publication has been developed by the American Academy of Pediatrics. The contributors are expert authorities in the field of pediatrics. No commercial involvement of any kind has been solicited or accepted in the development of the content of this publication. Financial and conflict of interest disclosures for the authors of this book can be found at www.aap.org/cfp2026.

Please visit www.aap.org/cfp2026 or www.aap.org/errata for an up-to-date list of any applicable errata for this publication.

Special discounts are available for bulk purchases of this publication. Email Special Sales at nationalaccounts@aap.org for more information.

This publication has prior approval of the American Academy of Professional Coders (AAPC) for 4.0 continuing education units. Granting of this approval in no way constitutes endorsement by the AAPC of the publication content or publication sponsor.

Printed in the United States of America

11-35V 1 2 3 4 5 6 7 8 9 10

MA1192
ISBN: 978-1-61002-836-3
eBook: 978-1-61002-837-0
Print ISSN: 1537-324X
Online ISSN: 2833-4361

2025–2026 Committee on Coding and Nomenclature

2025–2026 AAP Coding Publications Editorial Advisory Board

AAP Staff

Consulting Editor

Disclaimer

Every effort has been made to include the new and revised 2026 *Current Procedural Terminology* (*CPT*®); *International Classification of Diseases, 10th Revision, Clinical Modification* (*ICD-10-CM*); and Healthcare Common Procedure Coding System (HCPCS) codes, their respective guidelines, and other revisions that might have been made. Because of our publishing deadlines and the publication date of the American Medical Association *CPT*, additional revisions and/or additional codes may have been published after the date of this printing. It is the responsibility of the reader to use this manual as a companion to the *CPT*, *ICD-10-CM*, and HCPCS publications. Vignettes are provided throughout this publication to illustrate correct coding applications. They are not intended to offer medical advice on the practice of medicine. Further, it is the reader's responsibility to routinely access the American Academy of Pediatrics website (www.aap.org/cfp2026 or www.aap.org/errata) for any errata in the published version. At the time of this publication, final changes for 2026 codes and Medicare payment policies were pending. Visit www.aap.org/coding for updates.

Copyright Acknowledgment

Contents

Foreword

This publication has prior approval of the American Academy of Professional Coders (AAPC) for 4.0 continuing education units (CEUs). Granting of this approval in no way constitutes endorsement by the AAPC of the publication content or publication sponsor. To earn your CEUs, complete the 40-question quiz online (www.aap.org/cfp2026). Click on "2026 AAPC CEU Quiz."

Online-Exclusive Content

The following online-exclusive content can be accessed at www.aap.org/cfp2026 by following the directions on the inside front cover of this book. (Readers who purchased this product as an eBook have automatic access to the content and do not need to redeem a code.)

- Asthma, Head Injury, and Laceration: Coding Continuums
- Care Management Tracking Worksheet Template
- Care Plan Oversight Billing Worksheet Template
- Centrally Inserted Central Venous Catheter: Codes for Insertion and Replacement
- Code Selection Requirements for Outpatient Evaluation and Management Service (Excluding **99211**)
- Coding Education Quiz/Continuing Education Units/Answer Key
- Common Emergency Department Procedures
- Common Office Procedures and Global Days
- Contraception: Codes for Long-Acting Reversible Contraceptives
- Contraception: Diagnosis Codes for Counseling, Initiation, and Surveillance by Method
- Critical Care Reporting in Outpatient Settings
- Echocardiography Code List
- Evaluation and Management Service Coding in Nursing and Residential Treatment Facilities
- General Documentation Checklist
- Global Per Diem Critical Care Codes: Direct Supervision and Reporting Guidelines
- Incident-to Services by Nonphysician Professionals and Clinical Staff: Medicare Requirements
- Medications for Pediatrics: Most Common
- Monthly Care Management and Care Plan Oversight Services: A Comparison
- Peripherally Inserted Central Venous Catheter: Codes
- Preventive Medicine Encounters: What's Included? (Letter Template)
- Primary and Additional Infusion Codes
- Relative Value Scale Update Committee (RUC) Times and Values for Pediatric Critical Care/Intensive Care Services
- Screening Laboratory Tests and Codes

At www.aap.org/cfp2026, you can also access links to the following American Academy of Pediatrics (AAP) coding resources:

- AAP/Bright Futures "Recommendations for Preventive Pediatric Health Care" (periodicity schedule)
- AAP Coding Hotline
- AAP coding webinars
- AAP Immunization Coding Table
- *AAP Pediatric Coding Newsletter*™
- AAP Position on Medicare Consultation Policy
- Coding fact sheets
- Coding for Standardized Assessment, Screening and Testing
- Prepare Your Office for a Payer Audit Site Visit
- Vaccine Financing and Coding
- When is it Appropriate to Report an Evaluation & Management Service During Immunization Administration?

The American Academy of Pediatrics (AAP) is pleased to publish the 31st edition of *Coding for Pediatrics*, an instructional manual and reference tool for use by primary care pediatricians, pediatric subspecialists, and others involved in the provision and reporting of care provided to children. This manual supports the delivery of quality care to children by providing the pediatric practitioner with the knowledge to best support appropriate business practices. This edition includes the 2026 *Current Procedural Terminology* (*CPT*®) code changes with guidelines for their application.

This edition introduces a range of new codes and guidelines, including new codes for reporting immunization counseling services when immunizations are not administered on the same date, remote physiologic monitoring treatment management services of 10 to 20 minutes, new and revised codes for immunization products including for clesrovimab (monoclonal antibody for passive immunization against respiratory syncytial virus), and percutaneous electrical nerve field stimulation of the cranial nerves, without implantation, used in treatment of functional abdominal pain disorders. In addition, this manual provides pediatric-specific guidance and examples of documentation and code selection using current coding guidelines for evaluation and management (E/M) and other procedural services.

For ease of reference, *Coding for Pediatrics 2026* is divided into the following parts:

- **Part 1, Coding Basics and Business Essentials**, includes information on code sets, modifiers, compliance, and business topics such as billing and payment methodologies.
- **Part 2, Primarily for the Office and Other Outpatient Settings**, includes information on coding and billing for services such as office visits, outpatient consultations, and preventive services.
- **Part 3, Primarily for Hospital Settings**, includes information on coding for facility-based services including emergency department and other hospital E/M services and surgical procedures.
- **Part 4, Digital Medicine Services**, includes discussion of the evolving codes for reporting telemedicine services and remote monitoring and interpretation of patient data.
- A quick reference to *International Classification of Diseases, 10th Revision, Clinical Modification* (*ICD-10-CM*) code changes applicable to pediatrics is provided in **Appendix I**.
- **A continuing education quiz** to earn 4.0 continuing education units from the American Academy of Professional Coders is included at www.aap.org/cfp2026.
- Supplemental material providing a wealth of information can be found on the *Coding for Pediatrics* website (www.aap.org/cfp2026).

Each chapter includes "Test Your Knowledge!" questions (answers are in **Appendix II**). Additionally, resources for more information on each chapter's contents can be located at the end of chapter.

The AAP is also pleased to offer *Coding for Pediatrics 2026* as an eBook on a searchable platform.

Coding for Pediatrics 2026 does not replace *CPT*, *ICD-10-CM*, or the Healthcare Common Procedure Coding System; rather, it supplements those manuals. Every effort has been made to include the 2026 codes and their respective guidelines; however, revised codes and/or guidelines may have been published after the date of this printing. Errata to this manual will be posted as appropriate on the *Coding for Pediatrics* website (www.aap.org/cfp2026) and www.aap.org/errata.

The AAP actively works with the American Medical Association (AMA) *CPT* Editorial Panel and the AMA/Specialty Society Relative Value Scale Update Committee (RUC) to develop pediatric specialty codes and assign them appropriate relative value units. Since 1995, the AAP has contributed to the process that evaluates and reviews changes to the Medicare Resource-Based Relative Value Scale (RBRVS). Pediatricians have been actively involved in the RUC process to develop work valuation and direct practice expense input recommendations for all existing codes. The AAP is also represented on the AMA *CPT* Editorial Panel and on the *ICD-10-CM* Editorial Advisory Board. The AAP continues to be involved in all areas of payment. The AAP Committee on Coding and Nomenclature oversees all areas of coding related to pediatrics, including *CPT* procedure coding, *ICD-10-CM* diagnosis coding, and the valuation of *CPT* services through the Medicare RBRVS.

The AAP will continue to request new code changes and attempt to expeditiously notify membership of changes through various means.

- The *AAP Pediatric Coding Newsletter*™, a monthly newsletter available in print and online formats, provides up-to-date coding and payment information. The newsletter and other online resources can be accessed through the *AAP Pediatric Coding Newsletter* website (https://publications.aap.org/codingnews).
- AAP coding seminars presented at the AAP National Conference & Exhibition (https://aapexperience.org).
- AAP coding webinars (https://publications.aap.org/codingnews/resources/27969).
- *AAP News*™, including the Coding Corner (https://publications.aap.org/search-results?f_ArticleTypeDisplayName=Coding+Corner).
- *Pediatric ICD-10-CM 2026: A Manual for Provider-Based Coding* (www.aap.org/Pediatric-ICD-10-CM-2026-11th-Edition-Paperback).

- *Pediatric Evaluation and Management Coding Revisions: Facility and Office Services* (www.aap.org/Pediatric-Evaluation-and-Management-Coding-Revisions-Facility-and-Office-Services-Paperback).
- AAP coding cards (www.aap.org/en/shopaap/shop-by-topic/coding).

Use of these resources should provide pediatricians with the skills needed to report their services appropriately. The AAP Pediatric Health Care Systems & Finance Transformation staff stands ready to assist with coding problems and questions not covered in this manual. The AAP Coding and Payment Hotline can be found at www.aap.org/en/practice-management/child-health-finance-payment-strategy/coding-payment-hotline.

Acknowledgments

Coding for Pediatrics 2026 is the product of the efforts of many dedicated individuals.

Our mission is to make coding easier to understand so pediatric providers can continue to serve children well. We have sought to make this book easier to understand by categorizing care areas and by using many examples (vignettes) of different coding situations. This knowledge is key to helping all pediatric providers stay in compliance and correctly code with confidence. We hope you enjoy reading this book, and we will continue to strive to always serve you with excellence.

This work has been made immeasurably easier and the final edition dramatically improved by the dedicated work of many collaborators. First and foremost, I must thank Cindy Hughes, CPC, CFPC, consulting editor, for her professional input. Additionally, I must thank the Committee on Coding and Nomenclature (COCN) support staff at the American Academy of Pediatrics (AAP), particularly Stefanie Muntean-Turner, CPC, CPMA, for her review of major portions of the project. Thank you also to Teri Salus, MPA, CPC, CPEDC, for her contributions and advice regarding new *Current Procedural Terminology* (*CPT*®) codes. I would also like to thank the members of COCN and the AAP Coding Publications Editorial Advisory Board. The members of these groups have each contributed extensive time in reviewing and updating content in the manual.

None of this work is possible without the support of the COCN members who work tirelessly to develop and value codes and fight for pediatrics "at the table." The committee strives to keep pediatrics at the forefront of coding and valuation. The excellent teams that follow are truly experts in these areas and are devoted to representing the AAP and its members:

***CPT* Editorial Panel Advisory Committee Team**
Renee F. Slade, MD, FAAP (*CPT* Advisor)
Kathryn B. Lalor, MD, FAAP (*CPT* Alternate Advisor)
Teri Salus, MPA, CPC, CPEDC (AAP Staff to *CPT*)

American Medical Association/Specialty Society Relative Value Scale Update Committee (RUC) Team
Steven E. Krug, MD, FAAP (RUC Advisor)
Margie C. Andreae, MD, FAAP (RUC Representative)
Eileen D. Brewer, MD, FAAP (RUC Alternate Representative)
Marsha Schofield, MS, RD, LD, FAND (AAP RUC Consultant)

***International Classification of Diseases* (*ICD*) Team**
Jeffrey F. Linzer Sr, MD, FAAP (AAP Representative to *ICD*)
Edward A. Liechty, MD, FAAP (AAP Alternate Representative to *ICD*)
Stefanie Muntean-Turner, CPC, CPMA (AAP Staff to *ICD*)

I am most grateful to the invaluable input of the following AAP committees and individuals:

- Committee on Medical Liability and Risk Management, specifically Steve Bondi, JD, MD; David Horowitz, MD; and AAP staff Teresa Salaway, senior health policy analyst, Child Health Finance & Quality
- Committee on Child Health Financing, specifically Alison Amidei Galbraith, MD, FAAP
- Section on Neonatal-Perinatal Medicine coding trainers

In addition, we reached out to other AAP members for their expertise on specific content areas.

This project would not have been completed were it not for the outstanding work of AAP staff. In Membership, Marketing, and Publishing, Laura Underhile, senior editor, professional/clinical publishing; Grace Klooster, editor, professional/clinical publishing; Jason Crase, senior manager, production and editorial services; Leesa Levin-Doroba, production manager, practice management; Amanda Helmholz, medical copy editor; Peg Mulcahy, manager, art direction and production; Soraya Alem, manager, digital publishing; and Mary Louise Carr, MBA, marketing manager, professional resources deserve special recognition for their outstanding skill and dedication to this project. I especially appreciate the support and professional expertise of AAP staff support to the AAP COCN, dedicated advocates for all of us who medically care for children.

These are challenging times for pediatric physicians, but this manual has been developed to provide guidance on coding that is necessary to gain payment, show quality, and demonstrate the value of pediatric care. We are deeply dedicated to serving children and would like to give a big thank-you to all our readers, billers, coders, medical team, and dedicated pediatric providers who work tirelessly around the clock to best care for all children. Your work inspires us to work very hard behind the scenes to provide you with the latest and most accurate coding information. We are always open to ideas to better serve you and welcome your suggestions. By all of us working together, we can accomplish the highest standards of care and be a voice for our children and their future.

Respectfully,
Linda D. Parsi, MD, MBA, CPEDC, FAAP
Editor in Chief, COCN Editorial Advisory Board

Quick Reference to 2026 *CPT*® Pediatric Code Changes

We have made every effort to include changes to procedures and services that apply to pediatric practices. Revisions and/or additional codes, however, may have been published after the date of this printing. This list does not include all changes made to *Current Procedural Terminology* (*CPT*) *2026*. Additionally, not all codes included in the quick reference table are further discussed in this publication, typically because of their limited use by most pediatricians. Always refer to *CPT 2026* for a complete listing of new codes, complete descriptions, and revisions. For questions or additional information on codes not discussed in this publication, please contact the American Academy of Pediatrics Coding and Payment Hotline (www.aap.org/en/practice-management/child-health-finance-payment-strategy/coding-payment-hotline). Any errata to *CPT 2026* will be posted to the American Medical Association website (www.ama-assn.org/practice-management/cpt/errata-technical-corrections). These changes take effect January 1, 2026. Do not report the changes or codes before that date.

Quick Reference to 2026 *CPT* Pediatric Code Changes	
In revised codes, use of underlined font (eg, first or only component of each vaccine administered) in a code descriptor indicates new text. Text that is shown with strike-through font (eg, ~~2 dose schedule~~) indicates a deletion of text from the code descriptor.	
2025	**2026**
Category III (Emerging Technology)	
No specific code	The following codes were released December 30, 2024; implemented July 1, 2025; and published in *CPT 2026:* ●**0973T** Selective enzymatic debridement, partial-thickness and/or full-thickness burn eschar, requiring anesthesia (ie, general anesthesia, moderate sedation), including patient monitoring, trunk, arms, legs; first 100 sq cm +●**0974T** each additional 100 sq cm ●**0975T** Selective enzymatic debridement, partial-thickness and/or full-thickness burn eschar, requiring anesthesia (ie, general anesthesia, moderate sedation), including patient monitoring, scalp, neck, hands, feet, and/or multiple digits; first 100 sq cm ●**0976T** each additional 100 sq cm
Immunization (Codes for vaccines, toxoids, and immunoglobulins are released in April, July, and October with implementation at ≤3 or 6 months following release or upon authorization for use by the FDA when approved for immediate release.)	
No specific code	The following code was released April 1, 2025; implemented July 1, 2025; and published in *CPT 2026:* ●**90382** RSV, monoclonal antibody, seasonal dose, 0.7 mL, for IM use
#▲**90480** IA by IM injection, of severe acute respiratory syndrome coronavirus 2 (SARS-CoV-2) (coronavirus disease [COVID-19]) vaccine, single dose	An errata to *CPT 2025* removed the symbol for resequenced code (#) from **90480**. ▲**90480** IA by IM injection, of severe acute respiratory syndrome coronavirus 2 (SARS-CoV-2) (coronavirus disease [COVID-19]) vaccine; first or only component of each vaccine administered #+●**90481** each additional component administered
No specific code	The following code was released October 18, 2024; implemented January 1, 2025; and published in *CPT 2026:* #●**90593** Chikungunya virus vaccine, recombinant, for IM use
#**90620** Meningococcal recombinant protein and outer membrane vesicle vaccine, serogroup B (MenB-4C), 2 dose schedule, for IM use	The following code revision was released April 1, 2025; implemented July 1, 2025; and published in *CPT 2026:* ▲**90620** Meningococcal recombinant protein and outer membrane vesicle vaccine, serogroup B (MenB-4C), 2 dose schedule, for IM use
No specific code	The following code was released April 1, 2025; implemented July 1, 2025; and published in *CPT 2026:* #●**90635** Influenza virus vaccine, H5N1, derived from cell cultures, adjuvanted, for IM use

Continued on next page

Quick Reference to 2026 *CPT* Pediatric Code Changes (*continued*)	
Immunization (*continued*)	
No specific code	⚡#●**90612** Influenza virus vaccine (IIV), H5, pandemic formulation, split virus, adjuvanted, for IM use
No specific code	The following codes were released April 1, 2025; implemented July 1, 2025; and published in *CPT 2026:* ⚡#●**90612** Influenza virus vaccine, trivalent, and severe acute respiratory syndrome coronavirus 2 (SARS-CoV-2) (coronavirus disease [COVID-19]) vaccine, mRNA-LNP, 31.7 mcg/0.32 mL dosage, for IM use ⚡#●**90613** Influenza virus vaccine, quadrivalent, and severe acute respiratory syndrome coronavirus 2 (SARS-CoV-2) (coronavirus disease [COVID-19]) vaccine, mRNA-LNP, 40 mcg/0.4 mL dosage, for IM use
No specific code	The following code was released April 1, 2025; implemented July 1, 2025; and published in *CPT 2026:* ⚡#●**91323** Severe acute respiratory syndrome coronavirus 2 (SARS-CoV-2) (coronavirus disease [COVID-19]) vaccine, mRNA-LNP, 10 mcg/0.2 mL dosage, for IM use
Immunization Counseling	
No specific code	★●◀**90482** Immunization counseling by physician or other QHP when immunization(s) is not administered by provider on the same date of service; 3 minutes up to 10 minutes ★●◀**90483** greater than 10 minutes up to 20 minutes ★●◀**90484** greater than 20 minutes
Integumentary	
10040 Acne surgery (eg, marsupialization, opening or removal of multiple milia, comedones, cysts, pustules)	▲**10040** Extraction (eg, marsupialization, opening or removal of multiple milia, comedones, cysts, pustules)
Laboratory	
No specific code	●**87812** Infectious agent antigen detection by immunoassay with direct optical (ie, visual) observation; severe acute respiratory syndrome coronavirus 2 (SARS-CoV-2) (coronavirus disease [COVID-19]) and influenza virus types A and B
No specific code	●**87494** Infectious agent detection by nucleic acid (DNA or RNA); *Chlamydia trachomatis* and *Neisseria gonorrhoeae*, multiplex amplified probe technique
No specific code	●**81354** Cytogenomic (genome-wide) analysis for constitutional chromosomal abnormalities; interrogation of structural and copy number variants, optical genome mapping
~~No specific code~~	~~●**86XX1** *Streptococcus pneumoniae* antibody (IgG), serotypes, multiplex immunoassay, quantitative~~
Mechanical Scalp Cooling Services	
Deleted for services on and after January 1, 2026 **0662T** Scalp cooling, mechanical; initial measurement and calibration of cap +**0663T** placement of device, monitoring, and removal of device	●**97007** Mechanical scalp cooling, including individual cap supply with head measurement, fitting, and patient education ●**97008** Mechanical scalp cooling, including hair preparation, individual cap placement, therapy initiation, and pre-cooling period +●**97009** scalp cooling provided after discontinuation of chemotherapy, each 30 minutes

Quick Reference to 2026 *CPT* Pediatric Code Changes (*continued*)	
Musculoskeletal	
No specific code	#●27458 Osteotomy(ies), femur, unilateral, with insertion of an externally controlled intramedullary lengthening device, including iliotibial band release when performed, imaging, alignment assessments, computations of adjustment schedules, and management of the intramedullary lengthening device
No specific code	#●27713 Osteotomy(ies), tibia, including fibula when performed, unilateral, with insertion of an externally controlled intramedullary lengthening device, including imaging, alignment assessments, computations of adjustment schedules, and management of the intramedullary lengthening device
27468 Osteoplasty, femur; combined, lengthening and shortening with femoral segment transfer	Deleted (Procedure is seldom provided. When performed, report distinct codes for each osteoplasty of bilateral femurs.)
Modifiers	
33 **Preventive Services:** When the primary purpose of the service is the delivery of an evidence-based service in accordance with a USPSTF A or B rating in effect and other preventive services identified in preventive services mandates (legislative or regulatory), the service may be identified by adding 33 to the procedure. For separately reported services specifically identified as preventive, the modifier should not be used.	33 **Preventive Services:** When the primary purpose of the service is the delivery of an evidence-based service in accordance with a USPSTF A or B rating in effect or is another preventive service identified in preventive services mandates (legislative or regulatory), the service may be identified by adding 33 to the procedure. For separately reported services specifically identified as preventive, the modifier should not be used.
Nervous System	
Deleted in 2026 0720T Percutaneous electrical nerve field stimulation, cranial nerves, without implantation	●64567 Percutaneous electrical nerve field stimulation, cranial nerves, without implantation
Pulmonary Medicine	
94662 Continuous negative pressure ventilation, initiation and management	Deleted in 2026
Remote Monitoring Services	
#99453 Remote monitoring of physiologic parameter(s) (eg, weight, blood pressure, pulse oximetry, respiratory flow rate), initial; set-up and patient education on use of equipment #99454 Remote monitoring of physiologic parameter(s) (eg, weight, blood pressure, pulse oximetry, respiratory flow rate), initial; device(s) supply with daily recording(s) or programmed alert(s) transmission, each 30 days	#▲99453 Remote monitoring of physiologic parameter(s) (eg, weight, blood pressure, pulse oximetry, respiratory flow rate); initial set-up and patient education on use of equipment #●99445 device(s) supply with daily recording(s) or programmed alert(s) transmission, 2–15 days in a 30-day period #▲99454 device(s) supply with daily recording(s) or programmed alert(s) transmission, 16–30 days in a 30-day period
#99457 Remote physiologic monitoring treatment management services, clinical staff/physician/other QHP time in a calendar month requiring interactive communication with the patient/caregiver during the month; first 20 minutes #✚▲99458 each additional 20 minutes	#●99470 Remote physiologic monitoring treatment management services, clinical staff/physician/other QHP time in a calendar month requiring 1 real-time interactive communication with the patient/caregiver during the calendar month; first 10 minutes #▲99457 first 20 minutes #✚▲99458 each additional 20 minutes (*unchanged from 2025*)

Continued on next page

Quick Reference to 2026 *CPT* Pediatric Code Changes (*continued*)

Remote Monitoring Services (*continued*)	
▲98975 Remote therapeutic monitoring (eg, therapy adherence, therapy response, digital therapeutic intervention); initial set-up and patient education on use of equipment	98975 is unchanged in 2026. #●98984 device(s) supply for data access or data transmissions to support monitoring of respiratory system, 2–15 days in a 30-day period
▲98976 device(s) supply for data access or data transmissions to support monitoring of respiratory system, each 30 days	▲98976 device(s) supply for data access or data transmissions to support monitoring of respiratory system, 16–30 days in a 30-day period #●98985 device(s) supply for data access or data transmissions to support monitoring of musculoskeletal system, 2–15 days in a 30-day period
▲98977 device(s) supply for data access or data transmissions to support monitoring of musculoskeletal system, each 30 days	▲98977 device(s) supply for data access or data transmissions to support monitoring of musculoskeletal system, 16–30 days in a 30-day period #●98986 device(s) supply for data access or data transmissions to support monitoring of cognitive behavioral therapy, 2–15 days in a 30-day period
▲98978 device(s) supply for data access or data transmissions to support monitoring of cognitive behavioral therapy, each 30 days	▲98978 device(s) supply for data access or data transmissions to support monitoring of cognitive behavioral therapy, 16–30 days in a 30-day period
	●98979 Remote therapeutic monitoring treatment management services, physician/other QHP time in a calendar month requiring at least 1 real-time interactive communication with the patient/caregiver during the calendar month; first 10 minutes
98980 Remote therapeutic monitoring treatment management services, physician or other QHP time in a calendar month requiring at least one interactive communication with the patient or caregiver during the calendar month; first 20 minutes	▲98980 first 20 minutes
+98981 each additional 20 minutes	+▲98981 each additional 20 minutes (*unchanged from 2025*)

Abbreviations: *CPT, Current Procedural Terminology*; FDA, US Food and Drug Administration; IA, immunization administration; IM, intramuscular; QHP, qualified health care professional; RSV, respiratory syncytial virus; USPSTF, US Preventive Services Task Force.

⚡ indicates pending US FDA approval.

How to Use This Manual

Step 1. Use the table of contents or the index to locate information on specific services, codes, or broader subjects. (If unfamiliar with codes and conventions, read **Chapter 1** to learn important information on the use of each code set.)	**Contents** An Introduction to the Official Code Sets........... 5 Telling the Encounter Story.......................... 6
Step 2. Use chapter content to review code descriptors and instructions for reporting. Before reporting, verify current codes and complete selection and reporting instructions in the appropriate code set manual or application.	**99238** Hospital inpatient or observation discharge day management; 30 minutes or less on the date of the encounter **99239** more than 30 minutes on the date of the encounter • Same date admission and discharge services for a patient stay of 8 hours or more, performed at 2 distinct encounters, are reported with **99234–99236**. • For admission and discharge services provided during a stay of less than 8 hours, report only **99221–99223**.
Step 3. Examples are used as guidance on meeting the criteria specified by codes and reporting instructions. However, note that codes must be assigned based on the service provided and supporting documentation.	➤ **A 14-month-old new patient presents following an ED encounter for complex febrile seizure.** ***Problem(s) addressed*** ➡ ***Moderate*** (undiagnosed new problem with uncertain prognosis) **Teaching Point:** Differential diagnoses for the complex febrile seizure include possibility of epilepsy resulting from a brain lesion or other life-threatening cause.
Step 4. Note highlights and takeaways in each chapter.	• The 4 code sets that are used for reporting professional services are *ICD-10-CM*, HCPCS, *CPT*, and the NDC.
Step 5. Resources for additional information are listed at the end of each chapter and are included at www.aap.org/cfp2026.	
Step 6. Although every effort is made to provide accurate and up-to-date coding guidance, changes do happen. Any corrections and code or instruction changes published subsequent to the date of this printing are included at www.aap.org/cfp2026 or www.aap.org/errata.	

Coding for Pediatrics 2026 Road Map

This road map was developed to help you quickly locate information in *Coding for Pediatrics 2026* by selecting your specialty and/or setting. Results are sorted into essential information and supplemental information to help find your relevant coding content.

Coding for Pediatrics 2026 Road Map

Find your applicable *CFP* chapters by specialty, and/or setting.

American Academy of Pediatrics
DEDICATED TO THE HEALTH OF ALL CHILDREN®

Part	1. Coding Basics and Business Essentials						2. Office and Other Outpatient Settings							3. Hospital Settings[a]					4. Digital Medicine		
Chapter	1. Coding Basics	2. Edits/ Modifiers	3. Quality/ Value	4. Payment Systems	5. Fraud/ Abuse	6. E/M Documentation	7. Non-Preventive E/M	8. Preventive Services	9. Chronic/ Complex Conditions	10. Mental/ Behavioral Health	11. Testing/ Therapeutic Services	12. NQHCP Services	13. Surgery/ Infusion/ Sedation	14. Emergency Dept	15. Newborn Care	16. Non-critical E/M	17. Critical/ Intensive Care	18. Surgery/ Sedation	19. Telemedicine Concepts	20. Outpatient Telemedicine/ Digital	21. Remote Data Collection/ Monitoring
Setting																					
Hospital[a]	◆	—	—	—	—	→								◆	—	—	—	→	◆	—	→
Outpatient	◆	—	—	—	—	→	◆	—	—	—	—	—	→				◆		◆	—	→
Specialty																					
Adolescent medicine	◆	—	—	—	—	→	◆	◆			◆		◆						◆	—	→
Allergy and immunology	◆	—	—	—	—	→	◆		◆	—	→								◆	◆	
Anesthesia/Pain	◆	—	—	—	—	→	◆						◆					◆			◆
Cardiology	◆	—	—	—	—	→	◆		◆		◆		◆		◆	—	—	→	◆	—	→
Dermatology	◆	—	—	—	—	→	◆		◆				◆						◆	—	→
Developmental and behavioral pediatrics	◆	—	—	—	—	→	◆	—	—	—	→								◆	◆	
Emergency medicine	◆	—	—	—	—	→							◆	◆			◆	◆	◆	◆	
Endocrinology	◆	—	—	—	—	→	◆		◆			◆							◆	—	→
Gastroenterology	◆	—	—	—	—	→	◆						◆			◆		◆	◆	—	→
General pediatrics	◆	—	—	—	—	→	◆	—	—	—	—	—	→		◆	◆			◆	—	→
Hematology-oncology	◆	—	—	—	—	→	◆		◆				◆		◆	◆		◆	◆	—	→
Hospital medicine	◆	—	—	—	—	→							◆		◆	—	—	→	◆	—	→
Infectious diseases	◆	—	—	—	—	→	◆		◆				◆			◆	◆		◆	◆	
Intensive care medicine	◆	—	—	—	—	→							◆			◆	◆		◆	◆	
Neonatology	◆	—	—	—	—	→							◆				◆	◆	◆	◆	
Nephrology	◆	—	—	—	—	→	◆		◆		◆				◆	—	—	→	◆	◆	
NQHCP[b]	◆	—	—	—	→					◆	—	→							◆		
Neurology	◆	—	—	—	—	→	◆		◆		◆		◆		◆	◆		◆	◆	◆	
Orthopedics	◆	—	—	—	—	→	◆		◆		◆					◆	◆		◆	—	→
Otolaryngology	◆	—	—	—	—	→	◆		◆		◆		◆			◆		◆	◆	—	→
Physical medicine/ Rehabilitation	◆	—	—	—	—	→	◆				◆	◆				◆			◆	—	→
Pulmonology	◆	—	—	—	—	→	◆		◆		◆	◆			◆	—	→		◆	—	→
Rheumatology	◆	—	—	—	—	→	◆		◆		◆		◆			◆			◆	◆	
Surgery	◆	—	—	—	—	→	◆						◆		◆	—	→	◆	◆	◆	
Urology	◆	—	—	—	—	→	◆		◆		◆		◆		◆	◆		◆	◆	◆	

Abbreviations: *CFP, Coding for Pediatrics*; dept, department; E/M, evaluation and management; NQHCP, nonphysician qualified health care professional.
◆ indicates the chapters that include coding content most relevant to specialty services. Find reference to specific codes and topics in the index.
[a] Hospital setting here references services commonly provided in emergency department, inpatient, and observation settings. This may also include surgery centers and stand-alone emergency facilities. This does not refer to physician services provided in clinician-based settings such as an outpatient clinic owned by a health system.
[b] NQHCPs include nonphysician clinicians such as dietitians, medical nutritionists, psychologists, clinical social workers, and other clinicians who may independently report services within their state-defined scope of practice.

Part 1

Coding Basics and Business Essentials

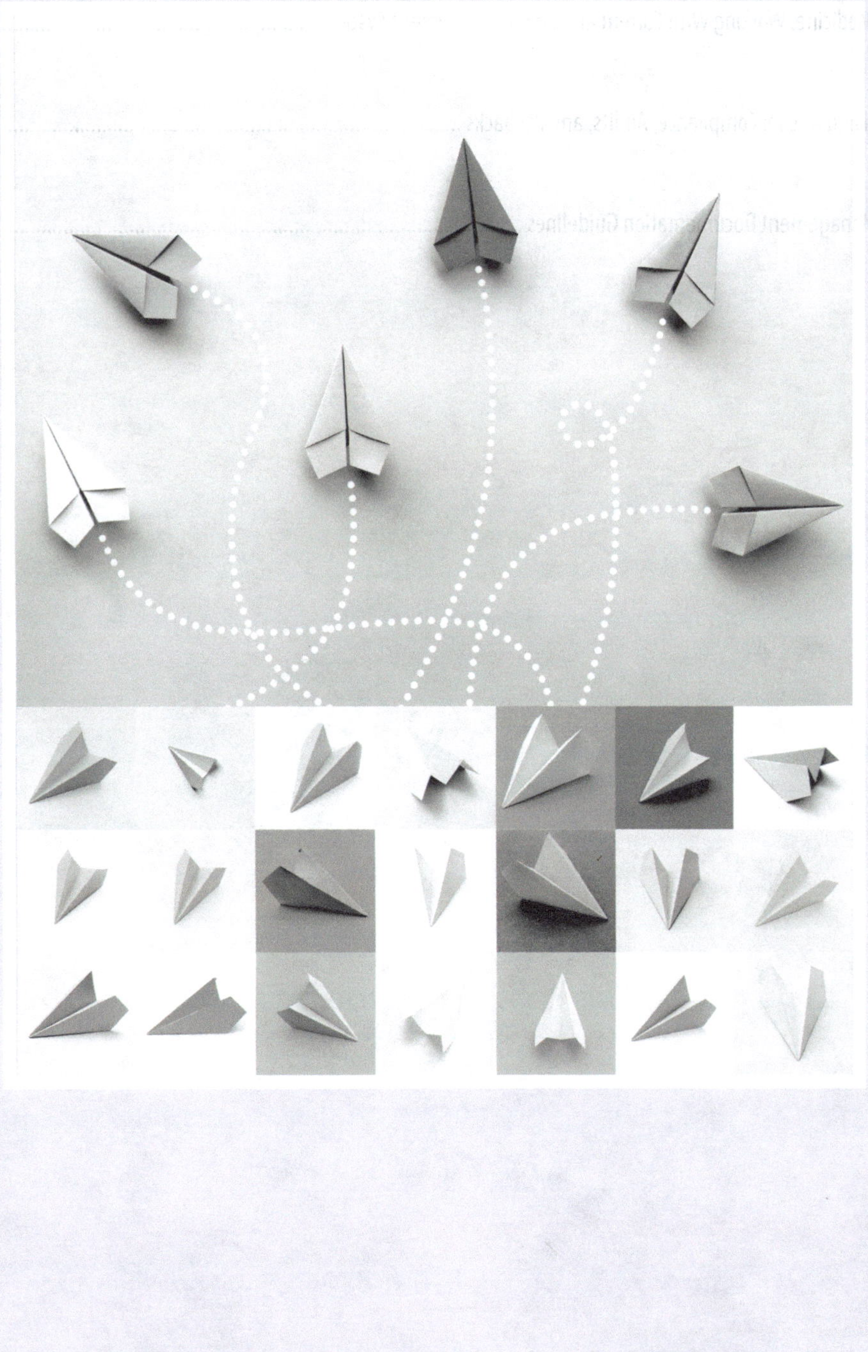

Part 1. Coding Basics and Business Essentials

CHAPTER 1

The Basics of Coding

Contents

Chapter Highlights

- The 4 code sets primarily used by physicians and other qualified health care professionals (QHPs) to report professional services
- Codes for conveying information to a payer in lieu of submitting actual documentation of an encounter or a service
- The structure and general conventions of each code set
- Important considerations for selecting and transferring codes to claims

An Introduction to the Official Code Sets

This chapter introduces the official code sets used for reporting pediatric professional services and briefly discusses the guidelines and conventions of each code set. Refer to *Pediatric Coding Basics: An Introduction to Medical Coding* for more information on each code set.

In the United States, the Health Insurance Portability and Accountability Act (HIPAA) of 1996 requires the use of 5 specific code sets for the purpose of health care transactions. The 4 code sets primarily used by physicians and other QHPs are listed in **Table 1-1**. The fifth designated code set, *Code on Dental Procedures and Nomenclature,* is primarily used to report dental procedures to dental insurance plans.

Table 1-1. Health Insurance Portability and Accountability Act of 1996 Code Sets

Code Set and Reporting Purpose	Examples	Code Set Implementation Schedule
ICD-10-CM Diagnoses and other reasons for encounters	**E66.811** Obesity, class 1 **Z68.54** Body mass index [BMI] pediatric, ≥95th percentile for age to less than 120% of the 95th percentile for age	Semiannually, April 1 and October 1
CPT[a] Most professional services, immunization products, and performance measurement tracking	**99470** Remote physiologic monitoring treatment management services, clinical staff/physician/other QHP time in a calendar month requiring 1 real-time interactive communication with the patient/caregiver during the calendar month; first 10 minutes **99457** first 20 minutes **99458** each additional 20 minutes **90382** RSV, monoclonal antibody, seasonal dose, 0.7 mL, for intramuscular use **3044F** Most recent hemoglobin A1c (HbA1c) level less than 7% (DM)	Category I—Annually January 1 except • Immunization—January 1, July 1, and October 1, or codes designated for rapid or immediate implementation • Proprietary laboratory analyses—January 1, April 1, and July 1 • Molecular pathology tier 2 and administrative multianalyte assays with algorithmic analyses—January 1, July 1, and October 1 Category II—January 1 Category III—January 1, July 1
HCPCS[b] Supplies, medications, some services and quality measures	**Q4010** Cast supplies, short arm cast, adult (11 years +), fiberglass **J0165** Injection, epinephrine, not otherwise specified, 0.1 mg	Annually—January 1—and quarterly for temporary codes January 1, April 1, July 1, and October 1
NDC Specific prescription drug, vaccine, and insulin products and dosages	49281-0575-00 Respiratory syncytial virus (RSV) monoclonal antibody, IgG1κ, (nirsevimab-alip), 0.5 mL, neonates and children to 24 months (Beyfortus, Sanofi Pasteur)	Required with any change to the product (eg, product name, dosage, composition, packaging)

Abbreviations: CMS, Centers for Medicare & Medicaid Services; *CPT, Current Procedural Terminology;* DM, diabetes mellitus; HCPCS, Healthcare Common Procedure Coding System; *ICD-10-CM, International Classification of Diseases, 10th Revision, Clinical Modification;* NDC, National Drug Code; QHP, qualified health care professional.

[a] Also known as Level I of the HCPCS code set.

[b] Refers to Level II HCPCS codes assigned by the CMS. HCPCS codes are reported for services only when a *CPT* code does not describe the service as covered by health plan benefits.

Code sets facilitate communication of standardized health information for purposes such as prior authorization of medical care and submission of health care claims in pediatric practice. Understanding the purpose and constructs of the 4 code sets used by physicians is important for successful interactions with health plans and supports accurate health care statistics.

New and revised codes are listed as quick references on **pages XIII to XVI** and in **Appendix I**.

- Quick Reference to 2026 *CPT* Pediatric Code Changes (effective with services provided on or after January 1, 2026)
- Quick Reference to 2026 *ICD-10-CM* Pediatric Code Changes (effective with services provided on or after October 1, 2025)

The place of service (POS) code set, maintained by the Centers for Medicare & Medicaid Services (CMS), is an additional code set that is required on claims. POS codes are 2-digit codes that identify the setting (eg, 11 office) in which a service was provided such that a claims system can differentiate sites of service to apply payer policies and payment differentials (eg, facility or non-facility relative value units [RVUs]). Practice management and billing systems often automatically assign POS codes based on the site of service selected during charge entry. Refer to **Chapter 4** for more information on POS codes.

Telling the Encounter Story

Because physicians do not submit full documentation, various code sets and other supportive information (eg, procedure code modifiers) tell payers what happened and what is represented by the fees listed on each claim line (**Table 1-2**).

Codes submitted on a claim tell the story of what happened during a patient encounter. Yet documentation of an encounter must support the codes assigned for each diagnosis and service and may be requested by a payer to support the accuracy of code assignment. The following 7 general principles of documentation apply to all services:

1. The medical record should be complete and legible.
2. The documentation of each patient encounter should include
   - Reason for the encounter and relevant history, physical examination findings, and prior diagnostic test results
   - Assessment, clinical impression, or diagnosis
   - Plan for care
   - Date and legible identity of the observer
3. If not documented, the rationale for ordering diagnostic and other ancillary services should be easily inferred.
4. Past and present diagnoses should be accessible to the treating and/or consulting physician.
5. Appropriate health risk factors should be identified. Social determinants of health (SDoH) should be documented.
6. The patient's progress, response to and changes in treatment, and revision of diagnosis should be documented.
7. The *Current Procedural Terminology* (*CPT*) and *International Classification of Diseases, 10th Revision, Clinical Modification* (*ICD-10-CM*) codes reported on the health insurance claim form or billing statement should be supported by the documentation in the medical record.

Table 1-2. The Encounter Story Told Through Codes

Code or Modifier	Information Provided
ICD-10-CM	Why were services rendered?
CPT/HCPCS	What services or supplies were provided?
Modifier	Was something about the service altered or not routine?
NDC	Which medicine or immunization product and dosage were administered?

Abbreviations: *CPT, Current Procedural Terminology;* HCPCS, Healthcare Common Procedure Coding System; *ICD-10-CM, International Classification of Diseases, 10th Revision, Clinical Modification;* NDC, National Drug Code.

International Classification of Diseases, 10th Revision, Clinical Modification

ICD-10-CM codes, which physicians use to assign diagnoses and other reasons for encounters, are used in payment and public health data.

Updates to *ICD-10-CM* are implemented each April 1 and October 1. New codes are published a few months before implementation.

The American Hospital Association (AHA) Editorial Advisory Board for *Coding Clinic for ICD-10-CM and ICD-10-PCS* performs oversight and resolution of coding questions related to *ICD-10-CM*. Public-private "cooperating parties" participate in this as well: the CMS, National Center for Health Statistics, AHA, and American Health Information Management Association. The granularity and specificity in *ICD-10-CM* is implemented at the specific request of certain medical societies. Clinical diagnosis codes are not added for payment purposes.

The American Academy of Pediatrics (AAP) holds a seat on the editorial advisory board. Findings are published quarterly by the AHA in *Coding Clinic. ICD-10-CM* codes and accompanying guidelines and findings by the editorial advisory board are part of the standard transaction code sets under HIPAA and must be recognized by all payers. For *ICD-10-CM,* the hierarchy of official coding guidelines and instructions is as follows:

1. *ICD-10-CM* alphabetical index and tabular list
2. *Official Guidelines for Coding and Reporting*
3. AHA *Coding Clinic* advice

Pediatricians who have suggestions for changes to new or existing *ICD-10-CM* codes related to pediatric care are encouraged to forward their suggestions to coding staff at the AAP headquarters. The AAP staff and advisor who are involved in the process can be of great assistance. To contact the AAP coding staff, complete the form at www.aap.org/en/practice-management/child-health-finance-payment-strategy/coding-payment-hotline.

The United States is currently evaluating implementation of *International Classification of Diseases, 11th Revision* (*ICD-11*), which has been adopted by more than 70 countries worldwide. The National Committee on Vital and Health Statistics (NCVHS) has formed a work group tasked with gathering information from a broad range of stakeholders (eg, physicians and QHPs, payers, medical software vendors) for full committee use in developing advice and recommendations to the US Department of Health and Human Services about adoption of *ICD-11*. To learn more about the NCVHS, visit www.cdc.gov/nchs/isp/isp_who.htm.

Effect of Diagnosis Codes on Payment and Patient Access to Care

Although the values assigned to procedure codes are generally the basis for amounts paid for services, payers are increasingly using *ICD-10-CM* codes when determining the appropriateness of services submitted on a claim (eg, level of evaluation and management [E/M] service). *ICD-10-CM* codes are also used in prior authorization of services. Use of the most specific code for the diagnosis known at the time of an encounter may facilitate both payment and approval of additional health care services. Diagnosis codes are also used to inform and measure the effectiveness of population health efforts.

Importantly, many payers now use automated prepayment claims analysis that compares the *ICD-10-CM* and procedure codes reported to determine whether certain services (eg, E/M services) will be paid at the level reported. Correct use of *ICD-10-CM* codes may prevent reduced payment.

Complete documentation of diagnoses and correct assignment of *ICD-10-CM* codes also support payment methods other than fee for service. These include value-based purchasing methodologies and payment for meeting quality and performance measures.

Correct and complete diagnosing is necessary to communicate to the health plan the disease burden of your patients, because the assigned diagnoses drive risk adjustment. Risk adjustment is used to set the expected cost of care for a patient panel. Failure to show the true nature of each patient's health status may have a short-term effect on rates paid per visit and long-term implications in contracting with health plans.

Refer to Chapters 3 and 4 for more information on coding to demonstrate quality, risk adjustment, and value-based payment methodologies.

ICD-10-CM Guidelines

The official conventions found in the *ICD-10-CM Official Guidelines for Coding and Reporting* are outlined in sections that include descriptions of symbols, abbreviations, and other instructional notes. The guidelines are organized into 4 sections. Only Sections I and IV pertain to reporting physician services. Sections II and III relate to hospital or facility technical services and are not discussed here. *ICD-10-CM* guidelines can be found in *ICD-10-CM* manuals or at www.cdc.gov/nchs/icd/icd-10-cm/files.html.

The following excerpts from *ICD-10-CM* guidelines provide an overview of the information pertinent to pediatric care as provided in each section of the guidelines.

Section I—Conventions, General Coding Guidelines, and Chapter-Specific Guidelines

A. Conventions

The conventions of *ICD-10-CM* include punctuation, notes, and terminology used throughout the code set.

Punctuation

- Dash

- Indicates that additional characters are required for code completion (eg, **R10.-**)
- Indicates incomplete codes that should not be reported without additional characters

[ ] Brackets

- Identify manifestation codes in the Alphabetic Index. For instance, otitis externa caused by impetigo directs to **L01.00** [**H62.40**]. This indicates that both impetigo (**L01.00**) and otitis externa in other diseases classified elsewhere (**H62.41**, right ear; **H62.42**, left ear; or **H62.43**, bilateral ears) are used to report this condition. Code **H62.40** is the code for otitis externa in other diseases classified elsewhere, unspecified ear, and is not reported when laterality is known.
- Enclose synonyms, alternative wording, or explanatory phrases in the tabular list (eg, **S04.811A**, injury of olfactory [1st] nerve, right side, initial encounter).

( ) Parentheses

- Enclose nonessential supplementary words that may be included in the medical record but do not affect code selection, for example, moderate persistent asthma with (acute) exacerbation, **J45.41**. Code **J45.41** is reported for any exacerbation of moderate persistent asthma without status asthmaticus (**J45.42**).
- If a nonessential modifier is mutually exclusive to a sub-term of the main term, *the sub-term is given priority.*

Example

➤ **Sepsis (generalized) (unspecified organism) A41.9**

- with
-- organ dysfunction (acute) (multiple) **R65.20**
--- with septic shock **R65.21**
- anaerobic **A41.4**
- candidal **B37.7**

The sub-term of sepsis, "candidal," directs to **B37.7** for a diagnosis of candidal sepsis, overriding the nonessential modifiers to the main term "sepsis (generalized) (unspecified organism)." For additional discussion of sub-terms and the preceding dashes that connect them, refer to the Indexes section later in this chapter.

Notes

Notes in the tabular list to assist with accurate code selection are as follows:

- *Includes:* Further defines or gives examples of the content of a category.
- *Excludes1:* Not coded here—used to indicate codes for conditions that would not occur in conjunction with the code category in which the note is found. An exception to the *Excludes1* definition is the circumstance when the 2 conditions are unrelated to each other. If it is not clear whether the 2 conditions are related, coders are instructed to query the physician or other QHP to determine applicability of the *Excludes1* note.

Example

➤ **Excludes1 notes apply to J06.9 (acute upper respiratory infection, unspecified) to prohibit reporting the code in conjunction with less specific acute respiratory infection not otherwise specified (J22) or more specific codes for influenza virus with other respiratory manifestations (J09.X2, J10.1, J11.1) or streptococcal pharyngitis (J02.0).**

Excludes1: Report only if an unrelated condition.

- ***Excludes2:*** Not included here—used to indicate codes for conditions that are not included in the code category in which the note is found and may be additionally reported when both conditions are present.

Example

➤ *Excludes2* **notes apply to J02.0 (streptococcal pharyngitis).** An *Excludes2* note that applies to all codes in subcategory **J02** (**J02.0–J02.9**) indicates that **J31.2** (chronic pharyngitis) is not included here but is separately reportable when applicable. An *Excludes2* note that applies to **J02.0** indicates that **A38.-** (scarlet fever) is not included here, allowing reporting of both **J02.0** and **A38.8** (scarlet fever with other complications).

Excludes2: Report both codes when present.

- *Code first:* A sequencing rule in the tabular list to first report a code for an underlying cause or origin of a disease (etiology), if known.
- *Code also:* An instruction that another code may be necessary to fully describe a condition. The sequence of the codes depends on the circumstances of the encounter.
- *See:* In the alphabetical index, this instructs that another term should be referenced to find the appropriate code.
- *See also:* In the alphabetical index, this instructs that another term may provide additional entries that may be useful.
- *Use an additional code:* A sequencing rule often found at the listing of an etiology code; this instruction directs to also report a code for the manifestation.

Terminology

- *And:* Means "and/or" when appearing in a title in *ICD-10-CM;* for example, **Q16.1** (congenital absence, atresia and stricture of auditory canal [external]) includes absence, atresia, or stricture.
- *Combination code:* A single code that represents multiple conditions or a single condition with an associated secondary process or complication. When a combination code describes 2 diagnoses, or a diagnosis and its associated manifestation or complication, report only the combination code. If a manifestation or complication is not identified in a combination code, it should be separately reported.
- *Default code:* A code listed next to a main term in the *ICD-10-CM* Alphabetic Index is referred to as a *default code* (eg, **E66.9**, obesity). Report the default code only if a more specific sub-term (eg, **E66.811**, obesity, class 1) is not available to describe the diagnosis.
- *First-listed diagnosis:* When reporting professional services, list first the diagnosis, condition, problem, or other reason for the encounter or visit shown in the medical record to be chiefly responsible for the services provided, followed by other conditions that affected management or treatment.
- *NEC:* Not elsewhere classifiable. Indicates a code for other specified conditions that is reported when the medical record provides detail that is not captured in a specific code. Alphabetical index entries followed by NEC lead to "other" codes in the tabular list.

Example

➤ **A newborn is diagnosed with sepsis due to viridans streptococci.** The alphabetical index for "sepsis, -newborn, --due to, ---Streptococcus" includes further sub-terms; group B (**P36.0**) and specified NEC (**P36.19**). Viridans streptococci are specified in the documented diagnosis, but they are not the same as group B streptococci, supporting **P36.19** (sepsis of newborn due to other streptococci).

- *NOS:* Not otherwise specified. Indicates a code for an unspecified condition that is selected when the medical record does not provide sufficient detail for assignment of a more specific code. Unspecified codes are appropriately reported when information to support a more specific code was unavailable at the time of the encounter (eg, type of pneumonia is unknown).

Example

➤ **A newborn is diagnosed with anemia due to isoimmunization without further specification.** The alphabetical index directs from the main term "anemia" to "-congenital" and "--due to isoimmunization NOS," directing to **P55.9** (hemolytic disease of newborn, unspecified). If the diagnosis were more specific (eg, due to Rh incompatibility), a more specific code (eg, **P55.0**, Rh isoimmunization of newborn) would be reported.

- *Sequela:* A late effect of an illness or injury that is no longer in the acute phase. There is no time limit on when a sequela code can be used. The residual may be apparent early, such as that caused by cerebral infarction, or it may occur months or years later, such as that caused by a previous injury. When reporting a sequela of an injury or illness, report first the current condition and then the sequela code.

Example

➤ **An adolescent who was previously treated for a displaced fracture of the proximal third of the scaphoid bone of the right wrist presents with stiffness and pain.** The diagnosis is post-traumatic arthritis of the right wrist due to prior (healed) scaphoid fracture. Codes are **M19.131** (post-traumatic osteoarthritis, right wrist) and **S62.031S** (displaced fracture of proximal third of navicular [scaphoid] bone of right wrist, sequela).

- *With, In:* The classification presumes a causal relationship between the 2 conditions linked by the terms *with* or *in*. These conditions should be coded as related even in the absence of provider documentation explicitly linking them, unless the documentation clearly states that the conditions are unrelated or when another guideline exists that specifically requires a documented linkage between 2 conditions (eg, sepsis guideline for "acute organ dysfunction that is not clearly associated with the sepsis").

For conditions not specifically linked by these relational terms in the classification or when a guideline requires that a linkage between 2 conditions be explicitly documented, provider documentation must link the conditions to code them as related.

B. General Coding Guidelines

- ✖ Do not report codes for conditions documented as "ruled out," "suspected," "possible," or "probable." Instead, report codes for signs or symptoms. Exceptions are influenza diagnoses from category **J11** that are assigned for diagnostic statements, such as "possible avian influenza" or "influenzalike illness."
- A confirmatory test is not always required to make a final diagnosis (eg, influenza, streptococcal pharyngitis, croup, or thrush may be based on clinical findings in lieu of laboratory findings).
- ✖ Do not report additional codes for symptoms or conditions that are integral or routinely associated with a disease process (eg, wheezing in asthma).
- When the same condition is documented as acute and chronic, codes for both conditions are reported if the alphabetical index lists the conditions at the same indentation level. The acute condition is sequenced first.
- If both sides of the body are affected by a condition and there is no single code for the bilateral condition, assign codes for right and left. When a patient has a bilateral condition and each side is treated during separate encounters, assign the bilateral code for each encounter during which the condition exists on both sides. Do not assign a bilateral code if the condition no longer exists bilaterally.
- Generally, coders may not assume a complication of care without documentation of the cause-and-effect relationship (eg, infection in a patient with a central venous catheter) and the condition must be clinically significant (ie, alter the course of care).

C. Chapter-Specific Guidelines

Refer to guidelines for specific diagnoses and/or conditions found in each chapter of *ICD-10-CM*. Chapter guidelines must be followed for appropriate code selection.

When selecting electronic coding applications, look for inclusion of chapter-specific guidelines when using the code search functionality. *Pediatric ICD-10-CM: A Manual for Provider-Based Coding* adds chapter-specific guidance to each chapter for easy reference.

Section IV—Diagnostic Coding and Reporting Guidelines for Outpatient Services

Selecting a Code

- The codes selected must be supported by the physician's or other QHP's documentation of the diagnoses, signs and symptoms, and/or reasons for an encounter as determined after evaluation. Each health care encounter should be coded to the level of certainty known for that encounter.
- Never assign a code for a condition that is unconfirmed (eg, probable or rule-out obstruction). Instead, assign a code for a confirmed but nonspecific condition (eg, viral pneumonia, unspecified) or sign or symptom (eg, vomiting, abdominal distension).

Examples

➤ **A patient presents with concern of sore throat.** A rapid streptococcal antigen test confirms streptococcal pharyngitis, which is reported with **J02.0**.

➤ **A patient presents with concern of sore throat.** A specimen is sent to an outside laboratory. Diagnosis at the time of code assignment is pharyngitis, reported with **J02.9** (acute pharyngitis, unspecified). If a definitive diagnosis is added to the record before claims submission (eg, test results are received and analyzed later on the same date), the code for the final diagnosis is reported.

As noted in the General Coding Guidelines section earlier in this chapter, a confirmatory test is not always required for diagnosis, and a physician's statement of a diagnosis is sufficient to support code assignment.

- Certain information documented by the patient and/or clinical staff (eg, body mass index [BMI]) may be used in code selection when the physician or QHP has documented an associated diagnosis (eg, overweight or obesity). Refer to the "Documentation by Other Than a Physician or Other Qualified Health Care Professional" box that follows for more information.

Documentation by Other Than a Physician or Other Qualified Health Care Professional

With few exceptions, code assignment is based on documentation by the physician or other QHP legally accountable for establishing the patient's diagnosis. Documentation by another clinician (eg, nurse, medical assistant, clinical social worker) supports reporting codes for the items on the following list when the associated diagnosis was documented by the patient's physician or QHP:

- **BMI with diagnosis of underweight, overweight, or obesity**
- **Depth of diagnosed nonpressure chronic ulcers or pressure ulcer stage**
- **Coma scale in acute medical or traumatic brain injury**
- **National Institutes of Health Stroke Scale**
- **SDoH of health classified to Chapter 21 of *ICD-10-CM***
- **Laterality of either a condition or an injury**
- **Blood alcohol level with alcohol-related disorders classifiable to category F10**
- **Underimmunization status**

Patient self-reported documentation may also be used to assign codes for SDoH, as long as this documentation is signed off on and incorporated into the medical record by a clinician or provider.

- The coding conventions and guidelines of Section I take precedence over Section IV outpatient guidelines.
- Use codes in categories **Z00–Z99** when circumstances other than a disease or an injury are recorded as the reason for the encounter.

Sequencing of Diagnosis Codes

- Physicians and other providers of professional services should first list the condition, symptom, or other reason for the encounter that is chiefly (mainly) responsible for the services provided. List also any coexisting conditions. Always defer to the *ICD-10-CM* manual to determine if sequencing is outlined in the guidelines.

Diagnosis codes must be appropriately linked to a service on a claim to support the medical necessity of that service. Refer to the Reporting Codes for Payment section later in this chapter for more information.

Reporting Previously Treated Conditions

✖ Do not code conditions that were previously treated and no longer exist. Personal history codes **Z85–Z87** may be used to identify a patient's historical conditions. Codes for family history that affects current care are also reported (**Z80–Z84**).

- Report codes for chronic or recurring conditions as many times as the patient receives care for each condition.

Reporting Diagnoses for Diagnostic Examinations

- The condition, symptoms, or other reason for a diagnostic examination or test should be linked to the service. For laboratory or radiology testing in the absence of related conditions, signs, or symptoms, report **Z01.89** (encounter for other specified special examinations).
- When diagnostic tests have been interpreted by a physician and the final report is available at the time of coding, code any confirmed or definitive diagnosis(es) documented in the interpretation. Do not code related signs and symptoms as additional diagnoses.
- The code that explains the reason for the test (ie, sign or symptom; diagnosis when known at the end of the encounter) should be reported. A screening code is reported only when a test is performed in the absence of signs or symptoms of a condition.

Examples

➤ **A chest radiograph is ordered because the result of purified protein derivative testing was positive.** Code **R76.11** (nonspecific reaction to tuberculin skin test without active tuberculosis) is assigned on the order to indicate the reason for testing.

➤ **A tuberculin purified protein derivative test is performed to screen for tuberculosis in a patient with no symptoms and no known exposure.** Code **Z11.1** (encounter for screening for respiratory tuberculosis) is assigned as the reason for the test.

➤ **A patient presents with symptoms suggestive of urinary tract infection (UTI).** After urinalysis and evaluation, the diagnosis is UTI. Assign a code for UTI (eg, **N39.0**, UTI, site not specified) and link to codes for the urinalysis and the E/M service.

Reporting Preoperative Evaluations

- When the reason for an encounter is a preoperative evaluation, a code from subcategory **Z01.81-** (encounter for preprocedural examinations) is reported first, followed by codes for the condition that is the reason for surgery and codes for any findings of the preoperative evaluation.

Refer to Chapter 8 for discussion of reporting routine health examinations (preventive care).

The Pathway to *ICD-10-CM* Code Selection

To correctly select codes in *ICD-10-CM,* it is important to recognize and follow instructions found in the alphabetical index and tabular list to locate the most specific code for documented diagnoses. These are the prevailing instructions for reporting that are supplemented by the guidelines and guidance published in the AHA *Coding Clinic.*

Indexes

Code selection begins in the alphabetical index, table of drugs and chemicals (eg, to report an adverse effect or poisoning), and/or table of neoplasms. The instructions (eg, instructions to see other terms) in the index will direct to the most specific code in the tabular list. An external cause of injuries index is also useful for locating codes to describe causes such as animal bites, falls, or motor vehicle accidents.

Dashes are used in the alphabetical index to create a path from a main term to specific sub-terms.

Example

➤ **Obesity E66.9**
- with alveolar hypoventilation **E66.2**
- adrenal **E27.8**
- class
-- 1 **E66.811**
-- 2 **E66.812**

-- 3 E66.813

The sub-term "class" is followed by entries for Class 1, Class 2, and Class 3 obesity. The initial sub-term is preceded by a single dash (-), and when applicable, additional dashes precede terms that further define the sub-term.

Tabular List

The tabular list is the end point for code selection. It is an alphanumeric list of *ICD-10-CM* codes structured as an indented list of 22 chapters with further divisions, including blocks, categories, subcategories, and codes.

Look for instructional notes at each division within the tabular list (ie, chapter, block, category, or code), as these give important guidance to correct code selection.

The indented format helps users identify complete codes (eg, Z20.822, contact with and [suspected] exposure to COVID-19) in each category (eg, Z20, contact with and [suspected] exposure to communicable diseases) or subcategory (eg, Z20.82-, contact with and [suspected] exposure to other viral communicable diseases). Only complete codes are reported.

Some code categories include instruction to add a seventh character. The most required seventh characters are A, D, and S. Categories for traumatic fractures have additional seventh character values (eg, C, initial encounter for open fracture type IIIA, IIIB, or IIIC).

- Assignment of the seventh character A (initial encounter) is *based on whether the patient is undergoing active treatment* (ie, services to establish a pattern of healing) and not on whether the physician or QHP is seeing the patient for the first time over the course of treatment of an injury or illness.
- Encounters *during the routine healing phase* are reported with seventh character D (subsequent encounter) even if the patient is new to the physician or QHP for this condition.
- Sequelae or *late effects* are reported with seventh character S.

When selecting a seventh character to indicate the type of encounter, a helpful mnemonic for this character is A as active treatment/management, D as during healing, and S as scars and other sequelae.

Examples

➤ A **(initial encounter): A physician repairs a facial laceration (active treatment) and reports S01.81XA (laceration without foreign body of other part of head, initial encounter).** This is active management.

➤ D **(subsequent encounter): A pediatrician removes facial sutures placed by an emergency department physician and reports S01.81XD (laceration without foreign body of other part of head, subsequent encounter).** This is care during the healing phase.

➤ S **(sequela or late effect): A pediatrician evaluates a concern of scar contracture that resulted from repair of a facial laceration.** Codes L90.5 (scar conditions and fibrosis of skin) and S01.81XS (laceration without foreign body of other part of head, sequela) are reported. This is care for a scar or other sequelae.

Teaching Point: A sequela (eg, scar) must always be listed before the sequela code (eg, L09.5 before S01.81XS).

Refer to *Pediatric Coding Basics* and *Pediatric ICD-10-CM* for more information on codes and code selection.

Diagnosis Coding Tips

- Specificity in coding is important to demonstrate the reason for a service or an encounter, including the nature or severity of conditions managed. For further discussion of this important topic, refer to the Appropriate Use of Unspecified Codes section later in this chapter.
- Physicians and other QHPs should be familiar with the documentation elements that are captured in *ICD-10-CM* code categories for conditions commonly seen in their practice.

Example

➤ **When documenting care for asthma (category J45), key documentation elements include whether the condition**
- Is classified as intermittent (mild), mild persistent, moderate persistent, or severe persistent
- Is or is not exacerbated
- Is complicated by status asthmaticus (when applicable)

Exposure to or use of tobacco is also reported in conjunction with asthma. Eosinophilic asthma (J82.83) is reported in addition to asthma codes in category J45, when present.

- Assign codes for SDoH (eg, homelessness, food insecurity, or lack of transportation) that increase the complexity and risk of management or treatment (eg, lack of transportation that increases the risk of not returning for necessary follow-up).
- Pay close attention to the terminology for nonspecific diagnoses. For example, the diagnosis "reactive airways disease" is coded as asthma per the guidelines. It may be more appropriate to report the signs or symptoms as the primary diagnosis in children treated for an asthma-like condition when they have not been diagnosed with asthma.
- After evaluation and study of a suspected condition, if there is no diagnosis or no appropriate signs or symptoms, report the codes for observation and evaluation for suspected conditions not found (eg, parent's concern regarding an injury that is not found). Codes for reporting observation and evaluation for suspected conditions not found in a neonate (Z05.0–Z05.9) are distinct from those for reporting suspected conditions not found in older children and adults (subcategory Z03.8-).
- Use aftercare codes (Z42–Z49, Z51) for patients who are receiving care to consolidate treatment or management to address residual conditions.
- Conditions that were previously treated and no longer exist cannot be reported. Therefore, it is correct coding to report care following completed treatment with Z09 (encounter for follow-up examination after completed treatment of conditions other than malignant neoplasm).
  - Personal history codes (Z86.-, Z87.-) may be used to provide additional information on follow-up care.
  - If a payer does not accept follow-up care codes as primary and requires that the service be reported with the diagnosis code that reflects the condition that was treated, report the follow-up care codes as secondary. However, get the payer's policy in writing and inquire why coding guidelines are not being followed.

Example

➤ **A patient is seen to follow up on otitis media with effusion, which has resolved.** The physician reports Z09 and Z86.69 (personal history of other diseases of the nervous system and sense organs) in lieu of the code for otitis media with effusion (no longer applicable).

- ✖ Do not select a diagnosis code that is "close to" the diagnosis or condition documented in the medical record. For example, do not report other disorders of bilirubin metabolism (hyperbilirubinemia) (E80.6) if the diagnosis is neonatal jaundice associated with preterm delivery (P59.0). Follow alphabetical index and tabular list instructions for selecting codes to ensure that the correct code is assigned.
- Pay attention to age factors within certain code descriptors. For example, report R10.83 for infantile colic and R10.84 for colic in a child older than 12 months. Use P00–P96 to report conditions that originate in the perinatal period from birth through the first 28 days after birth (discussed further in **Chapter 15**).
- There is no limit to the number of diagnosis codes that can be documented.
  - Space is only allotted for up to 12 codes on the 1500 claim form, and each service line may be connected to 1 to 4 of the included codes. You may submit as many claim forms as necessary to report all current diagnoses.
  - Electronic claims in HIPAA version 5010 may also include up to 12 diagnosis codes.
- "Recurrent" is not defined by *ICD-10-CM*. Therefore, to use a recurrent code, the documentation should reflect that a physician or QHP believes the condition to be a recurrence.
- "Confirmed" influenza, COVID-19, or other conditions do not require a positive result from a laboratory or other test. What is required is that the physician or QHP, through training and experience, believes that the patient has the condition, given the clinical assessment, and documents the condition in the medical record.
- ✖ Do not report suspected or rule-out diagnoses for physician services. Code to the nearest clinical certainty, which may be signs or symptoms. Exposure to communicable disease (category Z20) may be reported when a patient has known or suspected exposure or when a disease is endemic but ruled out after evaluation.

Appropriate Use of Unspecified Codes

Unspecified codes are valid *ICD-10-CM* codes used to report conditions for which a more specific diagnosis has not yet been determined and/or when testing to determine that a more specific diagnosis would not be medically necessary. Misuse of unspecified codes may result in claim denials, underpayment, and unnecessary delays in receiving prior authorizations for testing or procedures.

Do not report the default code (first code listed in the alphabetical index) when more detail about the patient's condition(s) should be documented to support another, more specific code. For example, do not report **J45.909** for unspecified asthma, uncomplicated, for reevaluation of asthma, which includes clinical classification of intermittent, mild persistent, moderate persistent, or severe persistent asthma. The diagnosis code reported should reflect what is known at the end of the current encounter. Unspecified codes are not appropriate when information to support a more specific code would generally be known (eg, laterality, type of attention-deficit/hyperactivity disorder).

Examples

➤ **Unspecified codes that may be acceptable are as follows:**
- Viral intestinal infection, unspecified (**A08.4**)
- Infectious gastroenteritis and colitis, unspecified (**A09**)
- Acute pharyngitis, unspecified (**J02.9**)
- Pneumonia, unspecified organism (**J18.9**)
- Unspecified convulsions (**R56.9**)
- Sprain of unspecified site of right knee (**S83.91X-**)

➤ **The following examples of unspecified codes indicate inappropriate coding caused by failure to document information (eg, location) that would typically be known at the time of the encounter and/or inappropriate code selection:**
- Acute suppurative otitis media without spontaneous rupture of eardrum, unspecified ear (**H66.009**)
- Otitis media, unspecified, unspecified ear (**H66.90**)
- Cutaneous abscess of limb, unspecified (**L02.419**)
- Extremely low birth weight newborn, unspecified weight (**P07.00**)

In short, unspecified codes are necessary and should be reported when appropriate. Physicians must document in enough detail to capture what is known at the time of the encounter, and codes selected must reflect the documented diagnosis(es). At the time of code selection, if documentation does not appear to include information that would be known at the time of the encounter, it is appropriate for coders to query the physician for more information and/or request an addendum to the documentation to more fully describe the conditions addressed at the encounter.

More About *ICD-10-CM*

You can find additional resources from the AAP on *ICD-10-CM* topics at www.aap.org/en/practice-management/child-health-finance-payment-strategy/coding-and-valuation/icd-10-cm-resources.

Pediatric ICD-10-CM 2026 (www.aap.org/Pediatric-*ICD-10-CM*-2026-11th-Edition-Paperback) is a condensed version of the entire *ICD-10-CM* manual and provides only the guidelines and codes that are applicable and important to pediatric physicians and QHPs. The manual was designed for use in conjunction with the complete *ICD-10-CM* code set. The *ICD-10-CM* codes and guidelines are found at www.cdc.gov/nchs/icd/icd-10-cm/files.html.

AAP Pediatric Coding Newsletter™ provides timely articles on diagnosis coding for pediatric conditions (www.aap.org/AAP-Pediatric-Coding-Newsletter).

Healthcare Common Procedure Coding System

The Healthcare Common Procedure Coding System (HCPCS) includes Level I codes (*CPT*) and Level II codes (CMS national codes). HCPCS Level II codes are the standardized coding system for describing and identifying health care services, equipment, medications, and supplies (eg, **E0114**, crutches underarm, other than wood, adjustable or fixed, pair, with pads, tips and handgrips) that are not identified by HCPCS Level I (*CPT*) codes. To differentiate discussion of *CPT* and HCPCS Level II codes, the abbreviation HCPCS is typically used in reference to Level II codes unless otherwise stated.

HCPCS procedure codes may be reported when no *CPT* code describes the service provided or when the narrative (code descriptor) differs from and more accurately describes the service provided than a similar *CPT* code. Payer policies, particularly Medicaid plan policies, often drive the decision between reporting with *CPT* and reporting with HCPCS.

Example

➤ **A physician provides critical care services to a pediatric patient via a real-time audiovisual telecommunications system.** *CPT* does not designate codes for critical care services (99291 and 99292, 99468–99472) as services reportable with modifier 95 (synchronous telemedicine service rendered via a real-time interactive audio and video telecommunications system). As an alternative, the payer has adopted policy requiring HCPCS codes for critical care provided via telemedicine.

G0508	Telehealth consultation, critical care, initial, physicians typically spend 60 minutes communicating with the patient and providers via telehealth
G0509	Telehealth consultation, critical care, subsequent, physicians typically spend 50 minutes communicating with the patient and providers via telehealth

Teaching Point: The physician reports either G0508 or G0509 based on the service provided (first or subsequent episode of critical care).

Reporting Medications Supplied by the Billing Provider

HCPCS J codes (eg, J0696, injection, ceftriaxone sodium, per 250 mg) represent only the medication and not the administration of the medication.

- The term *injection* is included in the descriptor to specify that the medication code is reported for the medication that is labeled for administration via injection or infusion. This does not limit reporting of these codes when delivered via an alternative route.

Example

➤ **A physician orders and clinical staff deliver an oral administration of 9 mL of injectable dexamethasone sodium phosphate (from a 10-mg/mL single-dose vial) diluted in a flavor solution to a concentration of 2 mg/mL to a patient in the office.** The physician reports J1100 (injection, dexamethasone sodium phosphate, 1 mg) with 9 units (1 unit per milligram administered). Also, they include a note on the claim (field 19 of a paper claim or the electronic equivalent) that the drug was orally administered. Additional codes are reported for other services (eg, office visit) provided on the same date.

When using a dexamethasone product labeled for oral administration, report J8540 with 1 unit per 0.25 mg (eg, 4 mg equals 16 units).

Refer to discussion of modifiers JW and JZ in **Chapter 2** for information on reporting provision of medications supplied in single-dose containers.

- Separate procedure codes, typically *CPT* codes, are used to report each medication administration by injection (96372) or infusion.
- HCPCS codes for drugs specify the unit of measure for each unit reported on the claim (eg, 250 mg of ceftriaxone sodium is reported with 1 unit on the claim line reporting provision of the medication).

Units reported with HCPCS codes often vary from those reported with a corresponding National Drug Code (NDC). Refer to the National Drug Code section later in this chapter for information on reporting units of service in conjunction with NDC reporting.

Example

➤ **A physician administers 1,250 mg of ceftriaxone sodium by 2 separate injections.** Code J0696 (injection, ceftriaxone sodium, per 250 mg) is reported with 5 units in addition to 96372 × 2 (therapeutic, prophylactic, or diagnostic injection; subcutaneous or intramuscular). Additional codes may be reported for E/M and other services provided at the encounter.

Teaching Point: Do not report the number of milligrams (mg) as the unit of service on a claim. Reporting 1,250 mg of ceftriaxone sodium with 1,250 units would be incorrect; 1,250 mg of ceftriaxone sodium is reported per 250 mg with 5 units. Refer to the National Drug Codes section later in this chapter for additional codes submitted in conjunction with medications and immunization products.

Current Procedural Terminology

CPT is published annually by the American Medical Association (AMA). *CPT* codes are Level I codes of HCPCS but are commonly treated as a separate code set. This is the primary procedural coding system for professional services by physicians and other QHPs. *CPT* codes are commonly included in electronic health record (EHR) systems, but instructions for reporting may not be included. *CPT* manuals and code applications or software provide important instructions for appropriate code selection.

CPT includes 3 categories of codes.

Category I *CPT* codes (commonly performed services and procedures with documented clinical efficacy) are divided into 6 sections of codes.

1. Evaluation and Management Services (**98000–98016**, **99202–99499**)
2. Anesthesia (**00100–01999**)
3. Surgery (**10004–66990**)
4. Radiology (**70010–79999**)
5. Pathology and Laboratory (**80047–89398**, **0001U–0438U**)
6. Medicine (**90281–99607**)

Category II *CPT* codes (supplemental tracking used for performance measurement) are reported on a voluntary basis, in addition to Category I codes, to describe clinical conditions, performance measure sets, and screening measures. Category II *CPT* codes are not directly tied to payment for services.

Refer to Chapter 3 for more discussion and illustration of Category II codes.

Category III *CPT* codes represent emerging technology, services, procedures, and service paradigms. Category III *CPT* codes are not assigned RVUs, and payment for these services is based strictly on payer policies. If you are performing any procedure or service identified with a Category III *CPT* code, work with your payers to determine their coverage and payment policies.

The AMA hosts a website devoted to *CPT,* www.ama-assn.org/practice-management/cpt, with information on code development and maintenance, summaries of recent *CPT* Editorial Panel actions, and newly released codes.

Current Procedural Terminology Code Updates

Although most *CPT* code updates are annual with implementation on January 1 of each year, certain codes are updated more frequently and published online ahead of implementation as follows. Refer to Table 1-1 for the frequency of updates to *CPT* codes.

- **Newly released immunization codes are posted to www.ama-assn.org/practice-management/cpt/category-i-immunization-codes.**
- **Proprietary laboratory analyses codes are released quarterly at www.ama-assn.org/practice-management/cpt/cpt-pla-codes.**
- **New molecular pathology tier 2 codes (www.ama-assn.org/practice-management/cpt/molecular-pathology-tier-2-codes) and codes for administrative multianalyte assays with algorithmic analyses (www.ama-assn.org/practice-management/cpt/administrative-multianalyte-assays-algorithmic-analyses-codes) are updated 3 times per year.**
- **Category II *CPT* codes (supplemental tracking used for performance measurement) are released online up to 3 times a year at www.ama-assn.org/practice-management/cpt/category-ii-codes.**
- **Category III codes, released biannually with an implementation date 6 months after the release date, are found at www.ama-assn.org/practice-management/cpt/category-iii-codes.**

CPT® Guidelines Applicable to All Services

Correct coding is critical to obtain correct claims payment. Always read the applicable guidelines and instructions before selecting a code.

The following general guidelines apply to selecting and reporting all *CPT* codes:

- *CPT* guidelines do not establish documentation requirements or standards of care.
- In the *CPT* code set, the term *procedure* describes services, including diagnostic tests. The section of the book in which a code is placed does not indicate whether the service is a surgery or not a surgery for insurance or other purposes.

- Select the code for the procedure or service that accurately identifies the service performed.
- ✖ Do not select a code that merely approximates the service provided.
  - If no specific code exists, report the service with the appropriate unlisted procedure code. Unlisted procedure codes are provided in each section of *CPT* (eg, **99429**, unlisted preventive medicine service). When reporting an unlisted procedure code, medical records need to be submitted to the health plan to identify the service rendered (attach the records to the claim to prevent delay caused by a health plan request for them).
  - In some cases, a modifier may be reported in conjunction with a procedure code to indicate a reduced (**52**), discontinued (**53**), or increased (**22**) procedural service. For more about procedure code modifiers, refer to **Chapter 2**.
- A single code may incorporate or bundle multiple components. For example, **90710** is used to report provision of a measles, mumps, rubella, and varicella combination vaccine product. It is not appropriate to report codes for the individual components when a single code represents a specific product administered or services provided.
- A code that is reported "per day" or for services "on the same date" is reported for all services on a single calendar date (ie, not for all services provided in a 24-hour period).

Example

➤ **Hospital care of the newborn is reported once per day for all work provided by the same physician or QHP (or multiple individuals of the same group and same specialty) on that date.**

99463	Initial hospital or birthing center care, per day, for E/M of normal newborn infant admitted and discharged on the same date
99468	Initial inpatient neonatal critical care, per day, for the E/M of a critically ill neonate, 28 days of age or younger

- Time is the physician's or other reporting provider's time unless otherwise stated. Time spent by clinical staff is reported only when specified in *CPT* or allowed under incident-to policy established by a payer.

Refer to Chapter 7 for information on reporting services that are incident to a physician's service.

- A midpoint time rule applies when codes are selected according to time *and no specific time requirement is provided* in the section guidelines, prefatory instructions, parenthetical instructions, or code descriptor.
  - A unit of time is attained when the midpoint is passed (eg, a code described as 30 minutes may be reported when service time of 16 minutes has elapsed).
  - When codes are ranked in sequential typical times and the actual time is between 2 typical times, the code with the typical time closest to the actual time is used. If the actual time of service falls exactly between the typical times of 2 codes, report the code with the lower typical time (ie, the midpoint must be passed to report the greater service).
  - The midpoint rule does not apply to codes for E/M services for which a specified total time on the date of the encounter must be met or exceeded.

Documentation of Time

Documentation of time spent providing services should be evident in the medical record for each service reported according to time (ie, total minutes of service or start and stop times).

- **Documentation of time may be automated in an EHR, but physicians should be able to demonstrate that the EHR functionality captures the correct time for code selection as specified by *CPT*.**
- **When multiple services are provided on the same date, time spent in time-based services must be clearly distinguished from time spent in provision of other services. For instance, time spent in any separately reportable procedure (eg, 31500, endotracheal intubation) is not included in the time of hourly critical care services (99291, 99292). Documentation should clearly reflect total times and activities of each service.**
- **In addition to documentation of total times or start and stop times of service, documentation should clearly support the service reported. For example, documentation of counseling should include discussion of diagnosis and treatment options, patient and/or caregiver questions and concerns that were addressed, shared decision-making for management, and any SDoH that affect care and were addressed (eg, advice to enroll in a prescription discount program).**
- **All documentation must be signed or electronically authenticated with the name and credentials of the physician or other provider of care and date of service (DOS).**

In addition, *CPT* includes not only specific guidelines that are located at the beginning of each of 6 sections but also additional prefatory instructions for subsections of codes throughout the *CPT* manual. Code-specific instructions often follow a code in parentheses (referred to as *parenthetical instructions*).

Example

➤ **Parenthetical instructions following 99238 and 99239 advise of other codes that may be applicable in lieu of the hospital discharge service codes.**

99238 Hospital inpatient or observation discharge day management; 30 minutes or less on the date of the encounter

99239 more than 30 minutes on the date of the encounter

(For hospital inpatient or observation care, including the admission and discharge of the patient on the same date, refer to **99234–99236**.)

(For discharge services provided to newborns admitted and discharged on the same calendar date, use **99463**.)

Teaching Point: Instructions preceding **99238** and **99239** provide more description of the services and restrict reporting to the discharging physician or QHP (eg, principal or attending physician). Services by other physicians or other QHPs that may include instructions to the patient and/or family and coordination of post-discharge services may be reported with a subsequent hospital care code (ie, **99231**, **99232**, or **99233**).

Additional guidance can be found in *CPT Assistant,* a monthly newsletter published by the AMA that provides information about the intended use of codes, related guidelines, and parenthetical instructions. Although widely considered authoritative, *CPT* instructions, guidelines, and *CPT Assistant* are not part of the HIPAA standard transaction code sets. All payers must accept *CPT* codes but are not required to adhere to the published *CPT* guidelines and instructions. When payer policy differs from *CPT,* payer contracts typically require adherence to payer policy.

Example

➤ **A health plan policy does not allow separate payment for vision screening in conjunction with a routine child health examination even though *CPT* instructs that the screening be separately reported.** Although the health plan may deny charges associated with a vision screening, the plan must not reject the claim when a vision screening code is included (eg, **99173**, screening test of visual acuity, quantitative, bilateral).

Provider Terminology

Throughout the *CPT* code set, the use of terms such as *physician, QHP,* or *individual* is not intended to indicate that other entities may not report the service. In select instances, specific instructions may define a service as limited to certain professionals or to other entities (eg, hospital, home health agency).

Identifying the providers included when terms such as *physician or other QHP* and *nonphysician qualified health care professional* are used in *CPT* and/or payer instruction is of particular importance to correct reporting of services that include clinical staff and other nonphysician providers (eg, clinical social workers, dietitians).

CPT defines health care professionals as follows:

- Physician or other QHP: an individual who is qualified by education, training, licensure/regulation (when applicable), and facility privileging (when applicable) who performs a professional service within his or her scope of practice and independently reports that professional service

Codes in the E/M section are reported only by a physician or QHP whose scope of practice includes E/M services (eg, nurse practitioner, physician associate). In contrast, assessment and management codes are found in the medicine section for reporting services by nonphysician QHPs (eg, physical or occupational therapists and speech pathologists) who may independently provide and report medical services. Coding for services by nonphysician qualified health care professionals whose scope of practice does not include E/M services is discussed in Chapter 12.

- Clinical staff member: a person who works under the supervision of a physician or other QHP and who is allowed by law, regulation, and facility policy to perform or assist in the performance of a specific professional service but does not individually report that professional service

Services performed by clinical staff under the supervision of a physician or QHP are reported by the supervising physician or QHP.

Note: CPT does not include any requirements for licensure but, rather, advises physicians to follow state regulations and the related scopes of practice defined by regulations (eg, regulations defining services that require a nursing license).

CPT Conventions

Symbols are used throughout *CPT* to indicate certain code characteristics. At the beginning of a code,

- ● A bullet indicates a new code for the current year.
- ▲ A triangle means the code descriptor has been revised.
- ✚ A plus sign means the code is an add-on code (AOC).
- Ø A null sign means the code is a "modifier **51** exempt" code and, therefore, does not require modifier **51** (multiple procedures) even when reported with other procedures.
- ⚡ The lightning bolt identifies codes for vaccines and immunoglobulins pending US Food and Drug Administration (FDA) approval.
- # The pound symbol identifies re-sequenced codes that are out of numerical sequence. Related codes are placed into an appropriate location, making it easier to locate a procedure or service.
- ◀ An audio speaker symbol means the service is included in Appendix T of the AMA *CPT* manual and may be reported with modifier **93** when provided via audio-only telecommunications technology (eg, telephone).
- ★ A star means the service can be reported as a telemedicine service and is included in *CPT* Appendix P as a code to which modifier **95** (synchronous telemedicine service) may be appended to indicate that the service was rendered via real-time telemedicine services using audiovisual technology.

CPT appendixes provide quick references to modifiers; a summary of new, revised, and deleted codes; add-on and modifier-exempt codes; and other procedure code references.

CPT includes an index of procedures used to find codes and code ranges to help guide the user to the correct section(s) of codes.

- Terms in the index cover procedures and services, organs and anatomical sites, conditions, synonyms, eponyms, and abbreviations (eg, *EEG* for *electroencephalography*).
- Codes should not be selected from the index without verification of the code descriptor and reporting instructions in the appropriate section of the manual (eg, Evaluation and Management section).
- Many diagnostic services require both technical and professional components.
  - It is important to understand that the technical component (eg, obtaining an electrocardiogram) leads to results or findings.
  - The interpretation and creation of a report of the results or findings are a professional service. Some services specifically require a professional's interpretation and report.
  - Other services include only a technical component and require only documentation of the results or findings (eg, scoring of a developmental screening instrument).
  - Codes and modifiers exist to report the technical or professional component when the complete service is not provided by the same individual or provider (eg, facility provides technical component and physician provides professional component).

Never report a code for a global service without a modifier when only the technical or professional component is provided. Refer to Chapter 2 for discussion of appropriate modifiers (eg, 26, TC).

- AOCs (marked with a ✚ before the code) are always performed in addition to a primary service and are never reported as stand-alone services. AOCs describe additional intraservice work and are not valued to include preservice and postservice work like most other codes.

Example

➤ **Code 99459 is never reported without one of the E/M codes listed in the parenthetical instruction having been provided and reported on the same DOS.**

#✚99459 Pelvic examination (List separately in addition to the code of the outpatient E/M service)

(Use **99459** in conjunction with **99202–99205**, **99212–99215**, **99242–99245**, **99345**, **99383–99387**, or **99393–99397**.)

Teaching Point: The inclusionary parenthetical notes following the AOCs are not all inclusive but, rather, include the typical base code(s) and not every possible reportable code combination. The parenthetical note in the descriptor of **99459**, however, instructs that this code is reported in addition to outpatient E/M service codes (ie, not codes in other categories).

National Drug Code

NDCs are universal product identifiers for prescription drugs, including immunizations and insulin products. Codes are 10-digit, 3-segment numbers that identify the product, labeler, and trade package size. Medicare, Medicaid, and other government payers (eg, Tricare), as well as some private payers, may require the use of NDCs when reporting medication and immunization product codes.

- The HIPAA standards for reporting NDCs do not align with the 10-digit format; they require an 11-digit code.
  - Conversion to an 11-digit code in 5-digit–4-digit–2-digit format is required.
  - Leading zeros are added to the appropriate segment to accomplish the 5-4-2 format, as illustrated in **Table 1-3.**

Table 1-3. National Drug Code Format Examples

Product	10-Digit NDC Format	11-Digit NDC in 5-4-2 Format (Added 0 [Zero] Underscored)
Gardasil 9 (human papillomavirus vaccine) carton of ten 0.5-mL single-dose prefilled syringes	0006-4121-02 (4-4-2 format)	00006-4121-02
Fluarix trivalent (influenza vaccine) prefilled syringe	58160-884-52 (5-3-2 format)	58160-0884-52
Ceftriaxone 250 mg per vial powder single-dose	60505-6151-4 (5-4-1 format)	60505-6151-04

Abbreviation: NDC, National Drug Code.

It is important to verify each payer's requirements for NDC reporting. A payer may require either of the following:

- The NDC that is provided on the outer packaging when immunization products or another drug is supplied in bulk packages
- The NDC from the vial or prefilled syringe that was administered

When reporting NDCs,

- A qualifier (N4) precedes the NDC number on the claim form (eg, N400006412102).
- The correct number of NDC units must also be included on claims.
  - The NDC units are often different from HCPCS or *CPT* units.
  - For most payers, NDC units are reported as grams (GR), milligrams (ME), milliliters (ML), or units (UN).
  - The qualifiers GR, ME, ML, and UN are reported before the number of NDC units on a claim to indicate the measure.

For examples of how NDC codes and units are reported on a claim, refer to **Figure 1-1**.

If you are not currently reporting medications with NDCs, be sure to coordinate the requirements with your billing company or billing software company. For more information and updates on NDCs, visit www.fda.gov/drugs/drug-approvals-and-databases/national-drug-code-directory.

Beyond Code Sets

Who Assigns the Codes?

- Diagnoses should be assigned by the physician or QHP indicating a principal (primary) diagnosis that best explains the reason with the highest risk of morbidity or mortality for the patient encounter, followed by other conditions that were managed or that affected management at this encounter. Code assignment may take place in conjunction with documentation or later, depending on the workflow processes of the practice.
- Assignment of the specific diagnosis code by clinical or administrative staff should be done under the physician's or reporting provider's supervision.

Figure 1-1. Example of a Completed 1500 Form

Example 1500 Claim Form

ABC Health Plan
123 Money St
Anywhere, AK 00000

CARRIER

HEALTH INSURANCE CLAIM FORM

APPROVED BY NATIONAL UNIFORM CLAIM COMMITTEE (NUCC) 02/12

PICA PICA

PATIENT AND INSURED INFORMATION

1. MEDICARE (Medicare#) MEDICAID (Medicaid#) TRICARE (ID#/DoD#) CHAMPVA (Member ID#) X GROUP HEALTH PLAN (ID#) FECA BLK LUNG (ID#) OTHER (ID#)

1a. INSURED'S I.D. NUMBER (For Program in Item 1): 123456789

2. PATIENT'S NAME (Last Name, First Name, Middle Initial): Smith, Patient

3. PATIENT'S BIRTH DATE MM DD YY: 08 22 2024 SEX M X F

4. INSURED'S NAME (Last Name, First Name, Middle Initial): Smith, Parent

5. PATIENT'S ADDRESS (No., Street): 123 Main St

6. PATIENT RELATIONSHIP TO INSURED: Self X Spouse Child Other

7. INSURED'S ADDRESS (No., Street)

CITY: Anywhere STATE: KS

8. RESERVED FOR NUCC USE

CITY STATE

ZIP CODE: 12345 TELEPHONE (Include Area Code): (555) 555-5555

ZIP CODE TELEPHONE (Include Area Code) ( )

9. OTHER INSURED'S NAME (Last Name, First Name, Middle Initial): Smith, Parent

10. IS PATIENT'S CONDITION RELATED TO:

11. INSURED'S POLICY GROUP OR FECA NUMBER: 98765432102

a. OTHER INSURED'S POLICY OR GROUP NUMBER: 45612378900

a. EMPLOYMENT? (Current or Previous) YES X NO

a. INSURED'S DATE OF BIRTH MM DD YY: 01 01 1994 SEX M F X

b. RESERVED FOR NUCC USE

b. AUTO ACCIDENT? YES X NO PLACE (State)

b. OTHER CLAIM ID (Designated by NUCC)

c. RESERVED FOR NUCC USE

c. OTHER ACCIDENT? YES X NO

c. INSURANCE PLAN NAME OR PROGRAM NAME: Good Health Plan

d. INSURANCE PLAN NAME OR PROGRAM NAME: Another Good Plan

10d. CLAIM CODES (Designated by NUCC)

d. IS THERE ANOTHER HEALTH BENEFIT PLAN? X YES NO *If yes,* complete items 9, 9a, and 9d.

READ BACK OF FORM BEFORE COMPLETING & SIGNING THIS FORM.

12. PATIENT'S OR AUTHORIZED PERSON'S SIGNATURE I authorize the release of any medical or other information necessary to process this claim. I also request payment of government benefits either to myself or to the party who accepts assignment below.

SIGNED Signature on file DATE 02/22/2026

13. INSURED'S OR AUTHORIZED PERSON'S SIGNATURE I authorize payment of medical benefits to the undersigned physician or supplier for services described below.

SIGNED Signature on file

PHYSICIAN OR SUPPLIER INFORMATION

14. DATE OF CURRENT ILLNESS, INJURY, or PREGNANCY (LMP) MM DD YY QUAL.

15. OTHER DATE QUAL. MM DD YY

16. DATES PATIENT UNABLE TO WORK IN CURRENT OCCUPATION FROM MM DD YY TO MM DD YY

17. NAME OF REFERRING PROVIDER OR OTHER SOURCE 17a. 17b. NPI

18. HOSPITALIZATION DATES RELATED TO CURRENT SERVICES FROM MM DD YY TO MM DD YY

19. ADDITIONAL CLAIM INFORMATION (Designated by NUCC)

20. OUTSIDE LAB? YES NO $ CHARGES

21. DIAGNOSIS OR NATURE OF ILLNESS OR INJURY Relate A-L to service line below (24E) ICD Ind. 0

A. Z00.129 B. Z29.11 C. Z23 D.
E. F. G. H.
I. J. K. L.

22. RESUBMISSION CODE ORIGINAL REF. NO.

23. PRIOR AUTHORIZATION NUMBER

24.

	A. DATE(S) OF SERVICE From MM	DD	YY	To MM	DD	YY	B. PLACE OF SERVICE	C. EMG	D. PROCEDURES, SERVICES, OR SUPPLIES (Explain Unusual Circumstances) CPT/HCPCS	MODIFIER	E. DIAGNOSIS POINTER	F. $ CHARGES	G. DAYS OR UNITS	H. EPSDT Family Plan	I. ID. QUAL.	J. RENDERING PROVIDER ID. #
1	02	22	26				11		99392	25	A	150 00	1		NPI	1234567890
2	02	22	26				11		96110		A	20 00	1		NPI	1234567890
3	N49281057415 ML1															
	02	22	26				11		90381	SL	AB	25 00	2		NPI	1234567890
4	N458160082543 ML05															
	02	22	26				11		90633	SL	AC	25 00	1		NPI	1234567890
5															NPI	
6															NPI	

25. FEDERAL TAX I.D. NUMBER: 12-4567897 SSN EIN X

26. PATIENT'S ACCOUNT NO.: 11111

27. ACCEPT ASSIGNMENT? (For govt. claims, see back) X YES NO

28. TOTAL CHARGE $ 220 00

29. AMOUNT PAID $

30. Rsvd for NUCC Use

31. SIGNATURE OF PHYSICIAN OR SUPPLIER INCLUDING DEGREES OR CREDENTIALS (I certify that the statements on the reverse apply to this bill and are made a part thereof.)
Signature on file
SIGNED DATE 02/23/2026

32. SERVICE FACILITY LOCATION INFORMATION
Pediatric Practice
111 Some St
Anywhere, US 99999
a. NPI b.

33. BILLING PROVIDER INFO & PH # (555) 555-5555
Pediatric Practice
111 Some St
Anywhere, US 99999
a. 01233456789 b.

NUCC Instruction Manual available at: www.nucc.org PLEASE PRINT OR TYPE APPROVED OMB-0938-1197 FORM 1500 (02-12)

Documentation of diagnoses, signs and symptoms, or other reasons for a service is not accomplished through code assignment. Per official guidance from *Coding Clinic,* selection of a code cannot replace a written diagnostic statement. Multiple clinical conditions may be represented by a single diagnosis code, and more than one code may be required to fully describe a condition. Codes should be assigned to the documented diagnostic statement.

- When codes are selected by physicians at the time of EHR documentation, it is advised to have trained administrative staff verify the levels of service, need for modifiers, and compliance with *ICD-10-CM*, *CPT,* and payer policies. EHRs may fail to show complete code descriptors and/or *ICD-10-CM* instructions (eg, exclusion notes).
- For practices that use a printed encounter form, including 50 to 100 of the most used diagnoses *and* their respective codes on the outpatient encounter form allows the physician or QHP to mark the appropriate code(s), indicating which is primary.
  - If a specific diagnosis code is not included on the form, write it in.
- ✖ Do not select a diagnosis code that is "closest to" the diagnosis.
  - *Pediatric Office Superbill 2026* is a convenient card that includes the most-reported *CPT* and *ICD-10-CM* codes (www.aap.org/Pediatric-Office-Superbill-2026).

Reporting Codes for Payment

In addition to standard code sets, HIPAA has established electronic transaction standards for patient benefit inquiries and submission of health claims and related reports.

- Claims for professional services are typically submitted electronically in a format known as 837P (professional claim) as currently configured in version 5010A1.
- Paper claim form submissions using the 1500 claim form, version 02/12, are allowed for providers who meet an exception to the HIPAA requirements for electronic claim submission (eg, provider with <10 full-time employees).
  - Paper claim submissions increase the length of time between submission and payment and the chance of error in either form completion or claims processing. It is advisable to submit electronic claims whenever possible.
  - The 1500 claim form contains the same information as an electronic claim and is valuable for demonstrating how codes and other information necessary for claims processing must be relayed to payers. An example of a completed 1500 claim form is found in **Figure 1-1**.

Linking the Diagnosis to the Service

- Every claim line for a physician service must be linked to the appropriate *ICD-10-CM* code that represents the reason for the service.
  - Each *ICD-10-CM* code is placed into a diagnosis field labeled "21A–L."
  - A diagnosis pointer in field 24E indicates which diagnosis codes relate to each service line by indicating the letter(s) of the related diagnosis field. Up to 4 diagnosis fields may be linked to a service line.
- The first-listed code on the claim should be the principal reason for the service unless the tabular instructions direct the user to "code first" another reason (eg, code first routine child health examination [**Z00.121**, **Z00.129**] when immunizations [**Z23**] are provided at the time of a preventive E/M service).
- When using an EHR, physicians should list the primary diagnosis first in the EHR and make certain that the software does not reorder the codes alphabetically or numerically. In addition, the EHR should be able to link diagnosis codes to the appropriate services.
- The diagnosis code may be the same or different for each service performed.

Example

➤ **When a child is diagnosed with a UTI, the *ICD-10-CM* code for UTI (N39.0) is linked to the E/M service (eg, 99213) and to an in-office dipstick urinalysis performed without microscopy (81002).**

Other Coding and Billing Information

Correct code assignment and claim completion are 2 important steps in compliant and effective practice management. But many other processes and policies are required. Refer to **Chapter 4** for additional guidance on coding and billing procedures.

To test your knowledge of the information presented in this chapter, complete the quiz found at the end of it, after the resources. Answers to each quiz are found in **Appendix II.** Add to your knowledge through the information provided in other chapters that discuss codes for specific types of service.

Chapter Takeaways

Readers of this chapter should generally know the code sets used to report professional services. Following are takeaways from this chapter:

- The 4 code sets that are used for reporting professional services are *ICD-10-CM*, HCPCS, *CPT*, and the NDC.
- To correctly select codes in *ICD-10-CM*, it is important to recognize and follow instructions found in the alphabetical index and tabular list to locate the most specific code for documented diagnoses.
- HCPCS procedure codes may be reported when no *CPT* code describes the service provided or when the narrative (code descriptor) differs from and more accurately describes the service provided than a similar *CPT* code.
- Use of *CPT* guidelines and full code descriptors is important in correct coding. Correct coding is critical to obtain correct claims payment.
- Every claim line for a physician service must be linked to the appropriate *ICD-10-CM* code that represents the reason for the service.

Resources

AAP Coding Assistance and Education

AAP Coding and Payment Hassle Hotline Form (www.aap.org/en/practice-management/child-health-finance-payment-strategy/coding-payment-hotline)

AAP *ICD-10-CM* resources (www.aap.org/en/practice-management/child-health-finance-payment-strategy/coding-and-valuation/icd-10-cm-resources)

Pediatric Coding Q&A: Expert Advice From the AAP Coding Hotline (www.aap.org/en/catalog/categories/coding/pediatric-coding-qa-expert-advice-from-the-aap-coding-hotline-paperback)

Pediatric ICD-10-CM 2026: A Manual for Provider-Based Coding (www.aap.org/Pediatric-ICD-10-CM-2026-11th-Edition-Paperback)

Pediatric Office Superbill 2026 (www.aap.org/Pediatric-Office-Superbill-2026)

AAP Pediatric Coding Newsletter

"Back to Basics: Reporting National Drug Codes," September 2023 (https://doi.org/10.1542/pcco_book233_document003)

"Coding Review: Preparticipation Physical Evaluations," July 2024 (https://doi.org/10.1542/pcco_book243_document003)

"*CPT 2024:* Reporting Unlisted Procedure Codes," December 2023 (https://doi.org/10.1542/pcco_book236_document004)

ICD-10-CM article collection (https://publications.aap.org/codingnews/collection/510/ICD-10-CM)

"Use Diagnosis Coding Conventions to Avoid Denied Claims," June 2024 (https://doi.org/10.1542/pcco_book242_document003)

"Understanding Age Ranges in *Current Procedural Terminology*," May 2023 (https://doi.org/10.1542/pcco_book229_document005)

Current Procedural Terminology

AAP *CPT* resources (www.aap.org/en/practice-management/child-health-finance-payment-strategy/coding-and-valuation/cpt-coding)

AMA *CPT* general information (www.ama-assn.org/practice-management/cpt-current-procedural-terminology)

Category I immunization codes (www.ama-assn.org/practice-management/cpt/category-i-immunization-codes)

Category II code descriptors and clinical topics listing (www.ama-assn.org/practice-management/cpt/category-ii-codes)

Category III codes (www.ama-assn.org/practice-management/cpt/category-iii-codes)

ICD-10-CM Code Files and Guidelines

CMS *ICD-10* (www.cdc.gov/nchs/icd/icd-10-cm/index.html)

National Drug Codes

FDA National Drug Code Directory (www.fda.gov/drugs/drug-approvals-and-databases/national-drug-code-directory)

Test Your Knowledge!

1. **Which code set is used for reporting most professional services?**
   a. *CPT*
   b. HCPCS Level II
   c. National Drug Codes
   d. Place of service codes
2. **Which *ICD-10-CM* note means "not coded here and not reported in conjunction with codes in this category"?**
   a. See also
   b. Excludes1
   c. Excludes2
   d. Code first
3. **Which of the following is accurate regarding diagnosis code selection?**
   a. Codes for observation and evaluation for suspected conditions not found should be reported when a patient's symptoms do not support a specific diagnosis.
   b. A timesaving tip is to always report the default code at the main entry in the alphabetic index.
   c. It is never appropriate to report an unspecified code.
   d. An unspecified code is appropriately reported when testing to determine a more specific diagnosis would not be medically necessary.
4. **The abbreviation HCPCS is typically used in reference to which of the following?**
   a. Healthcare Common Procedure Coding System Level I
   b. Healthcare Common Procedure Coding System Level II
   c. Current Procedural Terminology
   d. Telemedicine codes and modifiers
5. **Which of the following is true of linking *ICD-10-CM* and procedure codes on a claim?**
   a. Each *ICD-10-CM* code must be linked to only one procedure code per claim.
   b. It is not necessary to link *ICD-10-CM* codes to procedure codes.
   c. Up to 4 diagnosis fields may be linked to a service line.
   d. *ICD-10-CM* codes are listed on a claim but not linked to a service line.

CHAPTER 2

Coding Edits and Modifiers

Contents

Chapter Highlights

- National Correct Coding Initiative (NCCI) edits commonly used by payers in the claim processing system for physician services
- The 3 types of code edits commonly used by payers to prevent errors in claims payment
- When modifiers do or do not affect application of code edits
- Appropriate use of modifiers, including those from *Current Procedural Terminology* (*CPT*®) and the Healthcare Common Procedure Coding System (HCPCS)
- Distinguishing *CPT* modifiers that are used exclusively with evaluation and management (E/M) services or reported only with surgical or other procedures (eg, medical, laboratory, or radiological testing).

Coding Edits

Coding edits and modifiers are important tools for getting paid correctly. Coding edits are used by most payers in electronic claims adjudication to determine which reported services are payable when multiple services are provided on the same date by the same physician, qualified health care professional (QHP), or multiple individuals practicing in the exact same specialty and same group practice. Edits also determine what number of units are allowed based on common utilization (eg, typical medication doses) and payment policies.

Modifiers are used to communicate information to payer systems about the service described by a procedure code. Modifiers indicate either a change in the way a service was provided or additional information, such as laterality of a body site or certain circumstances (eg, a significant problem was addressed at an encounter for a routine child health examination). Correct modifier use can prevent inaccurate denials due to coding edits.

National Correct Coding Initiative Edits

NCCI edits were initially developed for use by the Centers for Medicare & Medicaid Services (CMS) in adjudicating Medicare claims. All Medicaid programs use a Medicaid-specific version of the NCCI edits. The NCCI edits may form the basis for proprietary claim editors used by private payers.

NCCI edits

- Have been developed based on *CPT* code descriptors and instructions, coding guidelines developed by national medical societies (eg, American Academy of Pediatrics [AAP]), Medicare billing history, local and national Medicare carrier policies and edits, and analysis of standard medical and surgical practice
- Are commonly used in claim processing systems for physician services and promote correct coding through publication of the edits and manuals that provide rationales for certain edits
- Include 3 types of edits: procedure-to-procedure edits, add-on code (AOC) edits (not included in the Medicaid NCCI), and Medically Unlikely Edits (MUEs)

Procedure-to-Procedure Edits

- Identify code pairs that should not typically be billed by the same physician or physicians of the same group practice and same specialty (*provider* is used in NCCI manuals) for the same patient on the same date of service (DOS).
- Include edits based on services that are mutually exclusive in code descriptor or anatomy, services considered to be inherent to each other, and edits based on coding instructions.
  - If 2 codes of an edit are billed by the same provider for the same patient for the same DOS without an appropriate modifier, only the column 1 code is paid.
  - If clinical circumstances justify appending the appropriate modifier *to the column 2 code*, payment of both codes may be allowed. (The Medicaid NCCI will allow payment when an NCCI modifier can override the edit and is appended to either code in a code pair, provided that the modifier is appropriately reported in conjunction with either code.)

The CMS allows physicians to append modifiers 59, XE, XP, XS, and XU to the column 1 or column 2 code when reporting 2 codes paired by NCCI edits. Other payers may adopt this policy or require that the modifier be appended to the code in column 2 of the NCCI edit file.

Modifier indicators are assigned to every code pair identified in the NCCI. They dictate whether modifiers are needed or will be accepted to override the edit. These indicators are

0 Under no circumstance may a modifier be used to override the edit.
1 An appropriate modifier may be used to override the edit.
9 This edit was deleted.

Refer to **Table 2-1** for examples.

Table 2-1. Examples of Medicaid National Correct Coding Initiative Edits

Column 1 Comprehensive Code	Column 2 Component Code	Modifier Indicator	Effective Date
Edits apply to services provided on the same date by one physician or QHP or multiple individuals of the same specialty and same group practice.			
99221–99223 Initial hospital care E/M, per day	99460 Initial hospital or birthing center care, per day, for E/M of normal newborn	0	10/1/2020
NCCI edits preclude any payment for the column 2 code because each code represents all hospital care on a single DOS.			
96110 Developmental screening, with scoring and documentation, per standardized instrument	96160 Administration of patient-focused health risk assessment instrument with scoring and documentation, per standardized instrument	1	10/1/2020
The component code (96160) would be denied by payers using Medicaid edits unless a modifier indicating a distinct procedural service (eg, 59) were appended (eg,96160 59). The opposite is true when a payer uses Medicare edits (ie, 96160 is in column 1 and 96110 is in column 2 and 96110 should be appended with modifier 59, when appropriate).			
99291 Critical care, E/M of the critically ill or critically injured patient; first 30-74 minutes	99281–99285 Emergency department visit E/M	1	10/1/2020
NCCI edits preclude payment for the column 2 component code (eg, 99285) except when a modifier is appropriately used to override the edit. When a physician provides emergency department E/M service prior to the patient requiring critical care on the same date, and appends modifier 25 to the component code (eg, 99285 25, indicating that the services were separate and distinctly documented), both services may be reported.			
90460 IA through 18 years of age via any route of administration, with counseling by physician or other QHP; first or only component of each vaccine or toxoid administered	99381–99384 or 99391–99394 Preventive E/M services	1	01/1/2013
The component code (eg, 99391) would be denied if modifier 25 were not appended to it. To report modifier 25, E/M services must include significant and separate MDM or time beyond that included in the preservice and postservice work of a procedure performed at the same encounter. *Be aware that the higher-valued service may be the component code and would be denied without the application of the correct modifier.*			
Abbreviations: DOS, date of service; E/M, evaluation and management; IA, immunization administration; MDM, medical decision-making; NCCI, National Correct Coding Initiative; QHP, qualified health care professional.			

Appropriate NCCI Modifiers

- Only certain modifiers can be used to override edits when the service or procedure is clinically justified, and they may be used only on the code pairs that are assigned the 1 indicator. Refer to **Box 2-1** for a list of modifiers that override NCCI edits.
- The appropriate modifier is typically appended to the code that appears in column 2 because that is considered the bundled or exclusive procedure.
- To append the appropriate modifier and override an edit, it is imperative that the conditions of that modifier are met (eg, **XE**, separate encounter [different session]).

Box 2-1. Modifiers That Can Be Used to Override National Correct Coding Initiative Edits

Modifier	Description	Modifier	Description
24	Unrelated E/M service by the same physician or other QHP during a postoperative period	F6	Right hand, second digit
25	Significant, separately identifiable E/M service by the same physician or other QHP on the same day of the procedure or other service	F7	Right hand, third digit
57	Decision for surgery	F8	Right hand, fourth digit
58	Staged or related procedure or service by the same physician or other QHP during the postoperative period	F9	Right hand, fifth digit
59	Distinct procedural service	LC	Left circumflex coronary artery
78	Unplanned return to the OR by the same physician or other QHP following initial procedure for a related procedure during the postoperative period	LD	Left anterior descending coronary artery
79	Unrelated procedure/service by the same physician or other QHP during the postoperative period	LM	Left main coronary artery
91	Repeat clinical diagnostic laboratory test	LT	Left side
E1	Upper left, eyelid	RC	Right coronary artery
E2	Lower left, eyelid	RI	Ramus intermedius coronary artery
E3	Upper right, eyelid	RT	Right side
E4	Lower right, eyelid	TA	Left foot, great toe
FA	Left hand, thumb	T1	Left foot, second digit
F1	Left hand, second digit	T2	Left foot, third digit
F2	Left hand, third digit	T3	Left foot, fourth digit
F3	Left hand, fourth digit	T4	Left foot, fifth digit
F4	Left hand, fifth digit	T5	Right foot, great toe
F5	Right hand, thumb	T6	Right foot, second digit
		T7	Right foot, third digit
		T8	Right foot, fourth digit
		T9	Right foot, fifth digit
		XE	Separate encounter (different session)
		XP	Separate practitioner
		XS	Separate structure (site/organ)
		XU	Unusual nonoverlapping service

Abbreviations: E/M, evaluation and management; OR, operating/procedure room; QHP, qualified health care professional.

Add-On Code Edits

AOC edits have been created by the Medicare program but are not part of the Medicaid NCCI. Individual payers vary in their use of AOC edits.

CPT includes AOCs (indicated by a plus sign [✚] preceding the code) that are reported in addition to a primary procedure code. Claim processing systems may apply AOC edits to limit the combination of AOCs and primary codes that are payable. The AOC is eligible for payment if an acceptable primary procedure code, as determined by the payer, is also eligible for payment to the same physician or QHP for the same patient on the same DOS.

Medicare NCCI includes 3 types of AOC edits.

1. Type 1 AOC has a limited number of identifiable primary procedure codes.
2. Type 2 AOC does not have a specific list of primary procedure codes. Payers develop their own lists of primary procedure codes for this type of AOC.
3. Type 3 AOC has some, but not all, specific primary procedure codes identified in *CPT.*

Some codes included in the Medicare AOCs are not designated as AOCs in *CPT*. For example, health risk assessment codes **96160–96161** are not AOCs but are included in the Medicare AOCs based on assignment of a global period indicator of ZZZ (service related to another service and always included in the global period of the other service). Payers adopting the AOC edits for **96160–96161** will not pay for the service in the absence of a related E/M service on the same date.

Payers may publish AOC edit policies and code lists online or in a private payer portal.

Example

➤ **Code 90472 (immunization administration [IA] by injection, each additional vaccine/toxoid product) is included as a type 1 AOC and has the following identifiable primary procedure codes (excluding 2 HCPCS codes unique to IA benefits under Medicare policy):**

90460 IA through 18 years of age via any route of administration, with counseling by physician or other QHP; first or only component of each vaccine or toxoid administered

90471 IA (includes percutaneous, intradermal, subcutaneous, or intramuscular [IM] injections); 1 vaccine (single or combination vaccine/toxoid)

90473 IA by intranasal or oral route; 1 vaccine (single or combination vaccine/toxoid)

Teaching Point: Code **90472** would be denied if submitted on a claim with just **90461** (IA through 18 years of age via any route of administration, with counseling by physician or other QHP; each additional immunization or toxoid component administered [List separately in addition to code for primary procedure]) and not one of the primary codes listed previously. Payment would also be denied for **90461** when primary code **90460** is not included on the same claim.

Medically Unlikely Edits

The *National Correct Coding Initiative Policy Manual for Medicaid Services* describes MUEs as unit of service edits that were established by the CMS to prevent payment for an inappropriate number or quantity of the same service (eg, unintentional reporting of 100 rather than 10 units). An MUE for a HCPCS or *CPT* code is the maximum number of units of service, under most circumstances, allowable by the same provider for the same beneficiary on the same DOS.

Medicaid MUEs

- Are applied separately to each line of a claim. If the unit of service on a line exceeds the MUE value, the entire line is denied.
- Are coding edits rather than medical necessity edits.
- May be established based on claims data.
- May limit the number of units of service based on anatomical structures.
- May limit the number of units of service based on *CPT* code descriptors or *CPT* coding instructions.
- Are published on the CMS Medicaid NCCI website at www.cms.gov/medicare/coding-billing/ncci-medicaid.
- Are published with an *edit rationale* for each HCPCS and *CPT* code.
  - The MUE value assigned for **96110** (developmental screening, per instrument) is 3 according to CMS NCCI policy. (No further explanation of this rationale is provided in the current Medicaid or Medicare NCCI manuals but may be based on historical claims data.)
  - The MUE value assigned to **96127** (brief emotional/behavior assessment, per instrument) is 3 given the nature of the service or procedure, typically determined by the amount of time required to perform a procedure/service or clinical application of a procedure/service.
- Are applied separately to each claim line for a service when modifiers (eg, **59**, **76**, **77**, anatomical) cause the same HCPCS or *CPT* code to appear on separate lines of a claim.

It is important to recognize that using modifiers to override the MUE must be justified through correct selection of the procedure code, correct application of the number of units reported, medical necessity and reasonableness of the number of services, and, if applicable, reason the physician's practice pattern differs from national patterns.

Keeping Current With the NCCI

Medicaid and Medicare NCCI edits are updated quarterly. Each Medicare NCCI version ends with .0 (point zero), .1, .2, or .3 indicating its effective dates.

- Versions ending in .0 (point zero) are effective from January 1 through March 31 of that year.
- Versions ending in .1 are effective from April 1 through June 30 of that year.
- Versions ending in .2 are effective from July 1 through September 30 of that year.
- Versions ending in .3 are effective from October 1 through December 31 of that year.

The CMS releases Medicare NCCI edits free of charge on its website (www.cms.gov/medicare/coding-billing/ncci-medicare). Medicaid NCCI files are published separately free of charge at www.cms.gov/medicare/coding-billing/ncci-medicaid/medicaid-ncci-edit-files.

- Many Medicaid edits mirror Medicare edits, but that is not always the case. The CMS has instructed that use of the appropriate NCCI file is important for correct coding.
- Online NCCI edits are posted in a spreadsheet form that can be sorted by procedure code and effective date.
- There is a "Find" tool that allows users to look for a specific code. The edit files are indexed by procedure code ranges for simplified navigation.
- Policy manuals explaining the rationale for edits and correct use of NCCI-associated modifiers are published to the web pages listed previously.
  - Updated manuals for the year ahead are published annually in late fall.
  - Changes in the manual are shown in red font for easy identification.
  - Be sure to update your NCCI edit files quarterly and review changes to the NCCI manual each year.

Practice management and electronic health record software may also contain tools for identifying codes affected by NCCI edits.

Private payers may also publish code edits or provide online tools for determining if 2 or more codes are affected by the payers' code edits.

Reviewing and Using These Edits

1. Be aware of all coding edits that apply to your specialty. It is important to review them quarterly because each update replaces the former edits. Always look for new or deleted edits. Updated files can be found at www.cms.gov/medicare/coding-billing/ncci-medicare.
2. Pay close attention to the modifier indicator because it may have changed from the last quarterly update. For example, a code set that would not initially allow override with a modifier may now subsequently allow one, or vice versa.
3. Pay attention to the effective and deletion dates of each code set. The edits apply only if they are effective. The effective date is based on the DOS, not the date the claim was submitted. Sometimes an edit is retroactively terminated. If so, you may resubmit claims for payment if the DOS is within the payer's filing time frame.
4. Use modifiers as appropriate.
   a. Modifiers should be used only when applicable according to coding standards, when medically justified or necessary, and when supported by medical record documentation (progress notes, procedure notes, diagrams, or pictures) or, as previously mentioned, when dictated by payers.
   b. Refer to the CMS written guidelines (which are explicit about billing surgical procedures) or to your payer's provider manual.
5. When billing surgical procedures, you may need to look at several different codes for possible edits. Be sure to always use the code that is reflective of the total service performed. When no existing code accurately describes the procedure as performed, report an unlisted procedure code and attach documentation of the procedure to the claim when submitted for payment.
6. Appeal denied payment for services for which there is no edit and the policy manual and/or payment policies do not preclude reporting, for which a reported modifier should have allowed payment, and/or for which the edit is inconsistent with *CPT* guidelines. Knowing how this system works benefits you when appealing the denial.

Refer to the Filing Appeals section in Chapter 4 for information on appealing a denied payment.

7. Some payers have developed or adopted coding edit programs that differ from (and are often more comprehensive than) the NCCI.
   a. If a payer policy differs from the CMS NCCI policy and is not clearly defined in its provider manual, refer to the payer's website.
   b. Make sure you get policies in writing for the services you commonly perform. Your contracts with health plans should be explicit regarding how you will receive initial and updated policies.
8. Report the services provided correctly according to *CPT* code guidelines unless a payer has clearly stated otherwise.

Practice Policies and NCCI Edits

Physicians should not inconvenience patients or increase patient risk by performing services on different dates of service to avoid MUE or NCCI procedure-to-procedure edits.

- This instruction comes from the Medicaid NCCI manual and prohibits practice policies that focus on achieving maximum payment.
- Delaying patient care to avoid code edits could be seen as an abusive billing practice. Policies or practices that might be perceived in this way should be avoided.

Modifiers

CPT defines a *modifier* as an indicator that a service or procedure has been altered by some specific circumstance but not changed in its basic code definition. Modifiers are also used to show compliance with payment policy. Medical record documentation must always support using the modifier.

CPT and HCPCS modifiers are used with *CPT* or HCPCS codes. Most state Medicaid programs and many commercial payers recognize HCPCS modifiers and *CPT* modifiers.

When are modifiers needed? A modifier or combination of modifiers is appended to a procedure code when it is necessary to add context of how or when the service was provided. Context often affects payment, such as when a bilateral procedure is reported with a code that is not described as unilateral or bilateral. By appending modifier **50** (bilateral procedure), the claim for services provides context allowing claims adjudication systems to process payment at a higher rate, typically 150% of the allowable amount for the unilateral service. Examples of information provided by modifiers include

- A service provided on the same date or within the global period of a previous service is unrelated, more extensive, performed on a different body area, or performed at separate encounters.
- A face-to-face service, not specifically described as a telemedicine service, was provided via telemedicine using real-time, interactive communication technology.
- The same service was repeated on the same date.
- An E/M service that might otherwise be considered part of another service is significantly beyond the typical preservice and/or postservice components of the other service.
- The units of services provided were medically necessary but exceed the payer's unit of service edits.
- A service that may be provided for either diagnostic or preventive purposes was provided for preventive purposes.

Payers use coding edits (eg, paired codes and/or unit of service limitations) to aid in automated claims adjudication. Modifiers play an important role in this process.

- When a modifier is appropriately applied to 1 code in a pair of codes reported by a physician on 1 DOS or to a code for services that exceed the units of service typically allowed by payer edits, the payer may allow charges that would otherwise be denied as bundled or noncovered.

The Health Insurance Portability and Accountability Act of 1996 requires recognition of all *CPT* and HCPCS modifiers, but payers may have their own payment and billing policies for the use of modifiers that can vary from *CPT* guidelines.

- Know and understand individual payer policies. Doing so is important in capturing all payments allowed under your contract.
- If payment is denied inappropriately because of nonrecognition or the incorrect application of a modifier, you should appeal the denied services.
- For additional assistance, contact the AAP Coding and Payment Hotline (www.aap.org/en/practice-management/child-health-finance-payment-strategy/coding-payment-hotline).

Current Procedural Terminology Modifiers

Some *CPT* modifiers are used exclusively with E/M services, and others are reported only with surgical or other procedures (eg, medical, laboratory, or radiological testing). Refer to **Table 2-2** to review modifiers used with E/M service codes and those used only for other services. Multiple modifiers can be appended to a single *CPT* or HCPCS code.

Table 2-2. Modifiers and Evaluation and Management Services

Modifier	E/M Services
24, 25, 57	E/M-only modifiers
22, 26, 47, 50, 51, 52, 53, 54, 55, 56, 58, 59, 62, 63, 66, 76, 77, 78, 79, 80, 81, 82, 91, 92	Procedure-only modifiers (Do not append to E/M services.)
32, 33, 93,[a] 95,[a] 96, 97, 99	Either E/M or procedures

Abbreviations: AMA, American Medical Association; *CPT, Current Procedural Terminology;* E/M, evaluation and management.

[a] Refer to Appendix T of the AMA *CPT* manual for codes reportable with modifier 93 and to *CPT* Appendix P for codes reportable with modifier 95.

Modifiers Appended Only to E/M Codes

24—*Unrelated E/M Service by the Same Physician or Other QHP During a Postoperative Period*

The global period (preoperative, intraoperative, and postoperative periods) for surgical procedures is assigned by the CMS, private payers, or Medicaid and not by the American Medical Association or *CPT*. For more information on global surgery guidelines, refer to Chapters 13 and 18.

- Modifier **24** is appended to an E/M code when the physician or other QHP who performed a procedure provides an unrelated E/M service during the postoperative period.
- The CMS has its own system for defining global periods, and many payers will follow those guidelines or assign a specific number of follow-up days for surgical procedures.

Link the appropriate *International Classification of Diseases, 10th Revision, Clinical Modification* (*ICD-10-CM*) code to the E/M visit to support that the service was unrelated to the surgical procedure. Do not report the surgical diagnosis code if it was not the reason for the encounter; however, a different diagnosis is not required, as further treatment of the underlying condition for which surgery was performed is not part of the postoperative work of the procedure and may be separately reported.

Example—Modifier 24

➤ **A physician sees a 10-year-old established patient for follow-up of stable mild persistent asthma and performs a level 3 established patient office or other outpatient E/M service.** The visit occurs within the 90-day global period assigned by the payer to **25600** (closed treatment of a distal radial fracture) for which the same physician is providing care. Modifier **24** is appended to the E/M code to indicate that the service is unrelated to care of the fracture.

ICD-10-CM	*CPT*
J45.30 (mild persistent asthma, uncomplicated)	**99213 24** (established office/outpatient E/M)

Teaching Point: The diagnosis code reported provides support for the unrelated nature of the E/M service provided during the 90-day global period of the fracture care.

25—Significant, Separately Identifiable E/M Service by the Same Physician or Other QHP on the Same Day of the Procedure or Other Service

- Modifier **25** is appended only to an E/M service and only when *all the following circumstances are true:*
  - A separate service identified by a separate procedure code is performed by the same physician or other QHP, or by a physician or other QHP of the same specialty and group.
  - The patient's condition requires a significant E/M service (**99202–99499**) above and beyond the other service provided or beyond the usual preoperative and postoperative care associated with the procedure that was performed.
  - The service is separately identifiable in the documentation of the encounter(s).
- Different diagnoses are not required for reporting the E/M service on the same date.
- The performed and documented E/M components must support the level of service reported and be separately identifiable from the procedure or other service documentation, whether documented in one combined note or separate notes.
- *CPT* procedure codes *include evaluative elements routinely performed before the procedure* and the routine postoperative care. An assessment of the problem with an explanation of the procedure to be performed is considered inherent to the procedure and should not be reported separately with an E/M service code.
- When appropriate, modifier **25** may be reported on more than one E/M service for a single encounter. An example follows this list.
- **DO *NOT* USE MODIFIER 25 WHEN**
  - ✖ **The medical record does not support both services.**
  - ✖ **A problem encountered during a preventive medicine visit is insignificant or incidental (eg, minor diaper rash, renewal of prescription medications without reevaluation) or did not require additional work to perform medical decision-making [MDM] or additional time that is distinct from the time spent providing the preventive E/M service.**
  - ✖ **The E/M service is a routine part of the usual preoperative and postoperative care.**
  - ✖ **Modifier 57 (decision for surgery) is more appropriate. The decision on whether to use modifier 25 or 57 requires knowledge of payer policies. (Refer to modifier 57—discussed later in this chapter.)**

Examples—Modifier 25

➤ **A physician orders and inserts or supervises insertion of a non-indwelling bladder catheter to obtain urine for urinalysis and culture as part of the evaluation of a sick child.** Documentation supports a level 4 established patient visit in addition to the procedure.

ICD-10-CM	*CPT*
Applicable codes for diagnosis or, when undetermined, signs and symptoms	99214 25 (established patient office visit with moderate level MDM) 51701 (insertion of non-indwelling bladder catheter [eg, straight catheterization for residual urine])

Teaching Point: Medical record documentation supports that a significant, separately identifiable E/M service was provided and is reported in addition to the catheterization procedure. Modifier 25 is appended to code 99214 to signify that it is significant and separately identifiable from the preservice and postservice work of the procedure.

➤ **A physician ordered and clinical staff administered the first dose of human papillomavirus (HPV) vaccine at a preventive medicine E/M encounter 6 months earlier.** The patient returns for the second vaccine administration. The physician reviews vital signs and a brief history of no current illness and no history of adverse reaction to the first dose of the vaccine. The physician provides appropriate counseling and obtains consent for the immunization. Clinical staff administer the vaccine. A brief history and examination were performed, and a decision to administer the second dose of the vaccine was reaffirmed. This decision does not, however, represent a significant and separately identifiable E/M service. No office E/M code is reported.

ICD-10-CM	*CPT*
Z23 (encounter for immunization)	90460 (IA with physician counseling, first or only component) 90651 (HPV types 6, 11, 16, 18, 31, 33, 45, 52, 58, nonavalent [9v HPV], 2 or 3 dose schedule, for IM use)

Teaching Point: An E/M service with modifier 25 is *not* reported. A separate charge for an E/M service is not indicated, as the physician's preservice evaluation and counseling are included in the IA reported with code 90460. Had the patient requested evaluation of a problem requiring a significant and separately identifiable E/M service, the E/M service would have been reported (eg, 99213 25).

Refer to Chapters 13 and 18 for more information on reporting an E/M service on the date of a procedure. Refer to Chapter 8 for examples and guidelines for reporting a preventive medicine visit and a problem-oriented visit on the same day of service.

57—Decision for Surgery

- Modifier 57 is appended to an E/M service that resulted in the initial decision to perform the surgery or procedure. Appending modifier 57 to the E/M service indicates to the payer that the E/M service is not part of the global period.
- An E/M code with modifier 57 is reported only by the physician or a physician of the same specialty and group practice of the physician who performs the procedure. Other physicians providing E/M services on the day before or day of a procedure would not append modifier 57.
- Many payers will follow the CMS Medicare payment policy that allows reporting of modifier 57 only when the visit on the day before or day of surgery *results in a decision to perform a surgical procedure* that has a 90-day global period (major procedure).
- Know commercial and state Medicaid policies, maintain a written copy of the policies, and adhere to the policies.

Example—Modifier 57

➤ **A 10-year-old is seen by the pediatrician for the evaluation of pain in her foot and arm after a fall.** The radiograph reveals a metatarsal fracture, and the decision is made to treat the closed fracture. Arm injuries are limited to bruising and abrasions.

Code 28470 (closed treatment, metatarsal fracture; without manipulation) has an assigned global surgery period of 90 days. The appropriate E/M code (99202–99215 57), based on the clinically indicated performance and documentation of the required MDM, would be reported in addition to 28470.

Modifiers Appended Only to Codes for Procedures, Not to E/M Services

22—Increased Procedural Services

- Modifier 22 is used to report procedures when the work required to provide a service is substantially greater than typically required.
- Modifier 22 is appended only to anesthesia, surgery, radiology, laboratory, pathology, and medicine codes.
- Documentation must clearly reflect the substantial additional work and the reason for the additional work (eg, increased intensity, time, technical difficulty of procedure, severity of patient's condition, physical and mental effort required).
  - It is important that documentation is specific. For instance, documentation that a procedure took longer than 1 hour is less supportive than documentation that the procedure took a total of 85 minutes or lasted from 9:15 to 10:40 am.
  - Report additional diagnosis codes to support the increased work, when applicable.
- Most payers will require that a copy of the medical record documentation be sent with the claim when modifier 22 is reported.
- For an electronic claim, indicate "additional documentation available on request" in the claim level loop (2300 NTE) or in the line level loop (2400 NTE) segment. If the payer allows electronic claim attachments, follow the payer's instructions to submit the procedure note and, if necessary, a physician statement about the increased difficulty of the procedure.

Examples—Modifier 22

➤ **The physician required 45 minutes to perform a simple repair of a 1-cm laceration on a 2-year-old because the child's behavior was combative and several stops and starts were necessary.**

12011 22 Simple repair superficial wound of face; ≤2.5 cm

➤ **A tonsillectomy with drainage of a peritonsillar abscess is performed.** The surgery is complicated, requiring extensive work to control bleeding.

42826 22 Tonsillectomy, primary or secondary; age 12 or over

Teaching Point: When appropriately documented, the increased work of procedure is reported by appending modifier 22. Note that drainage of the peritonsillar abscess at the time of tonsillectomy is included in the tonsillectomy and not separately reported.

26—Professional Component

Professional, Technical, or Global Services

Certain procedures (eg, cardiac tests, radiography, surgical diagnostic tests) are broken down into professional and technical components. *CPT* has a modifier for reporting the professional component (26) but does not have a modifier for reporting only the technical component. That falls under the HCPCS modifier set (modifier TC).

- Professional component only: The physician who does not supply the equipment but performs the written interpretation and report of a service with professional and technical components should report the service with modifier 26 appended to the appropriate *CPT* code.

The professional component includes the physician work (eg, interpretation of the test, written report).

- Technical component only: Most payers recognize modifier TC (technical component only). The facility or provider who owns the equipment and is responsible for the overhead and associated costs would report the same procedure code with modifier TC appended.
- Technical and professional components (global): If a service includes both professional and technical components and the physician owns the equipment, employs the staff to perform the service, and interprets the test, the procedure is reported *without a modifier.*

***Reporting Modifier* 26**

- When reporting the professional component of diagnostic tests, interpretation should be documented in a report similar to that which is typical for the physicians who predominantly provide the service. This report should include *all the following items:*
  - Indication(s) for testing
  - Description of test
  - Findings and any comparison to findings of prior tests
  - Limitations, when applicable
  - Impression or conclusion
- If the report of a physician's interpretation is included in the documentation of another service (eg, office visit), it is important that the report is distinct and complete.
- The professional component is not reported when a physician reviews a test and notes agreement with the interpreting physician or when only a quick read without formal interpretation is provided.
- Some codes were developed to distinguish between technical and professional components (eg, routine electrocardiogram [ECG] codes 93000–93010). Modifier 26 is not appropriate when reporting codes that distinguish professional and technical components and may result in a denial of the charge.

Examples—Modifier 26

➤ **A physician interprets the results of an attended polysomnography provided to a 6-year-old patient and creates a report of the findings. The tests were performed in a facility's sleep laboratory, and the facility will bill the technical component of the service.**

95810 26 Polysomnography; age 6 years or older, sleep staging with 4 or more additional parameters of sleep, attended by a technologist

The physician reports modifier 26, indicating professional component only, because the facility provided the technical component.

➤ **A pediatrician electronically accesses the image of a foot radiograph that was taken at the outpatient department of the hospital and will be interpreted by a radiologist at that facility. The pediatrician notes findings in the patient's records.**

The pediatrician's review of the radiograph is not separately reported when a radiologist provides a final interpretation and report. The pediatrician's independent review and interpretation of the image, however, increases the level of data to be reviewed and analyzed when determining the level of MDM in a related E/M service. (Refer to **Chapter 6** for more on how independent interpretation of tests affects the level of MDM for a visit.)

➤ **A cardiologist performs transthoracic echocardiography with spectral and color-flow Doppler echocardiography on a patient in the hospital.**

The cardiologist reports 93306 26 (echocardiography, transthoracic, real-time with image documentation [2D], includes M-mode recording, when performed, complete, with spectral Doppler echocardiography, and with color-flow Doppler echocardiography), and the hospital reports 93306 TC.

47—*Anesthesia by Surgeon*

- Modifier 47 is used only when a physician performing a procedure *also personally performs* the regional and/or general anesthesia. The physician performing the procedure may not report codes 00100–01999 for anesthesia services. Instead, modifier 47 is appended to the code for the procedure performed.
- When performed, a code for regional anesthesia (nerve block) may be reported to indicate the site of the block.
- Modifier 47 is considered informational by many payers and does not affect payment.
  - Medicaid considers all anesthesia (other than moderate conscious sedation) provided by the same physician performing a procedure to be included in the procedure.
  - Other payers may restrict use of modifier 47 to specific procedure codes and provide specific reporting instructions. Be sure to verify payer policy before reporting.
- **DO *NOT* USE MODIFIER 47 WHEN**
  - ✖ **Administering local anesthetic because it is considered inherent to the procedure**
  - ✖ **Performing moderate (conscious) sedation**

For more information on reporting moderate sedation, refer to Chapter 13.

Example—Modifier 47

➤ **The surgeon performs a nerve block on the brachial plexus (64415) and removal of a ganglion cyst on the wrist (25111).**

25111 47 and 64415.

The regional anesthesia is separate from the procedure.

50—Bilateral Procedure

- Modifier 50 is used to identify bilateral procedures that are performed at the same session.
- It is used only when the services and/or procedures are performed on identical anatomical sites, aspects, or organs.
- ✖ Do not append modifier 50 to a code with a descriptor that indicates the procedure includes bilateral, "one or both," or "unilateral or bilateral."
- The Medicare Physician Fee Schedule (MPFS) Relative Value Files (www.cms.gov/medicare/payment/fee-schedules/physician/pfs-relative-value-files) include a column (Column T, BILAT SURG) that identifies codes that may be reported with modifier 50. Procedures with a 1 indicator can be reported with modifier 50.

Some private payers also publish lists of codes that may be reported as bilateral procedures.

- When the *CPT* code descriptor indicates a bilateral procedure and only a unilateral procedure is performed, modifier 52 (reduced services) should be appended to the procedure code.
- For Medicaid claims that require use of modifier 50, report only 1 unit of service on the line item for the bilateral procedure. Other payers may have different instructions for reporting bilateral procedures.

Examples—Modifier 50

➤ **A physician performs bilateral tympanostomy with insertion of ventilating tubes while the patient is under general anesthesia.**

69436 50 Tympanostomy (requiring insertion of ventilating tube), general anesthesia

➤ **A physician performs bilateral nasal endoscopy.**

31231 Nasal endoscopy, diagnostic, unilateral or bilateral (separate procedure)

Teaching Point: Modifier 50 would not be appended to code 31231 because the code descriptor indicates a unilateral or bilateral procedure. Modifier 52 is also not required for reporting a unilateral service when the code descriptor includes the phrase "unilateral or bilateral," as the unmodified code represents a service that is either unilateral or bilateral.

Coding Conundrum: Modifier 50

The Medicaid NCCI edits require that bilateral surgical procedures (for which there is no code specifying a bilateral procedure) be reported with modifier 50 and 1 unit of service.

Example: Report removal of foreign bodies from both ears with 69200 50 with 1 unit.

Bilateral diagnostic procedures may be reported with any of the methods that follow:

Example: Report bilateral radiographs of clavicles with 1 of the following 3 methods:

2 units of service on 1 claim line: 73000 (radiologic examination; clavicle, complete) × 2

1 unit of service and modifier 50 on 1 claim line: 73000 50 × 1 unit

1 unit of service and modifier RT on 1 claim line plus 1 unit of service and modifier LT on a second claim line: 73000 RT × 1 unit and 73000 LT × 1 unit

51—Multiple Procedures

- Modifier **51** is most often used for surgical procedures that are performed during the same session and through the same incision. This modifier identifies potentially overlapping or duplicative relative value units (RVUs) related to the global surgical package or the technical component of certain services (eg, radiology services).
- Some payers, including Medicare administrative contractors, advise against reporting this modifier, as their systems automatically assign multiple service reductions to the appropriate services. In these cases, the system ignores modifier **51**. Follow payer guidance for reporting modifier **51**.
- When required, modifier **51** is appended to codes for each additional procedure or service when multiple procedures are performed at the same session by the same individual or individuals in the same group practice. The primary procedure or service is reported first without a modifier.
- Although many claims adjudication systems now automatically identify the primary procedure, it is advisable that the first-reported service is that with the highest relative value, followed by additional services appended with modifier **51**, when applicable.
- Modifier **51** does not override NCCI edits.

For information on multiple surgery indicators and payment adjustments, refer to Chapter 12, Section 40.6, of the *Medicare Claims Processing Manual* at www.cms.gov/Regulations-and-Guidance/Guidance/Manuals/Downloads/clm104c12.pdf or individual payer policies for multiple procedures performed on the same date.

- **DO NOT USE MODIFIER 51 WHEN**
  - ✖ **Reporting add-on procedure codes (identified with the ✚ symbol) that are exempt from modifier 51 because the services are always performed in addition to a primary service.**
  - ✖ **Reporting *CPT* codes identified with the Ø symbol (exempt from modifier 51) because they have no associated preservice or postservice valuation and are already reduced (refer to *CPT* Appendix E for a list of these codes).**
  - ✖ **Different providers perform the procedures.**
  - ✖ **Two or more physicians provide different and unrelated procedures (eg, multiple trauma) to the same patient on the same day, unless one of the physicians performs multiple procedures.**
  - ✖ **Reporting E/M services, physical medicine and rehabilitation services, or provision of supplies (eg, immunization products).**

Example—Modifier 51

➤ **A child undergoes adenoidectomy and bilateral myringotomy with tube placement at the same surgical session. The surgeon reports**

69436 50	Tympanostomy (requiring insertion of ventilating tube), general anesthesia
42830 51	Adenoidectomy, primary; younger than age 12

Teaching Point: Code **69436** is reported first because it carries the highest relative value when reported with modifier **50** (7.28 facility total RVUs [4.85 × 150%] vs 6.53 for code **42830**). Modifier **51** is appended to **42830**. If the myringotomy was a unilateral procedure, **42830** would be listed first (with no modifier) and **69436 51** would be listed second (with no modifier **50**).

52—Reduced Services

- Modifier **52** is used when a service or procedure is partially reduced or eliminated (ie, procedure started but discontinued) at the discretion of the physician or other QHP.
  - ✖ Modifier **52** is not used when a procedure is canceled before the induction of anesthesia and/or surgical preparation in the operating/procedure room (OR).
- The diagnosis code linked to the procedure reported with modifier **52** should reflect why the procedure was reduced.
  - ✖ When reporting a reduced service or a procedure code with modifier **52**, do not reduce your normal fee. Let the payer reduce the payment according to its policy.

For further discussion of modifier **52**, refer to the "Coding Conundrum: Are Modifiers **52** and **53** Indicated for All Reduced/Discontinued Services?" box later in this chapter.

Examples—Modifier 52

➤ **A physician begins a circumcision (54150) on a 3-day-old boy.** The physician elects to perform the circumcision without a dorsal penile or ring block. In this circumstance, modifier 52 would be reported with code 54150 to indicate that the service was reduced from its full descriptor at the physician's discretion.

➤ **A peripherally inserted central venous catheter (PICC) without a subcutaneous port is inserted with imaging guidance, but the tip location is not confirmed by imaging.**

ICD-10-CM	*CPT*
J13 (pneumonia due to *Streptococcus pneumoniae*)	36572 52 (PICC insertion without subcutaneous port, with imaging guidance; younger than 5 years of age)

Teaching Point: Code 36572 includes confirmation of the tip location. Therefore, modifier 52 would be appended when performed without confirmation of catheter tip location.

53—*Discontinued Procedure*

- Modifier 53 signifies that a procedure was terminated (ie, started but discontinued) because of extenuating circumstances or circumstances in which the well-being of the patient was threatened (eg, patient is at risk or has unexpected, serious complications, such as excessive bleeding or hypotension) during a procedure.
- It is not used to report the elective cancellation of a procedure before the patient's anesthesia induction and/or surgical preparation in the operating suite.
- The diagnosis code should reflect the reason for the termination of the procedure.
- Most payers will require that operative or procedure reports be submitted with the claim.

Examples—Modifier 53

➤ **A child presents with a foreign body of the right great toe.** The pediatrician incises the toe and tries to remove the foreign body. However, during the procedure, the pediatrician decided that the procedure must be stopped to avoid injury to the child, who was struggling against restraint.

10120 53 Incision and removal of foreign body, subcutaneous tissues; simple

Teaching Point: If the pediatrician performs a second procedure to remove the foreign body within the 10-day global period of code 10120, modifier 58 (staged or related procedure or service by the same physician or other QHP during the postoperative period) should be appended to the code for that procedure. Refer to modifier 58 (discussed later in this chapter).

➤ **In-office spirometry is ordered for a child. Despite multiple attempts, a satisfactory evaluation is not obtained.** If results of suboptimal testing provide information of clinical value, the interpreting pediatrician might append modifier 53 to the global procedure code.

94010 53 Spirometry, including graphic record, total and timed vital capacity, expiratory flow rate measurement(s), with or without maximal voluntary ventilation

Teaching Point: Physicians and QHPs must use clinical judgment in determining whether the data from an incomplete test were sufficient to support interpretation and report for use in E/M of the patient's symptoms/problem. When there is no valid result for interpretation by the treating pediatrician, no code is reported for the global or professional components of the service.

If the pediatrician bills for the technical component of the incomplete spirometry (staff time and overhead of attempted spirometry), 94010 TC 53 (spirometry, including graphic record, total and timed vital capacity, expiratory flow rate measurement[s], with or without maximal voluntary ventilation) might be reported. Modifier 53 is appropriate when testing has not been completed because of an extenuating circumstance (eg, patient's inability to complete testing). Documentation should support the number of attempts, testing errors noted (eg, poor effort), graphic data obtained, and reason for discontinuing the service.

Coding Conundrum: Are Modifiers 52 and 53 Indicated for All Reduced/Discontinued Services?

Despite a reduction in some component of a service, there are times when a modifier may not be indicated.

- When an insignificant amount of the typical work of the service is performed, it may be more appropriate to report an E/M service representing only the work completed (eg, MDM regarding the service).
- When the work of a procedure is minimally reduced because a portion of the procedure could not be completed, it may be appropriate to report the code for the completed procedure without a modifier.

× Do not report modifier 52 or 53 if an existing code describes the service as performed.

54—*Surgical Care Only*

Modifier 54 is appended to the surgery procedure code when the physician does the procedure but another physician or other QHP (not of the same group practice) accepts a transfer of care and provides preoperative and/or postoperative management.

55—*Postoperative Management Only*

Modifier 55 is appended to the surgical code to report that only postoperative care is performed because another physician or other QHP of another group practice has performed the surgical procedure and transferred the patient for postoperative care.

56—*Preoperative Management Only*

Modifier 56 is appended to the surgical code when only the preoperative care and evaluation are performed because another physician or other QHP of another group practice has performed the surgical procedure. This modifier is seldom applicable.

Coding Conundrum: Modifiers 54, 55, 56, and G0559

Modifiers 54, 55, and 56 are typically used to report surgical procedures that have a global period of 10 to 90 days. They are not reported with procedures that have 0-day global periods. It is important to learn which guidelines are followed by your major payers. When reporting these modifiers, coordination and communication between the physicians and their billing staff is imperative. The physician providing follow-up care must know that the physician who provided the surgical care reported modifier 54 to report modifier 55. Alternatively, the physician providing follow-up care may be limited to reporting E/M codes for each follow-up encounter that does not include a new procedural service.

Medicare created add-on code G0559 for reporting by a physician or QHP who did not perform the procedure (and is in a different group practice and different specialty than the physician who performed the procedure) when there has not been a formal transfer of care supporting modifier 55. G0559 reports the added complexity of providing an initial postoperative follow-up visit to a procedure performed by another physician or QHP and is reported once within the 90-day global period. (For the full code descriptor, refer to your HCPCS reference.) Other payers may or may not adopt policy to pay for G0559 in addition to an initial E/M visit for postoperative care. When reporting code G0559, do not append modifier 55 to the E/M visit code.

For more information on global surgery guidelines, refer to Chapters 13 and 18.

Example—Modifiers 54 and 55

➤ **An emergency department (ED) physician provides initial care for a Colles fracture of the right radius and instructs the patient to follow up with a primary care or orthopedic physician for care during the global period.** The ED physician reports an ED E/M service (99281–99285) with modifier 57 (decision for surgery) and code 25600 54.

25600 54 Closed treatment of distal radial fracture (eg, Colles or Smith type) or epiphyseal separation, includes closed treatment of fracture of ulnar styloid, when performed; without manipulation

The primary care or orthopedic physician who assumes management of the patient's fracture care will report 25600 55. The transfer of care should be documented and the 2 physicians must coordinate how the services will be reported so each reports the appropriate modifier.

Teaching Point: If a physician's initial fracture care is limited to stabilization pending referral for fracture treatment, only the E/M and any splinting or casting and supplies are reported. The physician who will provide fracture treatment will report a fracture care code without a modifier.

58—Staged or Related Procedure or Service by the Same Physician or Other QHP During the Postoperative Period

- Modifier **58** is used to indicate that a procedure or service performed during the postoperative period was planned or anticipated (ie, staged), was more extensive than the original procedure, or was performed for therapeutic purposes after a surgical procedure.
- Modifier **58** is a recognized modifier under the NCCI.
- Typically, payers recognize modifier **58** only when there is a global surgical period associated with the procedure code.
- **DO *NOT* REPORT MODIFIER 58 WHEN**
  - ✖ **Treating a problem that requires a return to the OR (eg, unanticipated clinical condition) (Refer to modifier 78—discussed later in this chapter.)**
  - ✖ **Reporting procedures that include as part of their *CPT* descriptor "one or more visits" or "one or more sessions"**

Example—Modifier 58

➤ **A physician replaces a cast during the global period of fracture care.**

29000–29799 58 Appropriate casting code

Teaching Point: Only the first cast is included in the code for fracture care. For more on fracture care, refer to **Chapter 13**.

For another use of modifier **58**, refer to the first teaching point in the examples for modifier **53** (discussed earlier in this chapter).

59—Distinct Procedural Service

Never use modifier 59 in place of modifier 25 or on an E/M service code.

- Modifier **59** is used to identify procedures or services, other than E/M services, that are not normally reported together but are appropriate under the circumstances.
- Report modifier **59** only when no other modifier better describes the reason for separately reporting a service that might otherwise be bundled with another procedural service on the same date.
  - ✖ Never append modifier **59** to bypass payer edits without clinical justification.
- Refer to HCPCS anatomical modifiers (eg, **F8**, right hand, 4th digit) and **XE**, **XP**, **XS**, and **XU** for potential alternatives to modifier **59**.
- Per *CPT*, modifier **59** represents one of the following conditions of a procedure, in that the procedure
  - Was provided at a different session from another procedure
  - Was a different procedure or surgery
  - Involved a different site or organ system
  - Required a separate incision or excision
  - Was performed on a separate lesion or injury (or area of injury in extensive injuries)

Example—Modifier 59

➤ **Four behavioral health assessment instruments are completed and scored during 1 encounter to assess symptoms of depression and to reevaluate the status of previously diagnosed attention-deficit/hyperactivity disorder (ADHD) (standardized instruments completed by 1 parent and 3 teachers).**

96127 × 3 (brief emotional/behavioral assessment [eg, depression inventory, ADHD scale], with scoring and documentation, per standardized instrument).

96127 59 × 1 (fourth assessment instrument).

Modifier **59** would be appended to the code for the fourth assessment instrument to reflect that 4 distinct assessment instruments were scored and documented. Medicaid NCCI MUEs limit units of **96127** to 3 units per claim, but modifier **59** may be appended to units on an additional line to indicate that additional instruments were necessary.

62—Two Surgeons

- Modifier **62** is used when 2 surgeons work together as primary surgeons performing a distinct part(s) of the same procedure. Do not use modifier **62** when one surgeon assists another.

- Co-surgeons may be of the same specialty or different specialties, although usually they are of different specialties. Individual payer policies may vary regarding coverage of co-surgery by 2 physicians of the same specialty.
- Each surgeon should report their distinct operative work by adding modifier 62 to the procedure code and any associated AOC(s) for that procedure as long as both surgeons continue to work together as primary surgeons.
- Each surgeon should report the co-surgery once with the same procedure code.
- If an additional procedure(s), including an add-on procedure(s), is performed during the same surgical session, a separate code(s) may also be reported without modifier 62 added.
- Simultaneous bilateral services are procedures during which each surgeon performs the same procedure on opposite sides. Each surgeon should report the simultaneous bilateral procedures with modifiers 50 and 62.
- Column AB (CO SURG) of the MPFS (Resource-Based Relative Value Scale [RBRVS]) identifies procedures that may or may not be performed by co-surgeons. Indicator 1 is assigned to procedures for which co-surgery is allowed under the Medicare program. Visit www.cms.gov/Medicare/Medicare-Fee-for-Service-Payment/PhysicianFeeSched/PFS-Relative-Value-Files.html.

Example—Modifier 62

➤ **A neurosurgeon and a general surgeon work together to place a ventriculoperitoneal shunt.**

Both physicians would report 62223 62 with the same diagnosis code. The operative note must include the name of each surgeon, specific role of each surgeon, and necessity for 2 surgeons. Each surgeon should dictate their own operative report.

Most payers will require authorization before the procedure.

63—*Procedure Performed on Infants Less Than 4 kg*

- Modifier 63 is used to report procedures performed on neonates and infants up to a *present body weight of 4 kg* that involve significantly increased complexity and physician work commonly associated with these patients.
- Unless otherwise designated, this modifier may be appended only to procedures or services listed in the *CPT* descriptor for modifier 63 (ie, the 20100–69990 code series and the following codes in Medicine section: 92920, 92928, 92953, 92960, 92986, 92987, 92990, 92997, 92998, 93312–93318, 93452, 93505, 93563, 93564, 93568, 93569, 93573–93575, 93580–93582, 93590–93598, 93615, and 93616).
- Use of modifier 63 may require submission of an operative note with the claim. The operative note should include the patient's weight. It is also beneficial to report the patient's weight on the claim.
- **DO *NOT* REPORT MODIFIER 63**
  - ✖ **When the code is included in *CPT* Appendix F, as codes in this appendix were valued to include the increased complexity and physician work associated with modifier 63**
  - ✖ **With any *CPT* codes listed in the E/M Services, Anesthesia, Radiology, Pathology/Laboratory, or Medicine sections (other than those previously identified from the Medicine/Cardiovascular section)**
  - ✖ **When the *CPT* code includes a parenthetical instruction prohibiting reporting modifier 63**

Example—Modifier 63

➤ **A surgeon performed right- and left-sided heart catheterization through normal native connections on a 4-week-old with a weight of 3.1 kg and positive findings of congenital anomalies.**

93596 26 63 Right and left heart catheterization for congenital heart defect(s) including imaging guidance by the proceduralist to advance the catheter to the target zone(s); normal native connections

Because the procedure may be performed on patients weighing more than 4 kg, the complexity and work associated with performing the procedure on an infant weighing up to 4 kg *was not* included in the valuation assigned to 93596. Modifier 26 indicates that the surgeon is reporting only the professional component of the catheterization. For more information, refer to modifier 26 (discussed earlier in this chapter).

66—*Surgical Team*

- Modifier 66 is appended to the basic procedure code when highly complex procedures (requiring the concomitant services of several physicians or other QHPs, often of different specialties, plus other highly skilled, specially trained personnel and various types of complex equipment) are carried out under the surgical team concept.
- Each surgeon reports modifier 66.

- Each surgeon should dictate their own operative report, and it should reflect the medical necessity for team surgery.
- Column AC (TEAM SURG) of the MPFS (RBRVS) identifies procedures that may or may not be performed by a team of surgeons. Indicator 1 is assigned to procedures for which team surgery is allowed under the Medicare program.
- The operative notes are usually required by the payer.
- If a surgeon were assisting another surgeon, modifier **80**, **81**, or **82** would be more applicable.

Example—Modifier 66

➤ **Multiple surgeons perform different portions of an organ transplant.**

Each physician would report their services with modifier **66** appended to the procedure code.

76—Repeat Procedure or Service by Same Physician or Other QHP

- Modifier **76** is used when the same procedure or service is repeated by the same physician or other QHP subsequent to the original procedure or service. Use of this modifier may prevent denial as a duplicate service line.
- When a procedure is repeated on the same date, it may be helpful to include the start times of each procedure in a narrative statement on the claim (eg, field 19 on a paper claim).
- The repeat procedure may be performed on different days. (Payer guidance may vary.)
- This modifier is appended only to non-E/M procedure codes and is not reported when the code definition indicates a repeat procedure.
- Use of this modifier advises the payer that this is not a duplicate service. (For a repeat clinical diagnostic laboratory test, refer also to modifier **91**—discussed later in this chapter.)
- The CMS recognizes this modifier only for ECGs and radiographs or for a procedure performed in an OR or another location equipped to perform procedures. Medicaid programs or other commercial payers may follow this guideline. Check with payers to determine their policy on use of the modifier.

Examples—Modifier 76

➤ **You see a patient in your office with severe asthma and give them 3 nebulized albuterol treatments and steroids over the course of the visit. You report**

94640 × 1 (pressurized or nonpressurized inhalation treatment for acute airway obstruction for therapeutic purposes and/or for diagnostic purposes such as sputum induction with an aerosol generator, nebulizer, metered dose inhaler or intermittent positive pressure breathing [IPPB] device).

94640 76 × 1 on 2 separate claims lines to support adjudication of each repeat service.

Teaching Point: Most payers will deny services reported as **94640 76** with 3 units on a single line because of the lack of an initial service (ie, code reported without modifier **76**). Report on a single claim line only when a payer policy instructs to do so. Note that some payers require you to *report each service on a separate line,* by using a quantity of 1 and appending modifier **76** to the subsequent procedures.

The Medicare and Medicaid NCCI manuals contradict *CPT* instruction for *CPT* code 94640, stating that 94640 be reported once during a single patient encounter regardless of the number of separate inhalation treatments that are administered. Follow individual payer guidance.

➤ **A patient presents to the pediatric clinic in the morning with a nosebleed. Cautery (anterior) and packing are used to control the hemorrhage (30901).** Later that day, the patient returns because the clot has dislodged and bleeding has resumed. Control of the hemorrhage is again achieved with limited cautery and packing by the same physician. The payer's MUE for **30901** is 1 unit and is applied per claim line.

30901 Control nasal hemorrhage, anterior, simple (limited cautery and/or packing) any method

30901 76 XE

Teaching Point: The second procedure is billed on a second claim line with modifier **76** to alert the payer to the repeat service and allow override of the MUE. Modifier **XE** (separate encounter, discussed later in this chapter) may also be appended to provide additional context.

77—Repeat Procedure or Service by Another Physician or Other QHP

- Modifier 77 is used when a procedure or service is repeated by *another physician or health care professional* subsequent to the original procedure or service. Be sure that the same code(s) is reported by each physician to prevent denials when reporting modifier 77.
- Payers may require documentation to support the medical necessity of performing the same service or procedure on the same day or during the global surgical period, if applicable.

Example—Modifier 77

➤ **An orthopedic physician performs re-reduction (closed treatment with manipulation) of radial and ulnar shaft fractures. The initial closed treatment of the fractures was reported by a physician of another specialty or another group practice.**

Re-reduction: 25565 77 (closed treatment of radial and ulnar shaft fractures; with manipulation).

78—Unplanned Return to the OR by the Same Physician or Other QHP Following Initial Procedure for a Related Procedure During the Postoperative Period

- Modifier 78 is used when another procedure is unplanned and related to the initial procedure, requires a return to the OR, and is performed during the postoperative period of the initial procedure by the same physician.
- The related procedure might be performed on the same day or at any time during the postoperative period. (For repeat procedures, refer to modifier 76, discussed earlier in this chapter.)
- Link the appropriate diagnosis code(s) that best explains the reason for the unplanned procedure.
  - ✖ Do not report modifier 78 for treatment of complications that do not require a return to the OR. Payers that use the Medicare description of the global period do not pay separately for additional services caused by complications that do not require a return to the OR.

Example—Modifier 78

➤ **A pediatric surgeon returns to the OR to stop bleeding following a tonsillectomy performed 2 days ago.**

42962 78 Control oropharyngeal hemorrhage, primary or secondary (eg, post-tonsillectomy); with secondary surgical intervention

Teaching Point: The second procedure will usually be paid only for the intraoperative service, not for the preoperative or postoperative care already paid for in the original procedure.

79—Unrelated Procedure/Service by the Same Physician or Other QHP During the Postoperative Period

- The physician may need to indicate that the performance of a procedure or service during the postoperative period was unrelated to the original procedure. This circumstance may be reported with modifier 79.
- The diagnosis must identify the reason for the new procedure within the global period. (For procedures repeated by the same physician on the same day, refer to modifier 76, discussed earlier in this chapter.)

Example—Modifier 79

➤ **An adolescent patient requires an emergency appendectomy within 90 days of undergoing left-sided laparoscopic inguinal hernia repair (49650).**

44970 79 Laparoscopy, surgical, appendectomy

80—Assistant Surgeon

- Modifier 80 is used when the assistant surgeon is actively involved throughout the procedure. *Note:* Modifier 62, not 80, is used when 2 surgeons work together as primary surgeons, each performing a distinct part(s) of a procedure.
- The primary surgeon reports the appropriate *CPT* code for the procedure, and the assistant surgeon reports the same code with modifier 80 appended. Some payers require modifier AS (assistant at surgery) in lieu of 80 when any other QHP (eg, nurse practitioner [NP]) acts as assistant surgeon.
- Payers vary on payment rules. The CMS establishes guidelines for payment of assistant surgery for each procedure code. Most payers, including the CMS, do not pay for nonphysician surgery technicians in this role.
- Many payers require documentation to support the necessity of an assistant surgeon.

81—*Minimum Assistant Surgeon*

- Modifier **81** is used when an assistant surgeon is required for a short time and minimal assistance is provided.
- The assistant surgeon reports the same procedure code as the surgeon with modifier **81** appended.
- Many payers require documentation to support the use of an assistant surgeon for only a portion of a procedure.

82—*Assistant Surgeon (When Qualified Resident Surgeon Not Available)*

- Modifier **82** is used to report an assistant surgeon's work in a teaching hospital when a resident surgeon is not available to assist the primary surgeon during a procedure for which assistance is indicated.
- The unavailability of a qualified resident surgeon is a prerequisite for the use of modifier **82** appended to the usual procedure code number(s).

Modifiers 80, 81, and 82

The MPFS includes in column AA (ASST SURG) indicators identifying procedures that may or may not be billed by an assistant surgeon. Indicator 1 is assigned to procedures for which an assistant surgeon is allowed to bill under the Medicare program. Other payers may adopt the same or different policies.

90—*Reference (Outside) Laboratory*

- Modifier **90** is used to indicate that a laboratory service is being billed by the physician but performed at an outside laboratory.
- Modifier **90** indicates pass-through billing in that the payer will pay the physician for the laboratory service and the laboratory will charge the physician.
- Many payers do not accept modifier **90** and require that the laboratory performing the service bill the health plan directly for the services. Check with your payers before using modifier **90**.

91—*Repeat Clinical Diagnostic Laboratory Test*

- Modifier **91**
  - Is used to indicate that it is necessary to repeat the same laboratory test on the same day to obtain subsequent test results
  - Is reported only when the laboratory test is performed more than once for the same patient on the same day
  - Cannot be reported when tests are repeated to confirm initial results, when testing problems occur with the specimen or equipment, or, for any reason, when a single reportable result is all that is required
- ✖ Do not substitute modifier **59** (distinct service) for modifier **91**.

Example—Modifier 91

➤ **In the course of treatment of hypoglycemia by administration of oral carbohydrate, a patient underwent 3 blood glucose determinations (82947) on the same day in the same office.**

82947 91 × 3 units of service.

Some payers will require separate claim lines for each test performed, with modifier **91** appended to the codes for repeat services. Refer to *ICD-10-CM* codes **E16.A1–E16.A3** to report levels of hypoglycemia.

92—*Alternative Laboratory Platform Testing*

- Modifier **92** is used to indicate that laboratory testing was performed with a kit or transportable instrument that wholly or partially consists of a single-use, disposable analytic chamber.
- This modifier is not required or acknowledged by all payers.
- *CPT* instructs to report this modifier with HIV test codes **86701–86703** and **87389**.

Modifiers Appended to Either E/M or Procedural Services

32—*Mandated Services*

- Modifier **32** is appended to services (eg, a second opinion) mandated by a third-party payer or by governmental, legislative, or regulatory requirements.
- The modifier may be reported with codes for E/M services (eg, for a second opinion required by a payer).

- Modifier 32 would be used when, for example, radiological services are requested from a worker's compensation carrier, when laboratory testing (eg, a drug test) is requested by a court system, or when a physical therapy assessment is requested by an insurer.

Example—Modifier 32

➤ **A managed care organization requires that a child's family obtain a second opinion before receiving prior authorization for the child's surgery.** A physician reviews the child's medical history, examines the child, and, after discussion with their parents/caregivers, recommends the surgery. The level of MDM for the visit is moderate.

ICD-10-CM	*CPT*
Diagnosis for which surgery is considered	99254 32 (outpatient consultation with moderate MDM or total time of ≥40 minutes)

Teaching Point: Health plan policies may vary in coverage of consultation codes. Some plans may require use of alternative E/M codes (eg, office and other outpatient E/M visit codes, either new patient codes 99202–99205 or established patient codes 99212–99215).

33—Preventive Services

CPT modifier 33 is used to communicate to payers that a preventive medicine service (as defined by the Patient Protection and Affordable Care Act provisions; the 4 categories follow) was performed on a patient enrolled in a health care plan subject to the preventive service coverage requirements of the Patient Protection and Affordable Care Act and, therefore, should not be subject to cost sharing.

- Appropriate use of modifier 33 reduces claim adjustments related to preventive services and facilitates correct payments to members.
- Modifier 33 should be appended only to codes represented in one or more of the following 4 categories:
  - Services rated A or B by the US Preventive Services Task Force
  - Immunizations for routine use in children, adolescents, and adults as recommended by the Advisory Committee on Immunization Practices of the Centers for Disease Control and Prevention
  - Preventive care and screenings for children as recommended by Bright Futures (AAP) and newborn testing (American College of Medical Genetics and Genomics)
  - Preventive care and screenings provided for women supported by the Health Resources and Services Administration
- **DO *NOT* USE MODIFIER 33**
  - ✖ **When the *CPT* code(s) is (are) identified as inherently preventive (eg, preventive medicine counseling)**
  - ✖ **When the service(s) is (are) not indicated in the categories noted previously**
  - ✖ **With an insurance plan that continues to implement the cost-sharing policy on preventive medicine services**
- Check with your payers before reporting modifier 33 to verify any variations in reporting requirements.

Example—Modifier 33

➤ **A 17-year-old established patient is seen for an office visit and requests contraception.** The physician determines that the patient is not pregnant but has been sexually active and would like contraception. The physician then spends approximately 15 minutes discussing contraception and risks of sexually transmitted infection (STI) with the patient. Point-of-care HIV-1 and HIV-2 testing is conducted with negative results. A specimen is collected for chlamydia and gonorrhea screening by an outside laboratory. The patient chooses oral contraception, which is prescribed.

ICD-10-CM	*CPT*
Z30.09 (encounter for other general counseling and advice on contraception) Z11.4 (encounter for screening for HIV) Z11.3 (encounter for screening for STI)	99401 (preventive counseling, approximately 15 minutes [includes 8–23 minutes]) 86703 33 92 (antibody; HIV-1 and HIV-2; single assay)

Teaching Point: Although recommended as a preventive service, the test reported with 86703 is also used for diagnostic purposes. Modifier 33 indicates that this test was performed as a preventive service. Modifier 92 (alternative laboratory platform testing) is reported to indicate use of the HIV test kit (not all payers recognize modifier 92).

Typically, health plans cover services related to contraception (eg, **99401**) without cost to the patient. When performed, a pregnancy test (eg, **81025,** urine pregnancy test, by visual color comparison methods) may be separately reported with **Z32.01** (encounter for pregnancy test, result positive) or **Z32.02** (encounter for pregnancy test, result negative).

93—Synchronous Telemedicine Service Rendered via Telephone or Other Real-Time Interactive Audio-Only Telecommunications System

Synchronous telemedicine service is defined as a real-time interaction through audio-only technology between a physician or QHP and a patient who is located at a distant site from the physician or QHP. The modifier is not reported for back-and-forth voice messaging.

- *CPT* Appendix T lists codes that may be reported with modifier **93**. Codes eligible for use with modifier **93** are preceded by an audio speaker symbol (◀).
- Verify payer policies for audio-only telemedicine services before provision of services.
- The totality of communication during the audio-only telemedicine service must be of an amount and nature sufficient to meet the requirements of the same service when rendered with face-to-face interaction.
- Note that modifier **93** is different from modifier **FQ** (audio-only service). Modifier **FQ** was created for the Medicare program and is reported *only by certain types of providers (eg, rural health centers)* unless otherwise specified by a health plan.

95—Synchronous Telemedicine Service Rendered via a Real-Time Interactive Audio and Video Telecommunications System

Modifier **95** is used to indicate that a service was rendered via a real-time (synchronous) interactive audio and video telecommunications system. This modifier is not applied if the communication is not real-time interactive audio and video.

Codes to which modifier **95** may be applied are found in *CPT* Appendix P and are preceded by a star symbol (★).

✖ Do not report modifier **95** with codes **98000–98007**, which are specific to telemedicine services.

For more information on reporting synchronous telemedicine services, refer to Chapters 19 and 20.

99—Multiple Modifiers

CPT instructs that modifier **99** be reported under certain circumstances when 2 or more modifiers are required to completely describe a service. Yet current paper and electronic claims allow listing of up to 4 modifiers per claim line, and payers often instruct coders to report modifier **99** only when more than 4 modifiers are required on a single code.

Follow individual payer instructions regarding use of modifier **99** and placement of additional modifiers on the claim (eg, in narrative field 19 of the paper claim form).

Healthcare Common Procedure Coding System Modifiers

The HCPCS modifiers are used to report specific information not conveyed in code descriptors or by *CPT* modifiers, such as

CR	Catastrophe/disaster related
E1	Upper left eyelid
QW	Performance of tests waived by Clinical Laboratory Improvement Amendments (CLIA)
RT	Right side
SL	State-supplied vaccine
TC	Technical component only
XE	Procedural services performed at separate encounters on the same date

Medicaid programs often use a variety of HCPCS modifiers for state-defined purposes. Refer to your Medicaid provider manual for information on HCPCS modifiers and definitions assigned in your state (eg, modifier **SY**, persons who are in close contact with member of high-risk population, may be used with codes for certain immunizations).

Anatomical Modifiers

An anatomical modifier may be reported to identify specific sites, such as right foot, fifth digit (**T9**). Payer policies may require use of anatomical modifiers even when reporting a single procedure and despite site identification that may be included in a reported *ICD-10-CM* code.

- The anatomical modifiers are designated as appropriate modifiers under NCCI edits.

- The Medicaid NCCI manual indicates that procedures performed on fingers be reported with modifiers **FA** and **F1–F9** and procedures performed on toes be reported with modifiers **TA** and **T1–T9**. Refer also to modifiers for eyelids (**E1–E4**) and coronary arteries (**LC**, **LD**, **LM**, **RC**, **RI**).

MUE values are 1 (one) for many finger and toe procedures. Use anatomical modifiers for clinical scenarios in which the same procedure is performed on more than one finger or toe. (Refer to the Medically Unlikely Edits section earlier in this chapter for more information.)

Example—Anatomical Modifiers

➤ **A physician performs nail avulsion (11730) on the patient's right ring finger and evacuation of blood under the nail (11740) on the patient's right middle finger.**

11730 F8	Avulsion, nail plate, partial or complete, simple; single—right hand, 4th digit
11740 F7	Evacuation of subungual hematoma—right hand, 3rd digit

Note: Some payers may require that modifier **59** (distinct procedural service) or **XS** (separate structure) also be reported on the code for a second or other subsequent procedure provided on the same date. Verify coding edits and payer policy before reporting.

X{E, P, S, U} Modifiers

Modifiers **XE**, **XP**, **XS**, and **XU** more specifically identify reasons for separate reporting of procedures or services that may otherwise be identified by *CPT* modifier **59**.

XE	Separate encounter (different operative session)
XP	Separate practitioner
XS	Separate structure (site/organ)
XU	Unusual nonoverlapping service

- Payer guidance on use of these modifiers may vary; verify individual payer policy before reporting. Although these modifiers are accepted by most payers, few resources are available to describe their appropriate reporting.
- Given that the **XE**, **XP**, **XS**, and **XU** modifiers are more specific, payers may require reporting in lieu of modifier **59**.
  - ✖ Modifiers **XE**, **XP**, **XS**, and **XU** should not be appended to an E/M code.
  - ✖ Do not append modifier **59** and the **XE**, **XP**, **XS**, and **XU** modifiers to the same service line of a claim (ie, single code).

CR—Catastrophe/Disaster Related

Modifier **CR** is used according to payer instruction during a federal- or state-declared disaster or public health emergency to indicate that a service was provided in a manner or under circumstances for which payment may otherwise be prohibited by government statute or payer policies.

Example—Modifier CR

➤ **A well-child examination is conducted via telemedicine on a patient in her home during a public health emergency.** Per payer policy, the service requires a comprehensive, unclothed physical examination. A waiver has been issued allowing billing for the incomplete preventive E/M service with modifier **CR** (eg, **99391 CR**). Payer policy may require an in-person visit within a specified period.

EP—Service Provided as Part of Medicaid Early and Periodic Screening, Diagnostic, and Treatment Program

Some Medicaid and private payers require the use of modifier **EP** to denote services that are provided to covered patients as part of the Early and Periodic Screening, Diagnostic, and Treatment (EPSDT) program services required in the state.

Modifier **EP** can be appended to the preventive medicine service (eg, **99392 EP**) or screening services, such as developmental screening (**96110 EP**).

Modifier **EP** can also be applied to services provided when a referral is prompted by findings of an EPSDT well-child examination (eg, **96112 EP**, developmental test administration [including assessment of fine and/or gross motor, language, cognitive level, social, memory and/or executive functions by standardized developmental instruments when performed], by physician or other QHP, with interpretation and report; first hour).

FQ—*The Service Was Furnished Using Audio-Only Communication Technology*

Modifier **FQ** is reported by certain providers (eg, rural health centers) in lieu of modifier **93** (discussed earlier in this chapter). Report modifier **FQ** only as instructed by payer policy.

FS—*Split or Shared E/M Visit*

This modifier indicates that a service was provided in a facility setting as a split or shared E/M service by more than one physician or QHP in the same group practice. Medicare requires the reporting individual to append modifier **FS** to an E/M code when the E/M service was performed as a split/shared service. Other payers may adopt Medicare policy for use of modifier **FS**.

FT—*Separate, Unrelated E/M*

The CMS created modifier **FT** for reporting critical care services provided within a 10- or 90-day postoperative period when the services are above and beyond and unrelated to the specific anatomical injury or general surgical procedure performed. Refer to individual health plan guidance before reporting this modifier.

- The Medicare program advises that modifier **25** (significant, separately identifiable E/M service) continue to be reported when 2 E/M services are provided to a patient by the same physician or QHP or another physician or QHP of the same specialty and same group practice on the same date but for different reasons (eg, hospital care before critical care).

GA—*Waiver of Liability Statement Issued as Required by Payer Policy, Individual Case*

GU—*Waiver of Liability Statement Issued as Required by Payer Policy, Routine Notice*

GX—*Notice of Liability Issued, Voluntary Under Payer Policy*

Modifiers **GA**, **GU**, and **GX** may or may not be required by Medicaid and private payers when reporting services that are not covered under the patient's benefit plan. Follow individual payer policies regarding provision and reporting of advance notice of noncoverage to patients/responsible parties. Instructions regarding use of these modifiers may be included in contract language, provider manuals, or payment policies.

- Failure to obtain a parent's/caregiver's written consent on an advance notice of noncoverage form prior to providing a noncovered service and/or failure to append modifier **GA** (when applicable) may result in contractual prohibition against billing to the patient or parent/caregiver.

GC—*This Service Has Been Performed in Part by a Resident Under the Direction of a Teaching Physician*

- Modifier **GC** indicates that a teaching physician certifies that the service was rendered in compliance with the CMS requirements for services reported by teaching physicians.
- Requirements for reporting modifier **GC** may vary among commercial health plans. This modifier is typically *informational,* meaning it does not affect the amount paid for a service.
- If the service was provided solely by the teaching physician, the claim should not be billed with the **GC** modifier.

GE—*This Service Has Been Performed by a Resident Without the Presence of a Teaching Physician Under the Primary Care Exception*

- Modifier **GE** indicates that a teaching physician certifies that the service was rendered in compliance with the CMS primary care exception rule. Refer to **Chapter 6** for discussion of this rule.
- Requirements for reporting modifier **GE** may vary among Medicaid and commercial health plans. This modifier is typically *informational*, which means it does not affect the amount paid for a service.

GT—*Via Interactive Audio and Video Telecommunication Systems*

Modifier **GT** indicates that a face-to-face service was provided via a telecommunication system that included audio and video components. This modifier preceded *CPT* development of modifier **95** (telemedicine via audiovisual technology) and is reported in lieu of **95** when specified in payer policy (eg, appended to a code not included in *CPT* Appendix P).

JW—*Drug Amount Discarded/Not Administered to Any Patient*

- Practice administrators may use this modifier as a tool to internally track wasted drugs and immunization products.
- This modifier is reported on claims only when allowed or required by certain payers.

- Medicare requires use of modifier JW on codes for the unused portion of a drug or biologic from a single-dose vial or package. Medicaid plans may also require reporting of modifier JW.
  - Report only when the full amount of a single-dose vial is not used because of patient indications (eg, patient requires a lower dose) and when required by a payer.
  - Report only when the amount of drug wasted is equal to at least 1 billing unit (ie, do not report wastage when 7 mg of a 10-mg vial is administered and the billing unit is 10 mg, as the remaining 3 mg is already accounted for in the billing unit).
- ✖ Never report for discarded amounts from a multidose vial.
- ✖ Never report modifier JW for overfill wastage (ie, an excess amount placed in the single-dose vial by the manufacturer to ensure that an adequate amount can be drawn into the syringe for use).
- Modifier JW is not applicable for reporting the following circumstances. Yet some practices use the modifier for internal tracking of drug waste.
  - A parent decided to forgo an immunization after the product was drawn up. Report on a claim only when specifically allowed by payer policy. Practices should keep a log of all wasted immunization products. There is no applicable modifier.
  - The vial is dropped, and the medication must be discarded.
  - An immunization product is discarded because the temperature was out of range during storage.

Example—Modifier JW

➤ **A 45.8-kg child receives an infusion of a medication provided in a dose of 5 mg per 1 kg (ie, 229-mg dose).** The medication is supplied in a single-dose vial containing 100 mg of medication. Three vials are used to provide the 229-mg dose, with 71 mg of waste left in the third vial. The child's health plan requires the exact number of units administered. The code for the medication describes 10 mg of medication, and the amounts provided and wasted are reported on 2 claim lines.

Medication code × 22.9 units.

Medication code JW × 7.1 units.

Appropriate infusion codes (96413, 96415, 96365, 96366) are reported based on the total infusion time.

Teaching Point: The waste from the single-dose vial is reported on a separate claim line with modifier JW.

There are ten 10-mg doses in a 100-mg vial; 229 mg was administered in this example.

Units administered: 22.9 (twenty 10-mg units from two 100-mg vials and 2.9 units from a third vial).

Units wasted: 7.1 (71 mg of 100 mg in the third vial).

The appropriate National Drug Code (NDC) and NDC units (eg, ML, milliliter) may be required by the payer to provide more specific product and dosage information. Follow the specific payer's instructions for reporting drug units and wastage.

JZ—Zero Drug Amount Discarded/Not Administered to Any Patient

- The opposite of the JW modifier, JZ indicates that there was no waste of a billable amount of medication administered from a single-dose drug container. An amount above the number of units included in the HCPCS code descriptor for the medication would be a billable amount as in the example for modifier JW (discussed earlier in this chapter).
- Medicare began requiring modifier JZ in July 2023. Some Medicaid and commercial health plans have since adopted policies requiring this modifier.

Example—Modifier JZ

➤ **A patient receives a 40-mg injection of a medication supplied in a 50-mg single-dose vial.** The code for the medication is described as up to 50 mg. The code for the medication is appended with modifier JZ to indicate that there was no wasted medication.

Teaching Point: The wasted medication is included in the amount reported with 1 unit as indicated by the code descriptor (ie, up to 50 mg). Reporting the code appended with modifier JZ results in payment for the full 50 mg.

KX—Requirements Specified in the Medical Policy Have Been Met

This informational modifier is used to inform a payer that the service reported was provided in compliance with the payer's policy. This modifier can be used to bypass gender-specific edits that may designate a procedure code as applicable to only a female or male patient when the patient has ambiguous genitalia or is transgender.

For a discussion and an example of use of the KX modifier, refer to the February 2023 AAP Pediatric Coding Newsletter™ article "Coding for Adolescent Health Care Services" (https://doi.org/10.1542/pcco_book226_document002).

QW—CLIA-Waived Tests

- CLIA-waived tests are commonly done in a laboratory or an office and are considered simple and low-risk (eg, 87880, rapid streptococcal antigen test).
- Laboratories and physician offices performing waived tests should append modifier QW to the CPT code for CLIA-waived procedures. A small number of codes for CLIA-waived tests are exempt from the requirement for modifier QW (eg, 81002, nonautomated urinalysis without microscopy; 81025, urine pregnancy test; 82272, occult blood by peroxidase for other than colorectal neoplasm screening).

For further discussion of CLIA-waived laboratory tests, refer to Chapter 11.

RT, LT—Right and Left Side

- Laterality modifiers RT and LT may be required by payer policy or accepted as information that does not affect payment. Practices should be aware of payer policies that may require use of laterality modifiers when reporting any procedure on a paired body site (eg, left ear or right ear).
- Some plans allow modifiers RT and LT in place of modifier 50, but be sure of payer policy for reporting bilateral diagnostic procedures.
- Some payers may require that modifier 59 (distinct procedural service) be reported in addition to or in lieu of the laterality modifiers.

Example—Modifiers RT and LT

➤ **Radiographs of the left elbow and wrist are ordered.**

73110 LT	Radiologic examination, wrist; complete, minimum of 3 views
73080 LT	Radiologic examination, elbow; complete, minimum of 3 views

SA—Nurse Practitioner Rendering Service in Collaboration With a Physician

- Modifier SA is typically appended to a procedure code to indicate that a physician is reporting a service provided by an NP under incident-to policy. Yet some payers require the modifier on all services provided by NPs.
- Some payers include physician associates/physician assistants (PAs) and other QHPs who can provide E/M services in policies requiring use of modifier SA. Other payers may use alternative modifiers for services performed by PAs and other QHPs.
- Not all payers require modifier SA, but where required, failure to include the modifier could result in overpayment or coding errors.

Example—Modifier SA

➤ **An NP provides a follow-up visit to reevaluate a patient's type 1 diabetes in continuation of a plan of care developed by the patient's physician.** The physician is in the office suite and available during the visit but does not directly participate in the visit. The service provided is a level 4 established patient office E/M service (99214). The physician reports 99214 SA.

To learn more about incident-to policy, refer to Chapter 7.

To test your knowledge of the information presented in this chapter, complete the quiz found at the end of it, after the resources. Answers to each quiz are found in Appendix II. Add to your knowledge through the information provided in other chapters that discuss codes for specific types of services.

Chapter Takeaways

Readers of this chapter should generally know coding edits and modifiers. Following are takeaways from this chapter:

- Payers use coding edits to promote correct coding and provide correct payment for services.
- When applicable, use of modifiers to override coding edits must be clinically indicated. Not all edits can be overridden with a modifier.
- To append the appropriate modifier and override an edit, it is imperative that the conditions of that modifier are met (eg, **XE**, separate encounter [different session]).
- *CPT* and HCPCS include modifiers that may be appended to procedure codes from either code set.
- Some modifiers are limited to use only with E/M codes or only with other procedure codes. Some modifiers apply to either an E/M code or other procedure codes.
- Modifier use may be affected by payer-specific policies, requiring knowledge of payer policies for modifier use.

Resources

AAP Coding Assistance and Education

AAP Coding and Payment Hotline (www.aap.org/en/practice-management/child-health-finance-payment-strategy/coding-payment-hotline)

AAP News™

"When to use, how to document modifier 25," May 1, 2023 (https://publications.aap.org/aapnews/news/24168)

AAP Pediatric Coding Newsletter

"Coding for Adolescent Health Care Services," February 2023 (https://doi.org/10.1542/pcco_book226_document002)

"Coding Challenge: Anatomical and Laterality Modifiers," January 2025 (https://doi.org/10.1542/pcco_book249_document003)

"Coding Challenge Answers: Anatomical and Laterality Modifiers," January 2025 (https://doi.org/10.1542/pcco_book249_document006)

"Coding Hotline," February 2024 ("*CPT*: 2 Distinct E/M Services") (https://doi.org/10.1542/pcco_book238_document005)

"Did You Know? The CLIA-Waived Test Modifier," February 2024 (https://doi.org/10.1542/pcco_book238_document003)

"Evaluation and Management Coding: Reporting Multiple Services on the Same Date," April 2024 (https://doi.org/10.1542/pcco_book240_document003)

"Procedural Services: Modifiers to Report Site and Laterality," January 2025 (https://doi.org/10.1542/pcco_book249_document005)

Assistant Surgeon Procedure Identification

MPFS Relative Value Files (www.cms.gov/medicare/payment/fee-schedules/physician/pfs-relative-value-files; refer to Column U [ASST SURG] in the file applicable to the DOS)

Bilateral Procedure Identification

MPFS Relative Value Files (www.cms.gov/medicare/payment/fee-schedules/physician/pfs-relative-value-files; refer to Column T[BILAT SURG] in file applicable to the DOS)

Clinical Laboratory Improvement Amendments–Waived Tests

CLIA test category database (www.accessdata.fda.gov/scripts/cdrh/cfdocs/cfCLIA/search.cfm)

Co-Surgery and Team Surgery Procedure Identification

MPFS Relative Value Files (www.cms.gov/medicare/payment/fee-schedules/physician/pfs-relative-value-files; refer to Column V [CO SURG] or Column W [TEAM SURG] in the file applicable to the DOS)

Multiple Surgery Indicators and Adjustments

Medicare Claims Processing Manual, Chapter 12, Section 40.6 (www.cms.gov/Regulations-and-Guidance/Guidance/Manuals/Downloads/clm104c12.pdf)

NCCI Edits

Medicaid NCCI website (www.cms.gov/medicare/coding-billing/ncci-medicaid/medicaid-ncci-edit-files)

Medicare NCCI website (www.cms.gov/medicare/coding-billing/ncci-medicare)

Test Your Knowledge!

1. **Which of the following modifier indicators for NCCI edits means an appropriately appended modifier may override an edit?**
   a. 0
   b. 1
   c. 9
   d. 10
2. **Which modifier may be appended only to a non-E/M service code?**
   a. EP (service provided as part of a Medicaid EPSDT program)
   b. 33 (preventive service)
   c. 32 (mandated service)
   d. 22 (increased procedural service)
3. **Which service best supports use of modifier 59?**
   a. A physician or QHP is reporting a procedure performed bilaterally.
   b. A physician performs a surgical procedure following an E/M service on the same date.
   c. The units of service provided were clinically indicated and exceed the MUE for the procedure.
   d. Procedures are provided to treat multiple fingers or toes.
4. **When is modifier 63 appropriately reported?**
   a. When the code is included in *CPT* Appendix F
   b. When any service is provided to a neonate with a present body weight of 4 kg or less
   c. When procedures or services described by codes listed in the *CPT* description of modifier 63 are provided to a neonate or infant with a present body weight of 4 kg or less
   d. When any procedure is provided during a stay in the NICU
5. **Which is true for reporting anatomical modifiers?**
   a. Anatomical modifiers never override a coding edit.
   b. Payer policies may require use of anatomical modifiers even when reporting a single procedure.
   c. Anatomical modifiers are *CPT* modifiers.
   d. Anatomical modifiers are not applicable when site identification is included in a reported *ICD-10-CM* code.

CHAPTER 3

Coding to Demonstrate Quality and Value

Contents

Chapter Highlights

- The impact of quality and performance measurement on pediatric physicians and patients
- How correct coding supports performance measurement and value-based payment initiatives
- Measures of patient satisfaction with care
- Important details of each measure (eg, patient population, exclusions), including providing care within the time frame of a measure and indicating why a patient was excluded from the activity of a measure (eg, not immunized because of patient history or a condition that prevents immunization)

Quality and Performance Measurement

Quality and performance measurement are important aspects of the pediatric medical home and the movement from payment by fee for service (FFS) alone to value-based payment. Performance measures developed by national organizations, including the National Committee for Quality Assurance, are based on quality indicators currently accepted and used in the health care industry. Physicians and other qualified health care professionals (QHPs) who have successfully participated in quality measurement may see incentive payments, such as per-member-per-month payments, annual incentives, or a percentage of savings.

For more information on value-based payment and other emerging payment models, refer to Chapter 4.

In January 2017, the American Academy of Pediatrics (AAP) published a policy statement, "A New Era in Quality Measurement: The Development and Application of Quality Measures" (https://doi.org/10.1542/peds.2016-3442). This policy statement includes the following recommendation to national policymakers:

> Quality measures, as much as possible, should be reportable by either *International Classification of Diseases, 10th Revision, Clinical Modification*...or *Current Procedural Terminology*...codes [or by Healthcare Common Procedure Coding System codes] to reduce burden on pediatric health care providers. However, the inclusion of measures that also capture patient-centered perspectives on care is essential.

Increasingly, clinical registries and other electronic data (eg, Systematized Nomenclature of Medicine—Clinical Terms [SNOMED CT]) are used in quality measurement. This may be in addition to or in lieu of codes assigned by physicians and QHPs. Codes are still, however, a primary mechanism for determining which patients are included in the population of a quality measure and whether the measure has been met.

In addition to discussing how codes may support specific performance measures, this chapter discusses the following aspects of performance measurement:

- The Healthcare Effectiveness Data and Information Set (HEDIS) and its effect on coding and payment
- Measures of patient experience in primary and specialty care settings
- Measures applicable to Medicaid and Children's Health Insurance Program (CHIP) plans

Code Sets Used in Quality Reporting

International Classification of Diseases, 10th Revision, Clinical Modification Codes

International Classification of Diseases, 10th Revision, Clinical Modification (*ICD-10-CM*) codes are used to determine that a patient is included in or excluded from the population of most quality measures.

Examples

➤ **The measure for developmental screening in the first 3 years after birth requires reporting of *ICD-10-CM* code Z13.42 (encounter for screening for global developmental delays) to specify that a developmental screening was conducted for global developmental delay in children up to 3 years old.** In contrast, reporting **96110** (developmental screening) with **Z00.121** or **Z00.129** (routine child examination with or without abnormal findings) or **Z13.41** (autism screening), while indicating a recommended preventive service, does not support global developmental screening.

➤ **Patient encounters are included in the measure for avoidance of antibiotic treatment of acute bronchitis/bronchiolitis when the patient encounter (eg, office visit, telemedicine visit) with an infant or child aged 3 months to 17 years results in a diagnosis for acute bronchitis/bronchiolitis reported with *ICD-10-CM* codes in categories J20 (acute bronchitis) and J21 (acute bronchiolitis).** When pharmacy claims data or medical record documentation demonstrates that an antibiotic was prescribed for patients with a condition reported with category J20 or J21 codes, the measure for avoidance of antibiotic treatment of acute bronchitis/bronchiolitis *is not met.*

Correct and complete diagnosing is also necessary to tell the health plan the disease burden of patients who routinely receive care from a practice. *ICD-10-CM* codes collected from the claims submitted to health plans are used to estimate a patient's risk for future health expenditures. Health plans offered to individuals under the Patient Protection and Affordable Care Act are subject to revenue adjustment based on the average risk of insured members based in part on diagnoses that indicate a higher risk (eg, chronic conditions that require frequent reevaluation and/or intervention). To learn more about the importance of complete and accurate *ICD-10-CM* coding, refer to the "What Pediatricians Should Know About Coding and Risk Adjustment" box in **Chapter 4**.

Current Procedural Terminology Category II Codes: Performance Measure Codes

When codes are used to collect quality and performance measurement data, one category of *Current Procedural Terminology* (*CPT*®) codes that is useful for conveying this information is *CPT* Category II. Category II codes were developed and are used by physicians and hospitals to report performance measures and certain aspects of care not yet included in performance measures.

Category II codes may or may not be used by payers in pediatric performance measurement. Assignment of Category II codes also allows internal monitoring of performance, patient adherence, and outcomes.

Category II codes

- Are intended for reporting purposes only
- Describe clinical conditions, including complete performance measurements sets, and screening measures
- Have no relative values on the Medicare Physician Fee Schedule Resource-Based Relative Value Scale
- Are reported on a voluntary basis
- Are reported in addition to, *not in place of,* Category I *CPT* codes
- Describe the performance of a clinical service typically included in an evaluation and management (E/M) code or the result of a laboratory procedure/test

Category II codes are included after the Category I procedure codes in the *CPT* manual and online at www.ama-assn.org/practice-management/cpt/category-ii-codes. Also available at this link are the alphabetical clinic topics listing, an overview of the performance measures, a listing of *CPT* Category II codes that may be used with each measure, and any applicable reporting instructions. Abbreviations (eg, *PV* for *preventive care and screening*) following code descriptors of Category II codes indicate the performance measure to which the code is associated.

Category II codes are reported with no charge ($0.00) or, when required by billing or payment systems, a charge of 1 cent ($0.01).

Example

➤ **An adolescent was advised by a psychiatrist to see their pediatrician for metabolic monitoring after being prescribed an antipsychotic medication.** The pediatrician counsels the patient and family/caregiver about the increased risks of metabolic health complications associated with antipsychotic medications and recommends annual blood glucose and cholesterol monitoring. Hemoglobin A1c and lipoprotein direct measurement tests are performed in the office and the results are reviewed. The patient is advised that their results are normal and that they are to return for their next preventive care visit, or sooner as needed.

Office or other outpatient visit (eg, 99213).

3048F	Most recent LDL-C less than 100 mg/dL (CAD) (DM)
3044F	Most recent hemoglobin A1c (HbA1c) level less than 7% (DM)
83036 QW	Hemoglobin; glycosylated (A1c)
83721 QW	Lipoprotein, direct measurement; LDL cholesterol

Teaching Point: Any abnormal result would be reported with code 3049F (most recent LDL-C 100-129 mg/dL), 3050F (most recent LDL-C ≥130 mg/dL), 3046F (most recent hemoglobin A1c level >9%), 3051F (most recent hemoglobin A1c [HbA1c] level ≥7% and <8%), or 3052F (most recent hemoglobin A1c [HbA1c] level ≥8% and <9%).

The CAD and/or DM abbreviations following **3048F** and **3044F** indicate that these codes are used to report measures associated with risk for *coronary artery disease* and *diabetes mellitus*. Modifier **QW** is appended to laboratory tests that have a waived status under the Clinical Laboratory Improvement Amendments.

Healthcare Common Procedure Coding System Codes

The Centers for Medicare & Medicaid Services (CMS) incorporates Healthcare Common Procedure Coding System (HCPCS) **G** codes into quality reporting, and these codes may be used by any health plan or program, such as Medicaid or CHIP. Refer to each payer's guidance for reporting quality measures to learn when HCPCS codes may be applicable.

Example

➤ **A physician provides depression screening and documents a negative result during an established patient preventive E/M service.**

99394	Periodic comprehensive preventive medicine reevaluation and management of an individual including an age and gender appropriate history, examination, counseling/anticipatory guidance/risk factor reduction interventions, and the ordering of laboratory/diagnostic procedures, established patient; adolescent (age 12 through 17 years)
96127	Brief emotional/behavioral assessment (eg, depression inventory, attention-deficit/hyperactivity disorder [ADHD] scale), with scoring and documentation, per standardized instrument
G8510	Screening for depression is documented as negative, a follow-up plan is not required

Teaching Point: No charge (or $0.01) is entered on the claim line for **G8510**, as this code is used for informational purposes rather than for direct payment. A positive depression screening result with creation of a plan for follow-up care would be reported with **G8431**, in lieu of **G8510**. When a patient is not screened for depression because of factors such as cognitive limitations, a current diagnosis of depression or bipolar disorder—either **G8433** (screening for depression not completed, documented patient or medical reason) or **G9717** (documentation stating the patient has had a diagnosis of bipolar disorder)—can be reported to indicate the patient's exclusion from this measure. Refer to the Reporting a Preventive Medicine Visit With a Problem-Oriented Visit section in **Chapter 8** for discussion of reporting a problem identified and addressed during a preventive medicine visit.

National Drug Codes

National Drug Codes (NDCs) that specify a specific product and dosage are also used in quality measurement.

Example

➤ **A physician provides long-acting contraception to a 16-year-old patient in the office.** In addition to the diagnosis and procedure codes for the service, the NDC for the implant is reported.
78206-0145-01 Etonogestrel 68 mg drug implant (Nexplanon)

Be sure to report the current NDC for the product. Learn more about NDCs in **Chapter 1**.

For additional examples of codes used in support of performance measurement, refer to the Coding and Documentation for Performance Measures section later in this chapter.

Healthcare Effectiveness Data and Information Set

Physicians and QHPs should be aware of the HEDIS. The National Committee for Quality Assurance describes HEDIS as a tool used by more than 90% of American health plans to measure performance on important dimensions of care and service. It is intended to allow purchasers and consumers to compare quality among health plans. The HEDIS measures are often incorporated into physician quality initiatives.

Altogether, HEDIS consists of more than 90 measures across the following 5 domains of care (not all measures apply to the pediatric population).

1. Effectiveness of Care

Examples of effectiveness of care measures are

- Childhood immunization status
- Immunizations for adolescents
- Appropriate testing for children with pharyngitis
- Follow-up care for children prescribed ADHD medication

2. Access/Availability of Care

- Use of first-line psychosocial care for children and adolescents prescribed antipsychotics

3. Utilization

Examples of utilization measures are

- Child and adolescent well-care visits
- Mental health utilization

4. Risk-Adjusted Utilization

- Emergency department (ED) utilization

5. Measures Collected by Electronic Clinical Data Systems

- Depression Remission or Response for Adolescents and Adults (DRR for short)
- Follow-up care for children prescribed ADHD medication

To ensure HEDIS stays current, the National Committee for Quality Assurance has established an annual update to the measurement set.

Each health plan reviews a select set of measures every year. Because so many plans collect HEDIS data and the measures are so specifically defined, it is important to become familiar with the HEDIS system as it relates to quality measures and pay for performance.

Why HEDIS Matters to Health Plans

Payment for health care services is increasingly linked to patient outcomes. There are large sums of money at stake for health plans. For example, for a health plan with just 100,000 members being evaluated by HEDIS, each quality measure could mean millions in payments from federal or state agencies. When you consider that there are 20 to 25 measures directly tied to payment (depending on the health plan and population served), this is a significant amount of money. Now consider what that might look like for larger managed care organizations that have 1 million or more members enrolled. This is what keeps health care plans running. But they cannot do it without physicians.

HEDIS data also contribute to health plan ratings (eg, 1–5 stars). Ratings are displayed on health plan marketplaces/exchanges (eg, www.healthcare.gov and state-based exchanges), potentially driving health plan purchasers to plans with higher ratings. Medicaid programs use plan ratings, which incorporate the plan's results on HEDIS and other quality measures, to determine which plans receive automatic assignment of Medicaid enrollees.

Why HEDIS Matters to Physicians and QHPs

Because health plans need the support of physicians and other QHPs to meet quality measures and earn revenue, the plans will often pay physicians to help them. However, these payments may be tied to how well individual physicians or a physician practice provides and documents care that supports the goals of quality measurement.

Payers may use physician- or practice-level data to determine qualifications for incentive programs that pay greater than FFS revenue (eg, pay-for-performance or a quality bonus) when care that aligns with quality measures is performed, documented, and appropriately reported. Scores or ratings may be based on HEDIS measurement data and other physician- or practice-specific data (eg, percentage of physicians who are board certified, external recognition [eg, National Committee for Quality Assurance Patient-Centered Medical Home Recognition], patient satisfaction surveys). These rates then serve as a basis for physician profiling (eg, network inclusion) and eligibility for incentive programs.

Employed physicians may also earn bonuses based on meeting the organization's quality measurement goals.

What Is a Physician's or QHP's Role in HEDIS?

Practices can help facilitate HEDIS process improvement by

- Providing appropriate care within the designated time frames.

Pay close attention to time frames for providing recommended screenings and services across the patient population.

Example

➤ **A practice uses a reminder system to track preventive medicine visits for children younger than 30 months.** Tracking includes 8 or more visits within 2 distinct time periods to prevent failure to provide

1. 6 or more preventive medicine visits to children who turned 15 months old and/or
2. 2 or more preventive medicine visits to children who turned 30 months old during the measurement year

Teaching Point: If patients reach 15 months of age without receiving 6 or more preventive medicine visits, this negatively affects the HEDIS score for the physician or QHP until the child turns 30 months old (ie, is no longer included in the patient count for the measure). Likewise, when a child who does not receive 2 or more preventive medicine visits between the ages of 15 months + 1 day and 30 months, the HEDIS score is negatively affected until the child is 36 months old and included in the measure for preventive visits provided to children, adolescents, and young adults 3 to 21 years old.

- Documenting all care in the patient's medical record.

When a measure is met during an inpatient or observation stay (eg, newborn immunization during the birth admission), supporting documentation may be required in the record of the primary care physician even if the care was ordered or provided by another physician or QHP.

- Understanding payer and HEDIS guidelines for specific documentation requirements (eg, documentation of specific body mass index [BMI] percentile rather than a BMI percentile range).

Many health plans provide specific information on documentation and codes that do or do not support HEDIS measurement.

- Recognizing that not all patients will be included in a physician's patient count for HEDIS purposes, as continuous enrollment in the health plan without a gap of more than a specified number of days may be required for inclusion.

Example

➤ **The measure for appropriate prescribing for pharyngitis includes members continuously enrolled without a gap in coverage from 30 days before the encounter date through 3 days afterward (34 days total).**

Many payers will automatically exclude any patient who has had a hospice claim or another indication of ineligibility within the measurement year from the population for HEDIS measures.

- Accurately coding all claims. Providing information accurately on a claim may reduce the number of records requested. Use a full spectrum of diagnosis, procedure, and NDCs to show that each measure is met. Health plans typically produce educational resources giving examples of codes that indicate a measure has been met.
- Responding to a health plan's requests for medical records in a timely fashion, typically within a week. This is required under many health plan contracts. Health plans typically include a specific turnaround time for providing records. The time frames are set each year.
  - January to May 15: Medical record requests will come in from the plans. All data must be gathered by the plan by May 15, with no exceptions.
  - June: The plans must report their results to the National Committee for Quality Assurance.

– July to October: The National Committee for Quality Assurance releases the new Quality Compass, a quality comparison tool, nationwide: commercial plans in July, Medicaid and Medicare in September and October.

Medical Record Requests

Some information cannot be captured through claims or other electronic data, so requests for medical records related to health plan HEDIS surveys are necessary.

- The Health Insurance Portability and Accountability Act of 1996 allows disclosure of protected health information to a health plan for the plan's HEDIS purposes as long as the period for which information is needed overlaps with the period for which the patient is or was enrolled in the health plan.
- Health plans may contract with outside vendors to conduct HEDIS record reviews.
- Providers are notified of record requests, which will include a member list, the measure being evaluated, and the minimum necessary medical record information needed.
- Data collection may vary by plan but may include fax, mail, on-site visits for large requests, remote electronic health record access, and electronic data interchange via a secure web portal.

Records may also be requested for use in auditing a health plan's risk adjustment calculations. Risk adjustment, which affects health plan financing, is based in part on the diagnosis codes assigned during a measurement year. To learn more about the importance of complete and accurate *ICD-10-CM* coding, refer to the "What Pediatricians Should Know About Coding and Risk Adjustment" box in Chapter 4.

Consumer Assessment of Healthcare Providers and Systems

The Consumer Assessment of Healthcare Providers and Systems (CAHPS) is a program developed by the Agency for Healthcare Research and Quality (AHRQ), part of the US Department of Health and Human Services. CAHPS uses surveys to capture and learn about patient experiences in primary care and specialty care settings, in hospitals, and with health plans. The surveys must be conducted by approved survey vendors under a specific framework that is designed to eliminate bias in sample selection and results.

The CAHPS Clinician & Group Survey may be used to measure patient experience in primary and specialty care settings in the following categories. A version of this survey may be used by accountable care organizations to meet a requirement to measure patient experience.

- Getting timely appointments, care, and information

To provide timely appointments, care, and information, consider offering same-day appointments for sick-child visits or for sick- and well-child visits and providing patients with written information addressing diagnosed conditions such as ADHD, headaches, and abdominal pain. Telemedicine is also an increasingly covered benefit that may provide patients with easier access to care while maintaining continuity of care in the medical home.

- How well providers communicate with patients

Communication can be improved through accommodations for patients with language barriers, such as assistive technology or use of the free nationwide teletypewriter relay network to call hard-of-hearing patients/caregivers. The use of appropriate language interpreters (eg, clinical staff, translation services) is also important in patient communication. Learn more about meeting patient needs for communication assistance in the December 2021 *AAP Pediatric Coding Newsletter*™ article "Coding and Use of Interpretation Services" (https://doi.org/10.1542/pcco_book212_document002).

- Providers' use of information to coordinate patient care

The use of information to coordinate patient care can be facilitated, at least for initial referrals to other providers, by practice staff assisting patients with scheduling and transfer of relevant clinical and demographic information.

- Helpful, courteous, and respectful office staff

Physicians and other QHPs seldom make the first and last impressions on patients/caregivers. Training all office staff to be professional, respectful, and empathic in response to patient/caregiver concerns is necessary to support a positive image of the practice.

- Patients' rating of the provider

A rating by a patient/caregiver can be influenced by anything from a clear understanding of a plan of care to the level of customer service received from the practice's billing staff or agency. Each of the previous recommendations, along with empathy for patients/caregivers who have concerns about their experience, can drive a positive rating.

Health plans use a HEDIS version of CAHPS for gathering, reporting, analyzing, and acting on patient experience (CAHPS) data for Medicaid and commercial health plan members. The surveys are required not only by the CMS but also for health plans to receive or maintain HEDIS accreditation. The health plan surveys are typically a retrospective random sampling of patients from the prior 6 or 12 months.

These surveys measure patient experience based on the following criteria:

- Getting needed care
- Getting care quickly (eg, asking parents how frequently their child was able to receive urgently needed care from the physician [ie, never, sometimes, frequently, always])
- How well doctors communicate
- Health plan customer service
- How people rated their health plans

Health plans rely on physician practices and other sites of service to participate in quality improvement initiatives focused on patient experiences and may offer incentives to adopt policies and procedures that support an improved patient experience of care (eg, more timely access to care).

To learn more about CAHPS, visit www.ahrq.gov/cahps/index.html.

Medicaid and Children's Health Insurance Program Quality Measures

Medicaid and CHIP plans select and report measures from the Core Set of Children's Health Care Quality Measures for Medicaid and CHIP (Child Core Set). The Child Core Set includes many HEDIS measures and a few measures developed by the CMS or other parties. Refer to the current set of quality measures at www.medicaid.gov/medicaid/quality-of-care/performance-measurement/adult-and-child-health-care-quality-measures/childrens-health-care-quality-measures/index.html.

Coding and Documentation for Performance Measures

Following are documentation and coding tips for some of the pediatric performance measures for 2025 (2026 measures were not finalized at the time of this publication). Refer to guidance from health plans in your area for more specific documentation and coding guidance.

Note that each measure includes a defined patient population (eg, children who turn 2 years of age during the measurement year).

HEDIS requires that measures be met within specific time frames (eg, before the second birthday). Catching up after the specified time will not be counted in the number of patients for whom the measure was met.

Physicians and group practices may also report performance measures as part of a pediatric medical home or other quality improvement initiative by using data pulled from internal administrative data (eg, number of preventive medicine service *CPT* codes reported for population of patients 3–21 years old). Pediatric medical home and quality improvement initiatives vary by state or region and may include a combination of HEDIS and other nationally recognized quality measures.

Some measures include criteria that exclude a patient from the population for the measure. For an example, refer to the Preventive Screening and Utilization Measures section that follows. Most measures exclude patients receiving hospice care.

Preventive Screening and Utilization Measures

Following are some examples of measures in the categories of preventive screening and utilization with tips for coding and documentation:

Well-Child Visits—First 30 Months of Life

Measurement is based on the age of the patient at 2 distinct points *during the measurement period,* with 6 visits occurring before the child turns 15 months old and 2 visits occurring between the child's turning 15 months old and their turning 30 months old.

- Children who turned 15 months—6 or more well-child visits

Health plans may count normal newborn care provided during the birth admission as 1 of 6 well-child visits before 15 months. Inclusion of history from a child's birth admission (eg, date and provider of initial hospital care, hepatitis B immunization) in the patient's medical record may support this and other measures.

- Children who turned 30 months—2 or more well-child visits

This measure can be met by completing each child's recommended well-child visits at 18 and 24 months or, if delayed, before the child reaches 30 months of age.

Annual Child and Adolescent Well-Care Visits

The measure applies to patients aged 3 to 21 years. To meet the measure, one comprehensive well-care visit must be provided during each calendar year. A comprehensive well-care visit provided in conjunction with a preparticipation physical evaluation for school or sports participation or a problem-oriented visit may also support this measure.

Documentation of a comprehensive well-care visit should include specific information such as the Tanner stage, assessed skills that support the child's developmental milestones, and context of anticipatory counseling (eg, discussed diet, screen time, sleep). Adoption of Bright Futures recommendations for age- and gender-appropriate preventive services supports the provision of comprehensive well-child care.

Developmental Screening in the First 3 Years of Life

This measure applies to children who reached age 1, 2, or 3 years in the measurement year and requires use of a standardized screening instrument for motor, language, cognitive, and social-emotional development (must include all skills). Developmental screening is counted in each measurement year and for the 3-year period (ie, measure counts 4 times).

ICD-10-CM code **Z13.42** (screening for global developmental delays) and *CPT* code **96110** (developmental screening) are typically reported for these services. Remember, **96110** alone is insufficient because this code is also reported for screening for specific conditions (eg, screening for autism spectrum disorder [ASD] reported with **96110** and **Z13.41**).

Child/Adolescent Weight Assessment and Counseling for Nutrition and Physical Activity

Percentage of patients aged 3 to 17 years whose BMI was measured and documented as a BMI percentile (eg, 70th percentile) and whose counseling for nutrition and physical activity was documented (a checklist of counseling topics may be acceptable).

Most health plans require physicians to report a code for the BMI percentile (**Z68.51–Z68.56**). The BMI value is reported as an additional code to counseling for nutrition (**Z71.3**) and codes for any related condition (eg, overweight, obesity).

A payer may specify use of Category II code 3008F (BMI, documented) linked to the appropriate diagnosis codes for the service provided (eg, routine child health examination and BMI codes). Codes for obesity (E66.-) and class of obesity (E66.811–E66.813) may be reported in conjunction with BMI percentile codes Z68.54–Z68.56.

Code **Z71.82** (exercise counseling) is used to report counseling for physical activity.

When obesity is diagnosed and at least 15 minutes is spent in counseling specific to the obesity, code G0447 (face-to-face behavioral counseling for obesity, 15 minutes) may be separately reportable in addition to a preventive E/M service (eg, 99383). Verify individual health plan policies to determine if benefits for counseling for obesity are separately paid on the same date as a preventive E/M service.

Immunization Status

These measures are as follows:

- Child: Patients who received all recommended immunizations on or before their second birthday.
- Adolescent: Percentage of patients who are fully immunized by their 13th birthday.

There are 10 different combinations of immunizations for children and adolescents that can be measured. Check with payers to determine which combination(s) they are using to understand how your practice will be evaluated. For example, **Table 3-1** shows some combinations for the childhood immunization measures. The measure may be calculated by counting rates of each completed immunization and the completed combination.

Table 3-1. Combinations for Childhood Immunization Status Measures

Combination No.	Vaccines
3	DTaP, IPV, MMR, HiB, HepB, VZV, PCV
7	DTaP, IPV, MMR, HiB, HepB, VZV, PCV, HepA, RV
10	DTaP, IPV, MMR, HiB, HepB, VZV, PCV, HepA, RV, flu

Abbreviations: DTaP, diphtheria, tetanus toxoids, and acellular pertussis; flu, influenza; HepA, hepatitis A; Hib, *Haemophilus influenzae* type B; HepB, hepatitis B; IPV, inactivated poliovirus; MMR, measles-mumps-rubella; PCV, pneumococcal conjugate; RV, rotavirus; VZV, varicella-zoster virus.

Documentation of immunizations that require a series of administrations (eg, 3 doses) should be documented as such (dose 2 of 2 or dose 2 of 3). This may be accomplished through the use of a chart/template that indicates each immunization product administered, doses required to complete the series, and the date that each dose is administered.

The following *ICD-10-CM* codes (not a comprehensive list) may indicate a patient's reason for exclusion from one or more recommended immunizations:

Z28.03 Immunization not carried out because of immune compromised state of patient
Z87.892 Personal history of anaphylaxis
Z88.7 Allergy status to serum and vaccine
B20 Human immunodeficiency virus (HIV) disease
Z21 Asymptomatic human immunodeficiency virus (HIV) infection status
D81.9 Combined immunodeficiency, unspecified
D81.31 Severe combined immunodeficiency due to adenosine deaminase deficiency
D84.9 Immunodeficiency, unspecified

Coding Conundrum: Quality Measurement and Immunization Refusal

Codes for patient or caregiver immunization refusal do not exclude a patient from the population for immunization measures. This creates a dilemma for physicians whose quality scores and payment may be affected by unimmunized patients within their patient panel. Does the physician continue providing care to patients whose parents refuse immunization despite any effect on quality scores?

The AAP clinical report "Responding to Parental Refusals of Immunization of Children" (https://doi.org/10.1542/peds.2005-0316) provides the following guidance:

> In general, pediatricians should endeavor not to discharge patients from their practices solely because a parent refuses to immunize his or her child. However, when a substantial level of distrust develops, significant differences in the philosophy of care emerge, or poor quality of communication persists, the pediatrician may encourage the family to find another physician or practice. Although pediatricians have the option of terminating the physician-patient relationship, they cannot do so without giving sufficient advance notice to the patient or custodial parent or legal guardian to permit another health care professional to be secured. Such decisions should be unusual and generally made only after attempts have been made to work with the family. Families with doubts about immunization should still have access to good medical care, and maintaining the relationship in the face of disagreement conveys respect and at the same time allows the child access to medical care. Furthermore, a continuing relationship allows additional opportunity to discuss the issue of immunization over time.

Lead Screening

This measure is of the percentage of children who turn 2 years old during the measurement year who had at least 1 capillary or venous blood test for lead poisoning (83655 QW). (Alternatively, SNOMED CT or Logical Observation Identifiers, Names and Codes [LOINC] codes that identify an order for screening and/or a screening result may be transmitted from electronic data.)

Example

➤ **A 23-month-old presents as a new patient for clearance to attend preschool/child care.** Records from the child's former physician indicate that the last preventive E/M service was provided when the child was 12 months old. Per immunization registry, immunizations are up to date, including 2 doses of influenza vaccine in the prior year. The physician identifies that screenings for lead, global development, and ASD have not been performed. These are performed (with parental permission) at this encounter in addition to the 24-month well-child examination. The patient is scheduled for another preventive E/M service prior to turning 30 months old, and parents are counseled on the importance of the child receiving all preventive services.

ICD-10-CM	*CPT*	Related HEDIS Measures
Z00.129 (encounter for routine child health examination without abnormal findings)	99392 (periodic comprehensive preventive medicine reevaluation and management, age 1–4 years)	*Well-Child Visits—First 30 Months of Life* Patients turning 30 months old during the measurement year ≥2 comprehensive well-care visits completed between 15 and 30 months after birth
Z13.42 (encounter for screening for global developmental delays [milestones])	96110 (developmental screening, with scoring and documentation, per standardized instrument)	*Developmental Screening in the First 3 Years of Life* Once within each of the first 3 years after birth
Z13.41 (encounter for autism screening)	96110 59 (developmental screening, with scoring and documentation, per standardized instrument)	Not applicable—the measure for developmental screening is limited to screening for global developmental delay.
Z13.88 (encounter for screening for disorder due to exposure to contaminants)	36416 (collection capillary blood specimen) 99000 (handling and/or conveyance of specimen) 83655 QW (lead)	*Lead Screening* Patients turning 2 years old during the measurement year At least 1 capillary or venous lead blood test completed on or before their second birthday

Teaching Point: The physician in this scenario proactively provided preventive care that is recommended for this patient and, in doing so, can report diagnosis and procedure codes demonstrating that quality measures have been met.

Code Z02.0 (encounter for examination for admission to educational institution) is not reported because an *Excludes1* note prohibits reporting codes in category Z02 with codes in category Z00.

Refer to Chapter 8 for more details on coding for preventive medicine services.

Effectiveness of Care

Certain measures are used to determine the effectiveness of care. Some of these measures use a combination of medical and pharmacy claims data to assess overuse or appropriate use of medications. Other measures are of the percentage of patients receiving follow-up care after new diagnoses, ED visits, or hospital stays. Following are examples of these measures:

Pharyngitis and Antibiotic Prescriptions

The percentage of patients 3 years and older diagnosed with pharyngitis who were tested for streptococcal infection and, only if appropriate, prescribed an antibiotic.

Physician, pharmacy, and laboratory claims may be used for this measure. Codes for testing for streptococcal infection (eg, **87880**, infectious agent antigen detection by immunoassay with direct optical [ie, visual] observation; streptococcus, group A) and *ICD-10-CM* codes (eg, **J02.0**, streptococcal pharyngitis) are indicative of appropriate prescribing.

Avoidance of Antibiotic Treatment of Acute Bronchitis/Bronchiolitis

Includes any patient encounter (eg, office visit, telemedicine visit) with an infant, child, or adolescent aged 3 months to 17 years that results in a diagnosis for acute bronchitis/bronchiolitis (includes *ICD-10-CM* codes in categories **J20**, bronchitis, and **J21**, acute bronchiolitis). Exclusions from the denominator for this measure are reportable with the following HCPCS codes:

G2176 Outpatient, ED, or observation visits that result in an inpatient admission

G2177 Acute bronchitis/bronchiolitis episodes when the patient had a new or refill prescription of antibiotics (table 1) in the 30 days prior to the episode date

(*Note:* "table 1" refers to a table of antibiotics included in the measure specification.)

G9712 Documentation of medical reason(s) for prescribing or dispensing antibiotic

G9713 Patients who use hospice services any time during the measurement period

Example

➤ **A physician sees a 14-month-old established patient for complaint of congestion, fever, and crying throughout the prior night.** The patient is diagnosed with acute suppurative otitis media of the right ear and respiratory syncytial virus (RSV) bronchiolitis. An antibiotic is prescribed for treatment of the acute otitis media, and the parents are counseled about home management of symptoms of bronchiolitis. The prescribing physician's total time on the date of the encounter is 35 minutes.

ICD-10-CM	*CPT*
H66.001 (acute suppurative otitis media without spontaneous rupture of ear drum, right ear) **J21.0** (acute bronchiolitis due to RSV)	**99214** (office E/M of an established patient); 30–39 minutes of total time is spent on the date of the encounter. (For the full code descriptor, refer to **Chapter 7**.)
H66.001	**G9712** (documentation of medical reason[s] for prescribing or dispensing antibiotic)

Teaching Point: When prescription of an antibiotic is indicated to treat another condition diagnosed or managed at the same visit during which bronchiolitis is diagnosed, specific use of the *ICD-10-CM* code for the condition for which an antibiotic was prescribed (eg, **H66.001**) may demonstrate appropriate use of antibiotics. Code **G9712** also supports exclusion from this measure.

Putting It All Together

This chapter has discussed several topics related to demonstrating the quality of care provided. To test your knowledge of the information presented in this chapter, complete the quiz found at the end of the chapter, after the resources. Answers to each quiz are found in **Appendix II**.

Chapter Takeaways

Readers of this chapter should understand how coding may support quality and performance measurement initiatives. Following are takeaways from this chapter:

- Physicians, payers, and accreditation organizations may use codes or claims data as a first line of quality measurement.
- A patient's reported experience of care can affect not only quality ratings but also contractual relations between physicians and payers.
- The details of each measure (eg, patient population, exclusions) are important in either providing care within the time frame of a measure or indicating why a patient was excluded from the activity of a measure (eg, not immunized because of patient history or a condition that prevents immunization).
- Performance measures change annually. Physician practices should maintain awareness of how health plans collect data for performance measurement and the documentation and coding practices that may reduce burdens associated with associated medical record reviews.
- Many plans publish their performance measures and supporting codes, as it is important to payers that physicians achieve optimal measurements.

Resources

AAP Coding Assistance and Education

AAP clinical report, "Strategies for Improving Vaccine Communication and Uptake" (https://doi.org/10.1542/peds.2023-065483)

AAP policy statement, "A New Era in Quality Measurement: The Development and Application of Quality Measures" (https://doi.org/10.1542/peds.2016-3442)

Consumer Assessment of Healthcare Providers and Systems

AHRQ CAHPS program (www.ahrq.gov/cahps/index.html)

CPT Category II Codes and Alphabetical Clinical Topics Listing

www.ama-assn.org/practice-management/cpt/category-ii-codes

Quality Measures

Medicaid Children's Health Care Quality Measures (www.medicaid.gov/medicaid/quality-of-care/performance-measurement/adult-and-child-health-care-quality-measures/childrens-health-care-quality-measures/index.html)

National Committee for Quality Assurance (www.ncqa.org)

Test Your Knowledge!

1. **Which codes are intended only for reporting performance measures?**
   a. *ICD-10-CM*
   b. *CPT* Category II codes
   c. HCPCS
   d. NDC
2. **Which statement is true of why HEDIS matters to physicians and QHPs?**
   a. Health plans will often pay physicians to help them meet quality measures and earn revenue.
   b. HEDIS measures do not matter to physicians and QHPs because only health plans benefit from HEDIS measurement.
   c. HEDIS measurement benefits only physicians who are self-employed.
   d. Reporting HEDIS measures is directly tied to FFS payment.
3. **Which of the following is true of quality and performance measures?**
   a. Only HEDIS measures are used in the core set of Medicaid and CHIP quality measures.
   b. Each measure is applicable to all children seen in a physician's or QHP's practice.
   c. Health plans may provide more specific documentation and coding guidance for reporting quality and performance measures.
   d. Most children are excluded from quality and performance measures.
4. **How many visits are included in the measure for well-child visits in the first 30 months of life?**
   a. 2
   b. 6
   c. 8
   d. 10
5. **True or false? Codes for patient or caregiver immunization refusal exclude a patient from the population for immunization measures.**
   a. True
   b. False

CHAPTER 4

The Business of Medicine: Working With Current and Emerging Payment Systems

Contents

Chapter Highlights

- How physicians and their staff can respond to changing payment systems and continually refine their practice management skills to maintain a viable practice
- How services are currently valued and how assigned values may be used to guide practice management and payer contract negotiations
- How data are leveraged to negotiate contract terms and payment
- Guidelines and tools that may be used to monitor and manage charge accumulation, claims filing, payments review, the appeals process, and the use of audits to protect against lost revenue and incorrect billing practices

Fee-for-Service Payment for Physician Services

Values Assigned to Physician Services

A fee-for-service (FFS) payment methodology based on both the Medicare Resource-Based Relative Value Scale (RBRVS) and submission of claims reporting physician services is the basis for a large portion of payment for physician services. Although other payment methodologies are growing, they are often built on an FFS payment structure. Before a claim is generated, a physician practice must establish fees for services that are greater than the cost of providing the service. A simple fee schedule methodology involves use of the RBRVS. An understanding of how values are assigned to the codes for services and how the values relate to payment contributes to a practice's financial viability and success.

The 3 components of the RBRVS are as follows:

1. *Physician work:* Physician work represents approximately 51% of the total relative value units (RVUs) assigned to most services. Work RVUs are commonly used in employment contracts as a factor in physician payment.
2. *Practice expense:* This component is an estimate of the following items:
   - Preservice, intraservice, and postservice clinical staff time
   - Medical supplies
   - Procedure-specific equipment and overhead

   Practice expense makes up approximately 45% of the total RVUs for most services. Practice expense varies by site of service (ie, facility vs non-facility). Refer to the Place of Service Codes section later in this chapter for more information about how place of service (POS) affects payment.
3. *Professional liability:* This smallest component (approximately 4% of the total RVUs) is based on medical malpractice premium data.

Components of Physician Work

Physician work is described as time required to perform the service, mental effort and judgment, technical skill, physical effort, and psychological stress associated with concern about iatrogenic risk to the patient.

For most services, physician work is further broken down into *preservice, intraservice,* and *postservice* components. Correct coding requires understanding these components of work, because preservice and postservice components should not be separately reported (ie, a single code includes all typical preservice, intraservice, and postservice work).

- *Preservice work:* For nonsurgical services, this preparatory non–face-to-face work includes typical review of records and communicating with other professionals. (Prolonged preservice work, such as extensive record review, may be separately reportable.) For surgical services, this includes physician work from the day before to the beginning of the procedure but excludes the encounter that resulted in the decision for surgery or unrelated evaluation and management (E/M) services.
- *Intraservice work:* For most nonsurgical services, this includes time spent by the physician or other qualified health care professional (QHP) in direct patient care activities. Surgical intraservice work begins with incision or introduction of instruments (eg, needle, scope) and ends with closure of the incision or removal of instruments.
  - A physician's intraservice time on the date of an E/M service for which the level of service is selected according to total time or medical decision-making (MDM) includes all time spent on the date of the encounter. Pre-visit planning and post-visit work, such as documenting the service provided, are included in intraservice time when performed on the date of the encounter.

  - Certain services (eg, chronic care management [CCM] 99487, 99489, 99490, 99439, 99491, 99437) are inclusive only of intraservice time of physicians and/or clinical staff and are not valued to include preservice and postservice work.
- *Postservice work:* Documentation of services provided is included in the postservice work of most services.
  - For nonsurgical services, postservice work includes arranging for further services, reviewing and communicating test results, preparing written reports, and/or communicating by telephone or secure electronic means. Separately reported services, such as CCM or care plan oversight, are not part of the postservice work of other services.
  - For surgical services, postservice work includes typical work in the operating/procedure room after the procedure has ended, stabilization of the patient in the recovery area, communications with family or other health care professionals, and visits on the day of surgery. Surgical services are also valued to include typical follow-up care for the presenting problem during a defined global period (eg, 10 or 90 days after the service).

For more on the global period for surgery, refer to Chapters 13 and 18.

Participation in Relative Value Scale Update Committee Surveys

Pediatricians can recommend values for services to the Centers for Medicare & Medicaid Services (CMS) by participation in American Academy of Pediatrics (AAP) surveys conducted through the American Medical Association/Specialty Society Relative Value Scale Update Committee (RUC). These surveys are conducted to estimate the time and complexity of performing a service in comparison with another service. AAP staff sends out requests for participation to AAP section members to allow completion by physicians who most typically perform the service being surveyed. To learn more about participation in RUC surveys, watch the "Understanding the RUC Survey Instrument: Physician Services without Global Period" video at www.youtube.com/watch?v=nu5unDX8VIs; for information on code valuation, RBRVS, and payment, visit www.aap.org/en/practice-management/child-health-finance-payment-strategy/coding-and-valuation/code-valuation-and-payment-rbrvs.

Refer also to the July 2024 *AAP News*™ article "AAP Members Play Key Role in Shaping New Code Values for Nirsevimab" (https://publications.aap.org/aapnews/news/29183/AAP-members-play-key-role-in-shaping-new-code) for an example of how pediatric participation in RUC surveys supports appropriate assignment of RVUs.

Fee Schedules and Calculations

Some codes are valued only for practice expense and professional liability because the service described by the code does not include physician work. For example, in 2025, 96110 (developmental screening with scoring and documentation, per standardized instrument) was assigned no work RVUs, 0.34 practice expense RVUs, and 0.01 professional liability RVUs. The physician work associated with interpretation of the test scores and related E/M are part of an E/M service (eg, preventive or problem-oriented).

Each RVU component may be independently adjusted slightly upward or downward as a function of geographic area. The CMS calculates Medicare payment for a procedure code by multiplying total adjusted RVUs by a dollar conversion factor that is set annually. Physician practices and health systems may agree to differing fee schedules when contracting with payers. Contracts may list a specific year of the Medicare Physician Fee Schedule (MPFS) and a set monetary rate/conversion factor that is multiplied times the RVUs assigned to a code.

Example

➤ **A payer uses the 2025 MPFS as a basis for physician payment with a conversion factor or contracted fee schedule amount of $40 per RVU.** A physician submits established patient office visit code 99214 to the payer.

The total MPFS non-facility RVUs (3.87) assigned to 99214 are a combination of RVUs for physician work (1.92), non-facility practice expense (1.80), and professional liability (0.15). The total non-facility RVUs (3.87) are multiplied by the $40 conversion factor to determine the allowed amount for the service.

(Total Medicare RVUs) × (Payer conversion factor) = Allowed amount

(3.87) × ($40) = $154.80

Actual benefit payment may vary depending on the patient's out-of-pocket obligation. For example, if the patient's plan requires a $20 co-payment, the plan might pay the balance of $134.80. Alternatively, if a patient has a high-deductible health plan, they may be responsible for the full amount of $154.80.

Medicaid fee schedules vary by state, and although they are often based on RVUs or the MPFS, state regulations may also designate amounts paid for specific services. Commercial plan payments for many procedure codes are often linked to a percentage of Medicare payment (eg, 140% of MPFS rate). In 2024, the estimated national commercial payment by private health plans for professional services was 143% of the Medicare MPFS rates (www.milliman.com/en/insight/commercial-reimbursement-benchmarking-medicare-ffs-rates), although this may vary significantly across specialties and geographic areas. Alternatively, payers may offer their own fee schedule (eg, a particular year's MPFS) for a practice's most used procedure codes.

If a health plan contract states that payment is based on the MPFS, it is important to verify the year of the MPFS used by the health plan because the schedule is not always current or may not be updated annually. Resetting payment according to the MPFS for the year of service may result in higher or lower payments.

Understanding how health plan rates in your area compare with the current MPFS rates can help inform contract negotiations.

- It is important to obtain the payer's fee schedule for all codes used or likely to be used by a practice, including codes for immunization products and administration, and compare these with the current year's MPFS and other published fee schedules. Although Medicare assigns a status of N (noncovered) to *Current Procedural Terminology* (*CPT*®) preventive medicine E/M codes **99381–99385** and **99391–99395** in the MPFS, component RVUs are published in the MPFS, allowing calculation of Medicare equivalent payments.

When reviewing a payer's fee schedule, make sure the payer also fully discloses its policies for paying for services that it considers to be ***bundled*** (ie, payment for ≥2 codes during the same encounter may be less than the sum of the individual payments) and policies that shift cost to the patient/family.

Inclusion of codes in a payer's fee schedule should not be assumed to indicate that all codes qualify for payment as covered services. Payers often outline coverage guidelines in policies separate from a fee schedule listing, including clinical policies, reimbursement policies, and administrative policies. There are, however, alternative ways to ensure coverage of commonly provided noncovered services, such as requesting a "carve-out" for specific codes, with a relevant payment rate.

- The same payer may be the administrator of multiple plans with differing contractual terms regarding what may or may not be billed to the patient/caregiver.
- Learn payer policies and, in particular, whether the practice must obtain a patient's/caregiver's written agreement to an advance notice of potential noncoverage prior to billing the patient/caregiver for a noncovered service.
- Practices must develop policies and procedures to effectively collect amounts owed by the patient/caregiver to avoid lost revenue.

The RBRVS payment methodology may be used with practice- and physician-specific data generated from a practice's accounting and practice management systems to estimate an approximate cost of providing each service. This should result in a list of services that are each assigned a share of the practice's overhead costs as well as the margin and actual cost of providing the service.

- From the accounting system, an administrator may calculate the total practice expenses for a period, subtracting billable services that are not paid by RVUs, such as immunization products and medications.
- From the practice management system, reports may be generated to provide a total number of services billed by code, RVUs for each service, and total RVUs billed by the practice for the same period.
- By dividing total practice expenses by total RVUs, an administrator can calculate the practice cost per RVU.
- Additional calculations may be used to compare payment per RVU or per service among contracted payers. (Calculations should be viewed in context of other factors, such as history of timely and correct payment.)

It may be important to consider several years of data to account for seasonal, year-to-year, or unusual circumstance (eg, natural disaster, limited availability of an immunization product) effects, which may significantly limit the accuracy of data to predict future service costs and volume.

Such calculations should be used to inform decisions regarding acceptance of contractual fee schedules, number of services necessary to break even or profit from provision of services, and return on investment potential for new equipment or services.

Keep in mind that some accountable care organizations (ACOs) have financial agreements that require certain services be paid with a single lump payment that is then distributed among all providers of the service. (For discussion of ACOs, refer to the Organizational Support for Entering Value-Based Payment Contracts section later in this chapter.) To negotiate a fair portion of that lump payment, you need to know the cost of providing the service. More accurate cost estimates may be determined on an actual cost basis. RVU calculations, however, are straightforward and typically provide a reasonably reliable result.

Alternative Payment Models

The movement away from traditional FFS payment and toward value-based care through the implementation of alternative payment models has been offered and reimagined many times over the years. Yet many alternative payment models are still built on an FFS payment structure.

Capitation is one payment model that varies from the FFS structure. In capitation arrangements, the health plan will pay a fixed amount per health plan member assigned to the physician or practice on a per-member-per-month basis. Amounts may vary by patient age, patient sex, patient clinical risk, and plan design. Under capitation plans, physicians and other QHPs provide sick- and well-child services that are included in the per-member-per-month payment. In addition to per-member-per-month payments, plans may pay separately for provision of immunization products and other specified services. Capitation arrangements may also include elements of other alternative payment models that are focused on value-based payment.

Value-based payment models offer physicians and other providers (eg, QHPs and other nonphysician qualified health care professionals [NQHCPs]) incentive payments based on the quality of care, outcomes, and cost containment attributable to their practices. The intent is to promote patient value and efficiency, but some risk is shifted to physician practices, and there could be a lack of clarity about how payments are calculated. Value-based payment models are widely variable in regional implementation but are growing in national importance and impact.

Although value-based payment models focus on high-value and reduced costs of care, achieving these goals may depend on recognizing and addressing provision of care that is of low value and increases cost. Some examples of potential low-value care are provided in the AAP Choosing Wisely campaign toolkit (www.aap.org/en/news-room/campaigns-and-toolkits/choosing-wisely) and in some quality measures (eg, avoidance of antibiotic treatment for acute bronchitis/bronchiolitis) as discussed in **Chapter 3**.

Under value-based payment models, practice viability depends on how well quality, cost, and efficiency are managed. Examples of some of these value-based payment models include bundled payments, shared savings/risk, and pay for performance. Physician payments may be based on a combination of FFS and alternative payment methodologies.

- *Bundled payments:* These are a type of prospective payment in which health care providers (eg, hospitals, urgent care clinics, physicians, and other health care professionals) share 1 payment that covers all services involved in a patient's episode of care, as opposed to each provider's being paid individually. The intent of bundled payments is to foster collaboration and accountability among multiple providers to coordinate services and control costs, thereby reducing unnecessary utilization.
- *Shared savings/risk:* Shared savings/risk models may include upside reward or both upside reward and downside risk. In an upside-reward–only arrangement, the provider shares only in any savings and does not experience risk for financial losses. Under reward-and-risk arrangements, the practice shares not only a reward if costs are less than budgeted but also the loss should actual total costs exceed budgeted costs.
  - The contractual arrangement among the payer(s) and providers specifies how savings and/or risk is to be calculated and distributed.
  - Shared savings should include an up-front agreement to additional payments for support of infrastructure at all stages, including future years when the payer may want to cut back on the shared savings margin as savings plateau.

The target or expected budgeted amount should be reviewed periodically and renegotiated to account for the current savings opportunity. After implementing many initiatives and achieving significant cost savings early in a contract, providers may then target maintaining cost performance and limiting increases in total cost of care.

  - Quality metrics are typically tied to payment of shared savings, with physicians not receiving a portion of savings when not meeting established quality benchmarks.

Refer to Chapter 3 for more information on coding to support quality and performance measurement.

- *Pay for performance:* In this arrangement, physician payments are based on a prospectively determined comparison of the provider's performance against acknowledged benchmarks. If the provider meets or exceeds those benchmarks, an enhanced payment or bonus is provided.

- Benchmarks are often like the National Committee for Quality Assurance Healthcare Effectiveness Data and Information Set (HEDIS) quality metrics (some common metrics for pediatrics include rates of immunizations; rates of patient adherence to Early and Periodic Screening, Diagnostic, and Treatment visits; and rates of appropriate prescription of asthma medications). These metrics should be relevant to pediatrics. Other potential pediatric-specific measures include the 2026 Core Set of Children's Health Care Quality Measures for Medicaid and CHIP (www.medicaid.gov/medicaid/quality-of-care/downloads/2026-child-core-set.pdf).

When entering into pay-for-performance agreements, a practice may request use of the same standardized measure set across all payers to simplify performance tracking.

- Benchmarks based on transparent rubrics allow providers to track their performance against the benchmark on an ongoing basis. In contrast, if benchmarks are based on comparison with peers, providers might not know whether they meet the metrics until the period is over.
- Payers should provide information on how benchmarks are defined and measured. Practices should also ensure that benchmarks come from pediatric peers with similar patients to avoid comparison with practices that treat only patients whose conditions or situations are less medically and/or socially complex. When benchmarks are not limited to pediatric peers, they should include adjustments to consider the lower expense to payers for pediatric-specific care.
- Practices should also provide quarterly data on provider performance against benchmarks. This way, providers are aware of their performance standing and have an opportunity to improve throughout the measurement incentive year.
- Providers should be rewarded for achieving incremental improvements and maintaining high levels of quality once achieved.

When considering whether to participate in one of these alternative payment models, practices need to determine expected costs and utilization and assess whether they can deliver services under the projected budget. Using *CPT* codes and their RVUs will aid in this assessment. Projections can be made from RVUs of the services currently provided and projected to be provided with consideration of changes such as decreased number or complexity of patient visits resulting from better-coordinated care. With these types of data, the practice can assess the effect of new payment methodologies on its bottom line.

Important Considerations Regarding Payer Ratings in Value-Based Care Models

In value-based payment programs, payers may publish ratings and cost-of-care comparisons of practices within a community to guide a family's selection of a practice or physician. In addition, some payers prefer to drive patients to high-value practices or have tiered co-payments based on individual physician or practice performance. Families interpret ratings to reflect a lower quality of care rather than a lower cost of care.

When discussing publication of practice ratings and/or cost comparisons with payers, practices should be aware of whether immunizations and preventive care are counted in the total cost of care. Otherwise, they may find that if they improve well-child visit and immunization rates, the costs of those services are counted against the practice in total cost-of-care calculations.

In some parts of the country, practices can earn additional incentives if the total cost of care for patients compares favorably with that of geographically and specialty matched peers. In addition, some payers incentivize around "care efficiency measures" (eg, avoidance of antibiotic treatment for acute bronchitis/bronchiolitis: ages 3 months to 17 years). Both of these are often risk adjusted according to claims data about the overall patient population of the practice. Payers should define measures (eg, what constitutes an avoidable emergency department [ED] visit) and data that can be used to improve performance. As with other quality or cost measures, these measures should be relevant to pediatrics.

Participating in Alternative Payment Models

Value-based payment models are already in place for pediatrics in some geographic areas and may soon be adopted in others. Whether your practice provides primary or specialty care, there are steps you should take to prepare for success. When payment is based on the costs of care and patient experience, practices must take responsibility for keeping costs low and keeping quality of care and patient experience high. Steps that practices may take include

- Learning more about value-based payment options
- Generating and using reports of your costs, quality measurement, and other data
- Learning who your active patients are and staying up to date through routine data analysis

- Obtain lists of patients attributed to your practice by payers (patient panels) and reconcile with your active patient list.
- Identify and agree on a methodology by which patients will be assigned and any disputes over attributed patient panels will be reconciled.
- Encourage and instruct patients on how to identify/choose/change their primary care physician with their insurer.

Assignment, Engagement, and Attribution of Patient Panels

Value-based payment may be based on the patients assigned and/or attributed to a practice (patient panel) by a payer. This may be limited to comparison of the cost of care for a physician's patient panel to other patients in a geographic area or to another subset of patients. The cost of care for all attributed patients may lead to additional payment based on shared cost savings or may limit the amount of payments that the practice retains. It is important to understand the distinction between what you view as your practice panel and how the insurer views it. It is also important to differentiate assignment from engagement and attribution.

- *Assignment:* The patients the insurance company lists on your panel roster.

  For Medicaid managed care, every patient must be assigned to a provider (or provider practice) when patients are enrolled in the health plan. These patients may choose your practice or can be automatically assigned through insurer algorithms.
- *Engagement:* Patients you have seen and with whom you have a medical home relationship.

  If you have an after-hours clinic and you see patients from other practices, it is essential you communicate to those patients that they are not part of your medical home (ie, they are part of another physician's or practice's panel).
- *Attribution:* Patients who fall into the denominator of a metric in which value (ie, payment) is assigned. Physicians should understand how health plans attribute patients to individual physicians and/or groups for purposes of performance measurement and cost of care.
  - Factors such as time of continuous enrollment with the health plan and number of visits to a provider may affect how patients are attributed.

To ensure you are engaging patients who are assigned to your practice, make sure you receive a panel roster monthly, preferably as an Excel file, through the payer's portal. Identify new patients assigned to your practice, and plan for the services they will need based on their age, including preventive services that are included in quality metrics.

- Use the roster at check-in to make sure all patients seen in your medical home are assigned to you, and develop procedures for educating and assisting patients with changing the payer's assignment of their medical home. This step is just as important as identifying those you are not seeing on your roster. It will ensure you are getting credit for the quality work your office is providing.

Know the payer's rules for requesting that a patient be removed from your roster. The payer may require specific documentation to fulfill your request, such as the number of unsuccessful outreach attempts by phone or mail to the family of a patient who has not presented for care or information regarding the family's selection of another medical home.

- Track the number of patients assigned to your office each month. If there is a large increase, a group of patients from another practice may have been shifted to your practice. Consider including language in your contract that specifies that no panel transfers can be done without prior authorization of your practice.
- If the insurer is nonresponsive in working to ensure that only patients who can be or are engaged are assigned, consider limiting the ages that can be assigned to your practice or closing your practice to auto-assignment altogether.

For HEDIS measures, patients must meet certain age-, utilization-, or encounter-based criteria to fall into your denominator. Knowing when they will be attributed (and show up on your "gaps in care" reports) is essential. For further discussion, refer to **Chapter 3**. For primary care physicians, the cost of preventive services should not negatively affect the physician's calculated cost of care per patient.

Remember, your practice will never have a 100% accurate assigned panel. The effort you put into reaching this perfection must be balanced by what is being measured and how much payment is at risk.

Steps to Support Value-Based Payment

Even practices that are not yet ready to enter a value-based payment program can take initial steps to prepare. These might include

- Embracing automation and alternatives to paper handling.

- Increasing access to care beyond traditional office-based care (eg, telemedicine, care management services, remote patient monitoring).
- Seeking to remove inefficiencies by reviewing routine tasks and patient flow. Provide staff with incentives and an expectation to create consistency and efficiency.
- When considering an alternative payment model contract, seeking expert consultation to help identify and, as necessary, negotiate points of concern within the contract.
- Learning about the communities of your patients (ie, school and community resources, school schedules, average income and education of caregivers, urgent and emergency care utilization patterns) and using that information in providing care.
- Considering options for adding nonphysician health care professionals to your practice, such as care coordinators, patient educators, and emotional/behavioral health specialists. (These clinicians may also add separately reportable services under FFS contracts.)

Steps that may increase successful participation in value-based payment include

- Setting shared goals and shared priorities with the payer
  - Evaluate your progress against goals and reevaluate targets each year with the payer. Targets might need to be adjusted depending on past achievements and future opportunities.
- Being aware of and collaborating with other health care providers who care for patients attributed to the practice
  - Recognize that every provider within and outside your practice must contribute to not only reducing the cost of care but improving the quality of care to reduce the practice's risk under new payment models.
  - Collaborate with other health care professionals to ensure that patients receive evidence-based and cost-effective care, including consideration of formulary and total cost of coordinated care.

Remember that care received in the ED and urgent care clinics and from subspecialists or NQHCPs (eg, physical therapists) is included in the cost of care attributed to your cost to care for your patients.

- Optimizing data systems
  - Embedding clinical guidelines into care delivery through protocols and reminders
  - Configuring and using your electronic health record (EHR) and other automated systems to promote efficiency (eg, display generic drugs first when a brand name is entered)

Other considerations for pediatricians include

- Recognizing that, depending on how the payment model is set up, managing a healthy population of patients may not result in significant cost savings.
- Having the ability to access and monitor patient population and performance metric data, which is important for successful participation in new payment methodologies. Physicians must be aware of not only the patients they are seeing but also those who are not receiving preventive and/or follow-up care.
- Making a plan with staff to perform post-payment follow-up and address inconsistencies between your records and the payer's record of services to ensure you are credited appropriately for services provided.
- For physicians, understanding the links between new payment methodologies and data collection to support quality metrics (eg, failure to report codes for screening services performed may result in negative performance measurement and lost opportunity for enhanced payment).
- Remembering that in states where the Children's Health Insurance Program (CHIP) operates independent of a Medicaid program, children covered by CHIP may or may not be included in new payment methodologies and/or performance measurement.

Organizational Support for Entering Value-Based Payment Contracts

Demonstrating that a practice provides care at a lower cost and higher value can significantly burden small practices. Entering into a contract to participate in a network or an organization with other physician practices, and sometimes hospitals or health care systems, can offer support on multiple levels. Through these contractual relationships, physicians may achieve objectives such as improved capitation rates, entrance into other risk-sharing contracts, and increased ability to demonstrate quality and cost reductions. There are multiple types of contractual entities that can influence success in value-based payment arrangements.

Various federal and state regulations (eg, antitrust regulations and price-fixing, physician self-referral, false claims) must be accounted for when entering into a contractual agreement that organizes multiple independent physicians into an organization that will influence health care referrals and health plan fee schedule negotiations.

- *Management services organization:* These organizations focus solely on administrative tasks such as provision of space, equipment, nonclinical staff, billing and compliance, accounts payable, insurance credentialing (not contract negotiation), and human resources.
- *Independent physician or practitioner association:* Joining these organizations of independent physician practices often includes entering into risk-sharing or capitation contracts that place the organization as an intermediary between payers and physician members. These organizations cannot negotiate FFS contracts.
- *Clinically integrated network:* A group of physicians and providers (eg, hospitals or health systems) who are integrated at the clinical level to be able to jointly contract with and participate in performance incentive programs. The practices continue *independent medical practice* and the clinically integrated network members work together to achieve and demonstrate better quality and lower cost. A clinically integrated network is much like an ACO (as follows) but is not governed by the Medicare/Medicaid rules for ACOs.
- *Accountable care organizations:* An ACO is an organization of health care professionals that agrees to be accountable for the quality, cost, and overall care of beneficiaries. The ACO is a legal entity with a management structure capable of delivering and reporting on evidence-based and informed care to a defined population, effectively engaging patients and receiving and distributing shared savings.
  - The Patient Protection and Affordable Care Act of 2010 included provisions that establish ACOs in Medicare, Medicaid, and CHIP. Federal regulations, such as anti-kickback and self-referral prohibitions, continue to be revised to allow more cooperation and technical support among ACO participants.
  - From a practical standpoint, an ACO is a community of physicians and other QHPs who work collaboratively to reduce health care costs and improve the quality of care for their patient population. Accountable care organization members typically focus on data sharing and care coordination to help deliver timely preventive and care management services to generate health care savings that are then shared by the ACO members.
  - Most pediatric ACOs are affiliated with children's hospitals and/or health plans. Commercial health insurers are actively exploring the development of ACOs and may support establishment of an ACO.

Small practices that are not yet participating in one of the entities discussed earlier may use a variety of other external resources, such as an external billing company, vaccine management programs, health care accountants, payroll processing, and human resource managers.

Contracting and Negotiating With Payers

Participating in a payer's network typically involves entering into a contract with the payer. Physicians should not sign contracts without reading them and considering the impact of entering into the contractual agreement. The payer is going to seek terms that are most favorable to its business. Negotiation is important to ensure that your practice is profitable and able to provide quality care without burdensome payer requirements (eg, panel attribution methodology and primary care provider reassignment, dispute process for quality or other pay-for-performance programs).

The Importance of Data and Leverage

Successful negotiation requires data and leverage. Negotiating payment with payers can be more successful if a practice is prepared to provide data on the complexity of its patient panel, its quality performance according to standard quality measures, and any current initiatives and future opportunities to influence total cost of care. Be prepared to demonstrate the cost savings that may be recognized by the plan, as well as the value the practice brings to the plan in quality of care and/or patient satisfaction.

Refer to Chapter 3 for more information on demonstrating quality and patient satisfaction.

Preparing for Negotiation

Successful negotiation requires preparation. The following suggestions can help.

Identify the Practice's Payer Mix

Current and accurate information on payer mix and potential value/loss to the practice is essential in making participation decisions.

- Know how many patients you have in each plan and what percentage of your total patients that represents. In addition, know what percentage of RVUs each payer pays for your most frequently used codes and how these percentages compare with each other in terms of payment.

Contract Transparency and Network Tiering

- Fully read and ask questions, as necessary, about the terms of the contract.
  - Initial term and any automatic renewal (evergreen) clause
  - Time frame and notice required for termination with/without cause
  - Payment methodology, annual conversion factor, and any automatic increases or updates (eg, whether payment updates align with Medicare updates or are tied to a specific year of the Medicare fee schedule)
  - Time frame for payer recoupment and claim appeals
  - Notice and consent required for amendments and material changes
  - Types of products (eg, health maintenance organization [HMO], preferred provider organization [PPO]) and health plans included and whether there is a requirement to accept all products
- Be aware of any accountability (eg, penalties or other effect on shared savings) that a plan attributes to the practice when patients receive care outside their plan's network without referral by physicians within the practice.
- Ask whether there is any tiering of network providers based on quality or cost-efficiency rankings and, if so,
  - Whether tiering is done at the provider or practice/group level
  - Whether newly added providers will carry over their previous ranking
  - How tiering affects provider payment and/or patient cost sharing

Why Health Plan Tiering Matters

Many health plans assign in-network physicians to tiers based on the cost and value of care provided by the individual physician or the group practice.

Tiering is often tied to patient cost sharing (eg, deductible, co-payments, and coinsurance), with patients being responsible for the highest cost sharing if they see providers in the non-preferred tier. This may affect how and whether a patient receives health care services.

Tiering may also affect both the number of patients who select a particular health plan (eg, a tiered plan in which their current physician is in a high tier) and how the health plan negotiates with a physician or group practice (eg, by offering a lower fee schedule as a larger number of patients enroll in the tiered health plan).

Becoming a contracted network provider might not place you into the preferred tier, as this depends on how tiering is determined. Language on tiering may or may not be in the contract, so there is value in requesting information about the payer's use of tiering and tier assignment methodology.

- When adding new physicians to your practice, be aware of each payer's fee schedule policies. Do not assume that the same fee schedule will be applied across all physicians in the practice (eg, a payer may assign a reduced fee schedule to new physicians or carry forward a physician's contract from a previous practice).
  - When this occurs, discussion with a health plan should include the potential effect of delayed care when the patient/family opts to wait to see a provider for whom the out-of-pocket costs are lower because of differing fee schedules (eg, a new physician's fee schedule is carried forward from their prior practice).

Payment Policies and Code Edits

- Know a health plan's policies and procedures and their effect on pediatric services. Develop a system to monitor all policy and procedure updates and to receive and review in detail any communications from the payer on changes to the physician contract. The payer may automatically amend the contract if no response is received to a notice of proposed amendment in the specified time frame. Be aware of updates to the provider manual, updates provided via periodic email bulletins, and information posted on a payer website that practices have been instructed to review periodically. Practices must be aware that these alternative ways of disseminating payment information are often considered legal and binding.

- Know a health plan's processes and time frame for adding new *CPT* codes/services and how each plan pays for new services reported before developing and updating their systems with payment policy and fee schedule amounts. This preparation is especially important for new immunizations to make sure you will get paid. (New codes are often paid at a low rate or a percentage of charges, if covered at all.)
- Verify payer rules about modifier use, because this may affect payment. For example, when preventive and problem-oriented E/M services are provided on the same date, modifier **25** (significant, separately identifiable E/M service) is appended to the code for the problem-oriented E/M service (eg, **99213 25**). Some payers reduce the payment to 50% of the fee schedule amount for that code.
- Know how the payer adopts and discloses code edits used in claims adjudication (eg, Medicare and Medicaid National Correct Coding Initiative [NCCI] as discussed in **Chapter 2**). Often, access to code edits is limited to the payer's provider portal.

Interacting and Negotiating With Payers and Employers

- Know *CPT* codes and modifiers and the guidelines for their use.
- Understand and be able to describe the scope of services provided and the time requirements for the service.
- Be prepared to demonstrate the cost savings that may be recognized by the plan as well as the value the practice brings to the plan in savings, quality of care, and/or patient satisfaction. *This is your leverage.*
- Monitor and know the use (distribution) of codes by each physician and, if in a group practice, for the practice as a whole.
- Know and understand the payment basis and process.
- Have specific codes or issues to discuss, not generalities (agreement with general ideas may not address specific issues).

In negotiations,

- Try to negotiate for coverage and adequate payment of services.
- If the plan does agree to cover a particular service, make certain you understand how the carrier will cover and pay for the service and if there will be any restrictions or limitations. When payers refuse to cover services, ensure there is language in your contract stating that you can bill the patient for noncovered services. If the plan allows billing the patient for noncovered services, you must advise your patients of this policy (a service-specific written notification is usually required before rendering the service). In addition, claim submission may be required with the appropriate modifier appended to the procedure (eg, **GA**, waiver of liability statement issued as required by payer policy, individual case).
- Keep notes during the discussion and be certain you understand answers to any of your questions. Any specific agreements should be in writing and signed by both parties with the effective date clearly stated.

Seeking Assistance in Negotiations

When seeking assistance in negotiations,

- Engage parents or employers to work in partnership to help you negotiate with a plan. Encourage parents to work through their human resources department to communicate and appeal with payers. Petitions from parents can be very effective. For health insurance education resources from HealthyChildren.org, refer to www.healthychildren.org/English/family-life/health-management/health-insurance/Pages/default.aspx.

It is important to recognize that the employers in your area may offer their employees a self-funded health plan and that it is the employer that may be in control of the plan's network, payment rates, and policies for coverage and payment of specific services, although a third party (eg, health insurance company) receives and determines payment of claims. In 2024, 63% of workers were covered under their employer's self-funded health plan.

- Many AAP chapters have developed pediatric councils that meet with payers to address pediatric issues. Advise your chapter pediatric council of specific issues you have experienced to see how it can work with the plan. (The AAP chapter pediatric councils are not forums for negotiating contracts, setting fees, or discussing payments.)
  - If your chapter does not have a pediatric council, this may be the right time to begin developing one. For more information, visit www.aap.org/en/practice-management/child-health-finance-payment-strategy/payment-and-finance-advocacy.

When Negotiations Fail

If the insurance company is not addressing your concerns satisfactorily, you should be willing to provide notice of intent to terminate your contract if unable to reach an agreement after negotiating in good faith. Check your contract for specifications on the days of notice and notification process required for termination of your provider contract with or without cause. Inform the payer and patients' families and even the state insurance commission why continued participation is not possible.

- Some reasons for withdrawal might be slow payment, excessive documentation requirements, and substandard payment compared with those of other plans.
- Many times, negotiation begins when you walk away from the table.

Steps to Getting Paid: Clean Claims to Correct Payment

Getting paid for services provided requires a practice-wide team effort. Even salaried physicians are affected by lost revenue and should take interest in the effectiveness of the practice's billing processes. Opportunities for lost revenue can occur anywhere between patient scheduling and posting of health plan payments (or denials). **Figure 4-1** shows steps in the revenue cycle.

An effective charge accumulation system, accurate billing of procedure codes, and an efficient claims filing system are necessary but not sufficient to achieve clean claim submissions. Although the physician is ultimately responsible for the accuracy of codes selected and claims submitted, it typically takes a team effort to create and maintain an effective accounts receivable system, including

- Regular review and updating of fees for services and supplies to avoid charging lower rates than the practice is eligible to be paid. For example, vaccine prices increase regularly, so fees must be increased to support adequate payment.
- Development and use of management tools.
  - Incorporation of claims-processing tools for analysis of your claims-processing procedures.
  - EHR and/or billing systems may include automated tools to help identify errors before billing, alert you to payments that do not align with contracted fees, and provide data for monitoring the time lapse from provision of service to payment.

Figure 4-1. Revenue Cycle

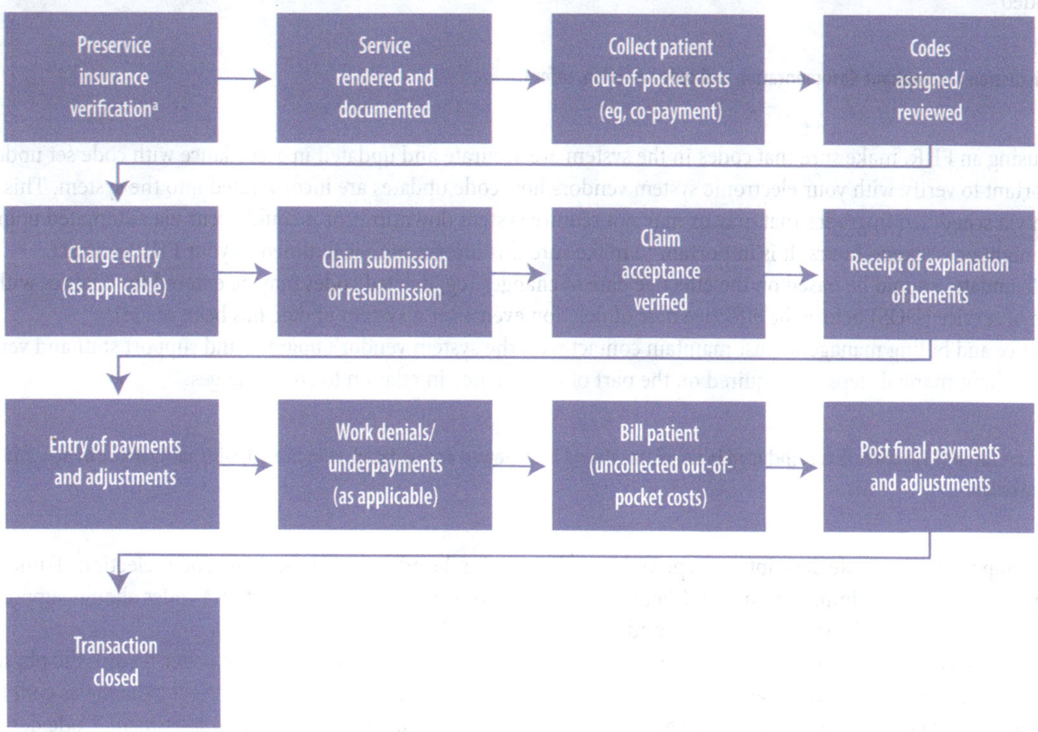

[a] Obtain prior authorization when required.

   - Provide access to and create policy for using payer resources such as online code-checking tools that alert to coverage limitations such as bundled services or services covered only in conjunction with specific diagnoses.
- Continuing provider and staff education with constant oversight and communication with staff, payers, and patients.
   - Policies and procedures support continual monitoring of payer communications and dissemination of information on benefit policy changes that affect coding and payment.
   - Assurance that staff assigned responsibilities related to correct coding and billing have access to current and authoritative resources on coding and documentation (eg, health plan provider portals, official coding guidelines).

Refer to **Chapters 2** and **5** for more information on code edits and compliant coding and billing.

- Regularly performing audits to identify potential corrective actions required to remain compliant with billing standards, coding guidelines, and federal rules and regulations (eg, Health Insurance Portability and Accountability Act [HIPAA] of 1996, Anti-Kickback Statute, False Claims Act). Audits benefit the practice by identifying
   - The number of timely and correctly submitted claims, resulting in faster and more appropriate payments and reduced practice cost of obtaining payment
   - The need for new or repeat physician and staff education on coding and documentation
   - Issues to be addressed in payer contract negotiations
   - Incorrect coding and related potential risk for charges of fraud or abuse
   - Areas that need written office policies and procedures (eg, preauthorization and referral processes, claims follow-up processes, control systems)
- Procedures for efficient review of payments and potentially inappropriate denials or reductions. Timely identification of payment errors is necessary to obtain redress because contracts often specify a time limit on appeals.
- Guidance for write-offs and initiation of appeals processes.

Capturing Charges in the Electronic Health Record

- Many physicians now capture encounter and billing information in the EHR. The basics of charge capture in the EHR include
   - Accurate listing of diagnoses
   - Selection of complete codes and access to a complete list of modifiers
   - Procedure code selection based on work performed and documented

Although integrating charge capture into the encounter documentation should create efficiency, there are pitfalls to be avoided.

For discussion of compliant documentation and code selection, refer to Chapter 5.

When using an EHR, make sure that codes in the system are accurate and updated in accordance with code set updates. It is important to verify with your electronic system vendors how code updates are incorporated into the system. This might happen via scheduled upgrades that may or may not require system downtime, or it could occur via automated upgrades during night or weekend hours. It is important to make sure this information is outlined in your EHR contract.

- Code updates should be based on the effective date of changes (eg, deleted codes may be entered for charges with a date of service (DOS) before the effective date of deletion even after a system update has been made).
- Practice and billing managers must maintain contact with the system vendor's upgrade and support staff and verify what, if any, manual steps are required on the part of the practice in relation to code changes.

Any codes saved to favorites lists or included in templates should be reviewed and updated, as indicated, with each release of new and revised codes.

It is also important that code descriptors displayed in code selection be adequate for accurate code selection. Truncated descriptors may omit key information that differentiates codes. For example, display of asthma codes should support selection based on severity and current status (eg, moderate persistent asthma with exacerbation).

Documentation of the diagnoses has been problematic in some EHR systems. As with the paper record, the physician must have the ability to fully describe patient diagnoses for each encounter (ie, not to merely select a diagnosis code).

- *Systems should not use diagnosis codes for populating the physician's diagnostic statement or assessment.* Code descriptors may be generalized and do not capture the physician's differential diagnoses, and many codes do not indicate when a condition is worsening or poorly managed.

Examples

➤ **Neonatal heart murmur; benign versus congenital heart disease (P29.89, other cardiovascular disorders originating in the perinatal period)**

➤ **Underachievement in school with grades dropping this semester (Z55.3, underachievement in school)**

➤ **Tachycardia, frequent headaches, fatigue, and lightheadedness on standing; postural orthostatic tachycardia syndrome suspected, return visit after receipt of laboratory results (R00.0, tachycardia, unspecified; R51.9, headache, unspecified; R53.83, other fatigue; R42, dizziness and giddiness)**

➤ **Delayed milestone in childhood—3 years old, late language emergence in speech therapy; possibly on the autism spectrum—makes little eye contact and likes to play alone (R62.0, delayed milestone in childhood)**

- List first the diagnosis and code most responsible for the encounter, followed by additional diagnoses, in compliance with coding guidelines.
- *The EHR should not reorder diagnoses entered by the physician.* An EHR that reorders documented diagnoses (eg, alphabetically) results in noncompliance with diagnosis coding guidelines and may fail to show support for the related services.

Sequencing instructions in *International Classification of Diseases, 10th Revision, Clinical Modification* (*ICD-10-CM*) are important for correct coding and for prevention of claim rejections. Refer to Chapter 1 for more on sequencing diagnosis codes.

- The patient problem list should not be pulled forward as the diagnoses for each encounter. Only those conditions addressed or that affected management or treatment of conditions addressed should be reported for that particular encounter.

Follow payer guidelines for reporting diagnosis codes for chronic conditions that may be reported annually (eg, evaluating problems at preventive service visits) for the purpose of risk adjustment (ie, projection of future health care costs for a patient). Documentation and coding to support risk adjustment are increasingly demanded by payers. Refer to the "What Pediatricians Should Know About Coding and Risk Adjustment" box that follows for discussion of appropriate coding to support risk adjustment.

Automated code selection is problematic. An EHR may be designed to determine the level of E/M service provided by using information documented. However, physicians must base the code determination on the medically necessary services provided and documented and the code selection criteria (eg, MDM or total time).

- Automatic population of records may result in documentation that overstates the level of work and intensity of the service provided.
- Failure to override suggested codes when appropriate may be considered an abusive practice.

Example

➤ **A child is evaluated for concern of ear pain and mild fever.** The EHR's coding algorithm selects 99214 because of the physician's documented diagnosis of acute otitis media with fever and prescription drug management, but the physician knows that the child was not very ill and that the acute, uncomplicated problem addressed, in combination with the moderate risk of prescription drug management, supports 99213, not 99214.

Teaching Point: The physician overrides the code suggested by the EHR and instead reports 99213. Consistent failure to override incorrectly assigned codes may lead to audits and/or a request for refund of amounts paid. It may also cause the physician to appear as a high-cost provider of services, which may affect health plan rankings, as discussed in the Preparing for Negotiation section earlier in this chapter.

What Pediatricians Should Know About Coding and Risk Adjustment

Multiple risk adjustment models are used in health care today for assessing and forecasting the costs of care for individual patients covered under a health benefit program. The primary goal of risk adjustment is to ensure that payment for providing coverage to a group of patients is based on the expected costs of care.

Risk adjustment is often accomplished through use of hierarchal condition categories or aggregated diagnosis groups (based on *ICD-10-CM* codes reported on claims) that are assigned weight values and used along with certain demographic and social factors, as well as claims data (eg, hospital claims, prescription drug claims), to assign a total risk score. Physicians and QHPs play a major role in documenting and assigning codes for diagnoses that may influence a patient's risk score.

- **Correct and complete diagnosing is necessary to share the disease burden of your patients with the health plan. Showing the true nature of your patient's health status may have not only a short-term effect on rates paid per visit but also long-term implications in contracting with health plans.**
- **Code assignment should accurately reflect the condition(s) documented, including identified social determinants of health that may alter treatment or management.**
- **Payment to physicians and QHPs may increasingly be based on quality and cost of care. Risk adjustment is used to set the expected cost of care for a patient panel. Physicians and QHPs will be affected, especially individuals whose employers may already gain or lose revenue based on risk factor adjustment.**
- **Patient access to care may be affected when conditions are undocumented or documented in insufficient detail.**
  - **Risk adjustment may also be used for stratifying patients into high-risk groups that are eligible for care management.**
  - **If risk adjustment results in lower revenue for health plans, health plan coverage and benefits will undoubtedly be affected.**

It is also important to know that

- **Like all health care payments, those based on risk adjustment are audited for accuracy. Medical records may be requested to validate *ICD-10-CM* codes supporting risk adjustment scores.**
- **Pediatric hierarchical condition categories, used in risk adjustment for health insurance marketplace and federally funded plans, apply to children younger than 2 years (ie, before their second birthday) or to those aged 2 through 20 years (ie, before their 21st birthday).**
- **Risk adjustment category values are cumulative, making documentation of all diagnoses that affect management important for accurate calculation of risk.**
- **Risk adjustment is also used in shared savings agreements with ACOs and value-based payment to hospitals.**

For more on compliant EHR documentation, refer to Chapter 5. Refer also to Chapter 20 for information specific to documentation and coding for telemedicine services.

Encounter Forms and Other Coding Tools

Encounter forms, which may be electronic or printed, are useful supplements to EHR-based code selection. They can also be used to convey codes to a billing office/system when systems are not integrated.

Designing and Reviewing the Encounter Form or Superbill

The encounter form, whether electronic or printed, should be designed to help physicians and clinical staff quickly find all codes for diagnoses and services common to the practice. An encounter form or superbill should prompt recognition of separately reported services and use of diagnosis codes that most accurately describe the patient presentation.

When developing the encounter form,

- Include clinical and billing staff in development and review to ensure that the form captures all necessary information to support billing and that the intended use of the form is clear.
- Include all levels of service for each category of E/M services (eg, 99211–99215, 99221–99223) and ensure that time is listed for coding based on time. List routine health examination codes by age and new or established patient.
- List procedures (eg, laboratory) to fit your practice's workflow. For example, group the codes together in the order of your workflow (eg, visit codes followed by immunization, laboratory, respiratory, and other procedures) to maximize efficiency and your workflow. Some codes may be listed in more than one section of an encounter form because of their different uses. For example, 96160 (patient-focused health risk assessment instrument) might be included as a preventive service for use of general health risk assessment instruments and along with respiratory testing codes for an instrument used to assess the patient's control of asthma symptoms.
- The printed encounter form should prompt staff for specific details of a procedure when required for code verification. For example,

  Code 120__________ Simple repair: body site __________ size __________

- Include the most reported diagnosis codes. Consider grouping diagnosis codes by organ system, and then alphabetically, within the system.
- Leave space on the form to allow reporting of the specific diagnosis and full *ICD-10-CM* codes.

Example

➤ **J45.2_** Asthma, mild intermittent
J45.3_ mild persistent
J45.4_ moderate persistent
J45.5_ severe persistent
Add fifth character: **0**, uncomplicated; **1**, w/ (acute) exacerbation; **2**, w/ status asthmaticus.

- Include the most frequently used modifiers.
- Leave open fields on forms to fill in any services or diagnoses that are not included.
- Include codes for prolonged and special services. For example,
  99358 Prolonged E/M service before and/or after direct patient care; first hour
  99051 Service(s) provided in the office during regularly scheduled evening, weekend, or holiday office hours, in addition to basic service
- Develop a separate encounter form for services performed in hospital or other facility settings. Make sure it includes all the services most commonly performed in the hospital setting. Access to a coding application or pocket-sized reference card with required elements of MDM and/or time of services also helps promote accurate code selection in facility settings.
- When quality initiatives depend on codes reported (eg, codes supporting HEDIS measures), be sure that these codes are clearly indicated on the encounter form, prompted by the EHR, or provided in an easily accessible quick reference.

Encounter forms and other coding tools should be reviewed periodically and updated at the time of each code set update to ensure that most of, if not all, the services and procedures commonly performed in the practice are included and the codes are accurate.

Refer to Chapter 1 for the timing of updates to code sets (eg, January, April, July, October).

Completing the Encounter Form

Every practice should develop a written policy of the requirements needed to complete an encounter form. Some points that should be part of the policy include

- The form is *not* part of the medical record. Information such as the need for follow-up care, diagnostic tests, or referrals must always be documented in the medical record even if written on the encounter form.
- If you are using a printed form, services must be clearly identified (eg, circle the procedure, use a check mark). Procedures or diagnoses must be written on a form if the form is not preprinted.

The person providing the service (eg, physician, laboratory technologist, medical assistant) should enter procedure codes or document that service on the encounter form to ensure that only the procedures performed are reported.

Example

➤ **A physician orders laboratory tests with in-office specimen collection and selects a code for venipuncture in addition to other codes for the encounter,** but the parents leave the office before clinical staff can collect the specimen(s).

Teaching Point: If the clinical staff (under supervision of the physician) are responsible for reporting the service when performed, it is not reported. The encounter form must provide space for the physician or QHP and clinical staff to indicate that a service was fully provided (eg, both counseling for and administration of immunization took place).

- The physician is ultimately responsible for the services reported and billed.
- Procedure codes must be linked to the diagnosis codes for the condition(s) or reasons the services were provided. Multiple diagnosis codes may link to one procedure code, when applicable.

Example

➤ **A 7-year-old boy is seen for an established patient preventive E/M service (99393), and evaluation and removal of a splinter of the right foot are performed with a small incision (10120).** The physician reports the following codes:

ICD-10-CM	*CPT*
Z00.121 (encounter for routine child health examination with abnormal findings) (field 21A) **S90.851A** (superficial foreign body, right foot, initial encounter) (field 21B)	**99393 25** with *ICD-10-CM* pointer A (**Z00.121**) and pointer B (**S90.851A**) in field 24E **10120** with *ICD-10-CM* pointer B in field 24 E

Teaching Point: If **Z00.121** were linked to **10120**, the claim line might be rejected or denied because the preventive diagnosis does not support the reason for the procedure. For more on *ICD-10-CM* code selection, refer to **Chapter 1**. For more on coding for preventive services, refer to **Chapter 8**.

Modifier **25** is appended to **99393** to indicate the significant and separately identifiable E/M service provided in conjunction with the splinter removal.

Refer to **Figure 1-1** for an example of how the linking of diagnoses to procedures appears on a claim form. An electronic claim form contains the same data.

- A system should be instituted to monitor and ensure capture of charges for all patient encounters on each day (eg, cross-reference to the patient check-in records).

Reviewing Assigned Codes

A staff member who understands correct coding and reporting guidelines should always review the assigned codes before the claim is submitted to ensure that all procedures and services are captured and accurate.

For example, the reviewer should check that

- An administration code is reported with immunizations and/or medication injections. Also, codes for medications administered via inhalation treatment should be reported in addition to codes for the treatment.
- Payer instructions for reporting National Drug Code (NDC) codes and units are followed.
- A venipuncture or finger stick is reported with a laboratory test, when applicable. The practice's Clinical Laboratory Improvement Amendments (CLIA) certificate number is included on claims for laboratory services, when required.

To learn more about requirements for in-office laboratory certification, refer to the July 2021 *AAP Pediatric Coding Newsletter*™ article "Coding for In-Office Laboratory Services" (https://doi.org/10.1542/pcco_book207_document009).

- A handling fee is reported when a specimen is prepared and sent to an outside laboratory.
- A modifier is appended when appropriate (eg, modifier **25** for significant, separately identifiable E/M services).
- The correct category of service (eg, new or established patient, initial or subsequent hospital observation or inpatient care) is reported.

Refer to Chapter 6 for more information on categories of E/M services.

- The diagnoses reported as primary and secondary are appropriate and are linked to the appropriate services or procedures.
- The documentation to support each service has been completed in a timely manner with required dates and signatures.

State Medicaid regulations may require completion of documentation, including written or electronic signature and date, within a specified period following completion of the reported service.

- Billing office staff should add or change a procedure or diagnosis code only with the agreement of the provider of the service.

Place of Service Codes

The POS is indicated on each claim by a *POS code* (often integrated into billing systems without need for manual entry with each charge). The POS may appear evident when reporting codes for services such as inpatient hospital care, but this is not always the case.

- It is important to report the correct POS because differences in practice expense in a facility versus a non-facility setting affect physician payment.

Chapter 4

Example

➤ **A physician provides an established patient office visit in a clinic that is an on-campus–outpatient hospital setting (POS code 22).** In this setting, the physician bills for a professional service and the hospital bills for the practice expense for each service. If the physician reports 99214 (established patient office visit with moderate level MDM or total time ≥30 minutes) with POS code 11 (office), payment may be based on total non-facility RVUs (3.87) rather than total facility RVUs (2.90), resulting in an overpayment.

Teaching Point: Physicians in provider-based practices (ie, the practices owned and operated as part of a hospital) should be aware that the POS code is especially important in this setting. Physician and practice expense portions of the patient's charges are often billed separately in provider-based practices.

- The same services provided in a facility-based practice are often costlier than those provided in an independent (physician-owned) practice. Facility fees charged by the provider are often significantly higher than the non-facility fees charged in independent practices.
- The Medicare program created POS code 19 to define an "off-campus" hospital practice to adopt site-neutral payment for many physician services conducted at provider-based practices. The rules and payment modifications have not been universally adopted, but it is important to know how your office is classified to ensure proper billing regardless. When considering purchase by a hospital system, it is important to consider the effect of billing with a different POS code.
- The increased number of high-deductible health plans has raised awareness of the greater costs to patients when services are rendered in provider-based facilities and has prompted Medicare and some states to take action to reduce the added costs. Practices should be aware of any such restrictions that apply to billing in their locality and under payer contracts or policies.

Other POS codes that may be commonly reported for pediatric services include 02 (telehealth provided other than in patient's home), 03 (school), 10 (telehealth provided in patient's home), 11 (office), 12 (home), 14 (group home), 19 (off campus—outpatient hospital), 20 (urgent care facility), 21 (inpatient hospital), 22 (on campus—outpatient hospital), and 23 (emergency room—hospital).

POS codes are further discussed for certain E/M services in chapters dedicated to those sites of service. For a full list of POS codes, refer to www.cms.gov/medicare/coding-billing/place-of-service-codes/code-sets. For further discussion of POS codes for telemedicine, refer to **Chapter 19**.

Submitting Clean Claims

Many states have enacted laws that require prompt payment of clean claims. In general, *clean claims* are those that contain sufficient and correct information for processing without further investigation or development by the payer (definitions may vary by state).

Although clean claims must be paid within a specified time, payer contracts also typically include a timely filing period (eg, within 90 days of the DOS). Claims submitted after the timely filing period may be denied and cannot typically be billed to the patient.

- Submitted claims must be accurate and in accordance with the process outlined in the executed carrier or health plan agreement. Knowing a payer's claim requirements will decrease chances of denied claims.
- Make sure the practice understands payer rules (eg, for billing for services provided incident to a physician's or other QHP's service). Rules may vary by health plan.

Refer to Chapters 7 and 12 for information on billing for services provided by clinical staff and health care professionals such as nutritionists, clinical psychologists, and social workers.

- Be aware of any updates issued by the carrier that affect billing and claims submission.

Generally, a clean claim should have the following information:

- Practice information (name, address, phone, National Provider Identifier [NPI], group tax ID number, and, if any laboratory tests are reported, CLIA certificate number)
- Patient information (patient name, birth date, policyholder, policy number, patient ID number, address)
- Codes (*CPT, ICD-10-CM,* Healthcare Common Procedure Coding System, NDC, POS), modifiers, and service dates
- Carrier information
- Secondary and, when applicable, tertiary insurance information
- Referring physician name and NPI, if applicable
- Facility name and address, as appropriate

If additional information is necessary to support a service or explain an unusual circumstance (eg, unlisted procedure code, unusual procedure, complicated procedure),

- Use the attachments feature of the electronic claims system, clearinghouse, or other claim attachment procedure as directed by the payer (eg, submission of attachments by online portal).
  - Health plans may have specific instructions for submission of claims attachments (eg, inclusion of a unique identifier [2–50 characters] or internal control number linking the claim and attachment).
- If necessary, send a hard-copy claim with a cover letter and a narrative report or copy of the appropriate part of the medical record (eg, progress note, procedure note) to facilitate claim processing.
  - Any documentation (eg, coordination of benefits information, letter of medical necessity, clinical reports) should include the patient's name, service date, and policy number on each page in case the documents become separated.
  - Keep a copy of the claim and supporting information for follow-up of payment.
- When filing claims for patients with coordination of benefits, make sure that all required information (ie, primary and secondary insurance information) has been obtained from the patient and claims are filed with the supporting information (eg, explanation of benefits [EOBs] or electronic remittance advice information), according to plan requirements.

Claims should be submitted for payment as soon as possible and before the deadline for timely filing specified in the agreement.

- The optimum time for filing outpatient claims is on the day of or the day after the service but no more than 2 to 3 days from the DOS.
- Codes for services to patients with prolonged hospitalizations may be collected for 7 consecutive days before billing; in this case, claims should be filed within 2 to 3 days of the end of the service week. It is not necessary to withhold claims until the patient is discharged. It is important to know whether your EHR and billing systems limit how data are captured and reported for services that extend over consecutive dates.

Practices should monitor lag time between completion of each service and submission of a claim for the service to identify and correct any cause of delayed submission. Timely finalization of documentation is necessary to make sure that codes are supported by the documentation before claims are submitted. Many practices adopt policies for timely completion of documentation.

Policy should be adopted requiring completion of medical record documentation within a specified period to support prompt billing of services. Physicians must understand that timely completion of documentation is required for appropriate code selection, claim filing, and, ultimately, prompt payment. New entries or corrections to documentation that occur after claim submissions may affect the accuracy of codes reported.

Special Consideration for Medicare Claims

Many health plans receive Medicare claims automatically when they are the secondary payer. In this case, the explanation of Medicare benefits will indicate that the claim has been automatically crossed over for secondary consideration. Physicians and providers should look for this indication on their EOBs and should not submit a claim to the secondary payer.

Monitoring Claim Status

An important aspect of billing operations is prompt and routine claim monitoring. A defined process for verifying that submitted claims were received and accepted by claim clearinghouses and/or payers should be included in the practice's or billing service's written billing procedures. Steps may include (refer to the last item in this list if billing is outsourced or centralized outside the practice)

- Identifying each type of report and/or dashboard feature of the practice's billing system for use in verifying claim submission and acceptance for processing, assigning follow-up activities for unpaid claims, and tracking average time from DOS and/or submission to receipt of payment.
- Assigning responsibilities for verifying that electronic claim submissions were received and accepted for processing as soon as possible after transmission. Failure to verify claim acceptance by the clearinghouse and payer often leads to unrecoverable revenue because of timely filing limitations.
  - Most clearinghouses will send a report indicating acceptance or rejection of a batch of claims within minutes of transmission and a report with individual claim-level detail within 24 hours of submission.
  - It is also necessary to log in to a payer's website or system to verify receipt of claims and monitor acceptance or rejection. Errors and omissions may occur in transmission.
- Electronic claim submission reports must be promptly reviewed for rejections or denials. All rejected or denied claims must be investigated to determine what corrections or payer contact is necessary to resubmit or return the claim for re-adjudication (eg, when a payer system error is corrected).
- Claims should not be resubmitted without investigation, as
  - Resubmission of a claim containing errors is unlikely to result in payment.
  - Resubmission of the claim with errors may reset the aging of the claim in the billing system and result in late follow-up or denial for lack of timely filing.

Claims that are rejected (without denial) should be corrected and resubmitted as new claims. Only denied or wrongly paid claims require submission of a corrected claim or appeal.

- Identify staff responsible for claims follow-up and establish standards for timely follow-up on unpaid claims. System-generated reports are useful in identifying the age of claims.
- Policies and procedures should address communication with patients and responsible parties when a payer requests additional information before claims processing (eg, many payers will request information on other coverage and/or details of where and how an injury was sustained).

Failure to respond to payer requests for information in a timely manner can result in delayed or denied claims payment.

- If centralized billing or an outsourced billing service is used, maintain oversight of performance by reviewing reports and acting on any areas in which potentially delayed or lost revenue are indicated. Examples of potential areas of concern include
  - Lag time between completion of documentation and submission of claims
  - Aging reports that show that the average number of days since claim submission for unpaid claims is more than 45 days
  - Amounts adjusted or written off

Monitoring Payments

Develop a process to monitor the timeliness of all payments. Tips for monitoring payments include

- Identify payers that do not pay clean claims within the time frame agreed on in your contract, and follow up on all late payments with the payer.
  - Check the provisions of your state prompt pay law and know the provisions for clean claims, timely filing, and penalties.
  - Report a payer's practice of late or delinquent payments to the proper agency, because your practice may be entitled to payment plus interest.
- Many electronic systems automatically apply payments and adjustments, but systems may apply incorrect adjustments based on payer remark codes. Staff should monitor all denials and reduced payments as appropriate and appeal incorrect adjustments when applicable.
- Review each EOB and/or remittance advice (electronic or printed) carefully to determine whether the payment is correct.
  - Identify any discrepancies, such as changes to codes (eg, down-coding), payments that are inconsistent with contracted fee schedule rates (specifically, reductions and/or a payer's failure to enter fee schedule rates into the claims adjudication system), or denials.
  - Familiarity with standard claim adjustment reason codes and remittance advice remark codes is essential in identifying denial reasons, such as a noncovered service, bundled payment, or provision of service not typical for physician specialty (not relevant for taxonomy code), and any patient responsibility for denied charges.

- Find claim adjustment reason code and remittance advice remark code descriptions online at https://x12.org/codes.
- Make certain that any denials or reductions in payment are not caused by practice billing errors (eg, incorrect modifiers, obsolete codes) or by an incorrectly applied NCCI edit that does not pertain to pediatrics. If errors are identified, correct them immediately and educate staff members as appropriate to ensure correct future claim submissions.

- Review all payer explanations, particularly reasons for denials or down-coding. If the service provided is not a benefit covered by the plan, the patient should be billed directly (a signed waiver form obtained prior to provision of service may be required).
  - Bill patients only for amounts deemed noncovered or patient responsibility by the payer and only in compliance with the health plan contract and/or policy manual.
- ✖ Do not bill patients for bundled services or other reduced payments resulting from the contract between your practice and the payer. Renegotiate your contract if payment is lower than the cost of providing care.

Billing staff must be aware of unique payment policies for health plans whose claims are processed by third-party administrators. For example, health plans A and B are employer-sponsored plans administered by insurance company A, but each plan has policies that may differ from those of health plans offered directly by insurance company A.

- If your system does not provide a variance report, compare the EOBs and/or remittance advice to a spreadsheet listing your top 40 codes and their allowable payments by carrier to monitor contract compliance. Make sure that the payment is consistent with the fee schedule, write-offs, and discounts agreed to by the practice and payer. Follow up with the payer on any discrepancies.

Health plans may enter contracted fee schedules for each physician or provider individually, resulting in inaccurate payment for one or more providers in a practice.

- Maintain a log of all denials or payment reductions. This can be used as a basis for future negotiations or education of the payer. (Identify 1 individual who has billing and coding expertise to monitor as well as accept or reject denials.)
- Review your fee schedule to see if your practice is paid at 100% of any billed charges. This is an indication that your fees are below the maximum payment amount established by the carrier. Payers often base the amount paid on the lesser of the billed charge or the contracted fee schedule amount for the service. This excludes services that are always patient responsibility (eg, form fees, cosmetic services).
- Review your fees annually and understand the Medicare RBRVS, using it to value the services you provide, as discussed in the Values Assigned to Physician Services section earlier in this chapter.

Tracking immunization product acquisition cost is very important. Costs may change during the course of the contract. Review the carrier contract for mid-contract immunization product cost changes (eg, some contracts will default to a percentage of billed charges during price transitions).

Review your payment to ensure that it exceeds your cost of providing that service (eg, total immunization costs), including time of clinical staff, supplies, tracking systems, and charges for electronic interfaces. When applicable, any non-FFS income based on provision of recommended services (eg, immunizations provided by ages specified in Centers for Disease Control and Prevention schedules) may be considered in determining the value of services.

Payment Options to Consider

When contracting with payers, be aware of any specified payment options (eg, paper checks, electronic fund transfers, virtual credit card payment).

- It is important to understand the pros and cons of each payment option (eg, credit card processing fees typically apply to card-based payment). Some health plans no longer offer payment by paper check and recommend electronic fund transfer.
- *Health plans must provide payment in compliance with HIPAA's electronic fund transfer standards rather than virtual card or wire transfer when requested by a physician.* Agreements to accept electronic fund transfers should not allow health plans to debit an account without notification and consent. Banks may offer additional protections against unauthorized withdrawals.

Appealing Denials

Do not assume that the carrier's denials or audits are accurate. Be prepared to challenge the carrier and request the specific policy on which the denial is based. If you are coding correctly and in compliance with coding conventions, you should appeal all inappropriately denied claims and carrier misapplication of *CPT* coding principles.

Knowing when to appeal a payer denial is just as important as knowing how to properly appeal. Appealing a claim denial requires confidence that the claim was correctly coded and supported by documentation. Ongoing coding education and internal compliance reviews are necessary to support compliant claim submissions. To learn more about coding compliance, refer to **Chapter 5**.

When claims are denied because of billing or coding errors, a corrected claim may be submitted in lieu of an appeal. To prevent potential denial of corrected claims caused by duplicate charges, a claim frequency code, placed in box 22 of a CMS-1500 form or loop 2300 of an electronic 837 format, is used to indicate that a claim is a corrected claim (code 7) or a voided one (code 8). Correcting or voiding a previously submitted claim typically results in either a complete replacement of a previously processed claim or voiding of the original claim from the health plan's record. Refer to specific instructions from the health plan when submitting a corrected claim.

- The AAP works directly with major insurance payers regarding policies that adversely affect pediatrics and pediatricians. If you receive inappropriate denials, we urge you to appeal them through the individual payer's processes and include documentation and any other coding support, such as information taken directly from the *CPT* or *ICD-10-CM* manuals.

You can alert the AAP to issues with payer policies that prohibit payment for correctly reported services by electronically submitting the AAP Coding and Payment Hassle Hotline Form (www.aap.org/en/practice-management/child-health-finance-payment-strategy/coding-payment-hotline).

Filing Appeals

Develop a system to monitor payer updates and any changes to the provider agreement so you are aware of the current payment policies and coding edits used by the payer.

- By accepting inappropriate claim denials, a practice may be setting itself up for charges of abusive billing practices.
  - If a practice recodes claims as a result of inappropriate claim denials, the resubmitted claim may not actually reflect the treatment the patient received.

Note that some payers have multiple appeal levels, with many initial appeals denied only because of the payer's electronic claim edits. Higher levels of appeal may be necessary for a denied claim to be reconsidered according to specific details about the service provided and the payer's contract or written policy.

Here is a summary of basic guidelines and tips for appealing payment determinations.

- When you contact a payer, always document the date, name, and title of the payer representative with whom you have talked and a summary of the details of the conversation.
  - If a payer requests that you submit a claim by using codes or modifiers that are not consistent with clean coding standards, ask for written documentation of the direction (preferably via fax or email).
  - Address issues with the person who has the authority to make decisions to overturn denials or reductions in payment.
  - Keep an updated file with names and contact information of the appropriate personnel with each of your contracted payers.
  - Always request a call reference number from the payer representative. This may be needed for secondary or tertiary levels of appeal.
  - Request an email or letter verifying the information provided, and archive written correspondence containing payer representative advice and payer policies. If the carrier does not provide written documentation, prepare a summary and send it to your contact, stating that it constitutes documentation of the discussion.
- Submit all appeals in writing.
  - Understand the payer's appeal process and appeal within its timeliness guidelines.
  - Format the letter to include the name of the patient, policy number, claim control number, and DOS(s) in question on each page of the letter.
  - The body of the letter should state the reason for the appeal and why you disagree with the payer's adjudication of the claim. Speak to the payer's rules/regulations regarding the decision and how your documentation supports payment.

  - Specify a date by which you expect the carrier to respond.
  - Support your case by providing medical justification (eg, clinical guidelines) and referencing *CPT* coding guidelines. If necessary, consult with the AAP Coding and Payment Hotline (www.aap.org/en/practice-management/child-health-finance-payment-strategy/coding-payment-hotline) for clarification of correct coding. It may be helpful to hire a certified coding expert with knowledge in pediatric coding to review your claims. (When hiring a full-time certified coding expert is not practical for a small practice, part-time employment or periodic consultation may be an option for access to coding and compliance expertise.)
  - Consider sending correspondence to the carrier by certified mail to verify receipt. Document and retain copies of all communications with the carrier about the appeal.
- Maintain an appeals-pending file.
  - If there is no response from the payer within 4 weeks of the date of the letter, send a copy of the appeal letter stamped "Second Request."
  - If there is no response within 2 weeks of the second request, or if the matter remains unresolved, contact the state department of insurance (or other appropriate agency in your state) to file a complaint or engage its assistance.
  - Contact your AAP chapter and pediatric council, if your chapter has one, to make them aware of the situation with the payer. AAP chapter pediatric councils meet with health plans to discuss carrier policies and practices affecting pediatrics and pediatricians.

Medicaid managed care payers are often required by their respective state Medicaid programs to respond to appeals within a certain time frame. Failure to adhere to payment or appeal timelines should be reported to the state Medicaid organization.

Subscribers to the *AAP Pediatric Coding Newsletter* can access resources for payer advocacy and appeal letters from the online AAP coding resources (https://publications.aap.org/codingnews/info-parent/27376/Coding-Resources). Refer to **Chapter 5** for information on preparing for a payer audit.

Documentation and Coding Audits

Medicare, Medicaid programs, and commercial payers will audit claims as well as monitor coding profiles, especially E/M coding. Physician practices should also adopt standards for conducting internal audits or reviews. Internal audits provide important information to inform practice policy and procedures, detect missed revenue, protect against erroneous billing and poor documentation habits, and prevent issues with payers and outside auditors. Some key benefits of internal auditing include

- Identification of negative billing and revenue trends, including
  - Increased lag time between encounter and billing (eg, delays in finalization of documentation, delayed coding or billing functions, technology issues)
  - Denial or underpayment of new services or new or revised procedure codes
  - Significant unexpected increased or decreased revenue
  - Inappropriate adjustments or write-offs of unpaid or underpaid claims that should be appealed
- Charge verification (eg, number of visit codes entered is equal to or greater than number of reportable encounters)
- Identification of incorrect billing and coding practices, especially overall accuracy of E/M coding based on visit documentation, which is often a focus of payer audits
- Identification of payment that does not align with a payer contract
- Identification of electronic system or workflow issues
- Identification of areas in which new or additional training is necessary

Refer to Chapter 5 for more detailed information on conducting internal audits and responding to payer audits.

Tools for Pediatric Practices

Working with third-party payers on coding and payment issues can be a difficult task. There is little uniformity between carriers, and frequently there are great inconsistencies within the same umbrella organization of carriers (eg, differing payment policies for commercial, health exchange, and Medicaid plans). The AAP Payer Advocacy Advisory Committee is charged with enhancing systems for members and chapters to identify and respond to issues with carriers.

The AAP has several available resources to assist the pediatric practice.

- AAP members are encouraged to use the AAP Coding and Payment Hotline to report payer issues. The AAP Coding and Payment Hassle Hotline Form (www.aap.org/en/practice-management/child-health-finance-payment-strategy/coding-payment-hotline) may be completed online to report insurance administrative and claim-processing concerns.

The information submitted is used to assist the AAP and chapters in identifying issues and facilitating public and private payer advocacy related to health plans, including discussion topics with national carriers by the AAP Payer Advocacy Advisory Committee and at chapter pediatric council meetings with regional carriers. AAP staff are also available to clarify coding issues.

- The AAP policy statement "Guiding Principles for Managed Care Arrangements for the Health of Newborns, Infants, Children, Adolescents, and Young Adults" (https://doi.org/10.1542/peds.2022-058396) provides key principles that are necessary for managed care plans to minimize patient underutilization and overutilization of services, as well as to enhance quality of care for children.
- AAP members and their staff are encouraged to attend AAP coding webinars (https://publications.aap.org/codingnews/resources/27969), presented by pediatric coding experts.
- The *AAP Pediatric Coding Newsletter*™ provides articles on coding and documentation of specific services and supplies (eg, immunizations) with updates on new codes and emerging issues affecting coding and billing practices. Subscribers can access current and archived issues and coding resources at https://publications.aap.org/codingnews.

The resources on this page and the next help address issues that arise in payer contracting and payment. To test your knowledge of the information presented in this chapter, complete the quiz found at the end of it, after the resources. Answers to each quiz are found in **Appendix II**. Add to your knowledge through the information provided in other chapters that discuss codes for specific types of service.

Chapter Takeaways

This chapter provided information on how professional services are valued, how physicians are paid, and how charges can be captured and clean claims for payment can be reported. Following are some takeaways from this chapter:

- The underlying basis for physician payment is the RBRVS, although alternative payment models focus largely on payment for demonstrating higher quality and lower costs of care.
- Physicians and QHPs should not enter into payer contracts without understanding the terms and negotiating for terms that are fair to the practice and the payer.
- Receiving appropriate payment depends on correctly capturing charges, assigning correct codes, and submitting clean claims. Monitoring for and appealing identified underpayments and denials are also an important part of revenue management.

Resources

AAP Coding Assistance and Education

AAP Coding and Payment Hotline (www.aap.org/en/practice-management/child-health-finance-payment-strategy/coding-payment-hotline)

AAP coding webinars (https://publications.aap.org/codingnews/resources/27969)

AAP payer contract negotiations and payment resources (www.aap.org/en/practice-management/child-health-finance-payment-strategy/payment-and-financial-resources/payer-contract-negotiations-and-payment-resources)

AAP pediatric councils (www.aap.org/en/practice-management/child-health-finance-payment-strategy/payment-and-finance-advocacy/aap-pediatric-councils)

Pediatric Office Superbill 2026 (www.aap.org/Pediatric-Office-Superbill-2026)

AAP Pediatric Coding Newsletter

"Beyond Codes: Electronic Claims Acknowledgement Reports," May 2023 (https://doi.org/10.1542/pcco_book229_document003)

"Coding and Payment in Pediatrics: The A, B, Cs of Being Paid for the Care You Give," June 2024 (https://doi.org/10.1542/pcco_book242_document002)

"Did You Know? Getting Paid for Denied or Rejected Services," May 2022 (https://doi.org/10.1542/pcco_book217_document006)

"Did You Know? Responding to an Untimely Filing Denial," May 2023 (https://doi.org/10.1542/pcco_book229_document004)

"Is Your Practice Experiencing Down-coding?" March 2023 (https://doi.org/10.1542/pcco_book227_document001)

"Responding to Inappropriate Code Edits," April 2022 (https://doi.org/10.1542/pcco_book216_document005)

"Spring Cleaning: Time to Tidy Up Coding and Billing Processes," April 2023 (https://doi.org/10.1542/pcco_book228_document002)

"Use Diagnosis Coding Conventions to Avoid Denied Claims," June 2024 (https://doi.org/10.1542/pcco_book242_document003)

"Using Documentation to Demonstrate the Value of Care," July 2022 (https://doi.org/10.1542/pcco_book219_document003)

Claims Processing

Remittance advice remark codes (https://x12.org/codes/remittance-advice-remark-codes)

Health Insurance

Health insurance education resources from HealthyChildren.org (www.healthychildren.org/English/family-life/health-management/health-insurance/Pages/default.aspx)

Payment/Relative Value Units

AAP News, "AAP members play key role in shaping new code values for nirsevimab," July 2024 (https://publications.aap.org/aapnews/news/29183/AAP-members-play-key-role-in-shaping-new-code)

AAP policy statement, "Guiding Principles for Managed Care Arrangements for the Health of Newborns, Infants, Children, Adolescents, and Young Adults" (https://doi.org/10.1542/peds.2022-058396)

AAP policy statement, "Pediatric Application of Coding and Valuation Systems" (https://doi.org/10.1542/peds.2019-2496)

Milliman *Commercial Reimbursement Benchmarking* (www.milliman.com/en/insight/commercial-reimbursement-benchmarking-medicare-ffs-rates)

"RBRVS: What Is It and How Does It Affect Pediatrics?" (www.aap.org/en/practice-management/child-health-finance-payment-strategy/coding-and-valuation/code-valuation-and-payment-rbrvs)

"Understanding the RUC Survey Instrument: Physician Services without Global Period" video (www.youtube.com/watch?v=nu5unDX8VIs)

Place of Service Codes

POS code set (www.cms.gov/medicare/coding-billing/place-of-service-codes/code-sets)

Value-Based Payment

AAP Choosing Wisely campaign toolkit (www.aap.org/en/news-room/campaigns-and-toolkits/choosing-wisely)

AAP policy statement, "The Unique Value Proposition of Pediatric Health Care," January 2023 (https://doi.org/10.1542/peds.2022-060681)

"Accountable Care Organizations (ACOs): General Information" (https://innovation.cms.gov/innovation-models/aco)

Hospital Pediatrics®, "How Will a Shift to Value-Based Financial Models Affect Care for Hospitalized Children?" February 2024 (https://doi.org/10.1542/hpeds.2023-007400)

Test Your Knowledge!

1. **How can pediatricians recommend values for services to the CMS?**
   a. Charge more for services in an effort to increase the average rate for a service.
   b. Pediatricians cannot influence values assigned by CMS.
   c. Complain about low payment rates to anyone who will listen.
   d. Participate in AAP surveys conducted through the AMA/Specialty Society RUC.
2. **Which is true of value-based payment?**
   a. Physician payments may be based on a combination of FFS and alternative payment methodologies.
   b. Small practices cannot participate in value-based payment models.
   c. Physicians must be part of an ACO to participate in a value-based payment model.
   d. Value-based payment always results in reduced FFS payment.
3. **Which is always true for all health plan contracts?**
   a. The same fee schedule will be applied across all physicians in the practice.
   b. Physicians should not sign contracts without reading and considering the impact of entering into the contractual agreement.
   c. Becoming a contracted network provider places a physician into the payer's highest (preferred) tier.
   d. If the plan does not agree to cover a particular service, a contracting physician can always bill the patient for the service.
4. **Which of the following promotes accuracy in documentation and charge capture in an EHR?**
   a. The physician must have the ability to fully describe patient diagnoses for each encounter (ie, not to merely select a diagnosis code).
   b. The EHR automatically reorders the diagnosis codes entered.
   c. Automated E/M code selection is recommended and more accurate than code selection by a physician or QHP.
   d. Deleted codes should be immediately unavailable for selection in the EHR or billing system.
5. **Which of the following is correct regarding health plan payments?**
   a. Health plans must provide payment in compliance with HIPAA's electronic fund transfer standards rather than virtual card or wire transfer when requested by a physician.
   b. Agreements to accept electronic fund transfers should not allow health plans to debit an account without notification and consent.
   c. Credit card processing fees typically apply to card-based payment.
   d. All of the above

CHAPTER 5

Preventing Fraud and Abuse: Compliance, Audits, and Paybacks

This chapter was contributed by the American Academy of Pediatrics Committee on Medical Liability and Risk Management.

Contents

Chapter Highlights

- The importance of safeguarding the health care system from fraud and abuse
- The importance of protecting a pediatric practice from the consequences of failing to recognize and appropriately respond to noncompliant activities within the practice
- How in-practice compliance programs can protect medical practices from unintentional billing errors and revenue loss
- How to respond to overpayment notices and inquiries from auditors

What Compliance Means in a Medical Practice

Compliance, when used in a medical setting, means actively working to be sure that all staff follow the requirements of federal and state regulations that govern medical practice and billing for medical services and supplies. It also means knowing and honoring the terms the practice has agreed to in contracts with various payers, including related payment policies. The opposites of compliance in physician practice include terms such as *fraud* and *abuse* (each defined later in this chapter). A compliance program is an effort to avoid fraud and abuse as well as errors that put the practice at risk legally or financially.

Whether practicing medicine as an employee of a large health system, in solo practice, or somewhere in between, physicians and other qualified health care professionals (QHPs) must actively support and promote compliance with all applicable regulations and contractual obligations. As discussed in more detail later in this chapter, compliance in a physician practice includes

- Educating oneself and practice staff on a significant number of federal and state regulations that affect how a practice operates
- Providing education on billing and coding in agreement with code set instructions, payer policies, and state regulations regarding patient billing and collection activities
- Dedicating resources (ie, a compliance program) to limit the practice's risk of inadvertent or intentional actions that do not support the practice's compliance with obligations under federal and state regulations and payer contracts
- Encouraging staff to alert administrators/managers of any activities that might put the practice at risk of noncompliance with regulations or contractual obligations
- Routinely assessing the practice's compliance by monitoring and conducting reviews of claims and documentation to verify coding and billing accuracy
- Responding to a discovery of noncompliant activity with corrective actions to resolve past issues and prevent recurrence
- Using the practice's compliance program to defend against external allegations of noncompliance

Although coding and billing compliance is a key topic in this book, practices can promote efficiency and avoid creation of conflicting policies by maintaining a comprehensive set of policies and procedures that include other areas of compliance (eg, privacy and security of protected health information).

The Importance of Compliance in Medical Practice

Most physicians and QHPs work ethically, provide high-quality care, and submit appropriate claims for payment. Unfortunately, however, some providers exploit the health care system for personal gain. These few "bad apples" necessitate laws to combat fraud and abuse and protect the integrity of the health care payment system. (For some examples, refer to the Can This Really Happen? section later in this chapter.)

Just as patients put enormous trust in physicians, so do payers. Medicare, Medicaid, other government-funded health care programs, and private payers rely on physicians' medical judgment to treat patients with appropriate services by appropriately trained (and licensed, when required) health care professionals. They depend on accurate and truthful claims for the services provided to patients. And most physicians and QHPs intend to do just that. But the process is made more difficult by the complex and dynamic nature of payer coding and billing procedures, which, despite standardization efforts, can vary from carrier to carrier, policy to policy, state to state, and month to month.

This complexity of delivering and receiving payment for medical services and potential penalties for noncompliance support physician practices needing to reduce the risk of noncompliance through knowledge, active monitoring, and, as needed, corrective action.

Defining Medical Fraud and Abuse

Fraud

Fraud is obtaining something of value through intentional misrepresentation or concealment of material facts. Examples of fraud in the physician's office may include

- Requiring that a patient return for a procedure that could have been performed on the same day
- Billing Medicare or Medicaid for services not provided, including no-shows
- Billing one member for services provided to another (noncovered) member
- Billing services under a different National Provider Identifier (NPI), except as allowed by payer guidance, to receive payment for services that would otherwise be noncovered or paid at a lesser rate
- Taking a kickback in money, in kind, or other valuable compensation for referrals
- Completing a certificate of medical necessity for a patient who does not need the service or who is not professionally known by the provider

Abuse

Abuse includes any practice that is not consistent with the goals of providing patients with services that

- Are medically necessary
- Meet professionally recognized standards
- Are fairly priced

Examples of actions that will likely be considered abusive are

- Charging in excess for services or supplies
- Billing Medicare or Medicaid according to a higher fee schedule than that used for other patients
- Providing medically unnecessary services
- Submitting bills to Medicare or Medicaid when they are the responsibility of another insurance plan (eg, failing to ask for information on other insurance or other liable entities, such as automobile insurance for injuries incurred in a crash)
- Waiving co-payments or deductibles, except as permitted for financial hardship
- Advertising free services
- Coding all evaluation and management (E/M) visits at the same level
- Unbundling claims (ie, billing separately for services that are correctly billed under 1 code)

Are Payers Held to the Same Standards?

When reading the lists of actions that might be considered fraud or abuse, one might wonder whether all payers are held to the same standards. For example, why do payers have policies that bundle services that are not bundled per *Current Procedural Terminology* (*CPT*®) instructions?

Unfortunately, coverage of services is typically outlined in the terms of the health plan document or health program policy, but the plan or program administrator (payer) usually determines which codes are used in determining payment for covered services and what is included in the service described by each code. The Health Insurance Portability and Accountability Act (HIPAA) that requires use of *CPT* codes in billing for and payment of physician services does not also require payers to follow *CPT* instructions. Additionally, payer contracts may require that the practice accept the payer's policies (eg, bundled service policies).

Federal Fraud and Abuse Laws

The federal government has more than a dozen laws in its anti-fraud and anti-abuse arsenal. The 5 most important laws that apply to physicians are the

- False Claims Act: Prohibits and establishes civil penalties for submitting claims for payment to Medicare or Medicaid that you know *or should know* are false or fraudulent. (Intentional fraudulent activity may be subject to the criminal code for health care fraud with risks of fines and incarceration.)

Who Can File a Civil False Claims Lawsuit?

The civil False Claims Act includes a whistleblower provision that allows a private individual (eg, employee, patient) to file a lawsuit on behalf of the United States and entitles that whistleblower to a percentage of any recoveries. Compliance programs that provide for internal complaint submission and resolution, without retribution, may offset the risk of a whistleblower case.

- Anti-Kickback Statute: Prohibits the knowledge and willful payment/acceptance of anything of value (eg, money, trips) intended to induce or reward patient referrals or the generation of business involving any item or service payable by the federal health care program.
- Physician Self-Referral Law (Stark Law): Prohibits physicians from referring patients to receive designated health services payable by Medicare or Medicaid from entities with which the physician or an immediate family member has a financial relationship, unless an exception applies. The following items or services are designated health services:
  - Clinical laboratory services
  - Physical therapy services
  - Occupational therapy services
  - Outpatient speech pathology services
  - Radiology and certain other imaging services
  - Radiation therapy services and supplies
  - Durable medical equipment and supplies
  - Parenteral and enteral nutrients, equipment, and supplies
  - Prosthetics, orthotics, and prosthetic devices and supplies
  - Home health services
  - Outpatient prescription drugs
  - Inpatient and outpatient hospital services
- Exclusion Authorities: Prohibits billing a federal health program (eg, Medicaid, Tricare) for any services furnished, ordered, or prescribed by an excluded individual (ie, an individual or entity that has been restricted from payment for any items or services furnished, ordered, or prescribed to a patient covered by a plan wholly or partially funded by the US government). Practices are also responsible for ensuring that they do not employ or contract with excluded individuals or entities that may furnish items or services that may be paid for by a federal health care program.
- Civil Monetary Penalties Law: Authorizes the US Department of Health and Human Services (HHS) to impose civil money penalties on and/or exclude from the Medicare and Medicaid programs physicians who commit various forms of fraud and abuse involving Medicare and Medicaid (eg, anti-kickback violations, false claims, or submission of false information on enrollment in a federal health program).

Abiding by these laws is not just the right thing to do; violating them, even (for some) unwittingly, could result in criminal penalties, civil fines, exclusion from federal health care programs, or loss of a medical license from a state medical board.

Fraud and Abuse and Private Payers

Health care fraud and abuse regulations are not limited to government-funded programs. HIPAA legislation established fraud or attempted fraud against a health care benefit program as a federal criminal offense (18 USC §1347). This law defines the term *health care benefit program* to include any public or private plan or contract.

Fraud and abuse against private payers may also be an offense under state law.

Kickbacks, Inducements, and Self-Referrals

The Centers for Medicare & Medicaid Services (CMS) advises providers to be cautious when investing in health care business ventures. Providers may invest in third parties, such as laboratories, imaging centers, equipment vendors, or physical therapy clinics, to expand patient care access. But referral patterns to these facilities could implicate a provider in an investigation.

The CMS states that "these business relationships can sometimes improperly influence or distort physician decision-making and result in the improper steering of a patient to a particular therapy or source of services in which a physician has a financial interest" (refer to the Medicare Learning Network booklet *Medicare Fraud & Abuse: Prevent, Detect, Report* at www.cms.gov/Outreach-and-Education/Medicare-Learning-Network-MLN/MLNProducts/MLN-Publications-Items/MLN4649244). Many of these investment relationships have serious legal risks under the Anti-Kickback Statute and Stark Law, according to the CMS.

To prevent allegations of possible illegal kickback schemes with investment partners, the CMS recommends that providers ask the following questions:

- Is the investment venture promising the provider high rates of return for little or no financial risk?
- Is the investment interest for a nominal capital contribution?
- Is the partner asking the provider to guarantee patient referrals or item orders?
- Does the provider believe they will be more likely to refer patients for services provided by the venture just because they made the investment?

- Will the provider's ownership share be greater than their share of the total capital contributions made to the venture?
- Is the investment venture, or any possible business partner, offering to loan the provider money to make their capital contribution?
- Will the venture have enough capital from other sources to fund its operations?

If the answer to any of these questions is yes, legal consultation is advisable before entering into an investment interest. Whenever health care vendors offer free samples, business opportunities, and incentives, providers should ask themselves similar questions.

When considering whether to engage in a particular billing practice, enter into a particular business venture, or pursue an employment, a consulting, or another personal services relationship, it is prudent to evaluate the arrangement for potential compliance problems. Use experienced health care lawyers to analyze the issues and provide a legal evaluation and risk analysis of the proposed venture, relationship, or arrangement.

Your state bar association may have a directory of local attorneys who practice health care law. The American Health Law Association is another resource (www.americanhealthlaw.org).

Anti-Fraud and Anti-Abuse Activities

Physician practices are subject to several levels of scrutiny for possible fraudulent activity, including the federal and state levels of government as well as private payers. These groups increasingly share information. This means that a provider under investigation by one government health care program will likely be contacted by another program and possibly by private payers.

- The HHS Office of Inspector General (OIG) has several anti-fraud campaigns under way.
- Many states have enacted anti-fraud and anti-abuse legislation, and Medicaid programs have established Medicaid fraud control units.
- The Medicaid program integrity provisions include activities such as
  - Increased fraud detection methods
  - Terminating providers previously terminated from other government health care programs
  - Suspending future payments when there are credible allegations of fraud
  - Applying National Correct Coding Initiative (NCCI) edits and prepayment claims review

Refer to Chapter 2 for more information on NCCI edits.

Increasingly, Medicaid and other health plans are conducting, or contracting with an organization (eg, Cotiviti, Optum) to conduct, prepayment claims review that targets claims based on computer analytics intended to identify potential up-coding, fraud, or other billing inaccuracies. Physicians may be targeted when their claims history does not align with that of peers (eg, frequency of billing high-level E/M codes). When prepayment claims are reviewed by payers, it presents an administrative burden and prolongs time from claims filing to payment. *Physicians must be able to provide documentation to support claims, but the possibility that someone will suspect wrongdoing should not prohibit appropriate reporting of codes for the services provided and documented.*

Areas of Specific Concern

Many findings and initiatives put physician practices under high scrutiny for miscoded services, failure to adequately document services, and operating in a manner that conflicts with anti-kickback and self-referral laws. To identify potential fraud and abuse, analysis of claim data is increasingly combined across payers and care settings to identify physicians and other providers who are outliers in their billing and referral patterns. Specific areas of concern that affect physicians include

- Billing for a higher level of service than was provided.
- Misuse of modifiers to override NCCI edits when not clinically indicated.
- Billing for services provided by clinical staff or other QHPs when payer policy for incident-to services (eg, direct supervision) is not met. See **Chapter 7** for information on incident-to billing.
- Participation by physicians and QHPs in speaker programs that potentially pay for increased prescribing, ordering, or use of a company's products that will be billed to a government payer (https://oig.hhs.gov/documents/specialfraudalerts/865/SpecialFraudAlertSpeakerPrograms.pdf).
- Provision and/or billing of telehealth services that is noncompliant with state regulation or payer policy.

The fraud and abuse control units of HHS and the US Department of Justice also continue to cross-reference enrollment information for physicians and providers when there is history of enrollment in multiple states and/or programs. By cross-referencing enrollment data, the agencies may discover conflicting information and/or evidence of prior revocation of eligibility to participate in federal programs.

In addition to fraud and abuse regulations, practices should include compliance with the privacy, security, and patient access to medical records requirements of HIPAA, the 21st Century Cures Act, and patient accessibility requirements of the Americans With Disabilities Act in compliance education and activities.

Compliance Programs

Does your practice have a fraud and abuse prevention compliance program? For many years, compliance programs for small practices were voluntary. They are now required. Section 6401(a) of the Patient Protection and Affordable Care Act requires physicians and other providers and suppliers who enroll in Medicare, Medicaid, or the Children's Health Insurance Program (CHIP) to establish a compliance program with certain "core elements." This applies even for small practices, but the compliance program can be designed to meet the needs and capabilities of the practice.

A compliance program establishes strategies to prevent, detect, and resolve conduct that does not conform to

- Federal and state law
- Federal, state, and private payer health care program requirements
- The practice's own ethical and business policies

Pediatric practices benefit from compliance programs in many ways. A compliance program should support

- **Billing and coding accuracy and avoidance of missed opportunities to appropriately collect earned revenue**
- **Improved documentation that may prevent malpractice**
- **A practice's defense against insurance company takebacks**
- **Billing and coding patterns that eliminate the practice as a target of fraud investigation**
- **Staff training, including sending a clear message to all staff that compliance with practice policies and procedures is required**
- **Guidance of any staff who may be unsure of compliance risks related to a situation (eg, responding to a patient's request to alter codes on a medical claim)**

Practices with written compliance programs report better control over internal procedures, improved medical record documentation, and streamlined practice operations.

The 7 Elements of the HHS OIG Compliance Program

The 7 core elements described in the HHS OIG guidance for compliance programs for small physician practices published in 2023 are

- Implement written compliance and practice standards.
- Designate a compliance officer, contact, or team.
- Conduct appropriate training and education.
- Conduct internal monitoring and auditing.
- Respond appropriately to detected offenses and develop corrective action.
- Develop open lines of communication.
- Enforce disciplinary standards through well-publicized guidelines.

It is also useful to consult the *United States Sentencing Commission Guidelines Manual* (www.ussc.gov/guidelines), which makes it clear that an organization under investigation may be given more sympathetic treatment if a good compliance program is in place. Compliance programs not only help prevent fraudulent or erroneous claims but also show that the physician practice is making a good faith effort to submit claims appropriately. However, that would require the program to be integrated into the daily operations of the practice; it cannot be a set of policies and procedures merely kept in a binder or on a computer unrelated to actual business operations.

Here are some reasons cited by the *United States Sentencing Commission Guidelines Manual* to implement an effective compliance program.

- It may save the practice money if it prevents costly civil suits and criminal investigations.
- It sends an unambiguous message to employees that fraud and abuse will not be tolerated.
- It decreases the risk of employees' suing the practice under the False Claims Act because employees will have an internal communication system for reporting questionable activities and resolving problems.

- It helps if an investigation occurs. Investigators may be more inclined to resolve the problem as a civil rather than a criminal matter, or it may lead to an administrative resolution rather than a formal false claim action.
- It may help reduce the range used for imposing fines under federal sentencing guidelines.
- It may influence an HHS OIG decision on whether to exclude a provider from participation in federal health care programs.
- It frequently results in improved medical record documentation.
- It improves coding accuracy, reduces denials, and makes claims and payment processes more effective.
- It educates physicians and employees on their responsibilities for preventing, detecting, and reporting fraud and abuse.
- It should meet governmental requirements for practices to have a formal compliance plan.

Steps to Developing a Compliance Program

The CMS has described the steps to create an effective compliance and ethics program. A key aspect is that the organization exercises due diligence to prevent and detect criminal conduct and promotes a culture that encourages ethical conduct and a commitment to compliance with the law. Small practices may structure their compliance program to encompass the 7 elements of a compliance program within the constraints under which the practice operates (eg, use a template developed by an external source to create policies and procedures).

The CMS specifies that in creating the compliance program, the practice

1. Develop and then distribute and/or notify staff of digital access to written policies, procedures, and standards of conduct to prevent and detect inappropriate behavior. (Physicians and QHPs working within hospital or health care systems should know whom to contact regarding compliance concerns.)

   The HHS OIG *General Compliance Program Guidance* as of November 2023 (https://oig.hhs.gov/compliance/general-compliance-program-guidance) also includes a code of conduct as an element of the compliance program. The code of conduct is described as a tool that communicates the organization's mission, goals, and ethical requirements central to its operations and that governs the conduct of its officers, employees, contractors, medical staff, and others who work with or on behalf of the organization.
2. Designate a chief compliance officer and other appropriate bodies (eg, a corporate compliance committee) charged with the responsibility of operating and monitoring the compliance program and reporting directly to high-level personnel and the governing body. (A small practice may appoint a compliance contact to work under the practice owner's supervision.)
3. Use reasonable efforts to not include any individual in the substantial authority personnel whom the organization knew, or should have known, had engaged in illegal activities or other conduct inconsistent with an effective compliance and ethics program.
4. Develop and implement regular, effective education and training programs for (a) the governing body; (b) all employees, including high-level personnel; and, as appropriate, (c) the organization's agents. (Compliance training resources from reliable sources, such as state medical societies, may be used in lieu of those developed by a practice.)
5. Maintain a process, such as a hotline, to receive complaints and adopt procedures to protect the anonymity of complainants and protect whistleblowers from retaliation. (In a small practice, a hotline could be replaced with an "anonymous compliance report box.")
6. Develop a system to respond to allegations of improper conduct and enforce appropriate disciplinary action against employees who have violated internal compliance policies, applicable statutes, regulations, or federal health care program requirements.
7. Use audits and/or other evaluation techniques to monitor compliance and assist in the reduction of identified problem areas.
8. Investigate and remediate identified systemic problems, including making any necessary modifications to the organization's compliance and ethics program.

Written Policies and Procedures

A compliance program should include the practice's written compliance standards, policies, and procedures. The standards and policies should specifically describe the lines of responsibility for implementing the compliance program.

- Standards, policies, and procedures should reduce the likelihood of fraudulent activity while helping identify any incorrect billing practices.
- Small practices may use policy and procedure templates and training resources from other entities, such as consultants or professional organizations. Such resources should be edited to address the practice's identified compliance concerns and support documentation and billing in compliance with current standards (eg, current telemedicine coding guidance).

Examples

➤ **Standard: It is a standard of XYZ Pediatrics to conduct business with vendors and/or referral sources in an ethical manner, avoiding any activity that may be perceived as an intention to influence or potentially influence purchasing, prescribing, or referral activities through gifts or business courtesies.**

Policy: XYZ Pediatrics never accepts gifts from vendors, physicians, or other referral sources in exchange for patient referrals or any other businesses. Gifts of nominal value (eg, notepads), as described in the definitions section of this policy statement, may be accepted with manager/administrator approval. The administrator maintains a record of all accepted gifts.

Procedure: XYZ Pediatrics personnel shall request approval from their manager/administrator before accepting any gifts or business courtesies offered to them from business vendors and other external organizations/individuals.

➤ **Standard: XYZ Pediatrics will maintain current and accurate health records for all patients with sufficient detail and accuracy to inform future health care needs of each patient and to support accurate code assignment and billing for services provided.**

Policy: XYZ Pediatrics requires each clinician to accurately and completely document patient health communications and services.

Procedure: XYZ Pediatrics personnel will complete documentation training prior to providing services to our patients and may be required to complete additional training, as indicated by changes in electronic health record (EHR) functionality, addition of new services, or changes in regulations.

Procedure: XYZ Pediatrics personnel will accurately document and attest to the accuracy and completeness of each entry into a patient's health record in a timely manner upon completion of services or within the state-mandated 72 hours after provision of services).

Note: Actual policies may vary depending on any state regulations for timeliness of physician documentation.

Procedure: XYZ Pediatrics will conduct reviews of documentation practices to determine the accuracy, completeness, and timing of documentation completion for services provided to individual patients. Any findings not consistent with practice standards and policy will result in corrective action.

- Policies and procedures should be updated periodically to address newly identified areas of risk, new regulations, or process changes in the practice.
- All staff should receive periodic education on policies and procedures to maintain up-to-date knowledge.

Designate a Compliance Officer or Compliance Contact

The practice should designate an individual responsible for overseeing the compliance program. More than one employee may be designated with the responsibility of compliance monitoring, or a practice may outsource all or part of the functions of a compliance officer to a third party. Not all practices can support the designation of a compliance officer. For more on this topic, refer to the Compliance Contact Alternative for Small Practices section that follows.

Attributes and qualifications of a compliance officer include

- Independent position to protect against any conflicts of interest between "regular" position responsibilities and compliance officer duties
- Experience in leadership and stature to interact as an equal with senior leaders of the entity
- Effective communication skills (oral and written) with employees, physicians, and carriers
- Demonstrated integrity, good judgment, assertiveness, an approachable demeanor, and the ability to elicit the respect and trust of employees

In large practices, the compliance officer must have sufficient funding to staff and operate the compliance program with capabilities of identifying, preventing, mitigating, and remediating the entity's compliance risk.

The primary responsibilities of a compliance officer include

- Overseeing and monitoring the implementation of the compliance program.
- Establishing methods, such as periodic audits, to improve the practice's efficiency and quality of services and reduce the practice's vulnerability to fraud and abuse.
- Revising the compliance program in response to changes in the needs of the practice or changes in the law and in the policies and procedures of government and private payer health plans.

- Developing, coordinating, and participating in a training program that focuses on the elements of the compliance program and seeks to ensure that training materials are appropriate.
- Coordinating or personally checking the HHS OIG Excluded Individuals and Entities List (https://exclusions.oig.hhs.gov) and the federal System for Award Management (https://sam.gov/content/exclusions) to ascertain that any potential new hires, current employees, medical staff, or independent contractors are not listed; advising management of findings; and seeing that appropriate action is taken as described in the compliance program.
- Informing employees and physicians of pertinent federal and state statutes, regulations, and standards and monitoring their compliance.
- Investigating any report or allegation concerning suspected unethical or improper business practices and monitoring subsequent corrective action, compliance, or both.
- Assessing the practice's situation and determining what best suits the practice for compliance oversight.
- Maintaining records of compliance-related activities, including meetings, educational activities, and internal audits. Particular attention should be given to documenting violations found by the compliance program and documenting the remedial actions.

In large practices, the compliance officer may advise a board or senior leadership on compliance risks related to strategic and operational decisions.

Compliance Contact Alternative for Small Practices

The HHS OIG includes advice to small practices that cannot support a full- or part-time compliance officer that allows the option of designating one person as the practice's compliance contact. The compliance contact will be responsible for ensuring that the practice's compliance activities (eg, documenting a compliance plan and conducting medical record reviews) are completed. The compliance contact will report at least quarterly to the practice owner(s) or administrator regarding the status of the practice's compliance activities. The owner remains ultimately responsible for the practice's compliance with health care regulations.

The compliance contact might also be tasked with either identifying potential risks associated with practice decisions such as purchase of equipment to perform a new service within the practice or adding a new type of health care professional to the practice's clinical staff.

Examples

➤ **Practice XYZ's front office manager, who is also the practice's compliance contact, finds a concern regarding potential improper documentation practices in the Practice XYZ compliance box.** The concern is that a physician has instructed billing office staff to report all services to established patients under the physician's name and ID number, even services provided by the practice's nurse practitioner. The front office manager reviews the practice's policy for addressing billing concerns and directs a question regarding the appropriateness of the physician's billing instruction to the American Academy of Pediatrics (AAP) Coding and Payment Hotline. After receiving a response from AAP coding staff, the manager determines that the physician's instruction to the billing office could put the practice at risk of billing inappropriately when the service does not meet incident-to billing policy that allows a physician to report services provided by another QHP working under the physician's direct supervision and in continuance of an ongoing plan of care. The manager meets with the physician to confirm that the billing staff correctly understood the physician's instruction and informs the physician of the AAP Coding and Payment Hotline's advice. The physician agrees to review Chapter 7 of *Coding for Pediatrics* to learn more about incident-to services and correct the instructions provided to billing office staff. The discussion is documented.

The front office manager also meets with the billing office manager to discuss the complaint, findings, and proposed resolution. The billing office manager advises that bills for recent services by the nurse practitioner will require review for billing compliance and possibly submission of corrected claims. The front office manager asks for a report of the results of the review and notification of any ongoing concern that may require additional corrective action.

➤ **Practice XYZ's owner physicians are considering addition of a new medical device to screen patients for a particular condition.** The salesperson for the product provided information on how the service is performed by clinical staff. The salesperson states that after brief training, the service can be reported with a code that promises significant revenue and quick return on investment. The owners approach the clinical staff team lead, who is also the practice's compliance contact, to inquire what compliance risks might be associated with adding this service.

The compliance contact reviews the product information, which includes secure transfer of patient data to an off-site facility for test interpretation and references the practice's HIPAA policy manual regarding potential privacy and security concerns and the need for a business associates' agreement with the off-site facility. The compliance contact also discusses the new service with the billing and coding manager and learns first that the proposed code is not appropriate (because it describes the physician work of interpreting and reporting test results, not to be provided by the practice) and second that an unspecified code would be indicated for the new service, with coverage and payment determined by individual payer policy. The compliance contact provides the information to the owners for use in their decision-making regarding the new service.

Topics to Address in a Compliance Program

Coding and Billing

The following billing risk areas are frequent areas of investigations and audits by the HHS OIG and should be addressed in a good compliance program:

- Billing for items or services not provided or not provided as claimed
- Submitting claims for equipment, medical supplies, and services that are not reasonable and necessary
- Double billing or billing separately for bundled services
- Billing for noncovered services as if covered
- Known misuse of NPIs, which results in improper billing
- Misuse of modifiers
- Consistently under- or over-coding services (eg, using only 1 E/M service code within a category of service)

Other areas that may trigger an audit include

- Profile of services reported differs from payer profiles of physicians of your specialty whose patient population has similar health care coexisting conditions.
- Repeated inappropriate use of unspecified diagnosis codes or use of codes that are not consistent with the service or your specialty.
- Surgical services not consistent with claims submitted by a facility.
- Number of procedures or services reported exceeds the hours in a day.
- High numbers of denials.

Medical Record Documentation

One of the most important physician practice compliance issues is the appropriate documentation of diagnosis and treatment. Patients and other providers must be able to trust that information within shared records is accurate and actionable for the care of the patient.

Compliant documentation must encompass not only what should be documented but also what must be safeguarded from inaccuracies and potential noncompliant access to or disclosure of information.

The written compliance plan should specify that medical record documentation should comply with the following documentation principles and guidelines:

- The medical record should be complete (and legible, when handwritten) and individualized for each patient encounter.
- ✖ Do not allow *cut-and-paste* functionality in the EHR. (Cutting information from a prior entry is not an acceptable practice.) Any use of copying and pasting, copying forward, macros, or auto-population should be regulated by office policies that address maintenance of record integrity and supplementation via free text, where indicated.
- Retain all signatures when there are multiple authors or contributors to a document so individual contributions are unambiguously identified. For additional information about documentation by multiple authors, refer to the "Coding Conundrum: Pitfalls of Electronic Health Record Coding" box.
- All clinical staff should receive initial and periodic education on compliant medical record documentation, including use of EHR functionality, use of individual sign-on, and appropriate access to records as applicable.
- Documentation should be completed at the time of service or as soon as possible afterward. State regulations or payer policy may limit the time for record completion, including authentication (signature and date application).
- The documentation of each patient encounter should include the reason for the encounter; any relevant history; physical examination findings; prior diagnostic test results, when pertinent; assessment, clinical impression, or diagnosis; plan of care; and date and legible identity of the observer.
- If not documented, the rationale for ordering diagnostic and other ancillary services should be easily inferred by an independent reviewer or third party.

Coding Conundrum: Pitfalls of Electronic Health Record Coding

One advantage to using EHRs is enhanced documentation of services. Documentation of an E/M service may be easier when templates or drop-down options are used and legibility is not an issue. But there are disadvantages to documenting in an EHR. When completing an audit, be aware of the following pitfalls:

- Templates may not accurately describe pertinent patient history or abnormal findings on examination. Some EHRs do not allow free texting, thereby prohibiting more detailed, appropriate documentation. If a system does not allow free texting, work with the vendor to add this capability, or add all abnormal findings that might be pertinent in the template so documentation can be complete and accurate.
- Avoid templates and documentation tools that feature predefined text that may include information not relevant to the patient presentation and/or services rendered. Review and edit all default data to ensure that only patient-specific data are recorded for that visit, while removing all other irrelevant data pulled in by the default template.
- Become familiar with the way the EHR constructs a note from the data entered into each field and how the system may be customized to enhance the final note.
- Include only the problems that are evaluated and managed in determining the level of medical decision-making (MDM). Diagnostic tests and treatment options that are considered but not selected after discussion with the patient/caregiver, however, *do count* toward amount and/or complexity of data to be reviewed and analyzed or the risk of management that contributes to the level of MDM. Therefore, physicians should document those options considered and discussed but not selected.
- The EHR usually captures all documentation, whether performed by ancillary staff or the provider. Make certain it is clear who documented each portion of a service. For example, when a nurse, a pediatrician, and an obstetrician each enter portions of a delivery summary, the work of each individual may not be clearly identifiable. (EHR systems include audit trails that may be used to prove who entered specific elements of documentation. It is important to understand how the practice's EHR system creates and produces an audit trail.)
- The EHR audit log should always be enabled to ensure it creates an accurate chronological history of changes to the EHR. Practice procedures should describe any exceptions, including who can disable the log and when this may be appropriate.
- Scribes are not providers of items or services. When a scribe documents an encounter, the CMS does not require the scribe to sign and date the documentation. The treating physician's or QHP's signature on a note indicates affirmation from the physician/QHP that the note adequately documents the care provided. Private payers may have different documentation requirements.
- Review any information that is automatically carried forward by an EHR (eg, previous problems, medication lists) to verify it is still accurate, and document the review of the pertinent information.
- List the diagnosis chiefly responsible for the services provided first. The EHR should capture the diagnoses in the order in which they are documented (ie, not reorder alphabetically or otherwise).
- To support management options, it may be necessary to document the diagnoses being considered. These suspected or rule-out diagnoses should not be reported on claims for services provided in the outpatient setting.
- Make certain that any separately reportable procedure or service has documentation to support that it was performed.
- *Each physician/QHP should document* their total time and the problems and activities that support the necessity of time spent providing an E/M service. (This documentation is especially important in facility settings in which split or shared E/M services may be provided.)

× Do not depend on the software vendor to add codes to the system. Review all new, deleted, and revised codes with each code set update. Notify the vendor if codes have not been revised, and educate physicians and staff on the appropriate use of codes.

- Past and present diagnoses and history should be accessible to the treating and/or consulting physician.
- Identify appropriate health risk factors. The patient's progress, their response to and any changes in treatment, and any revision in diagnosis should be documented.
- All pages in the medical record should include the patient's name and an identifying number or birth date.
- Prescription drug management should include the name of the medication, dosage, and instructions.
- A diagnosis code may be assigned for any documented social determinant of health (SDoH). It should be explicitly documented when an SDoH increases the risk of patient management or treatment decisions in the course of an E/M service.
- Clinically important telephone calls should be documented, including date, time, instructions, patient/parent understanding of and agreement with those instructions, and plan for follow-up.
- Anticipatory guidance, patient education, and counseling are best documented when performed.
- Any addenda should be identifiable with the author's signature and labeled with the date the addendum was made. The compliance plan should address what circumstances justify making changes to the EHR and identify who can make changes, requirements for amendments and corrections to an EHR, and what information cannot be changed (ie, author, date, and time of original note).
- Consent forms should be dated, the procedure should be documented, and the form should be signed by the patient or their legal representative. Documentation should include a summary of the discussion of the procedure and risks.
- All abbreviations used should be commonly understood and standardized in a document developed by the practice or a listing obtained from a published source.
- Patient nonadherence, including immunization refusal, should be documented, as well as discussion of the risks and adverse consequences of nonadherence.

The AAP offers a refusal-to-immunize form and template in addition to a letter providing additional background on documenting refusal of recommended childhood immunizations at www.aap.org/en/patient-care/immunizations/implementing-immunization-administration-in-your-practice/refusal-to-vaccinate.

- Allergies and adverse reactions should be prominently displayed.
- Immunization and growth charts must be maintained and current.
- Problem and medication lists should be complete and current, including over-the-counter medications.
- When a waiver or advance notice of patient responsibility is obtained because a service is anticipated to be denied as noncovered or not medically necessary, the document should specify the service and the reason for anticipated noncoverage. Payer manuals may have further requirements (eg, billing with modifier **GA**, waiver of liability statement issued as required by payer policy, individual case).

Retention of Records

Policies and procedures should be written to include the creation, distribution, retention, and destruction of documents. In designing a record-retention system, privacy concerns and federal and state regulatory requirements should be considered. In addition to maintaining appropriate and thorough medical records on each patient, the HHS OIG recommends that the system include the following types of documents:

- All records and documentation (eg, billing and claims documentation) required for participation in federal, state, and private-payer health care programs
- All records necessary to demonstrate the integrity of the physician practice's compliance process and to confirm the effectiveness of the program

The following record-retention guidelines should be used:

- Specify the length of time that a physician's medical record documentation is to be retained. Federal and state statutes should be consulted for specific time frames. In the event of a disparity between federal and state statutes, it is advisable to select the longer retention period.
- Consulting with an attorney or risk management department of a medical liability insurer is prudent to determine the appropriate retention period.
  - At a minimum, pediatricians may want to retain records until patients obtain the age of majority plus the statute of limitations in their jurisdiction. The age of majority varies from 18 to 21 years.
  - Longer retention periods may be prudent, depending on the circumstances.
- Medical records, including electronic correspondence, should be secured against loss, destruction, unauthorized access, unauthorized reproduction, corruption, and damage.
- Policies and procedures should stipulate the disposition of medical records in the event the practice is sold or closed.

Document Advice From Payers

A physician practice should document its efforts to comply with applicable federal, state, and private health care program requirements. For example,

- When requesting advice from a government agency charged with administering a federal or state health care program or from a private payer, document and retain a record of the request and of all written or oral responses.
- Maintain a log of oral inquiries between the practice and third parties.
- Keep copies of all provider manuals, provider bulletins, and communications from payers about coding and submission of claims. *Remember that payers may demand repayment of benefits up to 6 years after the date of service (DOS) (recovery period varies by state and type of payer). Copies of the payer's policies in effect at the time of service may be the best defense against repayment.*

Coding Compliance Information Sources

A compliance program should train all employees to seek an authoritative source (eg, *CPT* instructions, Medicaid NCCI manual) for coding guidance. Information obtained from coding discussion forums, webinars, conferences, and, especially, medical product vendors should be verified against authoritative sources. Additionally, payment policies established by health plans vary, and one plan's policy does not necessarily apply to charges billed to other plans.

The Self-Audit/Medical Record Review Process

Items 1 through 5 are steps to selecting the focus of a self-audit based on practice data. Items 6 through 8 include tools and questions for use in reviewing each selected service.

1. Obtain and review a productivity report from your billing system.
2. Calculate the percentage distribution of E/M codes within each category of service (new and established office or outpatient visits, initial inpatient or observation services, use of modifier **25**) for each physician and QHP in the practice. (Most billing software provides these calculations.)
3. Use data from a 12-month period to include seasonal trends and better reflect practice patterns.
4. Perform a comparative analysis of the distribution with each physician and QHP in the practice. Remember that data reflect only the billing patterns and not whether one is more correct than another. More frequent oversight and monitoring are necessary for services provided by physicians who are new to the practice and may use documentation or coding guidance that conflicts with practice policy.
5. Review the report to ensure that all procedures performed are being captured and reported appropriately. For example, are discharge visits (**99238** and **99239**) being billed and is the number proportionate to the number of initial newborn and other initial hospital visits performed?
6. Review the practice encounter form or code selection application to ensure that *CPT,* Healthcare Common Procedure Coding System (HCPCS), and *International Classification of Diseases, 10th Revision, Clinical Modification* (*ICD-10-CM*) codes are correct and match the corresponding description.
7. Review the actual encounter and claim form with the medical record to ensure that the claim is submitted with the appropriate codes and/or modifiers. (Refer to the Documentation and Coding Self-Audits section that follows.)
8. Review each medical record and encounter form, as applicable, with the following questions in mind:
   - Is the patient's name, ID number, and/or date of birth on every page in the medical record?
   - Does the medical record contain updated demographic information?
   - Are allergies noted and prominently displayed?
   - Is the DOS documented?
   - Was the service medically necessary?
   - Are all the documented services and/or procedures captured on the encounter form?
   - Does the documentation support the procedure billed (eg, level and type of E/M service, administration of injection, catheterization, impacted cerumen removal)?
   - Does the documentation for the preventive medicine visit meet the requirements of the Medicaid Early and Periodic Screening, Diagnostic, and Treatment program when applicable?
   - Does the documentation support the diagnosis code(s) billed? Were diagnosis codes assigned for all conditions that required or affected management or treatment?
   - If using an EHR, does the documentation support physician review and personal documentation? For example, if the EHR incorporates new test results, is there a clear indication that the physician reviewed the information? If not, it should not be counted as part of the service.
   - Is there a completed growth chart and immunization record?
   - Is handwritten documentation legible?
   - Does any order for medication include its specific dosage and use?
   - Is there documentation of a follow-up plan for each problem managed? Are plans specific, such as an order for "consultation for opinion on initiation of glucose pump" versus "endocrinology consultation"?
   - Does documentation include the name and credentials of each contributing author in a manner that reflects each author's individual contributions?
   - Was an appropriate modifier reported with sufficient documentation?
   - Is the documentation in compliance with Physicians at Teaching Hospitals guidelines, split/shared E/M service, and/or incident-to provisions as appropriate?

Documentation and Coding Self-Audits

Medicare, Medicaid programs, and commercial payers will audit claims as well as monitor E/M coding profiles. Although the specialty-specific E/M profiles published by the CMS provide helpful information, keep in mind that these distributions reflect only code use and not code accuracy. An atypical code distribution may result when one is caring for a more complex patient population than average (eg, patients with chronic diseases or with social and economic challenges) or when physicians and QHPs are more knowledgeable and confident in E/M code assignment. Correct coding appropriately identifies the risk stratification for your patients and may directly affect your payments.

Also, just because you were paid does not mean that payers will not retrospectively audit and demand repayment or withhold future payments, particularly if claims were processed incorrectly or in error according to your contract. Practices are advised to become familiar with state laws addressing retrospective audits and repayments and with payer procedures for repayment. Your AAP chapter or state medical society may be able to help you understand your state-specific laws.

Use of self-audits to identify and correct errors shows a good-faith effort to be compliant.

Preparing for the Self-Audit

Before using documentation and coding audits to reduce your practice's vulnerability to fraud and abuse, it is important to consider how your practice can best conduct and use findings of an internal audit. Individual practices must consider how to conduct audits in a manner that offers the most benefit and least disruption to the practice.

Figure 5-1 offers steps to consider when developing a medical record audit process.

Performing the Audit

Make certain that the reviewer has all appropriate and necessary tools, which may include

- Current *CPT, ICD-10-CM,* and HCPCS manuals.
- Access to or copies of all payer newsletters or information bulletins that outline coding and/or payment policies (increasingly requires access to a payer's provider portal).
- An audit worksheet. This may be one designed by your practice or one of many published templates. Be certain the audit form includes appropriate requirements for E/M code selection. The CMS does not endorse a specific audit form or coding template.

Electronic audit programs may be purchased and offer automated report and recordkeeping functions. The cost of these programs may be offset by the reduced time of manually documenting and creating reports of audit findings. However, compliance managers should carefully review the program's accuracy periodically (eg, when codes or coding instructions are revised).

- A general documentation checklist of elements of documentation applicable to all records (eg, having patient identification, date, and page numbers on each page of a record), which can help with identification of missing nonclinical documentation and record authentication (an example can be found online at www.aap.org/cfp2026).
- A log to document findings for each provider (**Table 5-1**). This log should include a summary detail of findings for each encounter reviewed. (Auditing software may generate a log based on the reviewer's entries during chart review.) The log and E/M audit worksheets can be used as teaching tools at the conclusion of the audit.

Table 5-1. Sample Audit Log

Physician:	Date:		Auditor:	
Patient ID No.	**Date of Service**	**Reported Code**	**Audited Code**	**Comments**
4494	2/5/25	99223	99223 FS	This visit was split/shared and the payer policy requires modifier FS (split [or shared] E/M visit). The service was appropriately reported by the physician who provided the substantive part of the MDM.
4494	2/5/25	J45.31 98006	J45.31 Z59.82 98006	Documentation indicates that the visit took place via telemedicine because of transportation insecurity (Z59.82). 98006 is supported by the documented MDM.
2973	6/4/24	24640	24640 RT	Documentation supports treatment of right nursemaid elbow. The payer requires use of anatomical modifiers when applicable.
43221	6/4/24	98013	Not applicable	Documentation does not support the time spent in medical discussion as required for an audio-only visit.

Abbreviations: E/M, evaluation and management; MDM, medical decision-making.

Figure 5-1. Preparing and Planning Medical Record Audits

Focus

- Focus audits on documentation and coding of the most commonly performed services, adherence to medical record standards, appropriate reporting of diagnosis codes, use of modifiers, and adherence to coding and federal guidelines (eg, Physicians at Teaching Hospitals guidelines, physician self-referral laws).

Agreement

- Make certain all physicians in the practice are in agreement with how any audit will be conducted and how results will be used.

Auditor

- The auditor (eg, physician, other clinician, coder or other administrative employee, outside consultant, a combination thereof) must be proficient at coding, understand payer guidelines and requirements, and know medical terminology. Consider a team approach (eg, nurse and coder). If a physician is not actually performing record reviews, one should be available to assist as necessary.

Legal

- Determine if audits should be performed under the direction of a health care attorney, who may offer assistance with developing an audit process and provide guidance on any internal compliance concerns discovered in the process.
- Attorney-client privilege may apply when audits are directed by an attorney.

Timing

- Determine if audits should be performed under the direction of a health care attorney, who may offer assistance with developing an audit process and provide guidance on any internal compliance concerns discovered in the process.
- Prospective reviews are recommended because any necessary corrections can be made before a claim is filed. Although a prospective review will delay claims submission and introduce additional practice expense, this practice may have a net positive financial effect.

Services

- Select the types of services to be included in the audit. For example, if the review will include only office or outpatient services, include services most frequently reported (eg, a sampling of new and established patient problem-oriented and preventive medicine visits, documentation of nebulizer treatments) and new services.
- Include newborn care, critical care, and initial and subsequent inpatient or observation services when performing an audit of facility-based services.

Number

- Determine how many records or encounters will be included in the audit. Most coding consultants recommend at least 10 records per physician or provider per baseline or subsequent review (may be less for part-time providers). If a more focused review is required, the sample size may need to be increased. Medical records should be randomly selected for each E/M level of service and from different dates of service.

Schedule

- Determine the frequency of audits. Large practices might consider conducting audits on a rotating schedule of 1 physician or provider per week or 1 physician or provider per month throughout the year. Small practices should conduct at least an annual audit and additional audits when indicated (eg, increase in payer down-coding or denials).

E/M indicates evaluation and management.

- Audit summary reporting forms—results by individual provider with encounter details (eg, levels of MDM assigned vs audit finding); results by individual with codes and variances (eg, level of service and/or relative value unit variances); and report of key findings (eg, practice accuracy rates; strengths; areas of concern, including historical comparisons; recommendations for education and correction/improvement).

Following the Audit

- Discuss audit findings with each provider.
- Educate providers and staff as necessary.
- If a problem is encountered (eg, inappropriate use of modifiers, miscoding), a more focused retrospective review should be conducted to determine how long the error has been occurring and its effect. This is especially important when reviewing claims for physicians new to the practice or when a particular coding guideline or code has changed.
- If overpayments have occurred because of miscoding or billing errors, the errors should be corrected and education of appropriate staff performed. For further discussion, refer to the Refunding Self-Identified Overpayments section later in this chapter.
- If necessary, document a corrective action plan with deadlines for completion (eg, completion of education, attainment of a specified accuracy rate) and administrative sign-off verifying completion.
- Schedule follow-up audits, if indicated, to determine if problems have been resolved (eg, improved documentation, capturing of procedures, correct use of modifiers).
- Determine if audits need to be performed on a quarterly or annual basis and follow through with audits on a routine basis.
- If changes need to be made to the EHR system, contact the vendor and discuss how these might be accomplished. Educate physicians and providers on the changes made or the need for additional physician documentation.
- Establish or update written policies and procedures to prevent future errors.
- Maintain records of your compliance efforts and training.

Audits are not onetime events. Depending on your practice's resources for conducting audits and education, your practice may choose to conduct small audits monthly (eg, 5 medical records per provider), larger audits quarterly (eg, 10 medical records per provider), or continual prospective audit of a small number of medical records weekly. There may be a period of trial and error to find what works best for your practice.

The HHS OIG states that small entities should conduct at least annual audits based on a risk assessment to determine which types of services are to be included. When, however, audit results indicate potential for systemic issues or potentially improper conduct, an expanded audit and engagement of outside assistance may be indicated.

Refunding Self-Identified Overpayments

Requirements (eg, contractual, regulatory) for refunding overpayments and disclosure of errors must be understood and included in practice procedures.

The Patient Protection and Affordable Care Act requires any person who has received an overpayment from certain defined government health programs, including Medicaid plans, to report and return the overpayment within 60 days of the date the overpayment is identified.

- Overpayment due to a billing error (eg, typographic error in number of units), without indication of an intent or willful ignorance of correct billing practices, requires only a refund and/or submission of a corrected claim based on the payer's policy.
- When an identified overpayment raises concern for related but undiscovered overpayments, the timeline for refunding may be delayed for up to 180 days while conducting an investigation for related overpayments.
- When overpayment is suspected to be due to abusive or fraudulent actions by someone in the practice, always seek advice from the practice's attorney before disclosure or repayment. An experienced health law attorney may be able to guide the practice's response to resolve the issue(s) in the most expedient and least costly manner.

States may have regulations regarding timely refund of overpayments and may include all payers (eg, commercial health plans).

Responding to Repayment Demands

To control costs and stamp out fraud, carrier claims processing and special investigative units use sophisticated software programs to identify providers with atypical coding patterns that could indicate erroneous coding and potential overpayments. For example, some carriers may flag the providers considered outliers in frequently reporting high-level E/M codes or frequently using modifiers. They then extrapolate the alleged overpayments over several years and demand across-the-board repayments. Worse, carriers will reduce payments on future claims to correct alleged overpayments on past claims. These requests require a swift and skilled response. Usually, several thousand dollars are involved. Given the compressed timeline and dollars at stake, seeking legal advice is invaluable in these situations.

Do Not Get Caught Without a Plan

Most practices will never have to deal with demands for paybacks or fraud audits. Nevertheless, all practices should have a plan just in case these communications occur. Because time is of the essence in responding to these communications, it would be a calamity to have a letter sit on someone's desk while precious days tick away. Often, a response must be received within 30 days of the date of the request, and the paperwork demanded is not insignificant.

The first communication may be a request for repayment based on payer software analysis of claims history to detect claims paid in conflict with payment policies. It is important for all staff to be trained to recognize these requests and get them to the compliance officer/compliance contact immediately. Then, qualified staff tasked with receiving all requests for paybacks can determine the veracity of the request and, if inaccurate, act in accordance with the payer's rebuttal and appeal processes in a timely manner. Likewise, requests for records must be handled carefully and expeditiously.

Here is some general guidance for your consideration.

- If a problem truly results from a billing error by the practice, take action to correct it and demonstrate to the carrier how it has been or will be corrected and the measures implemented to prevent the problem in the future.
- Reply in writing to inform the carrier that you are willing to work with it and to ask that it identify each of the claims in question as well as the specific criteria or standards it is applying to the audit.
- Make sure the practice and the carrier consistently apply current *CPT* guidelines. Reference *CPT* coding guidelines and have appropriate documentation for support. The AAP Coding and Payment Hotline can be a resource to you as well (www.aap.org/en/practice-management/child-health-finance-payment-strategy/coding-payment-hotline).
- Review your carrier contract's clauses on audits and dispute resolution as well as applicable state laws regarding audits and repayments with your attorney.
- Focus any overpayment recovery efforts on a case-by-case basis. Prevent unilateral takebacks by not allowing the carrier to extrapolate repayments on any or all future claims.
- Have the carrier provide documentation as proof of overpayment for each contested claim.
- Obtain and secure written documentation of all contacts with the carrier on this issue. Should a carrier payment policy require reporting that varies from *CPT* guidelines, obtain written, dated documentation from the carrier to verify that is the case. Keep this documentation permanently.
- Use legal counsel skilled in carrier contracting when negotiating contracts and confronted with repayment demands.

What If Your Practice Is Notified of an External Medical Record Audit?

- Contact legal counsel as soon as possible. Make sure the attorney or legal practice has experience with audits. If it is a Medicaid audit, it is preferable to have an attorney with Medicaid audit experience. An audit is a complex legal process with significant consequences. It is unwise to attempt to maneuver through this process without sound legal advice.
- Designate 1 physician or staff member to serve as the primary contact with the attorney and auditors. However, keep in mind that all physicians and staff members may need to work with auditors to some extent.
- Request that the auditor provide you with an opening and closing conference. At the initial meeting, ask for the individual's credentials and job title and ask them to summarize the purpose of the review or audit.
- Know how far back auditors may conduct reviews, the number of records a contractor may request, the amount of time allowed to respond to each request, any rebuttal process in place, and steps necessary to appeal adverse findings.
- If the time requirements for producing copies or gathering medical records are unmanageable, contact the auditing entity and request an extension in writing. Provide a clear justification for the extension request.
- Keep copies of all written communication (eg, letters, directives, memos, emails). Keep the postmarked envelopes of all letters, including the original notice.
- Fully document all verbal communication, including time, date, people involved, substance of the discussion, and conclusions and agreements.

- In response to requests for information, provide only the information requested and maintain copies of what you provide auditors. Before providing files, remove any information unrelated to the audit. For example, in a Medicaid audit, you could exclude information related to services provided when the patient was covered under a commercial plan or was uninsured.
- ✖ Do not alter any documents or medical records.
- Respond only to questions from the auditors; do not try to engage them in any conversations. If the auditors are conducting the review in your office, try to place them in a separate office away from patients, staff, and business operations.
- Be prepared to respond promptly to each request received. Keep a log of requests received by date, response due date, requesting party, any communication with the requester, date of response, and outcome.
- Know HIPAA privacy regulations, documentation principles, coding guidelines, and payment policies, and verify that all supporting documentation is included in each response.
- If legibility of the record is questionable, include a transcribed copy with attestation by the author of the original document stating that the transcription is accurate and provided to ensure legibility. Any unsigned entry should also be accompanied by a separate attestation by its author.
- Copied or scanned medical records should be carefully reviewed to be sure that all pages were legibly copied (front and back, if applicable) and are straight and within the margins on the page.
- Any questions about the sufficiency of medical record documentation should be addressed with the physician or provider who ordered or documented the service before responding to the request for records.
  - Any corrections to an entry should be performed in a manner that maintains legibility of the original content (eg, single-line strike-through) and should be signed and dated.
  - A summary of the service provided may be included to provide more information but should be distinctly labeled as such and not as part of the original record.
- Include any policy or correspondence from the payer that was used to guide your billing and coding practices related to the service. (Archived payer manuals supportive of claims from previous years may be available on Medicaid websites.) Clinical practice guidelines, policy statements, textbooks, and manuals may also support medical necessity.
- Send records in a manner that allows for confirmation of receipt.
- Secure a copy of auditors' contact information in case you need to follow up.
- Obtain, in writing, the expected date of a written summary of findings.

Can This Really Happen?

Conventional wisdom says that auditors will probably go after big organizations when it comes to investigating fraud and abuse, but the HHS OIG has said repeatedly that it has zero tolerance for fraud—so, technically, everyone is at risk. Because most of the software programs used to detect unusual coding and billing patterns are based on adult services, pediatricians may be identified as outliers. As a result, valid pediatric coding may be tagged as improper, and honest providers may have to respond to inappropriate recoupment requests or audits. The AAP works hard to minimize these problems and help chapters respond when payers target pediatric coding as inappropriate. This is an ongoing challenge.

Unfortunately, there are instances of fraud involving pediatricians. A review of past HHS OIG reports to Congress and press releases revealed the following cases:

- The *Medicaid Fraud Control Units Fiscal Year 2023 Annual Report* from the HHS OIG (most recent year available at the time of this publication) reports that 2 pediatricians reached a settlement or judgment and repaid a total of $193,025. Criminal fraud investigations continued for 45 pediatricians, and civil investigations continued for 15 pediatricians.
- A pediatric psychiatrist who operated a service tutoring children in addition to clinical therapy and psychiatric services was found guilty of submitting numerous claims to a Medicaid program for psychotherapy and medical services that were not provided. An investigation was prompted by an abnormal number of service hours that were billed each day. The psychiatrist faces a maximum of 30 years in prison with multiple sentences to be served concurrently.
- A pediatrician and pediatric practice entered a settlement agreement to pay $198,801 (at least in part from funds withheld by the state Medicaid and managed care organizations prior to the settlement) to resolve a case that involved findings of insufficient documentation to support claims paid over a 5-year period for tests of hearing (**92583**, **92587**) and visual evoked potential (**95930**). The settlement does not exclude the possibility of further investigations and legal actions by other authorities.
- Two pediatricians settled separate allegations of improper billing of both rapid direct optical observation and molecular tests for group A *Streptococcus pyogenes* either on the same date or within a 3-day period for the same patient. The combined settlements were over $1.8 million.

Explore the Need for Additional Insurance

Many medical liability insurers and insurance brokers offer products to provide additional coverage for the consequences of billing errors and omissions. Pediatric practices may want to contact their insurers to see whether their current medical liability policies cover any of the following problems. If they do not, it might be worthwhile to explore insurance options for obtaining that additional protection.

- Defense coverage for a Medicaid audit
- Qui tam action (False Claims Act)
- Unintentional billing errors and omissions
- Physician Self-Referral Law (Stark Law) violations
- Unintentional release of medical or financial data
- Breach of computers or network security
- Data recovery
- HIPAA fines or investigation costs

Health care fraud and abuse regulations will likely change as the health care system evolves to new care delivery and claims payment standards, such as value-based payment and accountable care organizations. Providers need to stay abreast of and comply with new regulations to prevent triggering fraud investigations.

To test your knowledge of the information presented in this chapter, complete the quiz found at the end of it, after the resources. Answers to each quiz are found in **Appendix II**.

Chapter Takeaways

Readers of this chapter should have a general knowledge of the importance of compliance in medical practice. Key takeaways include:

- Physician practices must understand the definitions of fraud and abuse in health care and the laws and regulations that govern financial arrangements and billing.
- Physicians and other providers who enroll in Medicare, Medicaid, or CHIP are required to establish a compliance program with certain core elements.
- One of the most important physician practice compliance issues is the appropriate documentation of diagnosis and treatment.
- Individual practices must consider how to conduct audits in a manner that offers the most benefit and least disruption to the practice.
- Overpayments identified by a practice must be refunded within time periods specified by legislation or payer contracts.
- Qualified staff should determine the veracity of requests for paybacks and, if inaccurate, act in accordance with the payer's rebuttal and appeal processes in a timely manner. Likewise, requests for records must be handled carefully and expeditiously.

Resources

AAP Coding Assistance and Education

AAP *Prepare Your Office for a Payer Audit Site Visit* (https://downloads.aap.org/AAP/PDF/PrepareYourOfficeforaPayerAuditSiteVisit.pdf)

AAP refusal-to-immunize form and template (www.aap.org/en/patient-care/immunizations/implementing-immunization-administration-in-your-practice/refusal-to-vaccinate)

AAP News™

"Keep calm and type on: importance of medical record-keeping," February 1, 2023 (https://publications.aap.org/aapnews/news/23124)

AAP Pediatric Coding Newsletter™

"Compliance Corner: Documentation Authentication," March 2024 (https://doi.org/10.1542/pcco_book239_document002)

"Compliance Corner: Refunds, Self-disclosure, and Investigations," March 2025 (https://doi.org/10.1542/pcco_book251_document003)

"Compliant Billing: Deductibles Coinsurance, and Copays," April 2025 (https://doi.org/10.1542/pcco_book252_document003)

"Fraud and Abuse: Learning from Mistakes of Others," March 2025 (https://doi.org/10.1542/pcco_book251_document002)

"Spring Cleaning: Time to Tidy Up Coding and Billing Processes," April 2023 (https://doi.org/10.1542/pcco_book228_document002)

CMS Medicare Fraud and Abuse Booklet

Medicare Fraud & Abuse: Prevent, Detect, Report (www.cms.gov/Outreach-and-Education/Medicare-Learning-Network-MLN/MLNProducts/MLN-Publications-Items/MLN4649244)

HHS OIG Excluded Individuals and Entities List and the Federal System for Award Management

https://exclusions.oig.hhs.gov and https://sam.gov/content/exclusions

HHS OIG *General Compliance Program Guidance* as of November 2023

https://oig.hhs.gov/compliance/general-compliance-program-guidance

HHS OIG Special Fraud Alert: Speaker Programs

https://oig.hhs.gov/documents/specialfraudalerts/865/SpecialFraudAlertSpeakerPrograms.pdf

Legal Advice

American Health Law Association (www.americanhealthlaw.org)

Medicaid Audits

Medicaid Recovery Audit Contractor program (www.medicaid.gov)

Online-Exclusive Content at www.aap.org/cfp2026

"General Documentation Checklist"

Test Your Knowledge!

1. **Under the Civil Monetary Penalties law, what penalty may apply to physicians who commit various forms of fraud and abuse involving Medicare and Medicaid?**
   a. Civil money penalties
   b. Exclusion from the Medicare and Medicaid programs
   c. Imprisonment
   d. Both a and b
2. **Which of the following is a key aspect of an effective compliance and ethics program?**
   a. Exercise of due diligence to prevent and detect criminal conduct.
   b. Only allow code assignment by certified professional coders.
   c. Limit the use of higher-level codes to only a specific percentage of patients.
   d. Require physicians to become certified professional coders.
3. **Which documentation function of an EHR system should be prohibited?**
   a. Copy and paste
   b. Cut and paste
   c. Macros
   d. Auto-population
4. **What is an advantage of performing self-audits/chart reviews of the codes assigned for services?**
   a. Detect which physician or QHPs are providing fewer services.
   b. Payers will not audit a practice that performs compliance self-audits/chart reviews.
   c. Self-audits/chart reviews show good-faith effort to be compliant.
   d. Self-audits/chart reviews offer a chance to alter records to support the codes assigned.
5. **How should a practice respond when a payer communicates an intent to extrapolate alleged overpayments over several years and demand across-the-board repayment?**
   a. Ignore the communication.
   b. Try to negotiate a settlement.
   c. Stop seeing any patients covered by that payer's plans.
   d. Ask the payer to identify each of the claims in question as well as the specific criteria or standards it is applying to the audit.

CHAPTER 6

Evaluation and Management Documentation Guidelines

Contents

Chapter Highlights

- General and specific evaluation and management (E/M) guidelines
- Concepts of new versus established patient and initial versus subsequent encounter
- Reporting single or multiple services when provided in the same setting or in 2 settings with different designations (eg, hospital and nursing facility)
- *Current Procedural Terminology* (*CPT*®) terms and definitions used in determining a level of E/M services based on a physician's or other qualified health care professional's (QHP's) total time on the date of an encounter or on medical decision-making (MDM)
- The Centers for Medicare & Medicaid Services (CMS) guidelines for reporting services provided as a teaching physician, when applicable

This chapter outlines the *CPT* E/M guidelines used in selecting codes for encounters to evaluate and manage a patient's health problems. The content of this chapter provides the basis for learning category-specific instructions for code selection discussed in later chapters.

Pediatric clinical vignettes are presented throughout this manual. These are only examples, and the associated *CPT* codes should not be used for every patient with the same or a similar diagnosis.

General Guidelines

The E/M guidelines in *CPT* are used to guide code selection and are neither documentation guidelines nor standards of care. The E/M guidelines section of *CPT* mostly applies to codes selected according to the physician's or QHP's total time on the date of an encounter (total time) or to the physician's or QHP's level of MDM. But the following portions of the E/M guidelines apply to many E/M services, including those not selected according to total time or MDM:

- Definitions of new versus established patients and initial versus subsequent visits
- Other services provided on the same date as an E/M service

Additional service-specific guidelines are found preceding E/M service categories (eg, telemedicine services) and subcategories (eg, 98000–98007, synchronous audio-video E/M services) and, in parenthetical instructions, following E/M codes.

Example

➤ **#★+99417 Prolonged outpatient E/M service(s) time with or without direct patient contact beyond the required time of the primary service when the primary service level has been selected using total time, each 15 minutes of total time (List separately in addition to the code of the outpatient E/M service)**

(Use 99417 in conjunction with 98003, 98007, 98011, 98015, 99205, 99215, 99245, 99345, 99350, 99483.)

(Do not report 99417 on the same date of service as 90833, 90836, 90838, 99358, 99359, 99415, 99416.)

(Do not report 99417 for any time unit less than 15 minutes.)

Refer to other chapters of this manual and your *CPT* coding reference for more detailed guidelines for reporting services such as normal newborn care in the hospital, hourly or daily critical care services, intensive care services, care plan oversight, care management services, and preventive medicine E/M services.

New Versus Established Patients

The categorization of new and established patients influences coding for the following services:

- Office or other outpatient E/M services (new patient, 99202–99205; established patient, 99211–99215)
- Synchronous audio-video visit (new patient, 98000–98003; established patient, 98004–98007)
- Synchronous audio-only visit (new patient, 98008–98011; established patient, 98012–98014)
- Home or residence services (new patient, 99341 and 99342, 99344 and 99345; established patient, 99347–99350)
- Preventive medicine services (new patient, 99381–99385; established patient, 99391–99395)
- Online digital E/M (established patient, 99421–99423)
- Brief communication technology-based service (established patient, 98016)

● indicates a new code; ▲, revised; #, re-sequenced; +, add-on; ★, audiovisual technology; and ◀, synchronous interactive audio.

About Documentation

Although *CPT* guidelines are not documentation guidelines, the information documented in the medical record must support the reported procedure codes.

When selecting a code level based on total time, *the total time* must be documented. The overarching criterion for payment is the medical necessity of the service provided. Documentation of a summary of the physician's or QHP's activities (eg, history and examination findings, counseling topics) during the total time of the visit provides support for the medical necessity of the visit and time spent.

When selecting a code level based on the MDM, the documentation should demonstrate the basis for the level selected. For instance, the record should include the signs, symptoms, and diagnoses that were addressed, including any conditions that were considered plausible but ruled out. It is also important to demonstrate review of external records or prior test results. The physician or other QHP might sign the external record or report of test results to indicate review or might document a brief notation of findings in the visit note. Conversations with external physicians and other health care professionals or sources (eg, social workers) should also be summarized in the documentation (eg, "Spoke with Dr X regarding management options for this patient").

When submitting documentation for an audit, be sure that notes from the electronic health record (EHR) include all documentation for each unique visit (eg, nursing notes, medication orders). Another clinician or coding auditor should be able to readily determine your basis for the level of service reported.

Timely completion of documentation, including the reporting individual's signature and date, is required to support billing and coding compliance. Physicians and QHPs should be aware of regulatory or contractual requirements for completion of all medical record documentation.

No distinction is made between new and established patients for emergency department (ED) services, for consultations, or for observation, inpatient, or nursing facility care. E/M services in these categories may be reported for any new or established patient. For E/M services provided to patients in observation or inpatient status or in a nursing facility, services are distinguished as initial or subsequent services during the same admission/stay, as discussed in the Initial and Subsequent Services section later in this chapter.

Following are the criteria for distinguishing between new and established patients:

- *New patients* have not received a face-to-face professional service from the physician or other QHP, or any physician or QHP of the same group practice and same exact specialty and subspecialty, in the prior 3 years.
  - Rules for new and established patients apply to physicians and QHPs whose charges are billed under a single tax ID number (eg, ABC Health System Physicians, tax ID number 48-1234567).
  - Medical subspecialties are defined by either a taxonomy code that designates a specific specialty or subspecialty (eg, 2084N0400X, neurology; 2084E0001X, epilepsy) designated during health plan credentialing or a payer's specialty identification code (eg, 13, neurology).
- *Established patients* have received, and were charged for, a face-to-face professional service from a physician or QHP of the same group practice and same exact specialty and subspecialty within the past 3 years.
- Per *CPT*, a QHP working with a physician(s) and who may report E/M services is considered to be working in the exact same specialty and subspecialty as the physician(s).
- When a physician is covering for another physician of the same specialty, the E/M service is reported as it would have been by the physician who is unavailable. A physician covering for another physician of a different specialty, however, determines whether a patient is new or established according to the rules listed earlier in this list for new and established patients (refer to the first 2 bulleted items).
- If the physician has moved to a different location or changed their tax ID number, patients would still be considered established if they were established patients before these changes took place.
  - When a new physician joins a group practice, patients who follow the physician to the new practice are considered established patients to any physician of the same specialty in the new practice because the patients were seen by a physician of the same specialty in the group within the past 3 years.

Examples

➤ **A pediatrician provides an office visit to an infant who received newborn hospital care from a pediatric QHP of the same group and same exact specialty (pediatric primary care).** The patient is considered established at the office visit.

➤ **A primary care pediatrician has provided an outpatient E/M service to a patient within the past 3 years.** A neurologist in the same group but *different specialty* is asked to provide an office or other outpatient E/M service to the patient. The patient is new for this service.

Initial and Subsequent Services

The following services are described as initial or subsequent services as opposed to services provided to a new or established patient:

- Hospital inpatient and observation care services (initial, 99221–99223; subsequent, 99231–99233)
- Nursing facility services (initial, 99304–99306; subsequent, 99307–99310)

Intensive and Critical Care Services

Refer to the prefatory guidelines for critical care (99291, 99292), inpatient neonatal and pediatric critical care (99468–99472; 99475, 99476), and neonatal intensive care services (99477–99480) for distinct instructions on reporting initial and continuing services.

As with new and established patients, differentiating between initial and subsequent encounters is based on the timing of the professional (face-to-face) services provided by a physician or other QHP to the patient during an admission/stay.

- Admission/stay: The duration of time from initiation of observation and/or inpatient care to discharge from a facility. For the purpose of determining initial versus subsequent encounters, an admission/stay that includes a transition in levels of care from observation to inpatient or between skilled nursing and nursing services in the same facility is one admission/stay.
- Initial service: During the inpatient or observation or nursing facility admission/stay, the patient has not received any professional services from the physician or QHP or another physician or QHP of the exact same specialty and subspecialty who belongs to the same group practice.
- Subsequent service: During the admission/stay, the patient has received professional service(s) from the physician or QHP or another physician or QHP of the exact same specialty and subspecialty who belongs to the same group practice.
- A physician or QHP who is on call for or covering for another physician or QHP reports the service as if provided by the physician or QHP who is not available. Unlike for new versus established patient status, there is no differentiation in selection of initial versus subsequent service when the covering physician or QHP is of a different specialty.

Examples

➤ **A physician provides hospital care to a patient who has not received prior care from the physician or any physician or QHP of the same group practice and same specialty during this admission/stay.** Initial hospital care is reported.

➤ **A physician provides hospital care to a patient who received observation care from a physician of the same group and same exact specialty on a prior date during this admission/stay.** The encounter is reported as subsequent hospital care.

➤ **A physician who is covering for a patient's attending physician who is unavailable sees the patient for the first time during an inpatient stay.** The encounter is subsequent hospital care.

Discharge Management and Readmissions on the Same Date

- When a patient is discharged and readmitted to the *same facility* (eg, readmission to inpatient hospital status) on the same date of service (DOS), this is considered a single stay for purposes of E/M code selection. The visit is reported as if the patient had not been discharged (eg, subsequent hospital care).

Multiple health care entities may colocate but operate separately (eg, nursing facility within a hospital) in compliance with regulations for each type of entity. When a patient is discharged from a hospital stay to a nursing stay within the same facility, the discharge and initial nursing facility care are considered 2 services in 2 facilities because there is a discharge from one entity to another. Time and MDM of each service are distinct, and one service does not affect code selection for another service.

- When a patient is discharged and readmitted to a *different facility* on the same DOS, this is considered a new stay for purposes of E/M code selection. A physician or QHP providing E/M services, including discharge (99234–99236; 99238, 99239) and initial E/M services, may separately report the services at each facility but, if reporting according to total time, may not count any time of the discharge service toward the time of service at the second facility.

When choosing between initial and subsequent E/M services provided in a facility setting, a single admission/stay includes any transfers from one level of care to another (eg, observation to inpatient). A transfer in the level of care is not a new admission/stay.

Separately Reported Services

Procedures and services described by *CPT* codes distinct from those of an E/M service provided on the same date may be separately reported except where specifically noted in *CPT* as included/bundled. For example, critical care E/M services include services such as electrocardiographic (ECG) collection and interpretation and vascular access procedures that are reported in addition to most other E/M services.

When an E/M service is caused or prompted by the symptoms or condition for which another diagnostic or therapeutic service (eg, ECG, injection of medication, surgery) is provided on the same date, different diagnoses are not required for reporting the 2 services on the same date.

Example

➤ **A physician provides an office E/M service to a patient who reports respiratory symptoms consistent with asthma.** After performing medically indicated history and examination, the physician orders spirometry, which is administered by clinical staff and interpreted by the physician. The physician diagnoses mild persistent asthma with exacerbation and initiates a care plan including prescription medication. The physician reports *International Classification of Diseases, 10th Revision, Clinical Modification* code J45.31 (mild persistent asthma with exacerbation) linked to a code for the E/M service (eg, 99214 25) and to 94010 (spirometry, including graphic record, total and timed vital capacity, expiratory flow rate measurement[s], with or without maximal voluntary ventilation).

Modifier 25 (significant, separately identifiable E/M service) is appended to an E/M code when an E/M service provided on the same date as a procedural service is significantly beyond the preservice work of the procedural service.

For more information on modifier 25, refer to **Chapter 2**.

E/M Guidelines for Use of Total Time or MDM

Applicability of E/M Guidelines for Use of Total Time or MDM

E/M guidelines used for selecting codes from the following categories are further discussed in this chapter:

- Office or other outpatient services (new patient, 99202–99205; established patient, 99211–99215)
- Synchronous audio-video visit (new patient, 98000–98003; established patient, 98004–98007)
- Synchronous audio-only visit (new patient, 98008–98011; established patient, 98012–98014)
- Hospital inpatient or observation care services (initial, 99221–99223; subsequent, 99231–99233; same date admission and discharge, 99234–99236; discharge day management, 99238–99239)
- Outpatient and inpatient consultations (outpatient, 99242–99245; inpatient, 99252–99255)
- ED services (99281–99285)
- Nursing facility services (initial, 99304–99306; subsequent, 99307–99310; discharge day management, 99315 and 99316)
- Home or residence services (new patient, 99341 and 99342, 99344 and 99345; established patient, 99347–99350)
- Prolonged service with or without direct contact on the date of an E/M service (99417, 99418)

Each of the listed code categories involves selecting a code based on the category of service (eg, telemedicine visit; hospital consultation) and a physician's or QHP's total time on the date of the encounter or the level of MDM associated with the encounter. All other E/M services are reported according to guidelines specific to the code category. The guidelines for these other E/M services are addressed elsewhere in this manual (eg, **Chapter 8**, **Chapter 17**). Refer also to **Chapter 1** for general guidelines for *CPT* code selection.

Generally, codes for E/M visits require a face-to-face encounter with a patient *and/or* family or caregiver. Telemedicine services are synchronous, real-time, interactive encounters between a physician or QHP and a patient and/or family or caregiver utilizing either combined audio-video or audio-only telecommunication. To learn more about coding for services provided via telemedicine, refer to Chapters 19 through 21.

Each of the categories and subcategories of E/M service to which these general guidelines apply may also have additional guidelines presented before the list of codes and/or as parenthetical instructions after the codes in *CPT 2025*. For instance, for audio-only codes 98008–98015, the total time of service must include more than 10 minutes of medical discussion. These additional guidelines, specific to each category of E/M code, are discussed in other chapters devoted to reporting these services (eg, **Chapter 20**).

History and Examination

History and examination are included components of all E/M services addressed by the E/M guidelines. The history and examination, although supporting the amount of time spent or the level of MDM, are not directly used in code selection. A medically appropriate history and/or examination, as determined by the reporting physician or QHP, should be documented for each E/M service.

History and examination are important elements of documentation to support that medical services provided were clinically indicated and to support quality initiatives (eg, verification of timely immunization and review of current medications and supplements). History documented by a patient, caregiver, or clinical staff member should be reviewed, expanded (when indicated), and authenticated by the reporting physician or QHP.

Code Selection Options

Once you have determined the correct code category (eg, outpatient consultation) or subcategory (eg, initial hospital inpatient or observation care), there are 2 options for selecting the appropriate codes based on these guidelines. However, ED services (99281–99285) are an exception, with selection based on MDM alone and no option for selection based on time.

- Select the code based on the reporting physician's or QHP's *documented total time* directed to care of the individual patient *on the date of the encounter.*
- Select a code based on meeting at least 2 of 3 elements of MDM.

Time and Emergency Department Services

Per *CPT*, time is not a descriptive component for the ED levels of E/M because ED services are typically provided on a variable-intensity basis, often involving multiple encounters with several patients over an extended period. The level of MDM determines the level of ED service.

Box 6-1 provides an overview of code selection based on total time or MDM. For each method of code selection, the documentation should support the clinical indication for the level of service reported.

Time Guidelines and Application

Time may be used to select a code level in the E/M services to which these guidelines apply *whether or not* counseling and/or coordination of care dominates the service.

- Time is the physician's and/or QHP's total time on the DOS, not their time in a 24-hour period.

The total time should be documented in the medical record when used as the basis for code selection. No specific verbiage is required by *CPT*. A documentation example is "My total time on this date was X minutes."

- Only time spent in activities directed to care of the individual patient is counted in total time on the date of a visit. Time before, during, and after the visit but on the same DOS is included in the total time used in code selection.
- Both face-to-face and non–face-to-face time or time on or off the unit/floor spent on the DOS are included in the time of the encounter.

Code Descriptors and Total Time

It is important to identify the time required in each code's descriptor to accurately assign codes based on total time. There are differences in how time is described across various categories of service.

For codes that may be selected according to a physician's or QHP's total time on the date of the encounter, a specific time must be met or exceeded.

Other codes, such as hourly critical care codes 99291 and 99292, have different guidelines and code descriptors that include only the time spent providing critical care services (ie, not the total time spent on the date of the encounter).

Box 6-1. Code Selection Based on Total Time or Medical Decision-Making

Select an E/M code level based on the pediatrician's or QHP's total time on the date of the encounter or on the MDM.

Time: May be used to select a code level whether or not counseling and/or coordination of care dominates the service.

- Time includes total time on the date of the encounter, face-to-face and non–face-to-face, personally spent by the physician and/or QHP focused on the care of 1 patient.
  - ✖ Do not include time in activities performed or normally performed by clinical staff (eg, rooming the patient).
  - Time does not need to be continuous. Total all time spent on 1 calendar date (ie, not all time in a 24-hour period).
  - Continuous time spanning 2 calendar dates (ie, before and after midnight) is reported as a single service on 1 calendar date inclusive of the total continuous time.
- The following activities are included when performed by a physician/QHP:
  - Preparing to see the patient (eg, reviewing previous test results)
  - Obtaining and/or reviewing separately obtained history
  - Performing a medically appropriate examination and/or evaluation
  - Counseling and educating the patient, family, or caregiver
  - Ordering medications, tests, or procedures
  - Referring to/communicating with other QHPs (when not separately reported)
  - Documenting clinical information in the electronic or other health record
  - Independently interpreting results (when not separately reported) and communicating results to the patient, family, or caregiver
  - Coordinating care (when not separately reported)

MDM: Four levels of MDM complexity are straightforward, low, moderate, and high.

Determine the level of MDM based on the highest 2 of 3 elements.

1. Number and complexity of problems addressed. Include problems addressed or managed by the reporting physician/QHP as part of the encounter.
2. Amount and/or complexity of data reviewed and analyzed. Data include
   - Tests, documents, orders, and/or requirement for an independent historian(s)
   - Independent interpretation of tests (not separately reported)
   - Discussion of management/test interpretation with an external physician, QHP, or appropriate source (not separately reported)
3. Risk of complications, morbidity, and/or mortality of patient management decisions made during the encounter, including decisions against a considered management option.

Abbreviations: E/M, evaluation and management; MDM, medical decision-making; QHP, qualified health care professional.

Examples

➤ **A physician spends 10 minutes reviewing laboratory results and consultation reports before an E/M visit with an established patient on the same date.** Later that day, a face-to-face visit with the patient and caregivers lasts 20 minutes. After the visit but on the same date, the physician spends 10 minutes in discussion with a consulting subspecialist and another 10 minutes in follow-up with the caregivers and in documentation. The physician's total time on the DOS is 50 minutes.

Teaching Point: The physician reports 99215 (40 minutes). All the physician's time spent in activities directed to the care of the single patient is counted. If the time had exceeded the required 40 minutes' total time assigned to 99215 by 15 minutes or more, 99417 (prolonged outpatient E/M service) would have been reported in addition to 99215.

***CPT* does not require documentation of each segment of time spent on the DOS or documentation in any specific format. But the physician must document the total amount of time spent on the date of the encounter and should be able to account for the time spent. Some physicians and QHPs elect to document each segment of time as advised by a consultant or based on practice policy.**

➤ **A physician spends 10 minutes reviewing laboratory results and medical records before an outpatient consultation on the same date.** Later that day, a face-to-face visit with the patient and caregivers lasts 20 minutes, and another 10 minutes is spent documenting the encounter and preparing a report to the QHP who requested the consultation. The physician's total time on the date of the face-to-face E/M service is 40 minutes. On the next day, the physician spends 10 minutes in discussion with the QHP who requested the consultation and another 10 minutes in follow-up with the caregivers and in documentation.

Code 99244 (40 minutes must be met or exceeded) is reported for the time on the date of the face-to-face visit.

Teaching Point: The time spent on the date following the visit date is not included in total time on the date of the encounter. But when a physician or QHP spends at least 30 minutes in patient care and coordination related to a previous or future face-to-face E/M service on a date other than the date of that E/M service, 99358 (prolonged E/M service before and/or after direct patient care; first hour) is reported. *CPT* instruction states that prolonged service code 99358 is not reported for less than 30 minutes' total duration on a given date.

➤ **On the second day of a patient's hospital stay, the attending physician spends 25 minutes on the unit/floor reviewing consultation reports and test results, reevaluating the patient, and discussing care with the patient and the patient's mother.** Another 10 minutes is spent entering orders and documenting the encounter. Later, when not on the patient's unit, the physician also spends 10 minutes on the phone with the patient's father explaining current findings and the plan for further E/M. Total time on the date of the encounter is 45 minutes, supporting subsequent hospital inpatient or observation care code 99232 (35 minutes). If the total time met or exceeded 50 minutes, 99233 would be reported.

Teaching Point: Total time on the date of the encounter includes time regardless of the location of the physician (eg, whether on or off the inpatient unit or in or out of the outpatient office). But the time must be directed to the care of that single patient and must require the skills of a physician or QHP.

- No time spent by clinical staff or time spent by a physician or QHP in activities typically performed by clinical staff is included.
- When the physician and a QHP of the same specialty and same group practice meet with a patient and caregiver at the same time (incident-to or split/shared encounter), only the reporting individual's time is counted. *Each minute of time is counted only once for overlapping or concurrent care time.*

Example

➤ **A nurse practitioner (NP) provides initial observation care to a patient.** After initially evaluating the patient, the NP spends 5 minutes discussing the patient with a physician in the same group practice and specialty and documents a total time of 25 minutes, including the time of the phone call with the physician. Later, on the same date, the physician of the same group practice and specialty reviews the patient's progress notes and test results since admission to observation and, after reevaluating the patient, agrees with continuing the current management overnight. The physician's total time is 20 minutes *not including the time of the phone conversation with the NP.*

Code 99221 (initial hospital inpatient or observation care; 40 minutes must be met or exceeded) is reported for the 45-minute service. The 5-minute conversation between the physician and NP is counted by only 1 of the providers.

Teaching Point: For further discussion of this example, refer to the Split or Shared Visits section later in this chapter.

MDM: Guidelines for Selecting a Level

Physicians and QHPs make medical decisions at each patient encounter. MDM includes the work of establishing or confirming a diagnosis, assessing the status of a condition, and selecting a management option. The complexity of MDM may vary with each encounter for the same patient even when the patient's condition remains the same. This complexity is determined by assessing the level at which 2 of 3 elements of MDM are performed and supported in the documentation of an encounter. The 3 elements of MDM are

1. The number and complexity of problem(s) addressed during the encounter
2. The amount and/or complexity of data to be reviewed and analyzed
3. The risk of complications, morbidity, and/or mortality of patient management choices and decisions made at the visit

Four levels of MDM complexity are recognized, as follows:

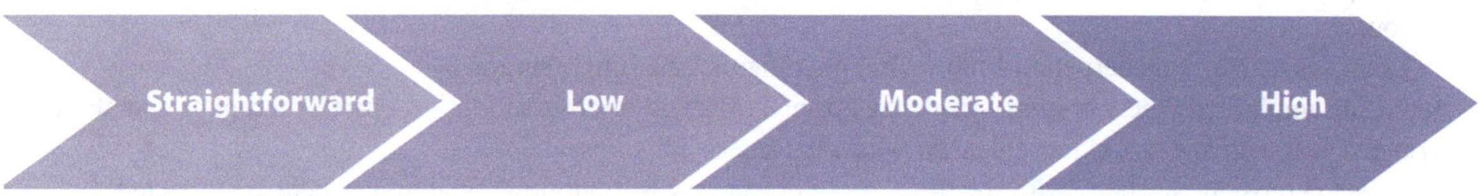

Each level of MDM is based on the same criteria whether the patient is new or established or the encounter is initial or subsequent.

Number and Complexity of Problems Addressed

The first step in determining the level of MDM for an encounter is identification of the number and complexity of problems addressed, with emphasis on the complexity. A problem is a disease, condition, illness, injury, symptom, sign, finding, concern, or other matter addressed at the encounter, with or without a diagnosis being established at the time of the encounter.

- Include all problems addressed at an encounter in the number and complexity of problems. Refer to the "Coding Conundrum: Addressed or Not Addressed" box that follows for guidance on problems considered to have been addressed.
- Complexity is determined by the type of problem(s) addressed. *CPT* instructs that
  - The final diagnosis for a condition does not, in and of itself, determine the complexity or risk of the problem, as extensive evaluation may be required to reach the conclusion that the signs or symptoms do not represent a highly morbid condition.
  - Manifesting symptoms that are likely to represent a highly morbid condition may drive MDM even when the ultimate diagnosis is not highly morbid.

Coding Conundrum: Addressed or Not Addressed

A problem is considered addressed or managed when evaluated or treated at the encounter by the physician or other QHP reporting the service.

- This includes consideration of further testing or treatment that may not be performed because of the risk-benefit analysis or choice of the patient, parent, guardian, or surrogate.
- When determining the level of MDM, do not consider the following addressed or managed by the physician or QHP reporting the service:
  - × A notation in the patient's medical record that another professional is managing the problem without additional assessment or care coordination
  - × Referral without evaluation (by history, examination, or ≥1 diagnostic studies) or consideration of treatment
  - × Problems listed in the medical record but not addressed at the current encounter

Defining Problems Addressed for Inpatient and Observation Services

For hospital inpatient and observation care services, select the complexity of the problem addressed according to the problem status on the date of the encounter, which may differ significantly from that on admission. For example, an encounter with a patient who was admitted in respiratory distress but who presents with no distress at the current encounter may include a lower number and complexity of problems addressed than that of prior encounters in the same admission. Likewise, a patient's condition may deteriorate such that problems at subsequent encounters are of higher complexity than at admission.

Problem(s) managed or comanaged by a reporting physician or QHP may not be the cause of admission or continued stay (eg, addressing a coexisting condition).

CPT does not provide examples of problems included in each level of MDM and instead leaves the determination to the reporting individual's clinical judgment. Examples included in this manual may not apply to all patient encounters.

The level of problem addressed for services reported with **99211** or **99281**, in which the presence of the physician or QHP is not required, is not defined because the concept of the level of MDM does not apply.

Following are definitions for the types of problems identified in each level of MDM:

Straightforward or minimal: Self-limited or minor. A problem that runs a definite and prescribed course, is transient in nature, and is not likely to permanently alter health status.

Low

- Two or more self-limited or minor problems.
- Acute, uncomplicated illness or injury. A recent or new short-term problem with low risk of morbidity for which treatment *is considered.*
  - Little to no risk of mortality with treatment and full recovery without functional impairment are expected.
  - The problem may be a self-limited or minor one that is not resolving consistently with a definite and prescribed course.
  - Examples may include herpetic whitlow, viral pharyngitis, or a simple sprain.
- Acute, uncomplicated illness or injury requiring hospital inpatient or observation-level care. A recent or new short-term problem with low risk of morbidity for which treatment *is required.*
  - Little to no risk of mortality with treatment and full recovery without functional impairment are expected.
  - The treatment required is delivered in a hospital inpatient or observation-level setting.

- Stable acute illness. A problem that is new or recent for which treatment has been initiated. The patient is improved and, although resolution may not be complete, is stable with respect to this condition.
- Stable chronic illness. A problem *with an expected duration of at least 1 year* or until the death of the patient, *for whom the risk of morbidity is significant without treatment.*
  - *Stable* is defined by the individual patient's specific treatment goals. A patient who is not at their treatment goal is not stable, even if the condition has not changed and there is no short-term threat to life or function.
  - Examples of stable chronic illness may include well-controlled attention-deficit/hyperactivity disorder, asthma, cystic fibrosis, allergic rhinitis, or diabetes.

Conditions are considered chronic whether or not stage or severity changes (eg, uncontrolled diabetes and controlled diabetes are a single chronic condition).

Moderate

- Two or more stable chronic illnesses.
- Chronic illness with exacerbation, progression, or side effects of treatment. Acutely worsening, poorly controlled, or progressing with an intent to control progression, *requiring additional supportive care or requiring attention to treatment of side effects.*
  - Examples include mild to moderate exacerbation of asthma, generalized anxiety disorder now with school avoidance, and attention-deficit/hyperactivity disorder with weight loss secondary to treatment.
- Acute, complicated injury. Requires evaluation of body systems that are not directly part of the injured organ, extensive injury, multiple treatment options, and/or association with risk of morbidity (eg, head injury with brief loss of consciousness).
- Acute illness with systemic symptoms. An illness causing systemic symptoms and *carrying a high risk of morbidity without treatment.*
  - For systemic general symptoms (eg, fever, body aches, fatigue) in a minor illness that may be treated to alleviate symptoms, refer to *self-limited or minor* or *acute, uncomplicated illness.*
  - Systemic symptoms may not be general but may be single system (eg, *Clostridioides difficile* colitis with just diarrhea).
  - Examples may include pyelonephritis or bacterial gastroenteritis.
- Undiagnosed new problem with uncertain prognosis. A problem in the differential diagnosis that represents a condition *likely to result in a high risk of morbidity without treatment.* Examples may include unexplained bruising, anterior neck mass, unexpected weight loss, and school failure.

Coding Conundrum: Acute, Uncomplicated, or Acute Illness With Systemic Symptoms

When a patient presents with a systemic symptom such as fever, the physician or QHP must determine whether the condition is an acute, uncomplicated illness (ie, a low-complexity problem) with systemic symptoms that are managed to alleviate the patient's discomfort or an acute illness with systemic symptoms that requires treatment because the risk of morbidity is high without treatment (ie, a moderate-complexity problem). For instance, when the problem addressed at the encounter requires medication to prevent complications, such as with pyelonephritis (when not requiring hospitalization), the problem meets the criteria for an acute illness with systemic symptoms. But fever in conjunction with a common cold with advice to use an appropriate over-the-counter medication to alleviate fever and discomfort does not change an acute, uncomplicated problem to an acute illness with systemic symptoms. When in doubt of the risk of morbidity and complexity of the problem addressed, a coder should seek the clinical judgment of the reporting physician or QHP.

Physicians and QHPs are not required to document risks commonly associated with a condition, but appropriate documentation of the assessment and plan of care supports the number and complexity of problems addressed at each visit. Factors that are unique to the patient presentation and that increase the risk of not treating a problem should be documented (eg, temporary change in asthma care to prevent exacerbation due to influenza, a congenital condition such as DiGeorge syndrome that influences management, severity of the problem [eg, moderate to severe bulging of tympanic membrane with temperature of 39.0 °C (102.2 °F) in otitis media]). Codes for complicating conditions should be included on the claim.

Fever has different indications based on factors such as a patient's age, developmental status, and medical history. To review an illustration of acute illness with fever across the spectrum of MDM, refer to the "Continuum Model for Fever in the Emergency Department" in **Chapter 14.**

Although the risk of morbidity without treatment is a consideration in determining the nature of the problem addressed, this problem-related risk is different from the separate element of risk of mortality or morbidity of management (ie, problem risk is distinct from patient management risk).

High

- Chronic illness with severe exacerbation, progression, or side effects of treatment. Severe exacerbation or progression of chronic illness or severe side effects of treatment with significant risk of morbidity that may require escalation in the level of care.
- Acute or chronic illness or injury posing a threat to life or bodily function. Acute illness with systemic symptoms or an acute, complicated injury, or a chronic illness or injury with exacerbation and/or progression or side effects of treatment, that poses a threat to life or bodily function in the near term without treatment.
  - Some symptoms may represent a condition that is significantly probable and poses a potential threat to life or bodily function. These may be included in this category when the evaluation and treatment is consistent with this degree of potential severity.
  - Examples may include severe respiratory distress, psychiatric illness with threat to self or others, acute renal failure, or an abrupt change in neurological status.

Determination of the type of problem addressed may require a pediatrician's clinical judgment. Coding staff should query the pediatrician when unsure of the appropriate types of problems addressed at an encounter (eg, self-limited vs acute, uncomplicated illness).

Table 6-1 provides a quick reference to the number and complexity of problems for each level of MDM.

Table 6-1. Number and Complexity of Problems Addressed at Encounter

Level of Medical Decision-Making	Problem(s) Addressed
Not applicable	(Refer to 99211, 99281.)
Straightforward	***Minimal*** 1 self-limited or minor problem
Low	≥2 self-limited or minor problems 1 acute, uncomplicated illness or injury 1 stable chronic illness 1 stable acute illness 1 acute, uncomplicated illness or injury requiring hospital inpatient or observation level of care
Moderate	2 stable chronic illnesses 1 chronic illness with exacerbation, progression, or side effects of treatment 1 acute, complicated injury 1 acute illness with systemic symptoms 1 undiagnosed new problem with uncertain prognosis
High	1 chronic illness with severe exacerbation, progression, or side effects of treatment 1 acute/chronic illness or injury posing a threat to life or bodily function

The following examples focus only on identification of the level of problem addressed. Can you identify the type of problem(s) addressed in each example?

Examples

➤ **Parents bring a newborn to the pediatrician with concerns regarding a rash on the newborn's face.** Examination reveals uncomplicated neonatal acne.

Problem(s) addressed ➡ *Minimal*

Teaching Point: The uncomplicated neonatal acne is a self-limited or minor problem.

➤ **A patient presents for follow-up evaluation of upper respiratory symptoms.** The patient's symptoms are consistent with a mild upper respiratory infection (URI).

Problem(s) addressed ➡ *Low*

Teaching Point: The cold is an acute, uncomplicated problem.

➤ **Hyperbilirubinemia requiring therapy is diagnosed in a neonate 30 hours after birth.**
Problem(s) addressed ➡ ***Moderate***
Teaching Point: The patient has an acute illness with systemic symptoms.

➤ **A patient presents to a pediatrician's office in moderate respiratory distress that worsens, requiring management before emergency transport.**
Problem(s) addressed ➡ ***High***
Teaching Point: The worsening respiratory distress in this patient represents a high-complexity problem.

➤ **A 16-month-old patient is admitted for E/M of new-onset neurological inflammatory disease with transverse myelitis, optic neuritis, and negative infectious disease workup.**
Problem(s) addressed ➡ ***High***
Teaching Point: The patient's injuries pose a threat to life or bodily function.

Amount and/or Complexity of Data to Be Reviewed and Analyzed

Data are divided into the following 3 categories:

1. Tests, documents, orders, or requirement for an independent historian(s) (Each unique test, order, or document is counted to meet a threshold number.)
2. Independent interpretation of tests not separately reported
3. Discussion of management or test interpretation with external physician or QHP or appropriate source when not separately reported

In straightforward MDM, minimal or no data review is performed. When data are used in support of higher levels of MDM, the requirements for either 1 or 2 categories of data must be met. Instructions are provided for each level of data. **Table 6-2** shows the data requirements for limited, moderate, and extensive amounts and/or complexity of data that correspond to low, moderate, and high MDM, respectively, when either the problems addressed or data reviewed support that level of MDM.

Note that Category 1 includes multiple types of data that may be combined to meet a limited, moderate, or extensive amount and/or complexity of data. Following are examples of data combinations that would support a limited level of data:

- Review of external notes from 2 unique sources
- Order or review of results of 2 unique tests (represented by separate *CPT* codes)
- Review of external notes from 1 unique source and order or review of results of 1 unique test

CPT E/M guidelines include definitions for these types of data. Most of these definitions are included in the examples provided later in this section.

It is important to understand how tests contribute to the amount and/or complexity of data to be reviewed and analyzed.

- Tests include imaging, laboratory, or psychometric/physiologic data. Pulse oximetry is not a test for purposes of the amount and/or complexity of data to be reviewed and analyzed.
- Each unique test is counted once toward the amount and/or complexity of data. Do not count both the order for and the review of the same unique test.
- When a test with multiple components can be reported with a single code (eg, **80047**, basic metabolic panel or a test with a specific number of images), count the test once for the purpose of data to be reviewed and analyzed.
- Any test for which the reporting individual or another individual of the same specialty and same group practice will separately report a code for interpretation and report is not counted toward the data analyzed at the encounter.

The following examples illustrate different levels of data to be reviewed and analyzed. Can you identify the amount and/or complexity of data to be reviewed in each example?

Examples

➤ **A 17-year-old presents with poison ivy.**
Data reviewed and analyzed ➡ ***Minimal or none***

Table 6-2. Amount and Complexity of Data in Medical Decision-Making

Limited *Must meet the requirements of 1 of 2 categories*	**Category 1: Tests and documents** Any combination of 2 from the following data: • Review of prior external note(s) from each unique source[a] • Review of the result(s) of each unique test[a] • Ordering of each unique test[a] **Category 2: Assessment requiring an independent historian(s)**
Moderate *Must meet the requirements of 1 of 3 categories*	**Category 1: Tests, documents, or independent historian(s)** Any combination of 3 from the following data: • Review of prior external note(s) from each unique source[a] • Review of the result(s) of each unique test[a] • Ordering of each unique test[a] • Assessment requiring an independent historian(s) **Category 2: Independent interpretation of tests performed by another physician/other QHP (not separately reported)** **Category 3: Discussion of management or test interpretation with external physician/other QHP/appropriate source (not separately reported)**
Extensive *Must meet the requirements of at least 2 of 3 categories*	**Category 1: Tests, documents, or independent historian(s)** Any combination of 3 from the following data: • Review of prior external note(s) from each unique source[a] • Review of the result(s) of each unique test[a] • Ordering of each unique test[a] • Assessment requiring an independent historian(s) **Category 2: Independent interpretation of tests performed by another physician/other QHP (not separately reported)** **Category 3: Discussion of management or test interpretation with external physician/other QHP/appropriate source (not separately reported)**

Abbreviation: QHP, qualified health care professional.

[a] Each unique test, order, or document is counted.

➤ **A 16-year-old established patient presents for follow-up of URI symptoms.** The patient was evaluated at an urgent care practice 2 days ago, but symptoms have increased. The physician reviews records of the urgent care visit, which include a diagnosis of a URI. An influenza test is ordered and its results are positive.

Data reviewed and analyzed ➡ ***Limited*** (Category 1)

Teaching Point: The combination of a review of external records from 1 source and an order for 1 test supports a limited amount and complexity of data to be reviewed and analyzed. If an independent historian were required (eg, to provide details of medical history that the patient cannot) in addition to the external records reviewed and test ordered, the level of data would be moderate.

External records, communications, and/or test results are those from an external physician, QHP, facility, or health care organization or from another appropriate source (eg, teacher, lawyer, case manager). *Review of all materials from any unique source counts once toward MDM.*

➤ **A 3-year-old patient presents with a splinter of the thumb.** The patient's mother advises that removal attempts at home were unsuccessful. The splinter is removed without incision.

Data reviewed and analyzed ➡ ***Limited*** (Category 2)

Teaching Point: Data are limited because assessment requires an independent historian.

An independent historian is an individual (eg, parent, guardian, surrogate, witness) who provides a history in addition to one provided by a patient who is unable to do so completely or reliably (eg, because of developmental stage or loss of consciousness) or because of a confirmatory history that is judged to be necessary.

If there may be conflict or poor communication between multiple historians and more than one historian is needed, the independent historian(s) requirement is met, but no higher level of data is met with multiple independent historians.

➤ **An established patient presents for follow-up regarding persistent headaches and fatigue.** Results of tests ordered at the previous visit were reviewed between visits, and 2 additional tests were ordered and completed before this visit. The physician reviews the results of the additional tests and discusses the findings and treatment recommendation with the patient and parents.

Data reviewed and analyzed ➡ ***Limited*** (Category 1)

Teaching Point: The review of 2 unique test results supports a limited level of data to be reviewed and analyzed. Even though 4 total tests were reviewed, the credit for ordering and reviewing the first 2 tests was applied to the initial visit and may not be counted again.

If obtaining history from the parents was required, the combination of 2 tests ordered and requirement for an independent historian would support a moderate complexity of data by meeting 3 items included in Category 1.

When tests are ordered *between encounters,* the new test results are counted toward the level of data reviewed and analyzed. Review of results for tests ordered at a prior E/M service is included in the order and not counted again at the next encounter.

➤ **A 5-month-old presents with suspected viral bronchiolitis.** The parents provide the patient's medical, family, and social history. Respiratory viral panel (eg, **87631**, infectious agent detection by nucleic acid [DNA or RNA]; 3–5 targets) and chest radiography with 2 views (**71046**) are ordered. A radiologist will interpret the radiograph and report the findings.

Data reviewed and analyzed ➡ ***Moderate*** (3 items in Category 1)

Teaching Point: A moderate level of data may be supported by any combination of 3 of the following Category 1 data: review of prior external note(s) from each unique source, order or review of the result(s) of each unique test, or assessment requiring an independent historian(s). In this example, the patient's parents are independent historians and the physician orders 2 unique tests (respiratory viral panel and chest radiography).

If the individual reporting the E/M service also reported the professional component of interpretation and report of the chest radiograph, the test would not be included in the amount and/or complexity of data for this encounter. When billing for interpretation and report of test findings, do not include the order or review of test findings in the data element of MDM.

If the individual reporting the E/M service independently reviewed the images and documented an impression to inform MDM prior to receipt of a radiologist's formal interpretation, the independent interpretation (Category 2 data) in combination with the Category 1 data would support a high amount and/or complexity of data.

The differentiation between single or multiple unique tests is defined in accordance with the *CPT* code assignment. Services reported with 1 code (imaging with multiple views) are 1 test.

Tests considered but not ordered or performed after shared decision-making with the patient/caregivers may be counted toward the amount and complexity of data. Shared decision-making includes soliciting preferences, providing education, and explaining risks and benefits associated with testing.

➤ **A patient is seen by an attending physician for initial care following admission the previous evening for altered mental status with history of headache for the past 4 days.** The parents provide the patient's history. The attending physician discusses the case with an infectious disease consultant before ordering a lumbar puncture and magnetic resonance imaging.

Data reviewed and analyzed ➡ ***High*** (Categories 1 and 3)

Teaching Point: A high level of data may be supported not only by Category 1 given the history from an independent historian and 2 tests ordered but also by Category 3 given the discussion of management or test interpretation with an external physician, other QHP, or other appropriate source when the discussion is not separately reported (eg, not reported as an interprofessional consultation [**99452**]).

External physicians or other QHPs are individuals who are not in the same group practice or are of a different specialty or subspecialty, including licensed professionals who are practicing independently. A facility or organizational provider such as a hospital, nursing facility, or home health care agency may also be an independent source.

Appropriate sources are professionals who are not in health care but may be involved in the treatment of the patient. Examples include lawyers, case managers, nonclinical social workers, or teachers. *Family or informal caregivers are inappropriate sources,* although they may be independent historians. Documents from an appropriate source may be counted for the purpose of documents reviewed.

Discussion requires all the following components: is an interactive and direct exchange between the reporting individual and external physician, QHP, or other appropriate source; may be asynchronous but completed within a short period; and is used in MDM for the encounter. Sending medical record notes (eg, consultation report) or a written exchange within medical record notes is not an interactive exchange.

➤ **A 15-year-old established patient presents for follow-up regarding type 1 diabetes with poor control.** The physician reviews results of 2 tests performed as a recurring order from a prior visit (eg, testing repeated 1 week before each visit). The parents provide the patient's medical, family, and social history since the previous visit.

Data reviewed and analyzed ➡ ***Moderate*** (3 items in Category 1)

Teaching Point: The review of 2 unique test results and use of an independent historian support a moderate amount and complexity of data. With a recurring order, only the initial result is included in the order. Count each additional result toward the level of data reviewed and analyzed in the visit in which it is analyzed. For example, an order for a blood glucose test to be performed every 2 months includes review of the initial test result, but future blood glucose test results count in the encounter at which the result is used in patient management.

Comparison of multiple results of the same unique test (eg, a new blood glucose test result is compared with previous results) is counted as review of 1 unique test result.

➤ **A 6-year-old new patient presents with fever, cough, and vomiting for 2 days.** The parents provide history of fever as high as 39 °C (102 °F) that started yesterday, coughing for 2 weeks, and now vomiting for 2 days. Chest radiography and an influenza test are ordered. The physician independently reviews the chest radiograph (pending receipt of the radiologist's report).

Data reviewed and analyzed ➡ ***Extensive*** (Categories 1 and 2)

Teaching Point: In this example, the requirements of categories 1 and 2 are met, supporting an extensive level of data. Category 1 is met with orders for 2 unique tests and an assessment requiring an independent historian. Category 2 is met by independent interpretation of a test reported by another physician or QHP. The order for and independent interpretation of the same test (eg, chest radiography) contribute separately to the amount and/or complexity of data.

Independent interpretation is the interpretation of a test for which there is a *CPT* code and an interpretation or report is included in the code descriptor. This does not apply when the same physician or QHP (or physician or QHP of the same group practice and same specialty) is providing or has previously provided an interpretation and report for the test.

Documentation of pertinent findings from review of an image or a tracing is sufficient, rather than the typical documentation completed when providing and billing for an interpretation and report.

Both independent interpretation of a test and discussion of the test result with the interpreting physician can be counted when both are performed for the same encounter.

➤ **A 12-year-old patient presents to a pediatrician with intermittent chest pain and pallor.** History is obtained from the patient's mother. A complete blood cell count and ECG are ordered. The ECG tracing is independently reviewed prior to formal interpretation and report by a cardiologist.

Data reviewed and analyzed ➡ ***Extensive*** (Categories 1 and 2)

Teaching Point: The extensive level of data reviewed and analyzed is based on 2 unique tests ordered, assessment requiring an independent historian, and independent interpretation of a test by a physician not reporting a code for the interpretation and report of the findings.

The independent history does not need to be obtained in person but does need to be obtained directly from the historian providing the independent information (eg, via telephone).

Risk of Complications and/or Morbidity or Mortality of Patient Management

Risk is the probability and/or consequences of an event. For the purpose of code selection, the level of risk considers the risk of morbidity from additional diagnostic testing or treatment considered at that encounter. Risk also includes MDM related to the need to initiate or forgo further testing, treatment, and/or hospitalization.

Morbidity is a state of illness or functional impairment that is expected to be of substantial duration during which function is limited, quality of life is impaired, or organ damage may not be transient despite treatment.

The risk of patient management criteria applies to the reporting physician's or QHP's patient management decisions associated with the diagnostic procedure(s) and treatment(s) during the reported encounter. *Although condition risk and management risk may often correlate, the risk resulting from the condition is distinct from the risk of the management.*

- Definitions of risk are based on the usual behavior and thought processes of a physician or QHP in the same specialty. That includes the risk of a decision regarding parenteral controlled substances that may or may not be associated with high risk of morbidity.
- Trained clinicians apply common meanings to terms such as *high, medium, low,* or *minimal risk* and do not require quantification for these definitions (quantification may be provided when evidence-based medicine has established probabilities).

***CPT* provides some examples of risk for purposes of code selection. However, these are examples only and are not requirements or restrictions on the physician's or QHP's assessment of risk.**

***CPT* does not include examples of minimal or low risk. Coders should seek guidance from a physician or QHP if unsure of the risk associated with a treatment or management option. For example, a decision to use an over-the-counter medication for a patient who is younger than the age indicated on the product label may carry higher risk than a decision to use it in a patient who is within the indicated age range.**

- Assessment of the level of risk is affected by the nature of the event under consideration. For example, a low probability of death may be high-risk, whereas a high chance of a minor, self-limited adverse effect of treatment may be low-risk. *Social determinants of health (SDoH) may also influence the risk of management decisions.*

SDoH are economic and social conditions that influence the health of people and communities. Examples may include food, housing, or transportation insecurity.

- Risk includes the possible management options selected, and those considered but not selected, after shared decision-making with the patient and/or family. For example, a decision about hospitalization includes consideration of alternative levels of care.

Shared decision-making is soliciting patient and/or family preferences and patient and/or family education and explaining risks and benefits of management options.

Risk levels are minimal, low, moderate, and high. **Table 6-3** lists examples of each level of risk.

The following examples provide information to identify a level of risk of management or treatment decisions made at an encounter. Can you identify the level of risk for each example?

Table 6-3. Examples of Levels of Risk

Minimal	Rest and plenty of fluids Diaper ointment Superficial wound dressing
Low	Over-the-counter medication(s) following directions as labeled Removal of sutures Physical, speech, or occupational therapy
Moderate	Prescription drug management or recommendation for off-label use of an over-the-counter medication Decision about minor surgery with identified patient or procedure risk factors Decision about elective major surgery without identified patient or procedure risk factors Diagnosis or treatment significantly limited by SDoH
High	Drug therapy requiring intensive monitoring for toxicity (eg, monitoring for a cytopenia in the use of an antineoplastic agent between dose cycles) Decision about hospitalization or escalation of hospital level of care Decision regarding elective major surgery with identified patient or procedure risk factors Decision about emergency major surgery (immediately performed or minimally delayed to allow for patient stabilization) Decision not to resuscitate or to de-escalate care because prognosis is poor Decision regarding parenteral controlled substances

Abbreviation: SDoH, social determinants of health.

[a] Examples are subject to clinical judgment for each individual patient and encounter.

Examples

➤ **A patient presents for follow-up after treatment of impetigo.** The patient appears well and the parents have no concerns but need clearance to return to child care. Clearance to return to child care is provided. The patient is to return as needed or at the next scheduled preventive visit.

Risk of patient management ➡ *Minimal to none*

➤ **A 6-year-old patient presents with resolving chronic constipation.** A pediatrician recommends continued daily use of an over-the-counter laxative until regular bowel movements are established.

Risk of patient management ➡ *Low*

➤ **A physician sees a 6-year-old patient who presents with an injury to their left leg.** A fracture is diagnosed, and repair under general anesthesia is recommended. The parents agree to proceed with the procedure.

Risk of patient management ➡ *Moderate or high*

Teaching Point: Decision for major surgery supports moderate risk when elective or high-risk when performed immediately or with minimal delay to allow for patient stabilization.

Risk of Surgery

In determining risk associated with a decision about surgery, the surgical package classification does not determine whether the procedure is minor or major. *CPT* states that the classification of surgery into minor or major is based on the common meaning of such terms when used by trained clinicians. Risk factors are those relevant to the patient and the procedure.

➤ **A 14-year-old presents for follow-up for asthma.** The patient's asthma is well controlled, and a refill of control medication is prescribed.

Risk of patient management ➡ *Moderate*

Teaching Point: The prescription medication presents a moderate risk.

➤ **A 6-year-old patient is evaluated for symptoms of acute gastroenteritis.** After examination, the pediatrician recommends hospitalization for management of dehydration.

Risk of patient management ➡ ***High***

Teaching Point: The risk associated with the decision to hospitalize the ill child is high. A decision for aggressive outpatient follow-up as an alternative to hospitalization may also support a high level of risk.

Selection of Codes Based on MDM

To select a code for E/M services based on MDM (rather than the physician's or QHP's total time), you must determine which code is supported by 2 of 3 elements of MDM. Refer to **Table 6-4** for an at-a-glance reminder of the levels of MDM.

Following are key points to remember in code selection:

- Examples given are not clinical recommendations, and levels of service supported may vary depending on documentation and patient age and presentation (eg, patient's immunization status).
- Select a code *on the basis of either* total physician and/or QHP time on the DOS or MDM.
- Use of new versus established patient codes is based on whether the patient has received any face-to-face professional service from the same physician or a physician in the same group practice of the same exact specialty and subspecialty in the 3 years before the DOS.
- Use of initial versus subsequent care codes is based on whether the patient has received any professional services from the physician or QHP or another physician or QHP of the exact same specialty and subspecialty who belongs to the same group practice during the current inpatient or observation or nursing facility admission/stay.
- Although *CPT* does not specify required documentation to support a level of MDM, the documentation should include the medically appropriate history and/or examination findings and support the diagnostic, management, and treatment decisions made during the encounter.

The following examples provide information sufficient to select a level of service according to the level of MDM. The actual code assigned will vary depending on the site of service. Can you identify the level of MDM in each example?

Examples

➤ **A patient encounter includes instruction to keep an uninfected bugbite clean and apply a simple bandage to prevent scratching.** No tests are ordered and no results are reviewed. History is obtained from the patient's mother given the patient's developmental status.

Problem(s) addressed ➡ ***Minimal*** (self-limited problem)

Data reviewed and analyzed ➡ ***Limited*** (independent historian)

Risk of patient management ➡ ***Minimal*** (simple wound cleansing and bandage)

Teaching Point: The level of MDM is straightforward. Although the amount and/or complexity of data to be reviewed and analyzed could support a low level of MDM, 2 of 3 elements must be met to support a level of MDM. The problems and risk at this encounter limit the level of MDM to straightforward.

➤ **A patient encounter includes addressing stable type 1 diabetes with history from parents, orders for and review of results for 2 unique tests (eg, hemoglobin A_{1c} level and urinalysis), reviewed insulin management, and renewed prescription of insulin.**

Problem(s) addressed ➡ ***Low*** (single stable chronic illness)

Data reviewed and analyzed ➡ ***Moderate*** (Category 1—independent historian and order/review of 2 tests)

Risk of patient management ➡ ***Moderate*** (prescription drug management)

Teaching Point: The level of MDM is moderate because both data reviewed and risk support this level of service.

➤ **Parents of a child with a life-threatening condition receive counseling regarding options for continuing hospitalization versus home care directed by a palliative care physician.** The parents elect palliative care, and the attending physician requests a palliative care consultation.

Problem(s) addressed ➡ ***High*** (1 acute or chronic illness or injury that poses a threat to life or bodily function)

Data reviewed and analyzed ➡ ***Not indicated in this scenario***

Risk of patient management ➡ ***High*** (decision to de-escalate care because of poor prognosis)

Teaching Point: The level of MDM is high given the problem addressed and the risk. Two of 3 elements are sufficient to support the level of MDM.

Table 6-4. Medical Decision-Making Requirements

	Medical Decision-Making (2 of 3 Required: Data,[a] Problems, Risk)		
Level of MDM	**Problems Addressed**	**Data Reviewed and Analyzed[b]**	**Risk**
Straightforward	1 self-limited or minor problem	Minimal or none	Minimal *Examples* • Rest and plenty of fluids • Diaper ointment • Superficial wound dressing
Low	Low—*Any 1 of* ≥2 self-limited or minor problems 1 stable chronic illness 1 acute, uncomplicated illness or injury 1 stable acute illness 1 acute, uncomplicated illness or injury requiring hospital inpatient or observation level of care	Limited (*Meet 1 of 2 categories*) Category 1: Tests and documents (*Any 2*) • Review of prior external note(s)—each unique source • Review of the result(s) of each unique test • Ordering of each unique test Category 2: Assessment requiring an independent historian(s)	Low *Examples* • Over-the-counter medication(s) • Removal of sutures • Physical, language, or occupational therapy • Decision regarding minor surgery without identified patient or procedure risk factors
Moderate	Moderate—*Any 1 of* ≥1 chronic illness with exacerbation, progression, or side effects of treatment ≥2 stable chronic illnesses 1 undiagnosed new problem with uncertain prognosis 1 acute illness with systemic symptoms 1 acute, complicated injury	Moderate (*Meet 1 of 3 categories*) Category 1 (*Any 3*) • Review of prior external note(s)—each unique source • Review of the result(s) of each unique test • Ordering of each unique test • Assessment requiring an independent historian(s) Category 2: Independent interpretation of a test performed by another physician/other QHP[b] Category 3: Discussion of management or test interpretation with external physician/other QHP/appropriate source[b]	Moderate *Examples* • Prescription drug management or off-label use of an over-the-counter medication • Decision about minor surgery with identified patient or procedure risk factors • Decision about elective major surgery without identified patient or procedure risk factors • Diagnosis or treatment significantly limited by SDoH
High	High—*Any 1 of* ≥1 chronic illness with severe exacerbation, progression, or side effects of treatment 1 acute or chronic illness or injury that poses a threat to life or bodily function	Extensive (*Meet 2 of 3 categories*) Category 1 (*Any 3*) • Review of prior external note(s) from each unique source • Review of the result(s) of each unique test • Ordering of each unique test • Assessment requiring an independent historian(s) Category 2: Independent interpretation of a test performed by another physician/other QHP[b] Category 3: Discussion of management or test interpretation with external physician/other QHP/appropriate source[b]	High *Examples* • Drug therapy requiring intensive monitoring for toxicity • Decision about hospitalization or escalation of hospital level of care • Decision regarding elective major surgery with identified patient or procedure risk factors • Decision about emergency major surgery • Decision not to resuscitate or to de-escalate care because prognosis is poor • Decision regarding parenteral controlled substances

Abbreviations: SDoH, social determinants of health; QHP, qualified health care professional.

[a] Each unique test, order, or document contributes to the combination of 2 or combination of 3 in Category 1.

[b] Do not count data review or communications reported with other codes (eg, test interpretation, interprofessional consultation).

Refer to other chapters discussing specific types of E/M services for more examples. For a quick reference to E/M coding, refer to the American Academy of Pediatrics (AAP) *Pediatric Evaluation and Management: Coding Quick Reference Card 2026* (www.aap.org/Pediatric-Evaluation-and-Management-Coding-Quick-Reference-Card-2026).

Split or Shared Visits

CPT guidelines define a split or shared visit as one during which physicians and QHPs act as a team providing an E/M service (all work performed on a single DOS). Unlike Medicare policy, the *CPT* guideline does not limit application of the split/shared visit guidelines to services provided in a facility setting. (Medicare applies an incident-to policy to split/shared visits in an office or other outpatient setting, as discussed in **Chapter 7**.)

The *CPT* guidelines apply to all split/shared E/M services. When physicians and QHPs work as a team providing an E/M service, the service is reported by the professional who performed the substantive portion of it. The substantive portion of the service is defined in either of the following ways:

- When code selection is based on time, the professional who spent the most time on that date in activities of an E/M service provided to the individual patient will report the service.
- When code selection for a split/shared visit is based on MDM, the professional who performed 2 of 3 elements of MDM has performed the substantive portion and reports the E/M service.
  - When the number and complexity of problems addressed at the encounter are one of the elements supporting the level of MDM, the professional who made or approved the management plan for the problem(s) addressed and who accepts the inherent risks of the management plan is considered to have performed the substantive portion of the service.
  - When the amount and/or complexity of data to be reviewed and analyzed is one of the elements by which the level of MDM is determined, the following guidance applies:
    - Consider the documented history from an independent historian and documented tests ordered or results/documents reviewed to have been used by the professional in formulating the management plan. The professional reporting the service does not have to personally perform these activities.
    - An independent interpretation of a test or discussion of management with an external physician is used only in selecting the amount and/or complexity of data to be reviewed and analyzed *when personally performed by the individual reporting the service.*

Modifier FS (split/shared E/M visit) must be appended to E/M codes when reporting to a payer that has adopted Medicare policy for split/shared visits. Modifier FS may not be required by all payers.

CPT does not address documentation of split/shared visits. A physician and QHP may each personally document their work in a split/shared visit; this may be 2 separate entries in the medical record or an initial entry with an addendum by the individual who provides services later on the same date. Medicare policy requires that documentation identify the physician and other QHP who performed the visit and that the individual reporting the service sign and date the documentation of the split/shared visit.

Examples

➤ **An NP provides initial observation care to a patient in the hospital.** After initially evaluating the patient, the NP spends 5 minutes discussing the patient's condition and management options with a physician in her same group practice and specialty and documents a total time of 25 minutes, including the time of the phone call with the physician. Later, on the same date, the physician of the same group practice and specialty reviews the patient's progress notes and test results since admission to observation and, after reevaluating the patient, agrees with continuing the current management overnight. The physician's total time is 25 minutes *including the 5 minutes of phone conversation with the NP earlier that day.*

Code **99221** (initial hospital inpatient or observation care; 40 minutes must be met or exceeded) is reported for the 45-minute total time of service.

Teaching Point: The 5-minute conversation between the physician and NP is counted by only 1 of the professionals for purposes of determining the combined total time of 45 minutes. If beneficial for the physician to report the service, adding the time on the phone call to the physician's time would support the substantive portion of the service (ie, 25 minutes vs the NP's 20 minutes) and support billing under the name and National Provider Identification number of the physician.

The individual providing the first visit may not document with an expectation that another visit will be provided by someone in the same specialty and same group practice later on that same date. Beware of overlap in separately documented total time.

Whether the physician or NP reports the service may depend on policy established by the individual payer or billing and compliance policies of the group practice.

➤ **An NP provides initial hospital care to a patient who is admitted from the ED under observation status for ongoing management of a moderate asthma exacerbation.** The NP reviews the ED record, including results of tests ordered in the ED, and documents history from the patient's parents. The NP orders inhalation treatments to be administered every 2 hours and continuation of oxygen and enteral steroids. The NP's documentation supports moderate MDM.

A few hours later, a physician from the same group practice and same specialty as the NP is called to see the patient, who is not responding adequately to treatment. The physician examines the patient, reviews the patient's hospital record, and decides to admit the patient to the pediatric intensive care unit for impending respiratory failure. The physician's documentation supports high MDM.

Teaching Point: A single initial hospital inpatient and observation care code for the service is reported according to the level of MDM supported in the combined documentation of the NP and physician.

Problem(s) addressed ➡ ***High*** (an illness that poses a threat to life or bodily function in the near term without treatment)

Data reviewed and analyzed ➡ ***Moderate*** (Category 1—based on the NP's documentation of history from the parents and review of multiple laboratory results)

Risk of patient management ➡ ***High*** (based on decision regarding escalation in the level of hospital care)

The physician reports 99223 because there is a high level of MDM supported by the problems addressed and risk of management decisions made at the physician's visit. Modifier FS is appended to indicate the split/shared visit, when required by the payer.

Payer policies for reporting split/shared visits may vary. Practices should learn and monitor updates to payer policies to support appropriate documentation and reporting.

Refer to **Chapter 17** for more information on reporting split/shared services in a hospital setting.

Teaching Physician Guidelines for Reporting E/M Services

Refer to Chapter 18 for the teaching physician guidelines for billing surgical, high-risk, or other complex procedures.

- Payment is made when a teaching physician involves a resident in providing care only if the teaching physician is present for the key or critical portions of the service except when a primary care exception, as discussed in the Primary Care Exception Rule section later in this chapter, applies.

For residency training sites of a teaching setting that are rural (outside a metropolitan statistical area), the CMS allows use of real-time audiovisual communication to interact with the resident to meet the requirement of being present for the key portion of a service, including telehealth services. This provision does not allow use of audio-only (eg, telephone) communication, and the communication must be real-time to allow the teaching physician to observe the resident providing the service.

- The level of service billed depends on the level of work performed and documented by the resident and the teaching physician in combination, or by the teaching physician if seen independent of the resident.
- The teaching physician, resident, or nurse must document that the physician not only was physically present (ie, in the same room as the patient) during the key or critical portions of the service performed by the resident but also participated in the management of the patient. The selected key or critical portion of the visit is at the discretion of the physician.

- Medicare requires that modifier **GC** (service performed in part by a resident under the direction of a teaching physician) be reported for each service unless the service is furnished under the primary care exception (reported with modifier **GE**). Other payers may or may not require a modifier.

- Only the teaching physician's total time is counted when total time is used to determine the E/M visit level, not including the time spent by the resident furnishing care without the presence of the teaching physician.
  - Only time spent by the teaching physician performing qualifying activities listed by *CPT* (with or without direct patient contact on the date of the encounter), including time the teaching physician is present when the resident is performing those activities, may be counted in selecting a level of service. This excludes teaching time that is general and not limited to discussion required for the treatment of a specific patient.

A resident may provide initial hospital or observation care without the teaching physician present; the teaching physician may then see the patient later, including on the next day. The date on which the teaching physician saw the patient is the teaching physician's DOS.

- Medicare guidelines stipulate that when documenting in an EHR, the teaching physician may use a macro (ie, entry of predetermined and unedited text by typing only a combination of keys such as Alt and A to add a predetermined attestation statement) as the required personal documentation if it is personally entered by the teaching physician. The resident or teaching physician must enter customized information to support medical necessity. The documentation is not sufficient if both the resident and teaching physician use only macros.

Examples

➤ **A resident admits a patient at 6:30 pm.** The teaching physician's initial visit is performed the following morning at 8:00 am. The teaching physician documents, "I saw and evaluated the patient. Discussed with resident and agree with the findings and plan as documented in Dr Resident's note except as per my addendum and edits within Dr Resident's note." *Note:* Edits should be distinguishable in the note.

The teaching physician reports an initial hospital care service based on the work personally performed that morning.

➤ **The teaching physician sees the same patient for follow-up inpatient care subsequent to the resident's visit.** The teaching physician documents, "I saw and evaluated the patient. Discussed with Dr Resident and agree with Dr Resident's findings and plan as documented in the resident's note."

➤ **The teaching physician and resident jointly admit the same patient.** The resident documents, "Dr Teacher was present during the history and exam. I discussed the case with Dr Teacher, who agreed with the findings and plan as documented."

Medical Student Documentation

- Any contribution and participation by a student to the performance of a billable service (other than obtaining history, which is not separately billable but is taken as part of an E/M service) must be performed in the physical presence of a teaching physician or resident in a service meeting the requirements set forth in this section for teaching physician billing.
- Students may document services in the medical record. However,
  - The teaching physician must verify in the medical record all student documentation or findings, including history, physical examination, and/or MDM.
  - The teaching physician must personally perform (or re-perform) the physical examination and MDM activities of the E/M service being billed but may verify any student documentation in the medical record, rather than re-documenting this work.

Primary Care Exception Rule

The primary care exception rule in the teaching physician guidelines allows teaching physicians to bill for services, without being present during the key or critical portions of the service, when provided by residents under their supervision who have completed at least 6 months of approved graduate medical education.

- To qualify for this exception, services must be provided in a teaching hospital or ambulatory care entity. If the services are provided outside a hospital, there must be a written agreement with the teaching hospital that includes a contract outlining the payment for the teaching services or written documentation that the services will be "donated." In general, this exception cannot be applied in a private physician's office or patient's home.
- The CMS includes its Medicare annual wellness visits in the primary care exception rule. However, because Medicare does not recognize the *CPT* preventive medicine visit codes, the CMS does not mention these codes in the primary care exception rule. Some Medicaid programs allow the primary care exception rule for preventive medicine services.
- No more than 4 residents can be supervised at a time by a teaching physician. Residents with less than 6 months in a graduate medical education–approved residency program may be included in the mix of 4 residents under the teaching physician's supervision. However, the teaching physician must be physically present for the critical or key portions of services furnished by the resident with less than 6 months in a graduate medical education–approved residency program. That is, the primary care exception does not apply to the resident with less than 6 months in a graduate medical education–approved residency program.
- Patients seen should consider this practice their primary location for health care.
- The teaching physician
  - Must be physically present in the clinic or office and immediately available to the residents and may not have other responsibilities, including supervising other personnel or seeing patients
  - Must review the care provided (ie, history, findings on physical examination, assessment, and treatment plan) during or immediately after each visit; the documentation must reflect the teaching physician's participation in the review and direction of the services performed

Example

➤ **The teaching physician is supervising a second-year resident in the clinic under the primary care exception rule.** An established patient is diagnosed with acute otitis media.

Unacceptable	Acceptable
Countersignature	"I reviewed Dr Resident's note and agree with Dr Resident's findings and plans as written." Signature "I reviewed Dr Resident's note and agree but will refer to ENT for consultation." Signature

- The exception applies only to low-level services, including **99202** and **99203** for new patient visits or **99211–99213** for established patient visits. If a higher-level E/M service is necessary and performed, the teaching physician must personally participate in the care of the patient as outlined in the guidelines.

E/M code selection is based only on MDM and not on total time when the service is provided under the primary care exception rule.

- Modifier **GE** (service performed by a resident without the presence of a teaching physician under the primary care exception) may be required by a payer that follows Medicare guidelines for teaching physician services.

The AAP continues to advocate for the preventive medicine service codes (99381–99385 and 99391–99395) to be included under the primary care exception rule. In some instances, Medicaid plans already consider preventive medicine service codes as part of their primary care exception, so be sure to check with your payers. Look for updates in the **AAP Pediatric Coding Newsletter™**.

You can access the current guidelines addressing the primary care exception rule in Chapter 12, Section 100.1.1c, of the **Medicare Claims Processing Manual** *(*www.cms.gov/Regulations-and-Guidance/Guidance/Manuals/Downloads/clm104c12.pdf*)*.

To test your knowledge of the information presented in this chapter, complete the quiz found at the end of it, after the resources. Answers to each quiz are found in **Appendix II**. Add to your knowledge through the information provided in other chapters that discuss specific categories of E/M service.

Chapter Takeaways

Readers of this chapter should generally understand the *CPT* E/M guidelines and the CMS teaching physician rules. Following are takeaways from this chapter:

- *CPT* provides general and specific E/M guidelines for many codes and code categories. It is important to recognize the guidelines that apply to each E/M service.
- Time must be documented when selecting a code on the basis of time. It is important to note the time required in a code descriptor (eg, time range, required minimum time for reporting).
- Each of the 4 levels of MDM is based on the same criteria whether the patient is new or established or the encounter is initial or subsequent.
- The level of MDM is determined by assessing the level at which 2 of 3 elements of MDM are performed and supported in the documentation of an encounter.
- *CPT* includes definitions of many terms used in selecting a level of MDM, as well as key instructions regarding what activities are counted toward MDM versus activities that are reported separately.
- The substantive portion of a split/shared E/M service is defined as either the greater portion of the total time of the service or the performance of 2 of 3 elements of MDM.
- Teaching physicians should maintain awareness of guidelines and primary care exception rules published by the CMS.

Resources

AAP Coding Assistance and Education

"Evaluation and Management" (www.aap.org/en/practice-management/child-health-finance-payment-strategy/coding-and-valuation/evaluation-and-management)

Pediatric Evaluation and Management: Coding Quick Reference Card 2026 (www.aap.org/Pediatric-Evaluation-and-Management-Coding-Quick-Reference-Card-2026)

AAP News™

"Understanding updated E/M coding guidelines can prevent underbilling, loss of revenue," August 1, 2024 (https://publications.aap.org/aapnews/news/29460)

"What constitutes 'acute illness with systemic symptoms?" March 1, 2023 (https://publications.aap.org/aapnews/news/23562)

AAP Pediatric Coding Newsletter

"Compliance Corner: Documentation Authentication," March 2024 (https://doi.org/10.1542/pcco_book239_document002)

"Compliance Corner: Incident-to Services," November 2024 (https://doi.org/10.1542/pcco_book247_document003)

Teaching Physician and Primary Care Exception

Medicare Claims Processing Manual, Chapter 12, Section 100.1.1c (www.cms.gov/Regulations-and-Guidance/Guidance/Manuals/Downloads/clm104c12.pdf)

Test Your Knowledge!

1. **To which category of service below does the concept of new or established patient apply?**
   a. Outpatient consultation
   b. Initial inpatient or observation care
   c. Office E/M services
   d. Emergency department services
2. **True or false? Two different diagnoses are required when reporting an E/M and another service provided by the same physician or QHP on the same date.**
   a. True
   b. False
3. **Which is true of a physician's and/or QHP's total time used in E/M code selection?**
   a. Time within 24 hours of the encounter is included in the total time.
   b. Total time includes only the time spent face-to-face with the patient and/or parent/caregiver
   c. Total time includes all time spent by a physician, QHP, and clinical staff on the date of the encounter.
   d. Only time on the date of the encounter is included in the total time.
4. **Which of the following is correct regarding how tests contribute to the amount and/or complexity of data to be reviewed and analyzed?**
   a. A test that is ordered with results reviewed at the same encounter counts twice, once for the order and once for the review of the result.
   b. Review of results of a test that was ordered by the same physician at a prior encounter contributes to the data of the current encounter.
   c. A test panel (eg, metabolic panel or complete blood count) is considered multiple tests for the purpose of the number of tests ordered.
   d. A test panel is considered a single test for the purpose of the number of tests ordered.
5. **Which of the following is true of determining the level of MDM of an E/M service?**
   a. 2 of 3 elements of MDM must support the level of MDM.
   b. 3 of 3 elements of MDM must support the level of MDM.
   c. 1 of 3 elements of MDM must support the level of MDM.
   d. The level of MDM is based solely on the number and complexity of problems addressed.

Part 2

Primarily for the Office and Other Outpatient Settings

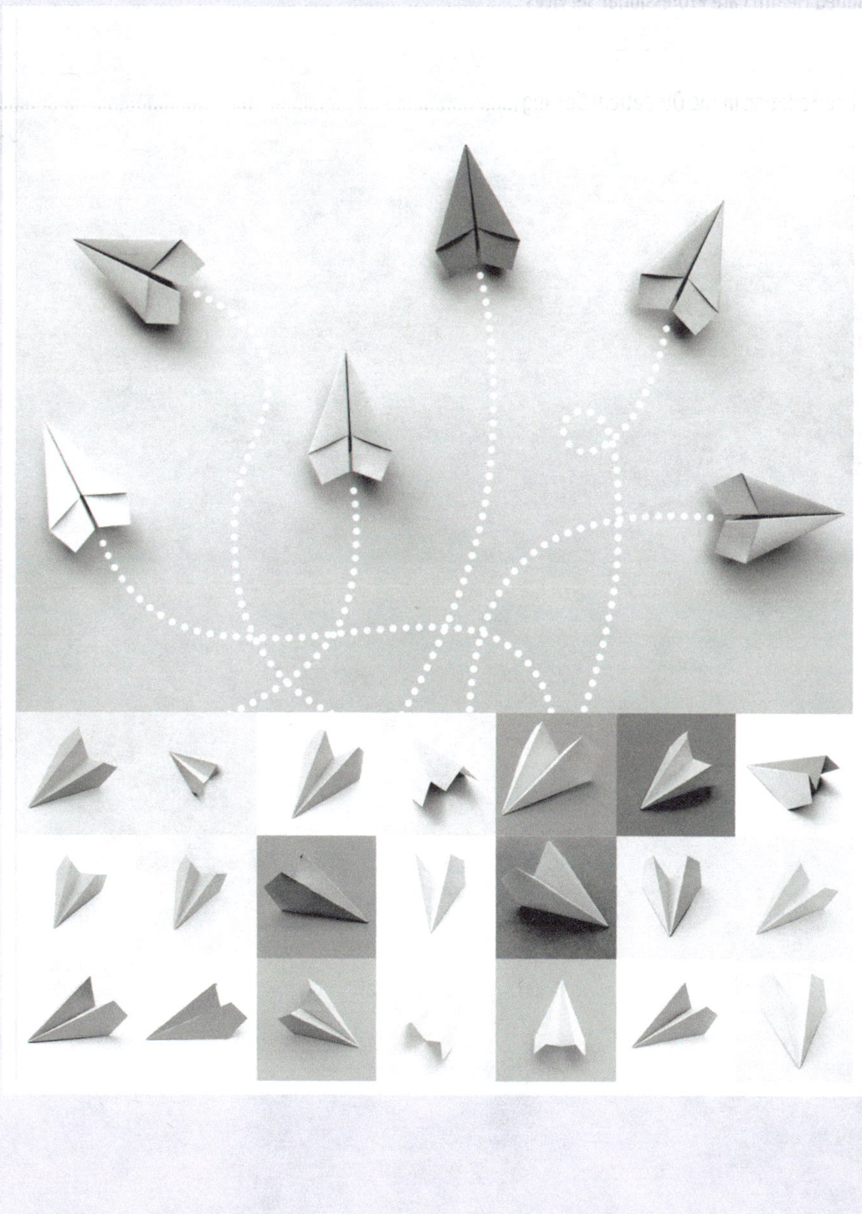

Part 2. Primarily for the Office and Other Outpatient Settings

CHAPTER 7

Non-Preventive Evaluation and Management Services in Outpatient Settings

Contents

Chapter Highlights

- Identifying evaluation and management (E/M) codes selected on the basis of guidelines for an outpatient site of service
- Determining when visit complexity code **G2211** is reported
- Distinguishing new and established patients, when applicable
- Reporting services provided under incident-to policy
- Using time in code selection for outpatient E/M services
- Selecting codes based on medical decision-making (MDM)
- Reporting prolonged or unusual E/M services

Outpatient Evaluation and Management Codes

This chapter addresses reporting problem-oriented E/M services when provided in outpatient settings other than the emergency department (ED) (discussed in **Chapter 14**). These codes are reported for most non-preventive E/M services in pediatric outpatient settings and urgent care facilities.

For information on non–face-to-face or indirect E/M services, refer to **Chapters 9, 19,** and **20**. For services provided in a nursing facility, psychiatric residential treatment facility, or intermediate care facility for individuals with intellectual disabilities, refer to "Evaluation and Management Service Coding in Nursing and Residential Treatment Facilities" at www.aap.org/cfp2026.

Current Procedural Terminology (*CPT*®) includes specific codes for reporting E/M services provided by synchronous audio-video or audio-only telemedicine and for a brief synchronous communication technology service. These codes are reported instead of outpatient E/M codes appended with telemedicine modifiers **93** and **95**. For the codes and discussion of appropriate reporting, refer to **Chapter 20.**

Codes and Sites of Service for Outpatient Services

This chapter provides important details and examples of how MDM and total time on the date of the encounter are used in code selection for the following services:

- Office or other outpatient E/M services (**99202–99205, 99211–99215**)
- Office or other outpatient consultations (**99242–99245**)
- Home or residence services (**99341, 99342; 99344, 99345; 99347–99350**)

Additionally, this chapter includes information on a Healthcare Common Procedure Coding System (HCPCS) add-on code (AOC), **G2211**, that is reported in addition to office E/M codes (**99202–99205, 99211–99215**) to indicate that the reported visit included the extra resources required to provide longitudinal care and/or care coordination for all the patient's health care needs or when providing longitudinal care for a patient's single serious or complex condition.

Outpatient sites of service for codes discussed in this chapter include the following sites:

- Private residence
- Temporary lodging or short-term accommodation (eg, hotel, campground, hostel, or cruise ship)
- Assisted living facility
- Group home (that is not licensed as an intermediate care facility for individuals with intellectual disabilities)
- Custodial care facility
- Residential substance abuse treatment facility

When a physician or qualified health care professional (QHP) provides E/M services to a patient in an outpatient setting (eg, office, home or residence, or ED) and later, on the same date, provides services to the same patient in an inpatient, observation, or nursing facility, refer to *CPT* guidelines for hospital inpatient and observation care services or nursing facility services for instructions. Refer also to **Chapter 16.**

Visit Complexity (G2211)

+G2211 Visit complexity inherent to E/M associated with medical care services that serve as the continuing focal point for all needed health care services and/or with medical care services that are part of ongoing care related to a patient's single, serious condition or a complex condition (AOC, list separately in addition to office/outpatient E/M visit, new or established, 99202–99205 or 99211–99215)

The Medicare program created and implemented AOC G2211 to provide additional payment for the work of building an effective relationship between a physician or QHP and a patient and/or caregivers for longitudinal care. This work has been previously unrecognized and unaccounted for in payment for office E/M visits.

The complexity described by G2211 is not condition complexity but, rather, relationship complexity. The key determinant for reporting G2211 is the intent for a long-term physician-patient relationship either as a focal point for all of a patient's health care needs or for management of a single serious or complex condition. Report G2211 for each office E/M service at which the criteria for reporting are met.

The following coding guidance for G2211 is based on Medicare policy at the time of this publication. Verify payment policies of individual payers before reporting this code.

G2211 is not reported

- ✖ In conjunction with an office E/M service provided in conjunction with management/treatment that is not expected to be of long-term duration (eg, preoperative visit, urgent care visit without a plan for longitudinal care).
- ✖ In conjunction with an E/M code that is appended with modifier 25 (significant, separately identifiable E/M service) except when reporting certain preventive services (eg, 90460–90461, immunization administration) on the same date. Otherwise, G2211 is not reported when modifier 25 is appended to the office E/M code (ie, when reporting other diagnostic or therapeutic services on the same date).

Important: Medicaid and private payer policies for payment of G2211 vary, and the benefit of pediatric physicians reporting G2211 may vary by locality and payer mix. Refer to payment policies of individual payers/plans and also consider the value of capturing the work relative value units (RVUs) of G2211 (eg, where physician and QHP pay is linked to work RVUs).

Examples

➤ **A child presents for an established patient visit with a cough and nasal congestion.** The pediatrician providing the E/M visit reviews the patient's medical history, including immunization history. After the patient is examined, the parents are counseled about upper respiratory infection (URI) and influenza immunization. The parents consent to immunization at this visit. An appointment for the child's next preventive medicine service is scheduled, and the parents are encouraged to call the pediatrician with any questions or concerns.

This visit meets the requirements for reporting G2211 (eg, 99213 25, G2211, 90460, and a code for the influenza vaccine). Although the problem addressed was not complex, the intent to establish an ongoing relationship in which the pediatrician will be the focal point for all the patient's health care needs is demonstrated by the instruction to call the pediatrician with any questions or concerns and scheduling of the preventive service.

➤ **An afebrile infant presents to an urgent care practice with a rash and history of fever a few days prior to the visit.** The urgent care pediatrician obtains pertinent history, examines the infant, and counsels the parents about roseola. The parents are advised to follow up with the patient's primary care physician.

This visit does not meet the requirements for reporting G2211. There is no indication of an intent to provide care on a longitudinal basis. Only the appropriate E/M code (eg, 99212) is reported.

➤ **A rheumatologist sees an established patient for follow-up care for juvenile idiopathic arthritis.** The visit includes an interval history, examination, and prescription drug management. The patient is scheduled for a follow-up visit in 3 months and instructed to contact the rheumatologist with any questions or concerns between visits.

This visit meets the requirements for reporting G2211 (eg, 99213, G2211). The visit is part of longitudinal care for a single complex condition.

E/M Services in Urgent Care Facilities

CPT does not include codes specific to E/M services provided at an urgent care facility. Office E/M codes (99202–99215) are typically reported.

The Centers for Medicare & Medicaid Services (CMS) describes an *urgent care facility* as a location, distinct from a hospital ED, an office, or a clinic, the purpose of which is to diagnose and treat illness or injury for unscheduled, ambulatory patients seeking immediate medical attention.

- ED codes 99281–99285 are not reported for urgent care E/M services.
- The site of service is differentiated by the place of service (POS) code (eg, 20 for urgent care facility, 11 for office).
- Other E/M codes that may apply to services in an urgent care facility include
  - After-hours service codes, discussed in the After-Hours Services section later in this chapter
  - HCPCS code S9088 (services provided in an urgent care center) that may be listed in addition to the codes for other services provided
  - Code S9083 (global fee urgent care centers) when an urgent care clinic contracts to bill all services under a global fee

Some physician practices operate as a primary care pediatric practice and an urgent care center in the same location but with different tax ID numbers and insurance contracts for each. Physicians should consult a health care attorney for assistance in establishing an urgent care practice and contracting with payers to cover the additional overhead costs often applicable to urgent care (eg, extended staffing, radiology, procedural services).

It is imperative to know your contractual agreements for coding and billing as an urgent care facility or clinic versus a primary care practice because rates of payment are typically higher for urgent care facilities, as are patient co-payments. Billing and payment also vary for urgent care facilities owned by hospitals. Guidance on billing and coding for these locations should be obtained from the compliance officer or other administrative personnel.

Office and Other Outpatient E/M Guidelines

Refer to **Chapter 6** for full guidelines that apply to all E/M services reported according to the level of MDM or total time on the date of the encounter.

New Versus Established Patients

The following criteria determine patient status when code descriptors designate whether a patient is new or established:

- *New patients* have not received a face-to-face professional service from the physician or QHP, or any physician or QHP of the same group practice and same exact specialty and subspecialty (eg, primary care, allergist), in any setting (eg, telemedicine, office, hospital) within the prior 3 years.
- *Established patients* have received, and a claim has been submitted for, any face-to-face professional service (eg, hospital care, immunization with physician counseling) from a physician or QHP of the same group practice and same exact specialty within the past 3 years.
- Per *CPT*, a QHP who is working with a physician(s) and who may report E/M services is considered to be working in the exact same specialty and subspecialty as the physician(s). Follow individual payer policies for reporting services by QHPs. A payer may use subspecialty designation in a notes field on claims to prevent claim denials within a multispecialty group practice.

Codes for outpatient consultations (99242–99245) apply to services provided to a new or established patient.

Examples

➤ **When a physician of a different specialty is covering for another physician (eg, pediatrician covering for a family physician) and has the first face-to-face contact with the other physician's established patient, the encounter is considered new.**

When a physician is covering for another physician of the same specialty, the patient's encounter is coded as it would have been by the physician who is unavailable. For example, an established patient for a pediatrician is seen by the on-call pediatrician. The on-call pediatrician should report that patient's service as established.

Per *CPT*, if a physician is covering for another physician of the same specialty, the patient's encounter is reported as it would have been by the physician who is unavailable.

➤ **When a physician has moved to a different location or changed their tax ID number, patients would still be considered established if they were established patients before these changes took place.**

When a new physician joins a group of other pediatricians, patients who follow the physician to the new practice are considered to be established patients to any of the pediatricians in the new practice because the patients were seen by a physician of the same specialty in the group within the past 3 years.

➤ **When a newborn or child is examined in the hospital (eg, nursery or ED care) and is subsequently examined in the office by the same physician or member of the same group and same specialty, the newborn or child is considered an established patient.**

Visits Not Requiring a Physician's or Qualified Health Care Professional's Presence

★99211 Office or other outpatient visit for the E/M of an established patient that may not require the presence of a physician or other QHP

Services by clinical staff, such as 99211 visits, are considered incidental to a physician's or QHP's services and are reported under the supervising physician's or QHP's name and National Provider Identifier (NPI). Generally, clinical staff, such as nurses and medical assistants, are not credentialed with payers and cannot independently provide and report these services.

Per *CPT*, a *clinical staff member* is a person who is working under the supervision of a physician or other QHP and is allowed by law, regulation, and facility policy to perform or assist in a specified professional service but who does not individually report that professional service.

Code 99211

- Is reported only for established patients
- Requires that services be provided according to a physician's or QHP's order
- Is reported for clinical staff assessments and other follow-up care not included in services described by other procedure codes (eg, face-to-face patient education not included in time billed as chronic care management services)
- ✖ Is not reported on the same date as another office E/M service by a physician or QHP of the same group practice
- ✖ Does not require the presence of a physician or QHP
- ✖ Does not require MDM by a physician or QHP
- ✖ Is not a time-based service

Do not report 99211 for non-E/M services such as venipuncture (36415, 36416) or injections (96372) or for demonstrating or teaching use of an inhalation device (94664). Do not report 99211 in conjunction with immunization administration (IA) (90471–90474) without separate and distinct nursing assessment and management. Do not report 99211 in conjunction with IA with counseling by a physician or other QHP (90460, 90461, 90480).

Code 99211 is not typically reported for an encounter solely for clinical staff to obtain a sample for laboratory testing. Report 99211 only for specimen collection when a payer has expressly provided guidance to report the code for this purpose.

Examples

➤ **An established patient presents for blood pressure and weight check by clinical staff.**

History: The patient is here per Dr A's January 28, 2025, order for follow-up on a weight loss plan for obesity and hypertension. The patient is following the recommended diet and began an exercise program at the local recreation center. The mother expresses more positive feelings about changing the family's diet and routines now.

Physical assessment: Blood pressure is 118/70 mm Hg, weight is 120 lb (down 7 lb since most recent visit), and body mass index (BMI) is now at 110% of the 95th percentile.

Plan: The patient is encouraged to continue diet and exercise and is already scheduled to follow up with her physician in 1 month. The patient and parent are instructed to call if there are any concerns before the follow-up visit.

Codes reported by Dr A or another supervising physician/QHP are **99211** linked to **I10** (hypertension), **E66.811** (obesity, class 1), and **Z68.54** (BMI pediatric, ≥95th percentile for age to <120% of the 95th percentile for age).

➤ **A nurse provides education to an established adolescent patient who wishes to assume responsibility for carrying a self-administered epinephrine kit and performing self-injection when necessary.**
The supervising physician reports **99211**.

➤ **An established patient is seen for evaluation of reaction to a tuberculin test.** A medical assistant assesses the site of the injection and finds no signs of reaction. The supervising physician reports **99211**. Note that **86580** (skin test; tuberculosis, intradermal) includes the work of administering the purified protein derivative but not the work of evaluating for potential reaction on a later date.

Incident-To Requirements: Services Provided Under Physician Supervision

Incident-to provisions apply only in the office or other outpatient setting in which the reporting physician or QHP is responsible for the practice expense of providing services (eg, labor costs for clinical and support staff, supplies, and other overhead expenses).

Incident-to policy is used by some payers to allow a physician or QHP to report services in 2 different circumstances:

1. Services that do not include direct care by the ordering physician or QHP (eg, nurse-only visit).
2. Services that include significant work by both a physician and a QHP who might otherwise provide and report the service individually. In a facility setting, this would be a split or shared service, but the Medicare split/shared service policy applies only to services provided in a facility setting (eg, hospital).

It is important to know whether a patient's health plan or other payer has adopted an incident-to policy, as this may affect billing and payment.

For payers that align with Medicare policy, refer to detailed requirements at www.aap.org/cfp2026 ("Incident-to Services by Nonphysician Professionals and Clinical Staff: Medicare Requirements"). Refer also to Chapter 12, Section 30.6, of the *Medicare Claims Processing Manual,* and Chapter 15, Section 60, of the *Medicare Benefit Policy Manual* at https://cms.gov/manuals (select "Internet-Only Manuals [IOMs]").

Billing for Services Performed by Clinical Staff Under Supervision

Under incident-to policy, a physician and QHP may bill under their NPI for services performed by clinical staff members who cannot independently provide and report E/M services, including nonphysician qualified health care professionals (NQHCPs) such as clinical social workers or pharmacists. This policy allows reporting of level 1 established patient E/M services (**99211**) and other services, as allowed under state regulations, when performed by clinical staff under the supervision of a physician or QHP.

The CMS defines *incident to* as "services incident to the service of a physician or other professional permitted by statute to bill for services incident to their services when those services meet all of the requirements applicable to the benefit."

- Incident-to services are always provided as a continuation of a physician's or QHP's services and do not address new problems (eg, a nursing visit performed at patient or caregiver request and not based on a physician's recommendation is not an incident-to service).
  - A treatment plan or order must be documented by a physician or QHP before provision of services billed incident to a physician or QHP.
- A supervising physician or QHP must be present *in the office suite* and available to assist, as needed, at the time of service. A payer that aligns with Medicare policy may allow availability of the supervising physician or QHP via real-time, audio-video communication technology rather than requiring "in the office suite" for certain services, including those reported with office E/M code **99211** and those that are designated as incident-to services (assigned PC/TC indicator 5 in the Medicare Physician Fee Schedule). (Incident-to supervision cannot be provided via audio-only communication under Medicare policy.)

Medicare makes an exception by not requiring the physician's presence in the office suite for certain activities of principal or chronic care management performed by clinical staff and for behavioral health services performed by licensed professionals. Private payers may also allow general rather than direct supervision when reporting these services.

- The individual providing the incident-to service must be an employee (direct or leased) or contracted to work with the physician practice (ie, paid as a practice expense).

Examples

➤ **A patient returns as directed by a pediatrician for evaluation of a tuberculin test result.** The physician is in the office suite at the time of service. A medical assistant evaluates the site of the injection (placed 48 hours earlier) and notes no reaction (0 mm). The medical assistant instructs the patient to notify the practice if any reaction occurs within the next 24 hours.

Code 99211 (established patient E/M, minimal level, not requiring a physician's presence) is reported by the supervising physician or QHP for this encounter. A best practice for clinical staff documentation is to include a reference to the pediatrician's prior order or standing order.

➤ **A medical assistant, as allowed under the state's scope of practice laws, administers an intranasal influenza vaccine that was ordered and directly supervised by the physician who documented counseling provided to the patient and/or caregivers.** Codes for the vaccine and administration (90672, 90460) are reported under the physician's NPI. If a pediatric nurse practitioner (NP) had ordered and supervised the treatment, the service would have been reported under that practitioner's NPI.

Incident-To Billing for Services by Qualified Health Care Professionals

Incident-to policy may also allow a physician to report services (eg, established patient visit, 99212–99215) provided by QHPs and NQHCPs who may otherwise bill for their services under their own NPI (within their state's scope of practice). The incident-to provision allows for reporting under the name and NPI of a supervising physician when the requirements of incident-to billing are met.

Examples

➤ **A patient returns for follow-up of attention-deficit/hyperactivity disorder (ADHD).** The patient's physician is in the office suite at the time of service, but the appointment was scheduled with a QHP in the same group practice. The patient and parents report improvement at home and in school. The physician may report the service when the payer has adopted an incident-to policy. The QHP's documentation should reflect the continuation of the physician's plan of care for the patient.

➤ **A patient returns for follow-up of ADHD.** The physician is in the office suite at the time of service, but the appointment was scheduled with a QHP in the same group practice. The QHP evaluates the patient and has concerns about the patient's report of side effects of medication. The QHP consults the patient's physician, who obtains additional history from the patient and decides to change the patient's medication. The QHP and physician each individually document the portion of the E/M service that they independently provided. The physician may report the total service when the payer has adopted an incident-to policy. Generally, where incident-to is applicable, guidelines for split/shared visits are not applicable.

The code for the established patient office E/M is selected according to the combined MDM or total time of service spent by the physician and QHP. No time is counted twice; any time that was spent simultaneously by the QHP and physician is counted only once. (Examples discussed in the Application of Time Guidelines section later in this chapter illustrate counting time when a physician and QHP each care for the same patient on the same date.)

- Nonphysician providers (eg, pharmacists, nonclinical social workers) without their own NPIs must report services incident to a physician and must meet all incident-to requirements, including physician supervision and continuation of a physician's previously established plan of care.

- Payment for QHPs and NQHCPs billing under the incident-to provision may be 100% of the physician payment versus 85% when reporting under the QHP's and NQHCP's individual NPIs.

Although Medicare and other payers reduce payment to 85% of the payers fee schedule amount when a QHP provides a service outside the incident-to requirements (eg, new patient visit), this is not the case for all payers. A physician billing for services provided by a QHP accepts responsibility for the accuracy of the code(s) reported.

- Not all services can be reported under incident-to policy. For example, the contract between the payer and physician may require that certain services (eg, medical nutrition therapy) be reported by the individual who provided the service.

Documentation Requirements and Tips When Reporting Incident-To Services

- Physicians and QHPs must document their order for a service or treatment (eg, continuing a series of injections of antibiotic) that will be performed as incident to or document their plan for a follow-up visit in the treatment plan (eg, follow-up visit within 1 week for a weight check).
- To demonstrate compliant incident-to billing, clinical staff providing services in continuation of a physician's plan of care *should, ideally, reference the date of the physician order for the service.* This may be documented in the chief complaint for the encounter (eg, "Patient is seen today per Dr Green's 1/2/2026 order for dressing change to left arm wound in 3 days").
- Documentation of incident-to services should fully describe the services provided, including date of service (DOS), assessment, concerns noted and addressed, details of care provided (eg, wound cleansed and new bandage applied), and education and/or instructions for home care and follow-up.
  - Inclusion of the supervising physician's name also supports that incident-to requirements were met.
  - Medical record documentation must reflect the identity, including credentials and legible or digital signature, of the person providing the service.

For Medicare purposes, the physician or QHP billing the service is not required to sign documentation prepared by the clinical staff. Other payer and state regulations may require authentication by the supervising physician or QHP. Documentation might be as simple as "Service performed/provided under the direct supervision of Dr X." When applicable, the signature must be legible.

Chapter 7

Code Selection Guidelines for Outpatient E/M Services

For all the outpatient visits discussed in this chapter except 99211, the level of service is determined by either

- The level of MDM alone
- The total amount of time (face-to-face and non–face-to-face) spent by a physician or other QHP on the DOS directed to care of the patient

It is not necessary to meet both the required MDM and required total time of service. For example, documentation supporting moderate MDM is sufficient to support new patient E/M code 99204 even if the total time on the date of the visit was less than 45 minutes. The inclusion of total time in the code descriptor does not indicate that the level of service always requires that much time.

Refer to **Box 7-1** for an overview of the key guidelines for code selection.

Application of Time Guidelines

- Time is the physician's and/or QHP's total time on the DOS, not the time in a 24-hour period, directed to the care of the individual patient.
- Both face-to-face and non–face-to-face time spent *on the DOS* are included in the time of the encounter. This may include time before, during, and after the visit.
- The total time should be documented in the medical record when it is used as the basis for code selection. No specific verbiage is required by *CPT.*

***CPT* does not require documentation of each segment of time spent on the DOS or any specific format of documentation. The physician must, however, document the total amount of time spent on the date of the encounter and be able to account for the time spent.**

Box 7-1. Key Office Evaluation and Management Coding Guidelines

History and examination: Each service includes a medically appropriate history and/or physical examination, when performed. Information supplied directly by the patient/caregiver or obtained by the care team may be reviewed and expanded on, as necessary, rather than re-documented.

Code selection: Select a code based on either MDM or the physician's or QHP's total time on the date of the visit.

MDM: Four types of MDM are recognized: straightforward, low, moderate, and high.
Determine the level of MDM based on the highest 2 of 3 elements of MDM.

1. Number and complexity of problems addressed. Include problems addressed or managed by the reporting pediatrician/QHP as part of the encounter.
2. Amount and/or complexity of data reviewed and analyzed. Data include
   - Tests, documents, orders, or independent historian(s)
   - Independent interpretation of tests
   - Discussion of management/test interpretation with external physician, QHP, or appropriate source
3. Risk of complications, morbidity, and/or mortality of patient management decisions made at the visit, associated with the patient's problem(s), and the diagnostic procedure(s) or treatment(s), including possible management options selected and those considered but not selected.

- **Time** includes the total time on the date of the encounter, face-to-face and non–face-to-face, personally spent by the physician and/or QHP focused on the care of 1 patient.
- ✖ Do not include time in activities performed or normally performed by clinical staff (eg, rooming the patient).
- ✖ Do not include travel time (eg, travel to a patient's home or residence).
- ✖ Do not count the same minute/period toward >1 service.
- ✖ Do not include time spent on a date before or after the DOS. (Refer to discussion of prolonged service code 99358 for time of ≥30 minutes.)
  - When >1 physician or QHP meet with a patient or discuss their care, only 1 individual counts that time toward an E/M service.
  - Time does not need to be continuous. Total all time on 1 date.
- Include the time of the following activities when performed by the reporting physician/QHP:
  - Preparing to see the patient (eg, medical record review)
  - Obtaining and/or reviewing separately obtained history
  - Performing a medically appropriate examination and/or evaluation
  - Counseling and educating the patient, family, or caregiver
  - Ordering medications, tests, or procedures
  - Referring to/communicating with other QHPs (when not separately reported)
  - Documenting clinical information in the medical record
  - Independently interpreting results (when not separately reported) and communicating results to the patient, family, or caregiver
  - Coordinating care (when not separately reported)

Abbreviations: DOS, date of service; E/M, evaluation and management; MDM, medical decision-making; QHP, qualified health care professional.

- When selecting a code based on time, it is important to verify the time required for the code selected. Codes include a specific time *that must be met or exceeded.* Time for all services discussed in this chapter is provided in **Table 7-1**.

Examples

➤ **An NP sees an established patient for a follow-up visit to address parent concerns about the child returning to sports after sustaining a concussion.** Five minutes is spent reviewing the patient medical record and accessing records from the emergency physician's initial management of the injury. History is obtained about the injury and ongoing signs and symptoms that may be related to the injury but have also occurred previously in relation to migraine headaches (10 minutes). The NP consults the pediatrician, who joins the practitioner in answering questions and counseling the parents for another 15 minutes. The patient and parents agree to neurological testing before a decision on clearance for sports. The NP spends another 10 minutes arranging the testing and documenting the encounter. Total time on the date of the visit is 40 minutes (5 + 10 + 15 + 10).

Code 99215 (40 minutes must be met or exceeded) is reported. Time spent jointly by the pediatrician and the NP (here, 15 minutes) is counted by 1 individual. Because the NP's time exceeded the physician's, the NP reports the service on the basis of the *CPT* guideline for split/shared visits. Note that *CPT* guidance on split/shared visits may vary from payer policies that may apply split/shared guidelines only to services in an inpatient or another facility setting. A payer may apply Medicare's incident-to policy to shared visits in non-facility settings.

Table 7-1. Code Selection Requirements for Outpatient Evaluation and Management Service (Excluding 99211)

Level/Codes/Total Time (min)[a]	Medical Decision-Making (2 of 3 Required: Data,[b] Problems, Risk)		
	Problem(s) Addressed	**Data Reviewed and Analyzed[c]**	**Risk**
Low *New patient* **99203** (≥30) *Established patient* **99213** (≥20) *Consultation* **99243** (≥30) *Home/residence* *New patient* **99342** (≥30) *Established patient* **99348** (≥30)	Low—*Any 1 of* ≥2 self-limited or minor problems 1 stable chronic illness 1 acute, uncomplicated illness or injury 1 stable acute illness 1 acute, uncomplicated illness or injury requiring hospital inpatient or observation level of care *Examples* • Acute gastroenteritis • Follow-up of stable ADHD • Uncomplicated hand-foot-and-mouth disease • Recheck of wound repaired by other physician/QHP • Resolution of URI with continued cough	Limited (*Meet 1 of 2 categories*) Category 1: Tests and documents (*Any 2*) • Review of prior external note(s)—each unique source • Review of the result(s) of each unique test • Ordering of each unique test Category 2: Assessment requiring an independent historian(s)	Low *Examples* • Over-the-counter medication(s) • Removal of sutures • Physical, speech, or occupational therapy
Moderate *New patient* **99204** (≥45) *Established patient* **99214** (≥30) *Consultation* **99244** (≥40) *Home/residence* *New patient* **99344** (≥60) *Established patient* **99349** (≥40)	Moderate—*Any 1 of* ≥1 chronic illness with exacerbation, progression, or side effects of treatment ≥2 stable chronic illnesses 1 undiagnosed new problem with uncertain prognosis 1 acute illness with systemic symptoms 1 acute, complicated injury *Examples* • Asthma with respiratory distress but not hypoxia • Stable asthma and stable anxiety disorder • Unexplained bruising • Acute gastroenteritis with dehydration • Intermittent headaches and confusion following concussion	Moderate (*Meet 1 of 3 categories*) Category 1: Tests and documents (*Any 3*) • Review of prior external note(s)—each unique source • Review of the result(s) of each unique test • Ordering of each unique test • Assessment requiring an independent historian(s) Category 2: Independent interpretation of a test performed by another physician/other QHP[c] Category 3: Discussion of management or test interpretation with external physician/other QHP/appropriate source	Moderate *Examples* • Prescription drug management or off-label use of over-the-counter medication • Decision about minor surgery with identified patient or procedure risk factors • Decision about elective major surgery without identified patient or procedure risk factors • Diagnosis or treatment significantly limited by SDoH
High *New patient* **99205** (≥60) *Established patient* **99215** (≥40) *Consultation* **99245** (≥55)	High—*Any 1 of* ≥1 chronic illness with severe exacerbation, progression, or side effects of treatment 1 acute or chronic illness or injury that poses a threat to life or bodily function	Extensive (*Meet 2 of 3 categories*) Category 1: Tests and documents (*Any 3*) • Review of prior external note(s) from each unique source • Review of the result(s) of each unique test • Ordering of each unique test	High *Examples* • Drug therapy requiring intensive monitoring for toxicity • Decision about hospitalization or escalation of hospital level of care • Decision regarding emergency major surgery

Continued on next page

• indicates a new code; ▲, revised; #, re-sequenced; ✚, add-on; ★, audiovisual technology; and ◀, synchronous interactive audio.

Table 7-1 (*continued*)

Level/Codes/Total Time (min)[a]	Medical Decision-Making (2 of 3 Required: Data,[b] Problems, Risk)		
	Problem(s) Addressed	**Data Reviewed and Analyzed[c]**	**Risk**
High (*continued*) *Home/residence* *New patient* 99345 (≥75) *Established patient* 99350 (≥60)	*Examples* • Asthma with respiratory distress with hypoxia • Infant with fever, tachycardia, lethargy, and dehydration • Epilepsy with increase in frequency of generalized tonic-clonic seizures	• Assessment requiring an independent historian(s) Category 2: Independent interpretation of a test performed by another physician/other QHP Category 3: Discussion of management or test interpretation with external physician/other QHP/appropriate source[c]	• Decision not to resuscitate or to de-escalate care because prognosis is poor • Decision regarding parenteral controlled substances

Abbreviations: ADHD, attention-deficit/hyperactivity disorder; QHP, qualified health care professional; SDoH, social determinants of health; URI, upper respiratory infection.

[a] Does not include time of clinical staff. Include only time spent by the physician or QHP directed to the individual patient's care on the date of the encounter.

[b] Each unique test, order, or document contributes to the combination of 2 or combination of 3 in Category 1.

[c] Do not count data review or communications reported with other codes (eg, test interpretation, interprofessional consultation).

➤ **A physician spends 10 minutes reviewing laboratory results and hospital records before a consultation on the same date.** Later that day, a face-to-face visit with the patient and caregivers lasts 20 minutes. After the visit but on the same date, the physician spends 10 minutes in discussion with the physician who requested the consultation and another 10 minutes in coordination of further treatment and in documentation. The total time on the DOS is 50 minutes.

The physician chooses to report the service based on total time on the date of the consultation service and reports 99244 (40 minutes). If the time on the DOS had met or exceeded 55 minutes, 99245 would have been reported.

Guidelines for Medical Decision-Making

Medical decision-making is the work of establishing diagnoses, assessing the status of a condition, and/or selecting a management option. The level of MDM is determined by assessing the level at which 2 of 3 elements of MDM are supported in the documentation of an encounter. The 3 elements of MDM are

1. The number and complexity of problem(s) that are addressed during the encounter
2. The amount and/or complexity of data to be reviewed and analyzed
3. The risk of complications, morbidity, and/or mortality of patient management decisions made at the visit, associated with diagnostic procedure(s) and treatment(s)

Four types of MDM are recognized: straightforward, low, moderate, and high. Each level of MDM is based on the same criteria whether the patient is new or established.

Number and Complexity of Problems Addressed

The first step in determining the level of MDM for an encounter is identification of the number and complexity of problems addressed.

- Include all problems addressed at an encounter in the number and complexity of problems.
- Complexity is determined by the types of problems addressed.

A *problem* is a disease, condition, illness, injury, symptom, sign, finding, concern, or other matter addressed at the encounter, with or without a diagnosis being established at the time of the encounter. The risk associated with a problem is distinct from the risk of morbidity and/or mortality associated with patient management decisions.

Refer to **Table 7-1** for the levels of problems in MDM. Expanded discussion of problem types is included in examples of outpatient E/M services, discussed in the Code Selection section later in this chapter. Use this table to identify the number and complexity of problems in the examples.

The guidelines for office E/M services provide definitions of the types of problems that are typically addressed at these encounters. Refer to the "Coding Conundrum: Addressed or Not Addressed" box in **Chapter 6**.

Amount and/or Complexity of Data to Be Reviewed and Analyzed

Data are divided into the following 3 categories:

1. Tests, documents, orders, or independent historian(s) (Each unique test, order, or document is counted to meet a threshold number.)
2. Independent interpretation of tests that are not separately reported
3. Discussion of management or test interpretation with external physician or other QHP or appropriate source

When data are used in support of low, moderate, or high MDM, the requirements for either 1 or 2 categories of data must be met. For example, Category 1 at the limited level of data is met when a physician orders 2 tests represented by separate *CPT* codes or reviews 1 test result and notes from 1 unique source (eg, hospital records from a recent admission). Instructions are provided for each level of data. Minimal or no data are required for straightforward MDM. **Table 7-1** shows the data requirements for limited, moderate, and extensive data.

A decision to not order a test that was considered is counted as a test ordered when the consideration and reason for not ordering the test are documented. For example, documentation may show that a test was discussed but determined to be unnecessary or that a test that is typically performed is not indicated because of patient risk or patient/parent decision to decline testing.

Risk of Complications and/or Morbidity or Mortality of Patient Management

Risk is the probability and/or consequences of an event. *For the purpose of code selection, the level of risk considers the risk of morbidity from additional diagnostic testing or treatment.* Risk also includes MDM related to the need to initiate or forgo further testing, treatment, and/or hospitalization.

The risk of patient management criteria applies to the patient management decisions made by the reporting physician or other QHP as part of the reported encounter.

Risk levels are minimal, low, moderate, and high. **Table 7-1** provides examples for minimal and low risk of morbidity from additional diagnostic testing or treatment that are not included in *CPT* and may vary depending on the individual patient presentation.

Code Selection

To select a code for an outpatient E/M service, you must determine which code is supported by 2 of 3 elements of MDM or the physician's or QHP's total time on the DOS. Refer to **Table 7-1** for an at-a-glance guide to the levels of MDM or time required for each level of outpatient E/M service.

The following sections provide an overview of a level of E/M service with time and MDM reporting criteria and examples of each level of service. Remember the following key points in code selection:

- Examples are not clinical recommendations, and levels of service supported may vary depending on documentation and patient age and presentation (eg, ill appearance beyond what is typical for the presenting problem).
- Select a code based on either total physician/QHP time on the DOS or MDM.
- The use of new versus established patient codes is based on whether the patient has received any face-to-face professional service from the same physician or a physician in the same group practice of the same exact specialty and subspecialty in the 3 years before the DOS.
- When selecting a code according to time, the total physician and/or QHP time spent devoted to the single patient's care must be documented in addition to the context of the care provided (eg, remarkable findings, counseling, care coordination, shared decision-making).
- When selecting a code level according to MDM, as described by *CPT,* the documentation should include the medically appropriate history and examination findings and all problems, diagnoses, management, and treatment options considered.

The American Academy of Pediatrics (AAP) *Pediatric Evaluation and Management: Coding Quick Reference Card 2026* (www.aap.org/Pediatric-Evaluation-and-Management-Coding-Quick-Reference-Card-2026) provides a quick reference for use in selecting E/M codes.

Category-Specific Instructions and Examples

Office and Other Outpatient E/M Services

Generally, a single office E/M code is reported per DOS when a patient receives more than one office E/M service by the same physician or QHP or physicians and/or QHPs of the same exact specialty and same group practice. An exception applies when a patient is seen at *2 distinct visits for distinct problems* (eg, follow-up of stable mild intermittent asthma [J45.20] in the morning and, later on the same date, care for a closed, non-displaced fracture of the right middle phalanx [S62.650A] incurred after the earlier visit). Although not required, separate billing may be preferred for the distinct visits (eg, to allow RVU credit to each physician or QHP). When reporting more than one office visit on the same date, append modifier 25 to the code for the later visit and link the distinct diagnosis code(s) for the problems addressed to the E/M code for each visit.

In each example, the physician may also report G2211 when serving as the focal point for all the patient's health care needs or when providing longitudinal care related to a patient's single, serious condition or a complex condition.

Office E/M (99202, 99212)

99202 Office or other outpatient visit for the E/M of a new patient, which requires a medically appropriate history and/or examination and straightforward medical decision making

When using total time on the date of the encounter for code selection, 15 minutes must be met or exceeded.

99212 Office or other outpatient visit for the E/M of an established patient, which requires a medically appropriate history and/or examination and straightforward medical decision making

When using total time on the date of the encounter for code selection, 10 minutes must be met or exceeded.

Example

➤ **A 3-year-old established patient presents with parent request for clearance to return to preschool after resolution of the patient's viral conjunctivitis.** A parent provides history of mild symptoms that resolved over the past 2 to 3 days. The physician performs a brief examination to determine that the problem is completely resolved. Clearance for return to preschool is provided.

Problem(s) addressed ➡ ***Minimal*** (resolved condition)
Data reviewed and analyzed ➡ ***Limited*** (independent historian required)
Risk of patient management ➡ ***Minimal*** (clearance for preschool)

Teaching Point: MDM is straightforward given the minimal number and complexity of problems addressed and minimal risk of morbidity. Although the data reviewed and analyzed are limited, this alone does not support a low level of MDM.

If an E/M service includes history from an independent historian and more than one self-limited or minor problem, documentation should typically support at least low MDM.

Office E/M (99203, 99213)

99203 Office or other outpatient visit for the E/M of a new patient, which requires a medically appropriate history and/or examination and low level of medical decision making

When using total time on the date of the encounter for code selection, 30 minutes must be met or exceeded.

99213 Office or other outpatient visit for the E/M of an established patient, which requires a medically appropriate history and/or examination and low level of medical decision making

When using total time on the date of the encounter for code selection, 20 minutes must be met or exceeded.

Examples

➤ **An established 7-year-old patient presents with low-grade fever, cough, and nasal congestion.** The child's parents provide history of symptoms for 3 days. Examination of the right tympanic membrane supports diagnosis of right acute suppurative otitis media in addition to URI. The parents are given a prescription for an antibiotic with counseling regarding the option to watch and wait for natural resolution of the ear infection or fill the prescription if symptoms worsen.

Problem(s) addressed ➡ ***Low*** (2 acute, uncomplicated illnesses)
Data reviewed and analyzed ➡ ***Limited*** (independent historian required)
Risk of patient management ➡ ***Moderate*** (prescription drug management)

ICD-10-CM	*CPT*
H66.001 (acute suppurative otitis media without spontaneous rupture of ear drum, right ear)	99213

Teaching Point: MDM is low given the 2 acute, uncomplicated illnesses addressed, limited data (independent historian), and moderate risk (prescription drug management). Although 2 problems were addressed, both were acute, uncomplicated illnesses that are not additive to the number and complexity of problems addressed. A more severe manifestation of otitis media might support a problem of higher complexity. If the total time on the date of the visit was 30 minutes or more and documented, 99214 would be reported according to total time.

➤ **A 5-year-old new patient presents with parental request for antibiotics for a URI.** Extended history is obtained from the child's parents, who state that the child has often required an antibiotic for respiratory infections in the past. The child is in kindergarten, and the parents feel that missing school is not an option. The parents are counseled regarding un-indicated use of antibiotic or over-the counter medication and appropriate home care and infection control precautions for their child. The pediatrician documents a total time of 35 minutes, which includes time spent completing documentation after the visit.

Problem(s) addressed ➡ ***Minimal*** (1 self-limited problem)
Data reviewed and analyzed ➡ ***Limited*** (independent historians required)
Risk of patient management ➡ ***Moderate*** (decision against prescription drug management)

ICD-10-CM	*CPT*
J06.9 (acute URI, unspecified) Z71.89 (other specified counseling)	99203

Teaching Point: Total time on the date of the encounter supports 99203 (≥30 minutes), as does the low level of MDM.

Office E/M (99204, 99214)

99204 Office or other outpatient visit for the E/M of a new patient, which requires a medically appropriate history and/or examination and moderate level of medical decision making

When using total time on the date of the encounter for code selection, 45 minutes must be met or exceeded.

99214 Office or other outpatient visit for the E/M of an established patient, which requires a medically appropriate history and/or examination and moderate level of medical decision making

When using total time on the date of the encounter for code selection, 30 minutes must be met or exceeded.

Examples

➤ **A 6-year-old child presents with a history of recurrent ear infections, bronchitis, and pneumonia as detailed in history from the child's parents and records from the child's primary care pediatrician.** A pneumococcal vaccine was recently administered. Follow-up levels of *Streptococcus pneumoniae* antibody (IgG) serotypes and total hemolytic complement (CH50) are ordered to assess for potential immunodeficiency. The patient will continue prophylactic antibiotics and return for follow-up in 1 week.

Problem(s) addressed ➡ ***Moderate*** (1 undiagnosed new problem with uncertain prognosis)

Data reviewed and analyzed ➡ ***Moderate*** (Category 1—independent historian, records from external source, and order for 2 tests)

Risk of patient management ➡ ***Moderate*** (prescription drug management)

ICD-10-CM	CPT
Z09 (encounter for follow-up examination after completed treatment for conditions other than malignant neoplasm) Z79.2 (long term [current] use of antibiotics) Z86.19 (personal history of other infectious and parasitic diseases)	99204

Teaching Point: MDM is moderate given the problem addressed, data to be reviewed and analyzed (≥3 items in Category 1), and risk of prescription drug management. A diagnosis of immunodeficiency is not made at this visit, so the diagnoses reported are those for follow-up examination and long-term antibiotic prophylaxis for a history of recurrent infection.

➤ **A 14-month-old new patient presents following an ED encounter for complex febrile seizure.** The neurologist obtains history from the patient's parents and reviews the ED visit note. The report of an electroencephalogram (EEG) that will be interpreted by an epileptologist at the hospital is not yet available. The neurologist independently reviews and interprets the EEG but does not separately bill for the service. The parents are counseled regarding risk of epilepsy related to a brain lesion or other cause. An abortive seizure medication is prescribed with counseling on use and possible side effects. Diagnosis is complex febrile convulsions.

Problem(s) addressed ➡ ***Moderate*** (undiagnosed new problem with uncertain prognosis)

Data reviewed and analyzed ➡ ***Moderate*** (Category 2—independent interpretation of tests)

Risk of patient management ➡ ***Moderate*** (prescription management)

ICD-10-CM	CPT
R56.01 (complex febrile convulsions)	99204 is supported by the physician's MDM to address a problem of moderate complexity with moderate risk of prescription management.

Teaching Point: Each element of MDM supports moderate MDM. Differential diagnoses for the complex febrile seizure include possibility of epilepsy resulting from a brain lesion or other life-threatening cause. In this example, data are moderate given the independent interpretation of the EEG. Although history from an independent historian was required and an external record reviewed, this does not meet the required combination of 3 items in Category 1 that, in conjunction with Category 2 data, would support extensive data. Given the 3 elements of MDM, the overall MDM is moderate.

Office E/M (99205, 99215)

99205 Office or other outpatient visit for the E/M of a new patient, which requires a medically appropriate history and/or examination and high level of medical decision making

When using total time on the date of the encounter for code selection, 60 minutes must be met or exceeded.

(For services ≥75 minutes, refer to prolonged services code 99417, discussed in the Prolonged Outpatient E/M Service, Physician or Other Qualified Health Care Professional, section later in this chapter.)

99215 Office or other outpatient visit for the E/M of an established patient, which requires a medically appropriate history and/or examination and high level of medical decision making

When using total time on the date of the encounter for code selection, 40 minutes must be met or exceeded.

(For services ≥55 minutes, refer to prolonged services code 99417, discussed in the Prolonged Outpatient E/M Service, Physician or Other Qualified Health Care Professional section later in this chapter.)

Examples

➤ **A physician provides an office visit to an established patient for possible depression associated with loss of interest in school and in activities previously enjoyed with family and friends.** The patient and their mother provide history of the patient's change in mood and interests. The patient completes a depression assessment instrument, the result of which is scored as positive. The patient admits to thinking about dying but not suicidal ideation. The patient's mother notes that an appointment with a psychologist was considered but no appointments were available within a month's time. The physician advises the patient and mother of general behavioral health integration services provided by a mental health counselor under the physician's supervision and obtains agreement to receive the services. An antidepressant is prescribed. The physician's total time on the date of the encounter is 50 minutes. Diagnosis is initial episode of major depressive disorder.

Problem(s) addressed ➡ ***Moderate*** (1 chronic illness that is not stable)

Data reviewed and analyzed ➡ ***Limited*** (review of score of the screening instrument and an independent historian)

Risk of patient management ➡ ***Moderate*** (prescription drug management)

ICD-10-CM	*CPT*
F32.9 (major depressive disorder, single episode, unspecified)	99215 is supported by 50 minutes of total time spent by the physician on the date of the visit. 96127 (brief emotional/behavioral assessment [eg, depression inventory, ADHD scale], with scoring and documentation, per standardized instrument)

Teaching Point: Although the MDM supports a level 4 E/M service, the physician's total time supports 99215.

The provision, scoring, and documentation of a depression assessment instrument is distinct from the E/M service. A physician's or QHP's review and analysis of the score of an assessment instrument is included in the amount and/or complexity of data reviewed.

➤ **A pediatrician reviews records from 3 unique sources for a new patient with complex medical history and later that day sees the patient to develop a plan of care and assists the parents with establishing subspecialty care.** Prescriptions are reviewed and prescribed, as needed. The physician's total time on the date of the visit is 60 minutes.

Problem(s) addressed ➡ ***Moderate*** (assumption of ≥2 chronic illnesses)

Data reviewed and analyzed ➡ ***Moderate*** (Category 1—review of records from 3 unique sources and independent historian)

Risk of patient management ➡ ***Moderate*** (prescription drug management)

ICD-10-CM	*CPT*
Appropriate codes for the diagnoses addressed at the encounter are reported.	99205 is reported according to the physician's total time on the date of the encounter.

Teaching Point: The documentation of this service must include the pediatrician's total time on the date of the visit and sufficient details to support the activities provided (eg, history obtained, data reviewed and analyzed, counseling provided, orders entered).

Outpatient Consultations (99242–99245)

CPT defines a consultation as a type of E/M service that is provided at the request of another physician, QHP, or appropriate source to recommend care for a specific condition or problem. Two major factors distinguish consultations from other E/M services.

1. The service is requested by another physician, QHP (eg, NP, clinical social worker, or psychologist), or appropriate source (eg, nonclinical social worker, educator, lawyer, insurance company) *to recommend care* for a specific condition or problem. *An E/M service requested by a patient or family member is not a consultation.*

2. The consultant's opinion and any services that were ordered or performed must also be *communicated by written report* to the requesting physician, QHP, or other appropriate source.

The consultant may initiate other services at the time of the consultation or at a subsequent encounter. Follow-up E/M services initiated by the consultant or patient/family are reported as established patient visits on the basis of the site of service (eg, established patient office visit).

Services that constitute transfer of care (ie, that are provided for the management of the patient's entire care or for the care of a specific condition or problem) are reported with the appropriate new or established patient codes for office or other outpatient visits or for home or residence services.

Services reported with codes 99242–99245 may be provided in an office or other outpatient site, including the home or residence or an ED.

When a Payer Does Not Accept Consultation Codes

Not all payers provide payment for services reported with consultation codes. Some payers have implemented policies that require reporting another E/M service code in lieu of consultation codes. The AAP supports payment for consultation codes as described in its position on Medicare consultation policy (www.aap.org/cfp2026; "AAP Position on Medicare Consultation Policy").

When consultation codes are not accepted, another E/M code reported is based on the site of service and whether the patient is new or established, as shown in **Table 7-2**.

Table 7-2. Coding Consultations Under Medicare Rules

New Patient	Established Patient
99202–99205 (office, outpatient hospital)	99212–99215 (office, outpatient hospital)
99341–99345 (home or residence visit)	99347–99350 (home or residence visit)

When a payer does not accept consultation codes, select the alternative E/M code based on the required level of MDM or total time on the date of the encounter.

Outpatient Consultation Services Examples

The following examples are intended to demonstrate how MDM or total time may be used to select each level of service for outpatient consultations. Refer to **Table 7-1** for an at-a-glance guide to the levels of MDM or time required for each level of outpatient E/M service. Each outpatient consultation code is followed by one or more examples.

★99242 Office or other outpatient consultation for a new or established patient, which requires a medically appropriate history and/or examination and straightforward medical decision making.

When using total time on the date of the encounter for code selection, 20 minutes must be met or exceeded.

Example

➤ **A pediatrician has requested a consultation by a dermatologist for evaluation of a nevus on the patient's right shoulder.** The patient presents to the dermatologist, who reviews patient and family history with the child's parents, evaluates the nevus, and recommends no treatment or follow-up. The patient and parents are reassured and counseled about sun protection behaviors. The diagnosis is melanocytic nevus of the right upper limb, including the shoulder. A report of the findings is sent to the pediatrician. Total time on the date of the encounter is 20 minutes.

Problem(s) addressed ➡ ***Straightforward*** (minimal—1 self-limited condition)
Data reviewed and analyzed ➡ ***Limited*** (independent historian)
Risk of patient management ➡ ***Minimal*** (routine follow-up by pediatrician)

ICD-10-CM	*CPT*
D66.21 (melanocytic nevi of right upper limb, including shoulder)	99242 is supported by straightforward MDM.

Teaching Point: The visit meets the requirements for reporting a consultation based on the pediatrician's request for advice and the consultant's written report to the pediatrician after evaluating the patient. The MDM is straightforward, based on the straightforward problem addressed, minimal data, and minimal risk of morbidity resulting from additional testing or treatment. The total time of 20 minutes also supports 99242.

If an E/M service includes history from an independent historian and either more than one self-limited or minor problem or low risk, documentation should typically support low MDM.

★99243 Office or other outpatient consultation for a new or established patient, which requires a medically appropriate history and/or examination and low level of medical decision making.

When using total time on the date of the encounter for code selection, 30 minutes must be met or exceeded.

Example

➤ **An adolescent ballet dancer is referred for evaluation and recommendation of treatment for pain and swelling to the posterior aspect of the ankle.** The physician reviews an encounter note provided by the physician who requested the consultation and independently interprets magnetic resonance imaging of the ankle. Diagnosis is posterior ankle tenosynovitis caused by os trigonum syndrome. Conservative treatment with rest and physical therapy is recommended, and an order for physical therapy is provided. A report of the encounter is sent to the requesting physician.

Problem(s) addressed ➡ ***Low*** (1 acute, uncomplicated illness or injury)
Data reviewed and analyzed ➡ ***Moderate*** (independent interpretation of tests)
Risk of patient management ➡ ***Low*** (decision for physical therapy)

ICD-10-CM	CPT
M65.871 (other synovitis and tenosynovitis, right ankle and foot) Q68.8 (os trigonum syndrome)	99243 is supported.

Teaching Point: The problem addressed and the risks of management support low MDM.

★99244 Office or other outpatient consultation for a new or established patient, which requires a medically appropriate history and/or examination and moderate level of medical decision making.

When using total time on the date of the encounter for code selection, 40 minutes must be met or exceeded.

Examples

➤ **A primary care pediatrician consults an otolaryngologist for opinion on adenoidectomy and tympanostomy with tubes.** The patient is new to the otolaryngologist, who reviews and summarizes records provided by the primary care pediatrician, noting management of perennial allergic rhinitis, chronic adenoid hypertrophy, and chronic serous otitis media over the past year. Results of tympanometry provided by an audiologist prior to the consultation are also reviewed. History is obtained from the patient's parents, who note that the patient finished a course of antibiotics 2 weeks ago for acute otitis media and is increasingly missing school and community events because of ear infections. Examination reveals enlarged adenoids and bilateral otitis media with effusion.

Assessment/plan: Diagnosis is bilateral chronic serous otitis media with chronic hypertrophy of adenoids and perennial allergic rhinitis. The otolaryngologist discusses treatment options with the parents, including tympanostomy with tube placement and adenoidectomy, and the parents agree to the surgery. The otolaryngologist sends a report to the primary care pediatrician advising that surgery be recommended.

Problem(s) addressed ➡ ***Moderate*** (≥2 chronic conditions)
Data reviewed and analyzed ➡ ***Moderate*** (independent historians, review of records from 1 source, and review of 1 test result)
Risk of patient management ➡ ***Moderate*** (decision for elective major surgery without known risk factors)

ICD-10-CM	*CPT*
H65.23 (chronic serous otitis media, bilateral) J35.2 (hypertrophy of adenoids) J30.89 (other allergic rhinitis)	99244 is supported.

Teaching Point: The moderate MDM is supported by all 3 elements, although only 2 are required.

➤ **An adolescent patient is seen in consultation for increasingly symptomatic mental health problems.** The patient's psychologist has requested evaluation and recommendation for treatment, as the patient has not adequately responded to current treatment. The physician reviews the patient's current medications and results of psychological tests. History is obtained mainly from the patient's mother, who is present. After extensive discussion, new medication is prescribed and a follow-up visit is scheduled in 1 week. The physician sends the psychologist a report with findings and recommendations. The physician's total time spent in medical management (not psychotherapy, which would be reported separately, when provided) is 50 minutes.

ICD-10-CM	*CPT*
Appropriate codes for problems addressed	99244 is supported by the time exceeding 40 minutes but not reaching the 55 minutes required for 99245.

★99245 Office or other outpatient consultation for a new or established patient, which requires a medically appropriate history and/or examination and high level of medical decision making.

When using total time on the date of the encounter for code selection, 55 minutes must be met or exceeded.

(For services ≥70 minutes, use prolonged services code 99417, discussed in the Prolonged Outpatient E/M Service, Physician or Other Qualified Health Care Professional section later in this chapter.)

Example

➤ **A neurologist is consulted by a primary care pediatrician to evaluate a patient who has Down syndrome and tingling of the hands possibly caused by atlantoaxial instability and is requesting clearance to participate in the Special Olympics.** The neurologist reviews the patient's history provided by the referring physician. Additional history is provided by the patient's parents, who state that the patient sometimes describes her hands as "tingling" after sleeping or playing a game on a tablet. Following examination of the patient, the neurologist orders radiography of the patient's cervical spine. Later that day, after receiving the radiologist's interpretation of the cervical spine radiographs, the neurologist views the images and then contacts the primary care pediatrician to discuss that there is no evidence of atlantoaxial instability on radiography and, after discussion, recommends clearing the child for participation. The neurologist's total time on the date of the encounter is 65 minutes.

Problem(s) addressed ➡ ***Moderate*** (1 undiagnosed new problem with uncertain prognosis)
Data reviewed and analyzed ➡ ***High*** (independent interpretation of tests and discussion of management)
Risk of patient management ➡ ***Low to moderate*** (decision for participation)

ICD-10-CM	*CPT*
Z03.89 (encounter for observation for other suspected diseases and conditions ruled out) R20.2 (paresthesia of skin) Q90.2 (trisomy 21, translocation)	99245 is supported.

Teaching Point: The physician's total time supports 99245, although the MDM for the encounter is moderate.

Home or Residence Services (99341–99350)

A home or residence may include the following sites for the purpose of reporting home or residence services. Each site is followed by the applicable POS code in parentheses.

- Private residence (12)

- Temporary lodging or short-term accommodation (**16** [eg, hotel, campground, hostel, cruise ship])
- Assisted living facility (**13**)
- Group home that is not licensed as an intermediate care facility for individuals with intellectual disabilities (**14**)
- Custodial care facility (**33**)
- Residential substance abuse treatment facility (**55**)

To report services provided in an intermediate care facility for individuals with intellectual disabilities and services provided in a psychiatric residential treatment center, refer to "Evaluation and Management Service Coding in Nursing and Residential Treatment Facilities" at www.aap.org/cfp2026.

Medicaid plans may vary in sites of service reported as home visits. Verify payer policies for E/M services provided in a patient's home or residence before provision of services.

E/M services provided in a patient's home by a nonphysician provider who does not have their own NPI may not be billable unless the physician provides direct supervision. Refer to **Chapter 12** for information on reporting services by professionals such as therapists, clinical social workers, and nutritionists.

Any procedures performed by the physician may be separately reported.

Home or Residence E/M Service Examples

Refer to **Table 7-1** for an at-a-glance guide to the levels of MDM or time required for each level of outpatient E/M service.

99341 Home or residence visit for the E/M of a new patient, which requires a medically appropriate history and/or examination and straightforward medical decision making.

When using total time on the date of the encounter for code selection, 15 minutes must be met or exceeded.

99347 Home or residence visit for the E/M of an established patient, which requires a medically appropriate history and/or examination and straightforward medical decision making.

When using total time on the date of the encounter for code selection, 20 minutes must be met or exceeded.

Example

➤ **A physician or QHP visits the home of a newborn whose parents are concerned that the newborn is not breathing normally.** On examination, the newborn is breathing normally and is free of any signs or symptoms of illness. The parents are reassured. The total time directed to care of this patient on this date is 10 minutes.

Problem(s) addressed ➡ ***Minimal*** (1 self-limited problem)
Data reviewed and analyzed ➡ ***Limited*** (independent historians required)
Risk of patient management ➡ ***Minimal*** (home care)

ICD-10-CM	*CPT*
Z05.3 (observation and evaluation of newborn for suspected respiratory condition ruled out)	**99341** if the patient is new or **99347** if the patient is established

Teaching Point: In this example, the physician's or QHP's total time did not meet the minimum required for code selection. However, straightforward MDM is the highest level supported by 2 of the 3 elements of MDM.

If an E/M service includes history from an independent historian and more than one self-limited or minor problem, documentation should typically support low MDM, at a minimum.

99342 Home or residence visit for the E/M of a new patient, which requires a medically appropriate history and/or examination and low level of medical decision making.

When using total time on the date of the encounter for code selection, 30 minutes must be met or exceeded.

99348 Home or residence visit for the E/M of an established patient, which requires a medically appropriate history and/or examination and low level of medical decision making.

When using total time on the date of the encounter for code selection, 30 minutes must be met or exceeded.

Examples

➤ **A physician or QHP visits the home of an autistic 5-year-old whose parents fear he has an ear infection.** The parents note that the child has been holding his right ear frequently for the past week. They have not seen him pulling at or trying to insert anything into his ear. The physician's examination of the patient takes 15 minutes because of extensive coaching to gain the child's cooperation. The child's ears are free of signs of infection and foreign bodies. The parents are counseled that this may be a self-comfort mechanism or habit and they are not to use cotton swabs to clean the ear canals and should try to dry the ear canals after showers. Diagnosis is suspected ear infection, ruled out; the behavior is likely a self-comfort measure, but the patient does not respond to questions about his ears. *Plan:* The parents will call if any fever or other concerns develop. The physician's total time on the date of the encounter is 30 minutes.

Problem(s) addressed ➡ ***Minimal*** (1 self-limited problem)
Data reviewed and analyzed ➡ ***Limited*** (independent historians)
Risk of patient management ➡ (home care)

ICD-10-CM	*CPT*
Z03.89 (encounter for observation for other suspected diseases and conditions ruled out) F84.0 (autistic disorder)	99342 if the patient is new or 99348 if the patient is established (based on a total time of 30 minutes)

Teaching Point: In this example, the physician's or QHP's total time on the date of the encounter supports a higher level of service than the straightforward MDM.

Inclusion of codes for conditions that limit the patient's ability to be seen in the office or outpatient clinic may help demonstrate the medical necessity of a home visit.

Travel time is not included in the time of service. But if escorting a patient to a medical facility becomes necessary, 99082 (unusual travel) may be appropriate.

➤ **A physician visits the home of a 3-year-old who is having infrequent, very hard stools.** Per the patient's mother, the child's stepbrother also has this problem. The physician reviews the patient's diet and level of activity with the mother. After examining the patient, the physician recommends a diet higher in fiber and lower in processed foods and the replacement of milk and other dairy products with plant-based products. Total time on the date of the encounter is 20 minutes, including time spent documenting the encounter.

Problem(s) addressed ➡ ***Low*** (1 acute, uncomplicated illness)
Data reviewed and analyzed ➡ ***Limited*** (independent historian)
Risk of patient management ➡ ***Minimal*** (dietary recommendations)

ICD-10-CM	*CPT*
K59.00 (constipation, unspecified)	99342 if the patient is new or 99348 if the patient is established

Teaching Point: The problem addressed and level of data to be reviewed support low MDM.

99344 Home or residence visit for the E/M of a new patient, which requires a medically appropriate history and/or examination and moderate level of medical decision making.

When using total time on the date of the encounter for code selection, 60 minutes must be met or exceeded.

99349 Home or residence visit for the E/M of an established patient, which requires a medically appropriate history and/or examination and moderate level of medical decision making.

When using total time on the date of the encounter for code selection, 40 minutes must be met or exceeded.

Example

➤ **A pediatrician agrees to provide medically necessary services at the infirmary of a youth ranch where an established 16-year-old patient lives.** The patient presents with concern of increased asthma symptoms. The patient-provided history and an examination are documented in addition to a decision to change the patient's control medication and update the patient's asthma control plan. Diagnosis is moderate persistent asthma with exacerbation.

Problem(s) addressed ➡ *Moderate* (1 chronic condition with exacerbation)
Data reviewed and analyzed ➡ *Minimal*
Risk of patient management ➡ *Moderate* (prescription drug management)

ICD-10-CM	*CPT*
J45.41 (moderate persistent asthma with [acute] exacerbation)	99349 (established patient)

Teaching Point: The problem addressed and risk associated with management support moderate MDM. If the patient were new, 99344 would be reported.

99345 Home or residence visit for the E/M of a new patient, which requires a medically appropriate history and/or examination and high level of medical decision making.

When using total time on the date of the encounter for code selection, 75 minutes must be met or exceeded.

99350 Home or residence visit for the E/M of an established patient, which requires a medically appropriate history and/or examination and high level of medical decision making.

When using total time on the date of the encounter for code selection, 60 minutes must be met or exceeded.

Example

➤ **A physician visits the home of an established patient who has cystic fibrosis.** The patient's mother notes that she requested the appointment because the patient is experiencing diarrhea and progressive, cramping abdominal pain in the right lower quadrant. The physician recommends admission to the hospital for further E/M of possible intestinal blockage. The physician arranges for the patient to be admitted to the local hospital through the ED, as required by the facility.

Problem(s) addressed ➡ *High* (1 chronic illness with severe exacerbation)
Data reviewed and analyzed ➡ *Limited* (independent historian)
Risk of patient management ➡ *High* (decision regarding hospitalization)

ICD-10-CM	*CPT*
E84.19 (cystic fibrosis with other intestinal manifestations)	99350

Teaching Point: The MDM is high, given an illness that poses a threat to life or bodily function and the decision to hospitalize. A decision to hospitalize and a decision to not hospitalize but to closely monitor would each support high risk in this scenario.

Prolonged Office E/M Service

Prolonged Outpatient E/M Service, Physician or Other Qualified Health Care Professional

★✚99417 Prolonged outpatient E/M service(s) time with or without direct patient contact beyond the required time of the primary service when the primary service level has been selected using total time, each 15 minutes of total time

Code 99417 is reported only when the code for the primary service was selected according to time. The time requirement for the highest-level code for the primary service must be met and exceeded by at least 15 minutes.

● indicates a new code; ▲, revised; #, re-sequenced; ✚, add-on; ★, audiovisual technology; and ◀, synchronous interactive audio.

Code **99417** is used to report prolonged total time (ie, combined time with and without direct patient contact) provided by the physician or QHP on the same date as one of the following outpatient E/M services. Prolonged total time is time that is 15 minutes beyond the time required to report the highest-level primary service (eg, level 5 office E/M service).

- Office or other outpatient services reported with **99205** or **99215**
- Synchronous audio-video services reported with **98003** or **98007**
- Synchronous audio-only services reported with **98011** or **98015**
- Office or other outpatient consultation reported with **99245**
- Home or residence service reported with **99345** or **99350**
- Assessment of and care planning for a patient with cognitive impairment reported with **99483** (not typically a pediatric service)

Refer to **Chapter 20** for information on reporting **99417** in conjunction with codes for synchronous audio-video or audio-only E/M services.

For prolonged services on a date other than the date of a face-to-face E/M encounter with the patient and/or family/caregiver, report **99358** or **99359**, discussed later in this chapter. For E/M services that require prolonged clinical staff time and may include face-to-face services by the physician or QHP, report **99415** or **99416**. Do not report **99417** in conjunction with other codes for prolonged service (eg, **99358**, **99359**; **99415**, **99416**; **99418**).

There is no limit on the number of units of **99417** reported per encounter. However, each unit must represent a full 15-minute period beyond the time included in a previous unit of time reported with **99417** (**Table 7-3**).

Table 7-3. Time Requirements for Prolonged Service Reported With 99417

Only time spent by a physician or QHP in providing care directed to the individual patient is included in total time on the date of the encounter.

Type of Service and Code	Assigned Time (min)	Minimum Time (min) Required for Reporting 99417	Minimum Time (min) Required for Reporting Additional Units of 99417[a]
Office E/M new patient 99205[b]	≥60	75–89 99205 × 1 and 99417 × 1	90–104 99205 × 1 and 99417 × 2
Office E/M established patient[c] **99215**	≥40	55–69 99215 × 1 and 99417 × 1	70–84 99215 × 1 and 99417 × 2
Outpatient consultation 99245	≥55	70–84 99245 × 1 and 99417 × 1	85–99 99245 × 1 and 99417 × 2
Home or residence, new patient 99345	≥75	90–104 99345 × 1 and 99417 × 1	105–119 99345 × 1 and 99417 × 2
Home or residence, established patient 99350	≥60	75–89 99350 × 1 and 99417 × 1	90–104 99350 × 1 and 99417 × 2

Abbreviations: E/M, evaluation and management; QHP, qualified health care professional.

[a] Each unit of service for 99417 is reported only for a *full 15-minute* period beyond the most recent unit reported. Although times for up to only 2 units are shown in this table, there is no limit on the number of units reported.

[b] Times in this row are also applicable to audio-video E/M new patient code 98003 and audio-only E/M new patient code 98011.

[c] Times in this row are also applicable to audio-video E/M established patient code 98007 and audio-only E/M established patient code 98015.

Do not report **99417**

- ✖ For prolonged service of less than 15 minutes on the date of the office E/M service
- ✖ For any additional increment of time that is less than 15 minutes from the last full 15-minute period
- ✖ For time spent performing separately reported services other than the E/M service
- ✖ In addition to codes for less than the highest-level service in a code category (eg, do not report with **99211–99214**)

Coding Conundrum: Healthcare Common Procedure Coding System Versus *Current Procedural Terminology*

Some payers may not accept 99417 for prolonged E/M services. The CMS developed HCPCS codes G2212 and G0318 (as follows) to require that the time of prolonged outpatient E/M services begin when all time included in the value of each E/M service is exceeded. For G0318, the CMS does not limit the time attributed to prolonged service to the time on the date of the encounter. Whereas 99417 is always based on total time on the date of the visit, the HCPCS codes vary depending on the duration of time included in the value of each service.

G2212 *Prolonged office or other outpatient E/M service(s)* beyond the maximum required time of the primary procedure, which has been selected using total time on the date of the primary service; each additional 15 minutes by the physician or QHP, with or without direct patient contact

G2212 is reported only in conjunction with 99205 (add G2212 for total time ≥89 minutes) or 99215 (add G2212 for total time ≥69 minutes) when the time requirement is met. The time included in prolonged service is only the total time on the date of the encounter.

G0318 *Prolonged home or residence E/M service(s)* beyond the total time for the primary service (when the primary service has been selected using time on the date of the primary service); each additional 15 minutes by the physician or QHP, with or without direct patient contact

G0318 is reported only in conjunction with 99345 (add G0318 for total time ≥140 min) or 99350 (add G0318 for total time ≥110 min). *The total time for G0318 includes time on the date of the visit and on 3 days before and 7 days after.*

In the absence of a contractual requirement to follow a payer's policy to report a HCPCS code in lieu of 99417, physicians should assign 99417 and follow *CPT* guidelines. Refer to the April 2023 *AAP Pediatric Coding Newsletter*™ article "Prolonged Services: *CPT* Guidelines and Medicare/ Medicaid Policy" (https://doi.org/10.1542/pcco_book228_document003).

Examples

➤ **A new patient is referred following discharge from observation care for asthma.** The patient has no usual source of care and has been seen in 3 EDs for a total of 4 visits in the past year. The pediatrician spends 20 minutes before the face-to-face visit, on the same date, reviewing observation and ED records for the child. At the visit, the pediatrician spends 45 minutes evaluating the patient, who also has behavioral issues in school; developing a plan of care; and counseling the patient and caregiver on the plan. After the visit, the pediatrician spends 20 minutes on the same date providing instructions to the school nurse about the patient's use of a rescue inhaler and arranging for teachers to complete rating scales for ADHD. Another 10 minutes is spent in documentation. The pediatrician reports 99205 and 99417 × 2 for the 95 minutes devoted to the patient's care on the date of the encounter.

➤ **An adolescent patient and her parents are scheduled for an outpatient consultation to evaluate the patient's treatment options for newly diagnosed Crohn disease.** The physician documentation of the consultation supports moderate-level MDM. Total time is not documented. Later, on that same date, the physician receives a call from the patient's parents with additional questions and concerns and spends 30 minutes communicating on the call and completing the documentation. The outpatient consultation is reported with 99244.

Teaching Point: Total time on the date of the encounter might have supported 99245 and possibly prolonged service, but the total time was not documented and the consultation code was selected according to MDM.

Prolonged Service Without Direct Patient Contact (99358, 99359)

99358 Prolonged E/M service before and/or after direct patient care; first hour
✚99359 each additional 30 minutes (Use in conjunction with 99358.)

Prolonged service without direct patient contact (ie, non–face-to-face) is reported when a physician provides prolonged service *on a date when no face-to-face E/M service has been or will be provided.* The prolonged service must relate to a service to a patient for whom direct (face-to-face) patient care has occurred or will occur and to ongoing patient management.

Refer to 99417 and 99418 for prolonged service on the date of a face-to-face E/M service.

Only time spent by a physician or other QHP may be counted toward the time of prolonged service. Prolonged service of less than 30 minutes on a given date is not separately reported. Report 99359 for 15 or more minutes beyond the first hour or the last full 30-minute period of prolonged service.

Codes 99358 and 99359 are not limited to specific sites of service.

Example

➤ **A physician provides an office or other outpatient consultation to a patient to evaluate whether surgery is indicated.** After the consultation, the physician requests records from a prior surgery. The following day (next date), the physician spends 30 minutes reviewing the old records, plans a surgical approach, and speaks with the referring physician about perioperative management. The total time of service is 45 minutes. The physician reports 99358 for the first hour of prolonged service (reported for services of ≥30 minutes).

Teaching Point: Payers may or may not allow payment for 99358 and 99359. Code 99359 may be reported for the first and each additional 30 minutes of service time, including a period of 15 minutes or more beyond the first hour or beyond the last 30-minute period.

Prolonged Clinical Staff Service (99415, 99416)

+99415 Prolonged clinical staff service (the service beyond the typical service time) during an E/M service in the office or outpatient setting, direct patient contact with physician supervision; first hour (List separately in addition to code for outpatient E/M service.)

+99416 each additional 30 minutes

Codes 99415 and 99416 are used to report 30 minutes or more of prolonged clinical staff time spent face-to-face providing care to a patient and/or parent or caregiver under the direct supervision of a physician or other QHP who has provided an office or other outpatient E/M service at the same session.

- Report prolonged clinical staff service 99415 and 99416 only in addition to office or other outpatient E/M codes 99202–99205 or 99211–99215.
- The starting point for 99415 is 30 minutes beyond the typical clinical staff time that is included in the value assigned to the office or other outpatient E/M code reported for the encounter. This time is not included in the code descriptors in *CPT* but, rather, in a table like **Table 7-4**.

While 99417 is reported for prolonged physician or QHP service only when the base E/M code is selected based on total time, base E/M codes 99202–99205 or 99212–99215 may be selected on the basis of either MDM or total time when reporting 99415 or 99416.

Table 7-4. Time Requirements for Prolonged Clinical Staff Service (99415, 99416)

Only time spent by a physician or QHP in providing care directed to the individual patient is included in total time on the date of the encounter.

Office E/M Code	Typical Clinical Staff Time (min)	Time Range (min) for +99415	Time Range (min) for +99416 (1st Unit)[a]
99202	29	59–103	104–133
99203	34	64–108	109–138
99204	41	71–115	116–145
99205	46	76–120	121–150
99211	16	46–90	91–120
99212	24	54–98	99–128
99213	27	57–101	102–131
99214	40	70–114	115–144
99215	45	75–119	120–149

Abbreviations: E/M, evaluation and management; QHP, qualified health care professional.

[a] Each unit of service for 99416 is reported only when the time included in 99415 or the prior unit of 99416 is exceeded *by at least 15 minutes*. There is no limit on the number of units reported, but documentation must support the time spent and the clinical indication for prolonged clinical staff service.

Example

➤ **A physician documents an office E/M service with moderate MDM supporting 99214.** At the same visit, clinical staff spent a total of 75 minutes monitoring the patient (face-to-face), under the physician's supervision, following administration of a medication that was previously associated with an allergic reaction. The physician reports 99214 for the office E/M service and 99415.

Teaching Point: The time requirement for 99415 is 30 minutes or more beyond the typical clinical staff time of the related office E/M service. The typical clinical staff time for 99214 is 40 minutes. The total clinical staff time of 75 minutes exceeds the 40-minute typical time by 35 minutes, supporting 99415. Although the office E/M code was selected based on MDM, rather than total time, the clinical staff time supports reporting 99415.

Documentation should support the clinical indication(s) for the prolonged service and the specific amount of time spent by clinical staff providing face-to-face services to the individual patient. If face-to-face time is discontinuous, each segment of time should be added together to support 99415 and, when applicable, 99416.

- ✖ *Never report both* prolonged office E/M service by a physician or other QHP (99417) and prolonged clinical staff services together.
- ✖ Do not include time spent providing separately reported services, such as intravenous medication administration or inhalation treatment, in the time of prolonged service.
- ✖ Do not include any time that is not face-to-face with the patient and/or family/caregiver.
- ✖ Do not report more than one unit of 99415 for service to the same patient on the same date. Report 99415 and 99416 for a cumulative time of 75 minutes or more beyond the typical clinical staff time.
- Codes 99415 and 99416 may be reported for *no more than 2 simultaneous patients,* and the time reported is the time devoted to only a single patient.
- Codes 99415 and 99416 were assigned RVUs (2025, 0.69 and 0.29, not geographically adjusted) based only on clinical staff's intraservice time, as the preservice and postservice times were included in the value of the related E/M service. RVUs for 2026 services were unavailable at the time of this publication.

The following guidelines apply to reporting of prolonged clinical staff services:

- A physician or other QHP must supervise the duration of prolonged clinical staff service.
- The total clinical staff time (whether continuous or segmented) and clinical indication(s) for the services must be documented.
- When not continuous, document and include the face-to-face time of each episode of clinical staff time.
- Report 99416 for each additional 30 minutes of clinical staff time beyond the first hour and for the last 15 to 30 minutes of prolonged clinical staff service. Do not report 99416 for a period of less than 15 minutes.

Outpatient Critical Care (99291, 99292)

Regardless of the patient's age, critical care services provided in outpatient settings are reported with hourly critical care codes (99291, 99292).

99291 Critical care, E/M of the critically ill or critically injured patient; first 30–74 minutes
+99292 each additional 30 minutes

Refer to Chapter 17 for further discussion of guidelines for critical care services and a listing of services included in critical care (ie, not separately reported).

A full 30 minutes of critical care service is required to support reporting 99291. For critical care services of less than 30 minutes, report the appropriate outpatient E/M code (eg, 99215).

If the same patient required outpatient and inpatient critical care services on the same day, the physician or a physician of the same group and specialty would report their services according to where the services were provided and the patient's age. Refer to "Critical Care Reporting in Outpatient Settings" at www.aap.org/cfp2026 for a decision tree for selecting codes for critical care provided in the outpatient setting.

Examples

➤ **A patient presents to an urgent care clinic with a respiratory illness and has become increasingly short of breath following coughing spells.** During the examination, the patient goes into respiratory failure with hypoxia, and her vital signs deteriorate. The physician provides critical care. An ambulance is called, and the physician continues critical care services until the transport team accepts care of the patient. The total time for critical care services provided by the physician is 40 minutes. The physician provides no further care to the patient and reports outpatient critical care services with a diagnosis of acute respiratory failure with hypoxia. Documentation includes the critical nature of the patient's condition, the care provided, and the total time spent in critical care dedicated to this patient.

ICD-10-CM	*CPT*
J96.01 (acute respiratory failure with hypoxia)	99291 (critical care, first 30–74 minutes)

Teaching Point: If the same physician or physician of the same specialty and group practice provided hourly critical care services in an inpatient setting on the same calendar date and the total critical care time was 75 minutes or more, 99292 would be reported with 1 unit for each block of time of up to 30 minutes beyond the first 74 minutes in addition to 99291 (eg, 99291 × 1, 99292 × 1).

➤ **A new patient experiences a seizure during intake by clinical staff in the neurology clinic.** Clinical staff summon a neurologist from another examination room and treatment is initiated, but the seizure continues. The physician provides critical care to the child for 20 minutes before an ambulance team assumes management. The physician documents a diagnosis of pharmaco-resistant juvenile myoclonic epilepsy with status epilepticus.

Problem(s) addressed ➡ ***High*** (1 acute or chronic illness or injury that poses a threat to life or bodily function)
Data reviewed and analyzed ➡ ***Limited*** (independent historian documented)
Risk of patient management ➡ ***High*** (decision regarding hospitalization)

ICD-10-CM	*CPT*
G40.B11 (juvenile myoclonic epilepsy, intractable, with status epilepticus)	99205 is supported by the problems addressed (ie, illness with threat to life or bodily function) and risk (ie, hospitalization). 99058 (service provided on an emergency basis in office, disrupting other scheduled services)

Teaching Point: Although the physician provided outpatient critical care services, the 30-minute minimum time for reporting 99291 (critical care, first 30–74 minutes) was not met. The office encounter is separately reported in addition to initial hospital care when a physician or QHP of the same specialty and same group practice provides both services on the same date. Modifier 25 is appended to the code for the office E/M service. For discussion of 99058, refer to the Codes for Reporting Special Circumstances section that follows.

Codes for Reporting Special Circumstances

The codes discussed in this section are reported in addition to the code(s) for an E/M service when there are special circumstances such as a service provided after the practice's normal business hours to allow care in the practice as opposed to an urgent care clinic or ED.

After-Hours Services (99050–99058)

After-hours codes are used to report services that are provided after hours or on an emergency basis and are always reported in addition to the primary service (eg, E/M service).

After-hours service codes 99050–99058 are used by physicians or other QHPs (under their state scope of practice when billing with their own NPI) to identify the services that are adjunct to the basic services rendered. These codes

- Describe the special circumstances under which a basic service is provided
- Are reported only in addition to an associated basic service (eg, E/M, fracture care)
- Are reported without a modifier appended to the basic service because they only further describe the services provided

Third-party payers will have specific policies for coverage and payment.

- Some carriers pay practices for extended hours because they recognize the cost benefit realized from decreased urgent care and ED visits.
  - Communicate with individual payers to understand their definition or interpretation of the service and their coverage and payment policies.
  - As part of this negotiation and education process, it is important to demonstrate the cost savings recognized by the payer for these adjunct services.
- If appropriate, more than one adjunct code may be reported on the same day of service (eg, **99058** and **99051** for services provided on an emergency basis during regularly scheduled evening or weekend hours).

Many payers will pay only for the use of a single special services code per encounter and may manually review, question, or deny payment for a claim with multiple after-hours codes.

Follow individual payer policy when reporting after-hours codes in conjunction with a service provided via telemedicine. Codes **99050** and **99051** are neither preceded by a telemedicine symbol (★ or ◀) nor included in Appendix P or T of the American Medical Association *CPT* manual. Therefore, these codes are not reported with telemedicine services.

Services Provided When the Office Is Normally Closed

99050 Service(s) provided in office at times other than regularly scheduled office hours, or days when the office is normally closed (eg, holidays, Saturday, Sunday), in addition to basic service

- Office hours must be posted. *CPT* does not define a holiday or posted office hours. Although most commonly applied to evening, weekend, or holiday hours, **99050** could be applied to services provided at the patient request on a weekday if the office is typically closed on that day.
- Code **99050** is *not* reported when a physician or other QHP is behind schedule and sees patients after posted office hours.
- The service must be requested by the patient, and the physician or other QHP must agree to see the patient.
- Documentation must indicate the time and date of the encounter and the request to be seen outside of normal posted hours.

Services Provided During Regularly Scheduled Evening, Weekend, or Holiday Hours

99051 Service(s) provided in the office during regularly scheduled evening, weekend, or holiday office hours, in addition to basic service

- Regularly scheduled office hours must be posted.
- Documentation must include the time and date of the encounter.
- Evenings and holidays are not defined by *CPT,* but holidays can generally refer to national and/or state holidays, and evenings are generally 6:00 pm and later. Check with payers for coverage and/or ability to bill patients these charges under the health plan contract.

Example

➤ **A pediatric clinic offers urgent care appointments 3 evenings a week with staffing by QHPs (eg, NPs, physician associates) working under general supervision.** A patient who has been seen at the clinic by Dr A within the past year is seen in the evening clinic by an NP who documents a clinically indicated history and examination with low-level MDM with diagnosis of URI.

ICD-10-CM	*CPT*
J06.9 (acute URI, unspecified)	**99213** (established office E/M) **99051** (service provided in office during regularly scheduled weekend hours)

Teaching Point: Because the office offers regularly scheduled evening hours, **99051** is reported. The patient is established because *CPT* instructs that QHPs are to be considered of the same specialty as the physicians with whom they work in a group practice. If the practice operated an urgent care clinic under a separate tax ID number, **99051** would not be applicable.

Services Provided on an Emergency Basis in the Office

99058 Service(s) provided on an emergency basis in the office, which disrupts other scheduled office services, in addition to basic service

- Report when an office patient's condition, in the clinical judgment of the physician, warrants the physician's interrupting care of another patient to deal with the emergency.
- Code **99058** may not be reported when patients are simply fit into the schedule or for walk-ins.
- Document that the patient was seen immediately and the reason for the emergent care.

Example

➤ **A pediatric practice offers scheduled appointments on Saturday mornings from 8:00 am to noon.** A child is scheduled for evaluation of increased symptoms of moderate persistent asthma on a Saturday at 9:00 am. The child arrives 30 minutes before the scheduled time with severe exacerbation and is immediately taken to an examination room by the triage nurse, and the physician disrupts his schedule to see the child urgently.

ICD-10-CM	*CPT*
J45.42 (moderate persistent asthma with status asthmaticus)	**99202–99215** (new or established office E/M) **99058** (service provided on an emergency basis in office, disrupting other scheduled services) **99051** (service provided in office during regularly scheduled weekend hours)

Teaching Point: If the Saturday hours were for walk-in visits only (ie, no scheduled appointments), **99058** would *not* be reported. If a physician or QHP of the same specialty and same group practice provides inpatient or observation care to the patient on the same date, modifier **25** (significant, separately identifiable service) is appended to the office E/M code. Check individual payer policy for reporting 2 E/M services on the same date.

Out-of-Office Service (99056–99060)

Codes **99056–99060** are used to report services provided after hours or on an emergency basis and are an adjunct to the basic E/M service provided.

Third-party payers have specific policies for coverage and payment. Communicate with individual payers to understand their definition or interpretation of the service and their coverage and payment policies. As part of this negotiation and education process, it is important to demonstrate the cost savings recognized by the payer for these adjunct services. After-hours service codes are used by physicians or other QHPs (under their state scope of practice when billing with their own NPI) to identify the services that are adjunct to the basic services rendered. These codes

- Describe the special circumstances under which a basic procedure is performed
- Are reported only in addition to an associated basic service (eg, home visit)
- Are reported without a modifier appended to the basic service because they only further describe the services provided

99056 Service(s) typically provided in the office, provided out of the office at request of patient, in addition to basic service

Documentation should include the patient's request to be seen outside the office.

99060 Service(s) provided on an emergency basis, out of the office, which disrupts other scheduled office services, in addition to basic service

Documentation should indicate that the physician was called away during scheduled office hours to attend to a patient in another location (eg, a nursing facility).

Example

➤ **A physician is seeing patients in the office when a parent calls and asks the physician to provide a house call for her child who would otherwise require specialized transport. The child has a fever and appears quite ill.** The physician agrees and, later that day, arrives at the patient's home to find that the patient is more withdrawn than typical. The physician spends a total of 40 minutes providing the home visit, which includes examining the child, diagnosing streptococcal sore throat based on clinical signs and symptoms, and prescribing an antibiotic.

ICD-10-CM	CPT
J02.0 (streptococcal pharyngitis) Assign codes for conditions that limit mobility.	99349 (established home or residence E/M requiring moderate MDM or total time of 40 minutes or more) 99056 (service[s] typically provided in the office, provided out of the office at request of patient, in addition to basic service)

Teaching Point: Payers may or may not allow payment for 99056 when services are rendered in a patient's home or residence or when a physician meets a patient in the ED. But it is appropriate to report 99056 when a service is provided at an alternative location at the request from the patient and/or caregiver. It is inappropriate to report 99056 when a physician instructs a patient to meet at a location other than the office. The POS on the claim should reflect where the encounter took place (eg, 12, patient's home).

To test your knowledge of the information presented in this chapter, complete the quiz found at the end of it, after the continuums and resources. Answers to each quiz are found in **Appendix II**.

Asthma, Attention-Deficit/Hyperactivity Disorder, and Otitis Media: Coding Continuums

Continuum Model for Asthma			
Code selection at any level above 99211 may be based on the level of MDM or the total time spent on the DOS by the reporting physician or other QHP. The extent of history and examination documented does not affect code selection.			
***CPT* Code and Vignette**	**Medical Decision-Making (2 of 3 Elements Required)**		
99211 Nurse visit for a well 10-year-old established patient	*Time and MDM do not apply. Must indicate continuation of physician's plan of care, medical necessity, assessment, and/or education provided.* Chief complaint: Review asthma care plan as ordered at last visit with doctor. Current medications documented, peak expiratory flow measured, education topics reviewed, and questions answered		
***CPT* Code With Total Physician Time and Vignette**	**No. and Complexity of Problems Addressed**	**Amount and/or Complexity of Data Reviewed and Analyzed**	**Risk of Complications and/or Morbidity or Mortality of Patient Management**
99212 (≥10 minutes) An 8-year-old with stable asthma presents with a single patch of poison ivy rash on her forearm.	**SF:** 1 self-limited or minor problem	**SF:** None	**SF:** Minimal risk of morbidity resulting from treatment
99213 (≥20 minutes) A 7-year-old with stable persistent asthma who is using a metered dose steroid inhaler with β-agonist as needed returns for follow-up.	**Low:** 1 stable chronic illness	**Limited:** Assessment requiring an independent historian(s)—Mother provides history of asthma symptoms and medication adherence since most recent visit.	**Moderate:** Prescription drug management
99214 (≥30 minutes) An 8-year-old with asthma is examined because of an acute exacerbation of the disease.	**Moderate:** ≥1 chronic illnesses with exacerbation, progression, or side effects of treatment	**Limited:** Assessment requiring an independent historian(s)—Mother provides history. *Note: Spirometry and pulse oximetry provided are separately reported and not counted toward data reviewed and analyzed.*	**Moderate:** Prescription drug management
***CPT* Code and Vignette**	**Medical Decision-Making (2 of 3 Elements Required)**		
***CPT* Code With Total Physician Time and Vignette**	**No. and Complexity of Problems Addressed**	**Amount and/or Complexity of Data Reviewed and Analyzed**	**Risk of Complications and/or Morbidity or Mortality of Patient Management**
99215 (≥40 minutes) An 8-year-old with unstable asthma presents with severe exacerbation of the disease and poor response to inhaler treatments at home. Oral steroids are administered with significant improvement. Hospitalization is discussed, but a decision is made for continued treatment at home with close monitoring.	**High:** 1 chronic condition with severe exacerbation	**Limited:** Assessment requiring an independent historian(s)	**High:** Decision regarding hospitalization

Abbreviations: *CPT, Current Procedural Terminology;* DOS, date of service; MDM, medical decision-making; SF, straightforward; QHP, qualified health care professional.

Continuum Model for Attention-Deficit/Hyperactivity Disorder

Code selection at any level above 99211 may be based on the level of MDM or the total time spent by the physician or other QHP on the date of the encounter.

CPT Code With Total Physician Time and Vignette	Medical Decision-making (2 of 3 Elements Required)		
	No. and Complexity of Problems Addressed	**Amount and/or Complexity of Data Reviewed and Analyzed**	**Risk of Complications and/or Morbidity or Mortality of Patient Management**
99211 Nurse visit to check growth or blood pressure before renewing prescription for psychoactive drugs	*Time and MDM do not apply. Must indicate continuation of physician's plan of care, medical necessity, assessment, and/or education provided.* Chief complaint: Check growth or blood pressure as ordered at last visit with doctor. Documentation: Height, weight, and blood pressure. Existing medications and desired/undesired effects. Assessment: Doing well. Obtained physician approval for prescription refill. Advised to keep appointment with physician in 1 month.		
99212 (≥10 minutes) 4-year-old whose parents are concerned about ADHD symptoms (ADHD is not diagnosed; parents are reassured.)	**Minimal:** 1 self-limited problem	**Limited:** Assessment requiring an independent historian	**Minimal:** Parent education
99213 (≥20 minutes) Initial follow-up after initiation of medication, patient responding well	**Low:** 1 stable chronic illness	**Limited:** Assessment requiring an independent historian	**Moderate:** Prescription drug management
99214 (≥30 minutes) Follow-up for recent weight loss in patient with established ADHD otherwise stable when taking stimulant medication	**Moderate:** 1 chronic illness with side effects of treatment	**Limited:** Assessment requiring an independent historian	**Moderate:** Prescription drug management
99215 (≥40 minutes) Initial evaluation of a patient with ADHD and new onset of suicidal ideation. The patient and mother decide on no hospitalization because of cost. *Tip:* Add **99417** if time on the DOS is ≥55 minutes. Add **99058** if service(s) are provided on an emergency basis in the office, which disrupts other scheduled office services.	**High:** 1 acute or chronic illness or injury that poses a threat to life or bodily function	**Moderate:** Assessment requiring an independent historian; discussion with behavioral health specialist; psychiatric testing	**High:** Decision regarding hospitalization

Abbreviations: ADHD, attention-deficit/hyperactivity disorder; *CPT, Current Procedural Terminology;* DOS, date of service; MDM, medical decision-making; QHP, qualified health care professional.

Continuum Model for Otitis Media			
Code selection at any level above **99211** *may be based on the level of MDM or the total time spent by the physician or other QHP on the date of the encounter. (Code 99211 is not included because of lack of indication for follow-up by clinical staff.)*			
	Medical Decision-making (2 of 3 Elements Required)		
***CPT* Code With Total Physician Time and Vignette**	**No. and Complexity of Problems Addressed**	**Amount and/or Complexity of Data Reviewed and Analyzed**	**Risk of Complications and/or Morbidity or Mortality of Patient Management**
99212 (≥10 minutes) Follow-up for otitis media, uncomplicated	**Minimal:** Follow-up for otitis media, evaluation of effusion and hearing	**Limited:** Assessment requiring an independent historian	**Minimal:** Risk associated with diagnostic testing and treatment
99213 (≥20 minutes) 2-year-old presents with tugging at her right ear. Afebrile. Mild otitis media.	**Low:** 1 acute, uncomplicated illness or injury	**Limited:** Assessment requiring an independent historian	**Moderate:** Prescription drug management, delayed prescribing
99214 (≥30 minutes) Infant presents with fever, lethargy, and cough and suspected third episode of otitis media within 3 months.	**Moderate:** 1 acute illness with systemic symptoms	**Limited:** Assessment requiring an independent historian	**Moderate:** Prescription drug management
99215 (≥40 minutes) 6-year-old presents with fever, severe left ear pain, and protrusion consistent with mastoiditis.	**High:** 1 acute illness that poses a threat to life or bodily function	**Moderate:** Assessment requiring an independent historian	**High:** Decision about hospitalization

Abbreviations: *CPT, Current Procedural Terminology;* MDM, medical decision-making; QHP, qualified health care professional.

Chapter Takeaways

This chapter focused on outpatient services that are reported according to either MDM or the total time by a physician or QHP on the date of the encounter. Readers of this chapter should generally understand outpatient code categories and code selection. Following are takeaways from this chapter:

- Codes for outpatient E/M services are selected according to the site of service as directed by *CPT* guidelines.
- The key determinant for reporting **G2211** is the intent for a long-term physician-patient relationship either as a focal point for all of a patient's health care needs or for management of a single serious or complex condition.
- To be considered a new patient, the patient must not have received a professional service from a physician or QHP of the same exact specialty and same group practice within the past 3 years.
- Office E/M services provided solely by clinical staff may be reported with **99211**. Payer policy may limit reporting to services that meet an incident-to policy.
- For all the outpatient visits discussed in this chapter except **99211**, the level of service is determined by either the level of MDM alone or by the total amount of time spent by a physician or other QHP on the DOS directed to care of the patient.
- Prolonged service may be reported when the time requirements are met.
- Critical care provided in outpatient settings is reported with time-based codes **99291** and **99292**.
- Use **99050–99060** in addition to the code for services provided when special circumstances apply (eg, a service provided after the practice's normal business hours to allow care in the practice as opposed to an urgent care clinic or ED).

Resources

AAP Coding Assistance and Education

AAP Initial History Questionnaire documentation form for office or outpatient visits (www.aap.org/Initial-History-Questionnaire-Documentation-Form-Pack-of-50)

Coding for Visit Complexity for Office/Other Outpatient Services (https://downloads.aap.org/AAP/PDF/AAP%20Factsheet%20Complexity%20Add%20On%20G2211.pdf)

Pediatric Evaluation and Management: Coding Quick Reference Card 2026 (www.aap.org/Pediatric-Evaluation-and-Management-Coding-Quick-Reference-Card-2026)

AAP News™

"Understanding updated E/M coding guidelines can prevent underbilling, loss of revenue," August 1, 2024 (https://publications.aap.org/aapnews/news/29460)

AAP Pediatric Coding Newsletter

"Answers to Questions About Evaluation and Management Code Selection in 2023," January 2023 (https://doi.org/10.1542/pcco_book225_document002)

"Compliance Corner: Incident-to Services," November 2024 (https://doi.org/10.1542/pcco_book247_document003)

E/M 2021 and 2023 coding resources (https://publications.aap.org/codingnews/info-parent/27376/Coding-Resources)

Online-Exclusive Content at www.aap.org/cfp2026

"AAP Position on Medicare Consultation Policy"

"Critical Care Reporting in Outpatient Settings"

"Evaluation and Management Service Coding in Nursing and Residential Treatment Facilities"

"Incident-to Services by Nonphysician Professionals and Clinical Staff: Medicare Requirements"

Test Your Knowledge!

1. **Which statement is true for reporting G2211 to indicate an office E/M (99202–99205, 99211–99215) was part of longitudinal care?**
   a. Do not report G2211 when reporting an office E/M service to address a problem (eg, 99213 25) and an influenza vaccine administration (eg, 90460) on the same date.
   b. G2211 is reported in addition to an office E/M code only when no other codes are reported on the same date.
   c. Do not report G2211 in addition to code 99211.
   d. G2211 is reported in addition to an office E/M code appended with modifier 25 only when reporting certain preventive services (eg, 90460–90461, immunization administration) on the same date.
2. **True or false? A service provided by clinical staff under the supervision of a physician or QHP who is immediately available via real-time audio-video telecommunications technology may be reported with 99211.**
   a. True
   b. False
3. **Which is true of the total time included in an office E/M code descriptor?**
   a. The time included in the code descriptor is the maximum time reported with the code.
   b. The time included in the code descriptor must be met or exceeded.
   c. The time included in the code descriptor includes only a physician's or QHP's face-to-face time with the patient and/or caregiver.
   d. Total time includes all time in a 24-hour period.
4. **Using Table 7-1 to guide code selection, which code is supported by documentation of a new patient office visit including 12 minutes, total time and straightforward MDM?**
   a. 99202
   b. 99212
   c. The visit cannot be reported because the code descriptor for 99202 requires at least 15 minutes of total time.
   d. The information in the question is insufficient for code selection.
5. **What information is necessary to support selection of prolonged clinical staff service code 99415?**
   a. The amount of clinical staff time that is beyond the total time spent by the reporting physician or QHP
   b. Only the total time spent by the reporting physician or QHP
   c. The office E/M code selected by the physician or QHP, based on MDM or total time, and the total face-to-face clinical staff time
   d. Only the total clinical staff time including both face-to-face and non-face-to-face time

CHAPTER 8

Preventive Services

Contents

Chapter Highlights

- Specific diagnosis and procedure codes for preventive evaluation and management (E/M) services, including sports preparticipation physical evaluations
- Coding for immunization administration (IA) services including vaccine/toxoid and immunoglobulin products
- Coding for immunization counseling without same-date administration
- Assigning and linking proper diagnosis and procedure codes for all preventive services provided at an encounter
- Reporting a significant E/M service to address a problem at the same encounter as a preventive E/M service

Preventive Care

Preventive care is the hallmark of pediatrics. A pediatric preventive visit (also known as a health supervision visit or well-child visit) typically includes a preventive medicine E/M service and recommended screenings, tests, and immunizations. In this chapter, we discuss coding for combinations of preventive services.

Payment for Recommended Preventive Care Services

The criterion standard of pediatric preventive care—the American Academy of Pediatrics (AAP) *Bright Futures: Guidelines for Health Supervision of Infants, Children, and Adolescents,* 4th Edition (www.aap.org/en/practice-management/bright-futures)—is recognized in the Patient Protection and Affordable Care Act as requiring coverage, *without cost sharing,* by most health care plans.

Coverage of and appropriate payment for these pediatric preventive services should, at a minimum, reflect the total relative value units (RVUs) outlined for the current year under the Medicare Resource-Based Relative Value Scale (RBRVS) Physician Fee Schedule, inclusive of all separately reported codes for these services. Section 2713 of the Patient Protection and Affordable Care Act includes the following 2 sets of services that must be provided to children without cost sharing:

1. The standard set of immunizations recommended by the Advisory Committee on Immunization Practices of the Centers for Disease Control and Prevention (CDC) with respect to the individual involved
2. Evidence-informed preventive care and screenings provided for in the comprehensive guidelines supported by the Health Resources and Services Administration, which include
   - The AAP/Bright Futures periodicity schedule, "Recommendations for Preventive Pediatric Health Care" (www.aap.org/en/practice-management/care-delivery-approaches/periodicity-schedule)
   - Recommendations of the Advisory Committee on Heritable Disorders in Newborns and Children

The AAP/Bright Futures periodicity schedule (refer to the insert in this book or visit www.aap.org/en/practice-management/care-delivery-approaches/periodicity-schedule) is a great tool for identifying recommended age-appropriate services, including many that may be reported with their own *Current Procedural Terminology* (*CPT*®) or Healthcare Common Procedure Coding System codes, when provided in conjunction with a comprehensive preventive service or on a separate date of service (DOS). The AAP *Pediatric Preventive Services: Coding Quick Reference Card 2026* (www.aap.org/Pediatric-Preventive-Services-Coding-Quick-Reference-Card-2026) combines these recommended services with the codes for each separately reportable service.

Although all recommended preventive services are covered, physicians and practice managers should be aware of health plan policies that may affect payment.

- Specific diagnosis codes may be required to support claims adjudication under preventive medicine benefits. Be sure to link the appropriate diagnosis to each service provided (eg, **Z71.3**, dietary counseling, may be linked to **99401** for a risk factor reduction counseling visit).
- Some payers bundle certain services when the services are provided on the same date. For instance, some plans will not allow separate payment for obesity counseling on the same date as a well-child examination (at a health supervision visit) but will cover obesity counseling when no other E/M service is provided on the same date.
  - It is beneficial to monitor and maintain awareness of the payment policies of the plans most billed by your practice.
  - Most policies are available on payers' websites with notification of changes provided in payer communications, such as electronic newsletters.

Preventive Medicine Evaluation and Management Services

Well-child or preventive medicine services are a type of E/M service and are reported with codes **99381–99395**. Most health plans provide a 100% benefit (no patient out-of-pocket cost) for the 30 recommended preventive medicine service encounters provided to patients from 3 to 5 days after discharge from the birth admission through adulthood when provided by in-network providers. Most health plans limit the benefits for preventive medicine E/M services covered in a year by patient age (eg, annually for patients aged ≥3 years).

Selection of the pediatric-specific codes **99381–99395** is based simply on the age of the patient on the date of the encounter and whether the patient is new or established to the practice (**Table 8-1**).

Table 8-1. New and Established Comprehensive Preventive Medicine Codes

Patient Age and Recommended Visits by the AAP/Bright Futures Periodicity Schedule	New Patient Code	Established Patient Code	Diagnosis Codes
Infant (age <1 year) 6 visits recommended at ages 3–5 days, by 1 month, and at 2, 4, 6, and 9 months	99381	99391	**Z00.110** (health examination for newborn <8 days) **Z00.111** (health examination for newborn 8–28 days old) **Z00.121** (routine child health examination [≥29 days] with abnormal findings) **Z00.129** (routine child health examination [≥29 days] without abnormal findings)
Early childhood (age 1–4 years) 7 visits recommended at ages 12, 15, 18, 24, and 30 months and at 3 and 4 years	99382	99392	
Late childhood (age 5–11 years) 1 visit recommended per year or per 12 months	99383	99393	
Adolescent (age 12–17 years) 1 visit recommended per year or per 12 months	99384	99394	
Age 18–39 years 1 visit recommended per year or per 12 months	99385	99395	**Z00.00** (encounter for general adult medical examination without abnormal findings) **Z00.01** (encounter for general adult medical examination with abnormal findings)

Abbreviation: AAP, American Academy of Pediatrics.

In brief, an established patient has received a face-to-face service (including via telemedicine) by the physician or another physician or other qualified health care professionals (QHPs; eg, advanced practice nurses, physician associates) of the same specialty and group practice within the past 3 years. Refer to **Chapter 7** for more information about *new* versus *established* patients.

A neonate who received hospital newborn care by the same physician or a physician of the same specialty and same group practice will be an established patient for post-discharge care in the office or other outpatient setting.

- The recommended newborn visit, within 3 to 5 days of birth and within 48 to 72 hours after discharge from the birth admission, may be called a weight check. A physician or other QHP provides this service to evaluate feeding, detect any signs of jaundice, and complete or review findings of neonatal screenings. This is a recommended preventive E/M service.

When a physician or QHP develops a plan of care that includes a return visit for a weight check by clinical staff because of feeding concerns, this visit is a problem-oriented visit typically reported with 99211 (office E/M not requiring the presence of a physician or QHP). Clinical staff documenting a 99211 service should reference the physician's or QHP's order for the service. A clinical staff visit to weigh a patient outside an established plan of care (eg, at the request of a parent/caregiver) is not an E/M service.

If the visit results in a face-to-face service by the physician or QHP on the same date, higher level E/M codes are typically appropriate (eg, level 3 established patient visit, 99213).

- Immunizations, laboratory tests, and other special procedures or screening tests (eg, vision, hearing, or developmental screening) that have their own specific *CPT* codes are reported separately *in addition to* preventive medicine E/M services.
- Most payers require reporting modifier **25** with the preventive medicine service when IA or other services are also performed and reported. Some payers do not pay for preventive screenings but may allow a physician to bill the patient. Contracts with payers may limit what may be billed to the patient.
- A comprehensive history and physical examination must reflect an age- and gender-appropriate history and examination.
- The comprehensive history performed as part of a preventive medicine visit requires a comprehensive age-appropriate review of systems with an updated past, family, and social history. The history should also include a comprehensive assessment or history of age-pertinent risk factors.
- Generally, the review of systems of a preventive medicine service is not a list of systems with pertinent positive and negative responses but, rather, a list of inquiries and patient responses for the areas of risk identified in preventive medicine guidelines as pertinent for patients of that age and gender. But some payers may require review of all systems regardless of age and gender (eg, required by some Medicaid plans under Early and Periodic Screening, Diagnostic, and Treatment benefits).

The AAP Initial History Questionnaire promotes documentation of preventive medicine services to support proper coding and appropriate payment. Forms can be ordered from the AAP by visiting www.aap.org/Initial-History-Questionnaire-Documentation-Form-Pack-of-50. Additionally, some Medicaid programs have developed documentation templates for preventive services delivered in their Early and Periodic Screening, Diagnostic, and Treatment program.

Chapter 8
Preventive Services

- Routine contraceptive counseling and management are considered part of the comprehensive preventive medicine E/M service when provided during the preventive visit. Contraceptive procedures (eg, insertion or removal of device or implant, injection) are separately reported as discussed in **Chapter 13.** Refer to *International Classification of Diseases, 10th Revision, Clinical Modification* (*ICD-10-CM*) category **Z30** for diagnosis codes for contraceptive counseling and/or management.
- A comprehensive physical examination is a multisystem examination that may include a routine pelvic and breast examination (when performed in the absence of specific symptoms of a problem) depending on the age of the patient and/or sexual history. Add-on code **99459** (pelvic examination) may be reported in addition to the preventive E/M code for the practice expense of performing the female pelvic examination. This code is not assigned work RVUs.
  - If the pelvic examination is performed to evaluate a gynecologic problem during a routine preventive medicine service, it may be appropriate to report a problem-oriented E/M service in addition to the preventive medicine service when additional physician work and requirements of the E/M code are met. Code **99459** may be reported in addition to codes **99202–99215** and **99242–99245**.

For further discussion of code 99459, refer to the December 2023 *AAP Pediatric Coding Newsletter*™ article "2024 *Current Procedural Terminology* Updates: Female Pelvic Examination" (https://doi.org/10.1542/pcco_book236_document002).

- Medicaid programs have requirements for performing, documenting, and reporting certain services in their Early and Periodic Screening, Diagnostic, and Treatment programs. Modifier **52** (reduced services) may be required when the complete Early and Periodic Screening, Diagnostic, and Treatment service cannot be completed. Review your Medicaid plan policies for the specific documentation and reporting requirements for services to patients in these programs.

ICD-10-CM Codes for Preventive Care Visits

ICD-10-CM well-care diagnosis codes should be linked to the appropriate preventive medicine code (**99381–99395**) as shown in **Table 8-1**. *ICD-10-CM* codes for well-child examinations include developmental, hearing, and vision screening. However, codes for screening for global developmental delays (**Z13.42**) and screening for autism (**Z13.41**) may be reported in conjunction with well-care diagnosis codes to identify the type of developmental screening performed.

- *ICD-10-CM* does not specify an age at which codes **Z00.00** and **Z00.01** are reported in lieu of childhood codes **Z00.121–Z00.129**. The age of majority varies by state and payer, which may or may not adopt the Medicare Outpatient Code Editor assignment of age limitations (29 days–17 years) to codes **Z00.121–Z00.129**, as indicated in many *ICD-10-CM* references.

- When assigning codes in category Z00, an *abnormal finding* is a newly discovered condition on screening or a known or chronic condition that requires attention because of exacerbation or inadequate control. Assign Z00.121 or Z00.01 and additional codes for documented abnormal findings. A stable chronic condition is not considered an abnormal finding, although a code for the condition may be reported as discussed in the next list item.
- When reporting a routine child health examination *without abnormal findings,* report Z00.129 or Z00.00 and a code for any stable or improving condition(s) addressed during the visit.
- An abnormal finding *ICD-10-CM* code (eg, Z00.121) can be linked to the procedure code for a normal screening test result; the abnormality will be identified with the appropriate *ICD-10-CM* code elsewhere on the claim so the payer will be aware that the abnormality is unrelated to the screening.
- Link routine child health examination codes (eg, Z00.129) and either Z23 (encounter for immunization) or Z29.11 (encounter for prophylactic immunotherapy for respiratory syncytial virus [RSV]), as applicable, to the IA and immunization product codes when immunizations are administered at a child's preventive medicine encounter. *ICD-10-CM* instructs to report Z00.1- first, followed by Z23. *ICD-10-CM* does not instruct to report first a code for any routine adult examination (Z00.0-); link only Z23 to codes for immunization services.

Preventive Services for Children With Chronic and Complex Health Care Needs

Like all children, children with chronic and complex health care needs must receive periodic preventive care visits. Preventive medicine E/M services may take longer for these children. But preventive E/M services are not reported according to time, and prolonged service does not apply. Only report a separate E/M service on the date of a preventive E/M service when a problem is addressed that requires significant physician work (ie, medical decision-making [MDM] or time) and is separately identifiable in the documentation. A chronic medical condition that is not separately addressed with documentation of the required MDM or time spent addressing the condition does not support reporting both preventive care and a separate E/M service (eg, 99213).

Refer to Chapter 9 for information on care management for children with complex health care needs.

Examples

➤ **A 9-year-old is seen for an established patient preventive medicine service.** The child was seen 1 month ago for mild persistent asthma and reports no increase in asthma symptoms. But the child's mother notes that the child's rescue inhaler, which is carried to and from school, is nearing the expiration date. An age- and gender-appropriate preventive service is provided and documented. A refill prescription is ordered for the rescue inhaler. Diagnoses are well-child visit and stable mild persistent asthma.

ICD-10-CM	*CPT*
Z00.129 (routine child health examination without abnormal findings) J45.30 (uncomplicated mild persistent asthma)	99393 (preventive medicine visit; age 5–11)

Teaching Point: Because the asthma is not newly identified or failing to respond adequately to treatment, this is not an abnormal finding. However, it is appropriate to report the code for the asthma that is still present in addition to Z00.129. In this example, the work of prescribing the asthma medication refill did not equate to a significant, separately identifiable E/M service.

➤ **A 9-year-old was diagnosed 8 weeks ago with mild persistent asthma.** The child presents today for a scheduled preventive service and follow-up visit. The child complains of increasing asthma symptoms and use of rescue inhaler. The patient's medications and asthma control plan are revised, and the physician provides counseling to reinforce the avoidance of asthma triggers and management adherence. The age- and gender-appropriate preventive service is also provided and documented. The diagnoses are well-child visit with abnormal findings and mild persistent asthma with increasing symptoms.

ICD-10-CM	*CPT*
Z00.121 (routine child health exam with abnormal findings) J45.31 (mild persistent asthma with acute exacerbation)	99393 (preventive medicine visit; age 5–11)
J45.31	99214 25 (established patient office visit with moderate level MDM)

Teaching Point: Because the asthma was inadequately controlled, the routine health examination included an abnormal finding. A significant E/M service was provided to address the patient's asthma control. For more on this topic, refer to Reporting a Preventive Medicine Visit With a Problem-Oriented Visit section later in this chapter. Code J45.31 is reported once on the claim but linked to each procedure code.

If an immunization had been administered at this encounter, modifier 25 would have also been appended to 99393 to signify that the preventive E/M service was significant and separately identifiable from the IA service.

Quality Initiatives and Preventive Care

Quality initiatives and measurement are standard practice in health care. In pediatrics, many quality measures are associated with preventive care.

Quality measurement is required of health plans funded by government programs or offered through health exchanges under the Patient Protection and Affordable Care Act. Plans collect a subset of the National Committee for Quality Assurance Healthcare Effectiveness Data and Information Set (HEDIS) measures and a Pharmacy Quality Alliance measure through claims data or medical records. Examples of HEDIS measures related to preventive care include

- Percentage of members who turned 15 or 30 months old during the measurement year and had 6 or more well-child visits with a primary care provider during the first 15 months after birth *and* 2 or more well-child visits from 1 day after the child turned 15 months old to the day the child turns 30 months old
- Percentage of members 3 to 21 years of age who had at least 1 comprehensive well-care visit with a primary care provider or obstetrician-gynecologist during the measurement year
- Members 3 to 17 years of age who had an outpatient visit with a primary care provider and who had the following services in the current year:
  - Body mass index (BMI) percentile documentation
  - Counseling for nutrition
  - Counseling for physical activity

Certain preventive services, such as anticipatory guidance on healthy diet (Z71.3) and exercise (Z71.82), are components of the preventive medicine service and require no additional procedure coding for payment purposes. Associated diagnosis and procedure codes, however, may be reported to support quality reporting initiatives.

Per *ICD-10-CM* guidelines, report BMI codes only when there is an associated, reportable diagnosis (eg, overweight, obesity). Some health plans, however, still require this code to support quality measures in lieu of *CPT* performance measurement code 3008F (BMI, documented). When reporting BMI in the absence of a related diagnosis, report the code secondary to the Z00 preventive visit code. Pediatric BMI codes in category Z68 include

Z68.51 BMI <5th percentile
Z68.52 BMI 5th–<85th percentile
Z68.53 BMI 85th–95th percentile
Z68.54 BMI ≥95th percentile for age to less than 120% of the 95th percentile for age
Z68.55 BMI 120% of the 95th percentile for age to less than 140% of the 95th percentile for age
Z68.56 BMI ≥140% of the 95th percentile for age

For additional discussion of BMI codes, refer to the September 2024 *AAP Pediatric Coding Newsletter* article "Important *ICD-10-CM* Changes to Reporting Obesity and Pediatric Body Mass Index" (https://doi.org/10.1542/pcco_book245_document003).

Any chronic conditions reported may also support quality measurement and/or risk adjustment. Refer to **Chapters 3** and **9** to learn more about HEDIS, quality reporting, risk adjustment, and reporting of chronic conditions.

Certain other procedure codes also support quality measurement. For example, reporting codes for meningococcal (eg, 90734, 90619); tetanus, diphtheria, and acellular pertussis (Tdap) (90715); and 2 or 3 doses of human papillomavirus (HPV) (90651) vaccines provided to an adolescent *before the patient's 13th birthday* is indicative of meeting the measure for the immunization of adolescents.

Some quality measures include information on reporting that a patient is ineligible for inclusion in the measure. For example, screening for depression (Z13.31) is recommended for patients 12 years and older who were seen during the measurement year. But patients already diagnosed with depression (eg, F32.1, major depressive disorder, single episode, mild) or bipolar disorder (eg, F31.81, bipolar II disorder) are not included in the measurement.

It is important to note that a request for medical records is less likely when claims are submitted with procedure and diagnosis codes associated with pediatric quality measures.

Sports/Camp Preparticipation Physical Evaluations

Preventive medicine service codes (99381–99395) most accurately describe physical evaluations performed to determine participation eligibility. The physical evaluations are preventive and age appropriate in nature, and physicians offer counseling on topics such as appropriate levels of exercise or injury prevention. Yet the need for these services often arises after the child has had a yearly preventive medicine service, thereby rendering this service noncovered by some health plans, which allow only 1 preventive service per year. In this case, the parent may be billed if the payer contract allows because the service is noncovered.

When reporting sports or camp preparticipation physical evaluations for patients who have already received a recommended preventive medicine service, check the health plan's policy on payment for these services and instructions for coding and billing. Under some plans, especially Medicaid plans, school and preparticipation physical evaluations may be covered even when the child has already had an annual preventive medicine service.

Office visit codes (99212–99215) may be used if the service is not comprehensive or a problem is evaluated during the service. Outpatient consultation codes (99242–99245) might be reported (when the health plan allows payment for these codes) if the coach or school nurse requested the physician's opinion of a suspected problem (eg, exercise cough associated with reduced performance in cold weather). The medical record must include documentation of the written or verbal request as well as a copy of the written report with the physician's opinion or advice that was sent back to the coach or school nurse when reporting a consultation.

If the preparticipation physical evaluation is incorporated into the annual health supervision visit, use Z00.121 or Z00.129. Report also any problems or conditions addressed during the visit. When a comprehensive preventive medicine service is not performed, report Z02.5 (encounter for examination for participation in sports) or Z02.89 (encounter for other administrative examination). Code Z02.89 includes an examination for clearance to attend a camp.

When reporting an examination for return to play after resolution of an illness or injury, report Z09 (encounter for follow-up examination after completed treatment for conditions other than malignant neoplasm) in addition to a code for the patient's history of illness or injury, when indicated, and the code for the examination for clearance (eg, Z02.5, Z02.89).

Example

➤ **A 15-year-old is seen at an established patient visit to evaluate fitness for return to play, specifically basketball, 3 months after diagnosis of infectious mononucleosis.** A comprehensive preventive medicine service is not indicated because the patient's most recent routine examination was 6 months before this visit. After evaluation and counseling, the physician completes the form releasing the patient to resume all activities, including basketball. Diagnoses are clearance for activities following resolved mononucleosis. A level 3 office visit is documented.

ICD-10-CM	*CPT*
Z09 (encounter for follow-up examination after completed treatment for conditions other than malignant neoplasm) Z86.19 (personal history of other infectious and parasitic diseases) Z02.5 (encounter for examination for participation in sports)	99213 (office E/M with low-level MDM or a minimum of 20 minutes' total time on the date of the visit)

Teaching Point: Because the determination to return to play required evaluation of the patient's health status following illness, the visit is reported as a follow-up after completed treatment. *ICD-10-CM* guidelines do not support reporting a code for a condition that no longer exists. However, a payer may require a code for a condition that prompted follow-up care (eg, B27.90, infectious mononucleosis, unspecified without complication) in addition to Z09.

Category Z02 codes are not reported in conjunction with codes for routine child health examination (category Z00). Report only the Z00 code when clearance for participation is provided in conjunction with a routine child health examination.

Immunizations

Vaccine, toxoid, and immunoglobulin services are reported with *CPT* codes to identify the product and for the services associated with administration of the product (IA). Exceptions apply when patients receive immunizations through the Vaccines for Children (VFC) program. Refer to the Vaccines for Children Program section later in this chapter for more details on VFC coding.

Implementation of New Immunization Product Codes

The *CPT* Editorial Panel, in recognition of the public health interest in immunization products, may publish new immunization product codes before US Food and Drug Administration (FDA) approval. The American Medical Association (AMA) uses its *CPT* site (www.ama-assn.org/practice-management/cpt/category-i-immunization-codes) to provide updates of *CPT* Editorial Panel actions on new products. Once approved by the *CPT* Editorial Panel, vaccine/toxoid/immunoglobulin product codes are typically made available for release on a triannual basis (April 1, July 1, and October 1) with implementation dates of July 1, October 1, and January 1 (eg, released 10/25, implemented 01/26). When a government agency has identified an urgent need for immunization services to address an emergent health issue and the FDA has granted the associated product an expedited review process, codes may be approved and released on an *immediate* (ie, outside the normal code consideration schedule) or *rapid* (ie, within the normal code consideration schedule but shortly after approval with an implementation date within 3 months of release) basis.

Codes for products pending FDA approval are indicated with a lightning bolt symbol (~) that will be removed once the FDA status changes to "approved." Refer to the AMA *CPT* site for the most up-to-date information on codes with this symbol.

In the rare event that (a) an immunization product enters the market this year and is FDA approved, (b) recommendations for use are published by the CDC or AAP, and (c) no code exists for the specific immunization product, use **90749** (unlisted vaccine/toxoid) and list the specific vaccine given. Code **90399** is reported for an unlisted immunoglobulin product.

Before administering any new product or an existing product with new immunization recommendations, make certain that the CDC, in the *Morbidity and Mortality Weekly Report,* or the AAP, in *Pediatrics*®, has endorsed the use or recommendations of the vaccine. Verification that individual payers have updated their systems and policies to pay for new immunization products is highly recommended.

It is also important to verify with a patient's health plan that a new immunization product and IA are covered.

National Drug Code

Medicare, Medicaid, other government payers (eg, Tricare), and some private payers, require the use of the National Drug Code (NDC) in addition to immunization product codes. The NDCs are universal product identifiers for medications, including immunization products. NDCs are found on outer packaging, product labels, and/or product inserts. Report the NDC from the outer packaging or product labels/inserts as required by the payer.

NDCs are 10-digit, 3-segment numbers that identify the product, labeler, and trade package size. The Health Insurance Portability and Accountability Act of 1996 standards require an 11-digit code. Refer to **Chapter 1** and **Table 1-3** for more information, including how 10-digit codes are converted to the 11-digit format for reporting.

Be sure to report the appropriate NDC (from outer or inner package) and number of units as required by the payer. The NDC units are often different from the units linked to the *CPT* code for the product. For example, when reporting a vaccine from a 0.5-mL single-dose vial, a payer may require that NDC units be reported with ML0.5 or, less frequently, with a single unit, UN1.0. (The units qualifier [eg, ML] is followed by the units administered without a space between the qualifier and units.)

If you are not currently reporting vaccines with NDCs, be sure to coordinate the requirements with your billing software company or external billing service, as applicable. For more information on NDCs, visit www.fda.gov/drugs/drug-approvals-and-databases/national-drug-code-directory.

Refer to the September 2025 *AAP Pediatric Coding Newsletter* article "Refresh Your Knowledge: Reporting National Drug Codes" (https://doi.org/10.1542/pcco_book257_document003) for more information on how NDCs are reported on claims.

Categories of Immunization Products and Associated Codes

Codes differentiate active immunization by administration of vaccine/toxoid products versus passive immunization via a monoclonal antibody product (eg, nirsevimab to immunize infants against RSV). The types of product codes for vaccines, toxoids, and immunoglobulins are linked to specific IA codes, as shown in **Table 8-2**.

Table 8-2. Codes for Immunization Administration by Type[a]

Pediatric Vaccine and Toxoid IA (90460–90461)[b]	General Vaccine and Toxoid IA (90471–90474)	COVID-19 Vaccine IA (90480 and 90461 or 90481[c])	RSV Seasonal IA (96380–96381)
Patients aged ≤18 years: Same-date counseling by physician or QHP is required.	Patients aged ≥19 years; also, those aged ≤18 years without same-date counseling by physician or QHP	All ages: includes counseling, when performed	0–19 months of age: IA codes distinguish with/without counseling by physician or QHP.
Product codes: 90476–90759	Product codes: 90476–90759	Product codes: 91304, 91318–91322	Product codes: 90380–90382
Report 1 unit per product. 90460 (first or only component of each vaccine or toxoid administered)	Report either 90471 or 90473 per DOS (not both). 90471 (initial IA by injection of 1 product) 90473 (initial IA by intranasal/oral route of 1 product)	Report with 1 unit per DOS. 90480 (IA by injection, COVID-19 vaccine; first or only component of each vaccine administered)	Report 1 code with 1 unit per DOS. 96380 (IA by injection, seasonal RSV product with counseling by physician or QHP) 96381 (without counseling)
90461 (each additional vaccine or toxoid component administered)	Report 1 unit per additional product administered (report per product, not per component). 90472 (each additional IA by injection) 90474 (each additional intranasal/oral IA)	Each additional component: 90461 or 90481[c] Refer to 90461, or 96380–96381, as applicable, for IA of separate products.	Refer to 90460–90461, 90471–90474, or 90480, as applicable, for additional IA.

Abbreviations: DOS, date of service; IA, immunization administration; QHP, qualified health care professional; RSV, respiratory syncytial virus.

[a] Report Z29.11 (encounter for prophylactic immunotherapy for RSV) in conjunction with codes for RSV seasonal immunization reported with 90380–90382 and 96380–96381. Report Z23 (encounter for immunization) in conjunction with all codes for vaccines and toxoids and for IA other than for RSV immunization.

[b] Includes IA by any route (eg, nasal, oral, or injection).

[c] Report 90461 for IA of additional components combined with a COVID-19 vaccine with counseling by the physician or QHP to patients ≤18 years of age. Report 90481 in lieu of 90461 for IA of additional components combined with a COVID-19 vaccine to patients ≥19 years or without counseling by a physician or QHP.

Immunization product codes and associated IA codes are discussed in more detail later in this chapter.

Immunization Administration With Counseling

IA codes are important for reporting the costs of physician supervision and practice expense associated with IA. Certain IA codes (90460–90461 and 96380) are reported only when immunization counseling is provided face-to-face with the patient by a physician or other QHP on the date of administration. Failure to report the appropriate IA codes can result in significant loss of revenue that is necessary to support IA in a pediatric practice.

Refer to the Coding for Counseling Without Same-Date Immunization section later in this chapter for discussion of new codes for reporting these services.

The following guidance applies to the selection of codes for IA with counseling versus IA without counseling (or to an adult patient):

- *CPT* defines a physician or other QHP as follows:

  A "physician or other qualified health care professional" is an individual who by education, training, licensure/regulation, facility credentialing (when applicable), and facility privileging (when applicable) performs a professional service within his/her scope of practice and independently reports that professional service. These professionals are distinct from "clinical staff."

- Clinical staff are not qualified to perform the counseling reported with **90460**, **90461**, or **96380**. Although state scope of practice may allow certain clinical staff to perform the service, it will not qualify them to report these codes. In the absence of counseling by a physician or QHP, IA services by clinical staff are reported with IA codes that do not require counseling. *CPT* defines clinical staff as follows:

  A clinical staff member is a person who works under the supervision of a physician or other qualified health care professional and who is allowed by law, regulation, and facility policy to perform or assist in the performance of a specified professional service, but who does not individually report that professional service. Other policies may also affect who may report specific services.

When a private payer contract does not allow QHPs to report services under their own name and National Provider Identifier, check with the payer to determine the eligibility of these professionals to report immunization counseling (**90460**, **90461**, and/or **96380**) under the name and number of the supervising physician.

- Documentation of immunization counseling should include a listing of all vaccine components with notation that counseling was provided for all listed components with authentication (electronic or written signature and date) by the physician or other QHP. Some payers require documentation of parent or caregiver questions or concerns that were addressed during counseling.
- The code for IA of a COVID-19 vaccine, **90480,** includes immunization counseling by a physician or QHP, when performed. Refer to the Codes **90480** and **90481** section later in this chapter for how to code IA of a vaccine that includes COVID-19 and another component.

The word *component* refers to an antigen in a vaccine that prevents disease(s) caused by 1 organism. For example, a measles-mumps-rubella (MMR) vaccine has 3 components, and HPV 9-valent vaccine has 1 component (although there are 9 HPV variants included, the vaccine prevents one disease).

Chapter 8

Preventive Services

✖ Do not report a code for IA with counseling for simply supplying the Vaccine Information Statement (VIS) without discussion of risks and benefits.

Reporting the correct IA code for pediatric IA with counseling by a physician or QHP should result in higher total payment based on the RVUs assigned to each code and the number of units reported. For further discussion, refer to the Vaccine and Toxoid Immunization Administration section later in this chapter.

Reporting Vaccine and Toxoid Products

Vaccine and toxoid product codes **90476–90759**, **91304**, and **91318–91322** are used to report the vaccine or toxoid product only. They do not include the administration of the product.

- The exact product administered needs to be reported to meet the requirements of immunization registries, vaccine distribution programs, and reporting systems (eg, Vaccine Adverse Event Reporting System), as well as for payment.
- Codes may be specific to the product manufacturer and brand, schedule (ie, number of doses or timing), chemical formulation, dosage, and/or route of administration. When a vaccine code descriptor includes "when administered to" patients of certain ages, this is not an indication of the ages for which the product is licensed.
- Codes for combination vaccines (eg, **90697**, diphtheria, tetanus toxoids, acellular pertussis vaccine, inactivated poliovirus vaccine, *Haemophilus influenzae* type b PRP-OMP conjugate vaccine, and hepatitis B vaccine [DTaP-IPV-Hib-Hep B]) are available, as are separate codes for single-component vaccines (eg, **90744**, Hep B).
- It is not appropriate to code each component of a combination vaccine separately with separate vaccine product codes when a combination vaccine is administered. But if a combination vaccine was commercially available and a physician elected to administer the component vaccines for clinical reasons (eg, separate IA of MMR vaccine and varicella vaccine to reduce the risk for seizures) or because of unavailability of a combination product, each vaccine product administered would be separately reported.

Vaccine and Toxoid Immunization Administration

CPT codes for vaccine IA are reported *in addition to* vaccine/toxoid code(s) **90476–90758**, **91304**, and **91318–91323**. There are 3 sets of codes for IA of vaccines and toxoids.

- **90460** and **90461** (IA with counseling by a physician or QHP to child from birth through 18 years of age)
- **90471–90474** (IA to adult or to a child, from birth through 18 years of age, without counseling by a physician or QHP)
- **90480** and **90481** (IA of COVID-19 vaccine or combination COVID-19/other vaccine product)

Reporting multiple IA codes does not typically require a modifier. Most payers advise reporting multiple units of the same service on a single line of the claim. Individual payer guidance, however, may vary.

Clinical staff performing IA should document the administration as required by the National Childhood Vaccine Injury Act and recommended by the AAP in the "7 Rights of Vaccine Administration" (www.aap.org/en/patient-care/immunizations/implementing-immunization-administration-in-your-practice/vaccine-administration).

Codes 90460 and 90461

90460 IA through 18 years of age via any route of administration, with counseling by physician or other QHP; first or only component of each vaccine or toxoid administered

+90461 each additional vaccine or toxoid component administered (report only in addition to **90460**)

When reporting **90460** and **90461**,

- Physicians or QHPs must provide *face-to-face* counseling to the patient and/or family (patient aged ≤18 years) on the date of the encounter for the administration of a vaccine.
- Report **90460** for the first (or only) component of each vaccine administered (whether single or combination) with vaccine counseling provided on the same date. *Every vaccine administered will include a first or only component.*
- Code **90461** is reported only in conjunction with **90460** or **90480** and is used to report the work of counseling for *each additional component(s) beyond the first* in a combination vaccine. (Refer to the Vaccines for Children Program section later in this chapter for reporting administration of vaccines containing multiple components to this program.)
- Combination vaccines are vaccines that contain multiple vaccine components.
- IA codes **90460** and **90461** include the physician or other QHP discussing risks and benefits of the vaccines, providing parents with a copy of the appropriate CDC VIS for each vaccine given, giving the vaccine, and observing and addressing reactions or adverse effects, as well as the cost of clinical staff time to record each vaccine component administered in the medical record and statewide vaccine registry and the cost of supplies (eg, syringe, needle, bandages).
- Higher total payment should result from reporting combination vaccines with **90460** and multiple units of **90461** for IA of the first and *each additional vaccine component* versus reporting IA without counseling or provided to a patient 19 years or older for the first and *each additional vaccine product* (**90471–90474**).
- Administration of vaccines provided through the VFC program is paid differently. For more about the VFC program, refer to the Vaccines for Children Program section later in this chapter.)

Append modifier **25** when a significant, separately identifiable E/M service (eg, office or other outpatient service, preventive medicine service) is performed in addition to IA. If vaccines are given during a preventive medicine E/M service and another E/M service, both E/M services will need modifier **25** if required by the payer. Refer also to the Reporting a Preventive Medicine Visit With a Problem-Oriented Visit section later in this chapter.

Examples

➤ **A 17-year-old presents with a request for an influenza immunization.** After a nurse practitioner counsels the patient, clinical staff administer an intranasal trivalent influenza vaccine (LAIV3) at the same encounter. IA code **90460** is reported with 1 unit in addition to product code **90660** (LAIV3). *ICD-10-CM* code **Z23** is linked to **90460** and **90660** on the health insurance claim.

Teaching Point: Code **90461** is not reported because the vaccine contains only 1 component (ie, protects against 1 disease).

➤ **An 11-year-old established patient presents for a routine health examination.** In the course of providing the routine examination, the pediatrician determines that immunization against influenza, HPV, meningococcal disease, tetanus, diphtheria, and whooping cough is indicated. After the pediatrician counsels the patient, clinical staff administer an intranasal trivalent influenza vaccine (LAIV3); the first of 2 doses of meningococcal conjugate vaccine (MenACWY-TT); Tdap vaccine; and the first of 2 doses of HPV vaccine (9vHPV) at the same encounter. The pediatrician documents the routine health examination (without abnormal findings) and counseling for the recommended vaccines.

ICD-10-CM	*CPT*
Z00.129 (routine child health examination without abnormal findings) **Z23** (encounter for immunization)	**99393 25** (preventive E/M; late childhood [age 5 through 11 years]) **90660** (intranasal trivalent influenza vaccine [LAIV3]) **90619** (MenACWY-TT) **90715** (Tdap) **90651** (9vHPV) **90460** × 4 (IA, first or only component) **90461** × 2 (IA, each additional component)

Teaching Point: Because counseling by a physician or QHP was provided to a patient younger than 19 years, IA is reported with **90460** and **90461**. Four vaccine products were administered, supporting 4 units of **90460**. The Tdap vaccine includes 3 components: tetanus, diphtheria, and acellular pertussis. Code **90461** is reported with 2 units for the second and third components of the Tdap vaccine. Only **90460** is reported for MenACWY-TT and HPV because these are single-component vaccines that protect against disease caused by one organism, although providing protection against multiple strains of each organism.

Payers that have adopted the Medicare National Correct Coding Initiative (NCCI) edits will require that modifier **25** be appended to **99393** to signify that it was significant and separately identifiable from the IA. (For more information on NCCI edits, refer to **Chapter 2**.) *ICD-10-CM* code **Z00.129** is reported first, followed by **Z23**.

The 2025 relative value units (RVUs, unadjusted for geographic locality) assigned to 90460 (total, 0.69; work, 0.24) and 90461 (total, 0.26; work, 0.18) are often the basis for the fee schedule amount determined by a payer. Total RVUs for the IA services in this example include 2.76 for 4 units of 90460 and 0.52 for 2 units of 90461 for a combined total of 3.28 RVUs.

When provided without counseling by a physician or QHP, and reported per product (not component) with codes 90471 (total, 0.62; work, 0.17) × 1, 90472 (total, 0.44; work, 0.15) × 2, and 90474 (total, 0.36; work, 0.15) × 1, the total RVUs for IA services would be 1.86. (2026 RVUs were not available at the time of this publication.)

Codes 90471–90474

90471 IA (includes percutaneous, intradermal, subcutaneous, or IM injections); one vaccine (single or combination vaccine/toxoid)

+90472 each additional vaccine (single or combination vaccine/toxoid) (List separately in addition to code for primary procedure.) (Use code **90472** in conjunction with **90460**, **90471**, or **90473**.)

90473 IA by intranasal or oral route; one vaccine (single or combination vaccine/toxoid)

+90474 each additional vaccine (single or combination vaccine/toxoid) (List separately in addition to code for primary procedure.) (Use code **90474** in conjunction with **90460**, **90471**, or **90473**.)

Codes **90471–90474** will be reported when criteria for reporting the 2 pediatric IA codes (**90460** and **90461**) have not been met. This occurs when either of the following circumstances are true:

- The physician or QHP does not counsel the patient or family or does not document that the counseling was personally performed for each component of the vaccines administered.
- The patient is 19 years or older.

When reporting codes **90471–90474**,

- Codes **90471–90474** are reported for each vaccine administered, whether single or combination vaccines.
- *Only 1* "first" IA code (**90460**, **90471**, or **90473**) may be reported per DOS, although multiple units of **90460** may be reported when multiple vaccine products are administered with counseling by a physician or QHP.

The first IA code can be either **90471** or **90473** depending on the route of administration (eg, when a patient receives an immunization via injection and a second one via intranasal route, IA services can be reported with **90471** and **90474** or with **90473** and **90472**).

- If a physician personally performs counseling on one vaccine but not on another when given during the same encounter, IA will be reported with 90460 (and 90461 if appropriate) and either 90472 (IA, each additional vaccine via injection) or 90474 (IA, each additional vaccine via intranasal or oral route). The Medicare NCCI edits pair 90460 with 90471 and 90473 and, therefore, do not allow codes from the pairs to be reported on the same day of service by the same physician or physician of the same group and specialty.

Refer to the Reporting Evaluation and Management Services With Immunization Administration section later in this chapter for information on distinguishing when it is appropriate to separately report an E/M service (eg, 99211, established patient office visit not requiring the presence of a physician or QHP) in conjunction with an IA service.

Examples

➤ **A 4-year-old patient who was recently seen as a new patient for clearance to attend preschool returns for influenza immunization, which was not available at the time of the previous visit.** The service is scheduled with clinical staff only. The patient is noted to be in good health with no contraindications to the immunization per CDC guidelines. Next, the VIS and the antipyretic dosage for weight are reviewed with a parent, who provides consent for the immunization. The influenza vaccine is administered, and the child is observed for immediate reactions before leaving.

ICD-10-CM	*CPT*
Z23 (encounter for immunization)	90656 (influenza vaccine [IIV3], preservative free, 0.5 mL, IM) 90471 (IA, first injection)

Teaching Point: Because counseling by a physician or QHP is not provided at this encounter, 90471 is reported in lieu of 90460.

➤ **A 5-year-old established patient presented 2 weeks ago for a routine health examination and vaccines.** At that appointment, a physician provided counseling for each recommended vaccine component and corresponding VISs. The patient's parent asked that the vaccines be split, so only the DTaP and IPV vaccines were given at that encounter. The patient returns today and sees a nurse for an immunization-only visit to get the MMR and varicella vaccines.

ICD-10-CM	*CPT*
First visit: Z00.129 (routine child health examination without abnormal findings) Z23 (encounter for immunization)	99393 (preventive E/M, ages 5–11 years, established patient) 90460 (IA with counseling by physician or QHP; 1st component) 90461 × 3 (each additional component) 90696 (DTaP-IPV)
Second visit: Z23 (encounter for immunization)	90710 (MMRV, live) 90471 (IA, first injection)

Teaching Point: Services at this second visit did not include physician counseling, which is required to support use of 90460 and 90461. Counseling for all vaccines occurred at the most recent encounter and all VISs were handed out, so only administration occurred today.

Alternatively, if the patient received IA of MMR and separate IA of varicella vaccine at this visit, codes 90471, 90472 (second injection), 90707 (MMR vaccine), and 90716 (varicella vaccine) would be reported at this visit. If separate DTaP and IPV products were administered at the first visit, the IA codes at that visit would include 90460 × 2 and 90461 × 2 in addition to 90700 (DTaP) and 90713 (IPV).

Only report 90460 and 90461 when physician counseling is provided on the date of vaccine administration. If vaccine administration is delayed to another date when physician counseling is not provided, report 90471–90474 as appropriate. Refer to the Coding for Counseling Without Same-Date Immunization section later in this chapter for guidance on reporting immunization counseling when IA takes place on the same date for some, but not all, immunizations discussed at the encounter.

➤ **A 19-year-old established patient presents for a routine health examination.** In addition to providing a preventive medicine service with no abnormal findings, the physician counsels the patient on the need for meningococcal serogroup B (MenB-4C) immunization. The vaccine is administered.

ICD-10-CM	*CPT*
Z00.00 (encounter for general adult medical examination without abnormal findings)	99395 25 (preventive medicine service, established patient, 18–39 years old)
Z23 (encounter for immunization)	90620 (MenB-4C) 90471 (IA, first injection)

Teaching Point: Because the patient is older than 18 years, 90460 cannot be reported even though the physician provided counseling for the vaccine provided. Code Z00.00 (encounter for general adult medical examination without abnormal findings) is reported for the age- and gender-appropriate preventive medicine E/M service. Code Z23 is reported for the encounter for immunization. Unlike for childhood examinations, *ICD-10-CM* does not instruct to report first a code for any routine adult examination.

Chapter 8 Preventive Services

Codes 90480 and 90481

The COVID-19 vaccine products have been assigned specific codes by product and dosage (91304, 91318–91322). Beginning January 1, 2026, 90481 may be used to report IA of an additional component of a vaccine that includes COVID-19 and another component (eg, combination COVID-19 and influenza vaccine). *Refer to the second example in this section for the limited application of 90481 to pediatric IA services.*

#▲90480 IA by intramuscular injection, of severe acute respiratory syndrome coronavirus 2 (SARS-CoV-2) (coronavirus disease [COVID-19]) vaccine; first or only component of each vaccine administered

#✚●90481 each additional component administered

- Report only 90480 for administration of a single-component COVID-19 vaccine.

Code selection for IA of a vaccine product that includes a COVID-19 component and an additional component(s) depends on the patient's age and whether immunization counseling was provided by a physician or QHP on the date of administration.

- Report both 90480 and 90461 when a vaccine containing a COVID-19 component and additional components (eg, combination COVID-19 and influenza vaccine) is administered to a patient 18 years or younger with same-date counseling by a physician or QHP.
- Report both 90480 and 90481 when a vaccine containing a COVID-19 component and an additional component(s) is administered to a patient 19 years old or older or administered without counseling by a physician or QHP.

✖ Never report 90481 without first reporting 90480.

Examples

➤ **A 6-month-old patient presents for an established patient well-baby visit.** The physician (or QHP) provides and documents the preventive medicine E/M service. The physician counsels the caregivers about recommended immunization with rotavirus vaccine (RV5, third dose); DTaP-IPV/Hib, third dose; pneumococcal vaccine (PCV20, third dose); and COVID-19 vaccine (Moderna, first dose). The parent/guardian is given the CDC VIS and consents; the nurse prepares the vaccines. The nurse administers each vaccine, documents the required information, and accesses and enters vaccine data into the statewide immunization registry. The nurse confirms that there are no serious immediate reactions before the patient leaves.

ICD-10-CM	*CPT*
Z00.129 (encounter for routine child health examination without abnormal findings)	**99391 25** (preventive E/M service, established patient; infant [age younger than 1 year])
Z00.129 **Z23** (encounter for immunization)	**90680** (rotavirus vaccine, pentavalent [RV5], 3 dose schedule, live, for oral use) **90698** (DTaP-IPV/Hib, for IM use) **90677** (PCV20, for IM use) **91321** (COVID-19, 25 mcg/0.25 mL dose, for IM use) **90460** × 3 **90461** × 4 **90480** × 1

Teaching Point: Because the physician personally performed the counseling, **90460** is reported for IA of the initial component of the DTaP-IPV/Hib vaccine and for the single-component RV5 and PCV20 vaccines. Code **90460** is appropriate regardless of the route of administration. Code **90461** is reported for the 4 secondary components of the DTaP-IPV/Hib vaccine. Code **90480** is reported for IA of a COVID-19 vaccine.

➤ **A 12-year-old established patient presents for a routine visit.** In addition to providing a preventive medicine service with no abnormal findings, the physician counsels the patient on the need for COVID-19 and influenza immunization and recommends a combination vaccine that protects against both diseases. The vaccine is administered.

ICD-10-CM	*CPT*
Z00.129	**99395 25**
Z23 (encounter for immunization)	No pediatric COVID-19 and influenza combination vaccine code was available at the time of this publication. When a combination vaccine is approved and administered, as in this hypothetical example, select the *CPT* code for the vaccine administered in addition to the following IA codes: **90480** (IA of COVID-19 component) **90461** (IA of additional component)

Teaching Point: Because the patient is younger than 19 years and the physician provided immunization counseling at the visit, **90461** is reported for the influenza component in lieu of **90481**. If the patient were 19 years or older or the physician did not provide immunization counseling, **90481** would be reported in lieu of **90461**.

Reporting Immunoglobulin Immunization

New in 2026! Code 90382 is added for reporting a seasonal RSV immunization using a product that requires only 1 dose.

Immunization with immunoglobulins is a passive immunization, meaning the administration of antibodies that provide long-acting protection rather than of a vaccine/toxoid that causes the body to produce antibodies (active immunization). Codes for seasonal doses of RSV monoconal antibody (RSV-mAb) are

90380 RSV, monoclonal antibody, seasonal dose; 0.5 mL dosage, for intramuscular use
90381 RSV, monoclonal antibody, seasonal dose; 1 mL dosage, for intramuscular use
●**90382** RSV, monoclonal antibody, seasonal dose, 0.7 mL, for intramuscular use

When a patient receives a 200-mg dose of nirsevimab (2 single-dose syringes of 100 mg/1 mL each), report 90381 × 2 units (ie, 2 × 1-mL dose).

RSV-mAb is recommended for infants in the following age-groups:

- Infants younger than 8 months who were born during or are entering their first RSV season and whose mothers did not receive an adult RSV vaccine between 32 and 36 weeks of pregnancy with a lapse of at least 14 days between vaccine administration and birth

An RSV vaccine (90678; brand name Abrysvo) is *administered to pregnant women* to prevent RSV in newborns and infants from birth to 6 months of age.

- Patients 8 to 19 months of age who meet high-risk criteria

When RSV-mAb is recommended to a child 8 to 19 months of age because of high-risk indications, documentation should support the indication on prior authorization requests, when required, and for diagnosis code assignment. Report diagnosis codes for the condition(s) or situation that places the patient at high risk (eg, when the patient has cystic fibrosis with pulmonary manifestations [E84.0], is underweight [R63.6], or has a BMI below the 5th percentile [Z68.51]) in addition to Z29.11 (encounter for prophylactic immunotherapy for RSV). Refer to the example and further discussion at www.aap.org/en/patient-care/respiratory-syncytial-virus-rsv-prevention/nirsevimab-coding--payment.

Report diagnosis code Z29.11 (encounter for prophylactic immunotherapy for RSV) in conjunction with any RSV-mAb (eg, nirsevimab, clesrovimab). Report additional codes for conditions to support high-risk indications, when appropriate.

Chapter 8

Preventive Services

RSV-mAb Immune Globulin Immunization Administration (96380–96381)

96380 Administration of RSV, monoclonal antibody, seasonal dose by intramuscular injection, with counseling by physician or other QHP

96381 Administration of RSV, monoclonal antibody, seasonal dose by intramuscular injection

Report administration of the RSV-mAb seasonal immunization (90380–90382) with 96380 for IA with counseling by a physician or other QHP on the date of IA or 96381 for IA without counseling by a physician or QHP on the date of IA.

- Report 1 unit of 96380 or 96381 for administration of a seasonal dose regardless of the number of injections.
- ✖ Do not report codes 90460–90461 for administration of the RSV-mAb immunization.

Examples

➤ **An infant receives an RSV-mAb (nirsevimab) vaccine (0.5-mL dose) after the parents are counseled regarding associated indications and risks.** The vaccine is provided in conjunction with a routine child health examination.

ICD-10-CM	*CPT*
Z00.129 (routine child health examination without abnormal findings) Z29.11 (encounter for prophylactic immunotherapy for RSV)	99391 25 (preventive E/M; age <1 year) 90380 (RSV-mAb 0.5 mL dose) 96380 (RSV-mAb IA with counseling by physician or QHP)

Teaching Point: Diagnosis code Z29.11 should be linked to codes 90380 and 96380.

➤ **An 18-month-old established patient with pulmonary manifestations of cystic fibrosis receives an RSV-mAb vaccine (2.0-mL dose).** Counseling was provided and a decision for immunization was made via a telemedicine visit 5 days ago. Prior authorization of the service was approved and the administration is provided by clinical staff without a face-to-face service by a physician or QHP.

ICD-10-CM	*CPT*
Z29.11 (encounter for prophylactic immunotherapy for RSV) E84.0 (cystic fibrosis with pulmonary manifestations)	90381 × 2 (RSV-mAb 1-mL dose) 96381 (RSV-mAb IA without counseling by physician or QHP)

Teaching Point: When a patient receives an RSV-mAb vaccine at 200 mg (2 separate injections of 100 mg each), report only 1 unit of **96380** or **96381** for administration of 1 seasonal dose. Although counseling was provided during the telemedicine visit, the service on the date of administration is without counseling. (Refer also to the Coding for Counseling Without Same-Date Administration section later in this chapter.)

Vaccines for Children Program

The VFC program makes immunization services available to children and young adults up to 19 years of age who meet any of the following criteria: are enrolled in the Medicaid program (depending on the Medicaid managed care plan), do not have health insurance, have no coverage of immunizations under their health plan, or are American Indian or Alaska Native peoples. Vaccines are provided at no cost to the participating physician or patient, and payment is made only for administration of the vaccine.

If reporting the VFC product with administration codes and not the product code, data for the vaccine products administered must be captured for registry and quality initiatives. That can be accomplished by entering the vaccine codes with a $0 charge, if your billing system allows, and appending modifier **SL** (state-supplied vaccine) to the product code. Follow individual payer rules for reporting.

Unless otherwise directed by the VFC program, report **90460** for administration of each immunization product provided with same-date physician or QHP counseling under the VFC program (also **90480** for COVID-19 and either **96380** or **96381** for RSV-mAb administrations). Some programs require and/or accept codes **90471–90474**. If **90461** is used for a vaccine with multiple antigens or components, it should be given a $0 or $0.01 value for a child covered under the VFC program. This guidance applies to Medicaid-enrolled VFC-entitled children as well as non–Medicaid-enrolled VFC-entitled children (ie, uninsured, underinsured, and American Indian or Alaska Native children) in certain circumstances. For more about VFC eligibility, visit www.cdc.gov/vaccines-for-children/about/index.html.

Be aware that some Medicaid programs have reporting rules that differ from those of VFC. *Be sure to get this policy in writing from your Medicaid program* and follow it to prevent denied payment. The AAP continues to advocate to the Centers for Medicare & Medicaid Services to allow for recognition of and payment for component-based vaccine counseling and administration (ie, **90461**). Under the current statute, administration can be paid only "per vaccine" and not per component.

Participants in the VFC program should be aware of program-specific guidance, including storage of VFC vaccines separate from privately purchased vaccines. For more information on the VFC program, visit www.cdc.gov/vaccines/programs/vfc/index.html.

Reporting Evaluation and Management Services With Immunization Administration

E/M services most often reported with the vaccine product and IA include new and established patient preventive medicine visits (*CPT* codes **99381–99395**), problem-oriented visits (**99202–99215**), and preventive medicine counseling services (**99401–99404**).

If a patient is seen only for vaccine administration, it is not appropriate to report an E/M visit if it is not medically necessary, significant, and separately identifiable. The E/M service must be clinically indicated.

Payers may require modifier **25** (significant, separately identifiable E/M service by the same physician on the same day of the procedure or other service) to be appended to the E/M code to distinguish it from the administration of the vaccine. Do not report *CPT* code **99211** (established patient E/M, minimal level, not requiring physician presence) when the patient encounter occurs only for vaccination because Medicare RBRVS relative values for IA codes include administrative and clinical services (ie, greeting the patient, measuring routine vital signs, obtaining a vaccine history, presenting the VIS and responding to routine vaccine questions, preparing and administering the vaccine, and documenting and observing the patient following administration of the vaccine). But if the service is medically necessary, significant, and separately identifiable, it may be reported with modifier **25** appended to the E/M code (**99211**). The medical record must clearly state the reason for the visit, any history and physical examination, the assessment and plan, and any other counseling or discussion items. Diagnosis codes reported may support a clinical indication for the E/M service. The progress note must be signed, and a physician's countersignature may be required. For more information and clinical vignettes on the appropriate use of E/M services during IA, refer to "FAQ: Immunization Administration" at www.aap.org/cfp2026. Payers that do not follow the Medicare RBRVS may allow payment of **99211** with IA. Know your payer guidelines, and if payment is allowed, make certain that the guidelines are in writing and maintained in your office. Be aware that a co-payment may be required when the "nurse" visit is reported.

The same guidelines apply to physician visits (**99202–99215**).

Coding for Counseling Without Same-Date Immunization

New in 2026! Codes 90482–90484 have been added for reporting immunization counseling for one or more immunizations that are not administered on the same date.

Pediatricians may counsel patients and caregivers on the need for immunization but not receive the patient's/caregiver's consent to immunize at the current encounter. Occasionally, pediatricians determine that immunization is contraindicated on the DOS (eg, during acute illness) and counsel in anticipation of the patient returning on another date when immunization is appropriate. Report codes 90482–90484 when a physician or QHP provides immunization counseling of *at least 3 minutes* for one or more immunizations that are not administered in the physician's or QHP's practice on the date of counseling.

★●◀90482 Immunization counseling by physician or other QHP when immunization(s) is not administered by provider on the same DOS; 3 minutes up to 10 minutes

★●◀90483 greater than 10 minutes up to 20 minutes

★●◀90484 greater than 20 minutes

Codes 90482–90484 are applicable for reporting counseling regarding immunization via vaccines, toxoids, or immunoglobulins (eg, clesrovimab, nirsevimab).

Codes 90482–90484 may be the only immunization-related service reported on a date when immunization counseling is provided without administration. When immunization counseling is provided for multiple immunizations, however, and some, but not all, immunizations are administered, multiple services are reported.

- Report 90482–90484 when at least 3 minutes was spent counseling the patient/family/caregiver about the immunizations *that were not administered*, and report appropriate IA codes (eg, 90460–90461) for IA that is provided on the same date.
- ✖ Do not include the time spent counseling for administered immunizations (reported with any IA code) in the time reported with codes 90482–90484.
- ✖ Do not report preventive medicine counseling codes 99401–99404 for time spent in immunization counseling without administration unless advised by a payer's written instruction. Codes 90482–90484 more specifically describe immunization counseling without administration.
- If a significant, separately identifiable E/M service (eg, 99381–99395, preventive medicine service; 99202–99215, office E/M service) is provided and supported by documentation, report an appropriate E/M service code in addition to the IA, immunization counseling, and/or vaccine and toxoid administration codes. Append modifier 25 to the E/M code.

As with any new procedure codes, it is recommended that practices verify inclusion of codes 90482–90484 in the coverage policies and fee schedules of frequently billed payers prior to providing and reporting services.

- Report *ICD-10-CM* code Z71.85 (encounter for immunization safety counseling) as the primary diagnosis. In addition, report the reason an immunization was not carried out, beginning with a code from *ICD-10-CM* category Z28 (immunization not carried out), and underimmunization status.
- Underimmunization is reported with codes in subcategory Z28.3-.

Z28.310 Unvaccinated for COVID-19

Z28.311 Partially vaccinated for COVID-19

Z28.39 Other underimmunization status

Codes in subcategory Z28.3- should not be used for individuals who are ineligible for the COVID-19 vaccines, as determined by the health care professional. Additional codes in category Z28 are reported to indicate the reason for underimmunization status.

- Contraindications to immunization are captured with codes in subcategory Z28.0-.

Z28.01 Immunization not carried out because of acute illness of patient

Z28.02 chronic illness or condition of patient

Z28.03 immune compromised state of patient

Z28.04 patient allergy to vaccine or component

Z28.09 other contraindication

Chapter 8

Preventive Services

● indicates a new code; ▲, revised; #, re-sequenced; ✚, add-on; ★, audiovisual technology; and ◀, synchronous interactive audio.

- Other codes in category **Z28** provide for reporting of immunization not carried out for patient reasons, caregiver refusal, or another specified reason.

Z28.1	Immunization not carried out because of patient decision for reasons of belief or group pressure
Z28.20	because of patient decision for unspecified reason
Z28.21	because of patient refusal
Z28.29	because of patient decision for other reason
Z28.81	due to patient having had the disease
Z28.82	because of caregiver refusal
Z28.83	due to unavailability of vaccine

If the patient has a permanent or long-term contraindication, it may not be appropriate to counsel at length. For a brief statement, such as "Vaccination with rotavirus, a live viral vaccine, is not appropriate today because of your child's immunocompromised status" without a longer discussion of at least 3 minutes, no code for immunization counseling is submitted. It is appropriate, however, to include the appropriate *ICD-10-CM* code, such as **Z28.03**.

The AAP offers additional resources for addressing refusal to vaccinate, including an AAP refusal-to-immunize form and template and a letter providing additional background on documenting refusal of recommended childhood immunizations (www.aap.org/en/patient-care/immunizations/implementing-immunization-administration-in-your-practice/refusal-to-vaccinate).

Examples

➤ **Parents of a 2-month-old established patient come to their physician's office to discuss immunizations.** To date, they have refused to have their infant immunized. Although the physician has discussed the need for vaccines during the infant's previous visits, the parents indicate they have further questions. The physician spends 20 minutes counseling the parents about current recommendations, safety and efficacy of vaccines, and their importance in preventing disease.

ICD-10-CM	*CPT*
Z71.85 (encounter for immunization safety counseling) **Z28.3** (personal history of underimmunization status) **Z28.82** (vaccination not carried out because of caregiver refusal)	**90483** (immunization counseling without administration; >10 minutes up to 20 minutes)

Teaching Point: Code **90483** includes up to 20 minutes. Report **90484** for greater than 20 minutes of immunization counseling without immunization administration.

For telemedicine services, append modifier **93** for synchronous audio-only telecommunication or modifier **95** for synchronous audio-video telecommunication.

➤ **A 12-year-old new patient presents to a pediatrician for a preventive medicine service.** In addition to the preventive E/M service with no abnormal findings, the physician discusses risks of the HPV and COVID-19 vaccines and the diseases for which these vaccines provide protection. The parent/guardian consents to immunization against HPV but refuses the COVID-19 vaccine. The parent/guardian is given the CDC VIS and the HPV vaccine is administered by clinical staff. Documentation includes counseling time of 5 minutes spent specifically discussing the risks and benefits of the COVID-19 vaccine.

ICD-10-CM	*CPT*
Z00.129 **Z23** (encounter for immunization)	**99384 25** **90651** (HPV types 6, 11, 16, 18, 31, 33, 45, 52, 58, nonavalent (9vHPV), 2 or 3 dose schedule, for intramuscular use) **90460** (IA through 18 years of age via any route of administration, with counseling by physician or other QHP; first or only component of each vaccine or toxoid administered)

Z71.85 (encounter for immunization safety counseling) **Z28.82** (vaccination not carried out because of caregiver refusal)	**90482** (immunization counseling without administration; 3 minutes up to 10 minutes)

Teaching Point: Code **90482** is reported for the time spent counseling the patient/family/caregiver about the declined COVID-19 vaccine in addition to the codes for the preventive medicine E/M, HPV vaccine, and IA of the HPV vaccine.

➤ **A 13-year-old new patient presents to a pediatrician for a preventive medicine service.** In addition to the preventive E/M service with no abnormal findings, for 2 minutes the physician discusses risks of the HPV vaccine and the disease for which it provides protection. The parent/guardian is given the CDC VIS. The parent/guardian consents; the nurse prepares to administer the vaccine. But the patient declines to be immunized. The physician returns to the examination room and provides additional counseling for 13 minutes, but the patient continues to decline the vaccine. The teenager does not sit still and struggles when staff attempt to give the injection. Given safety concerns for both patient and staff, the physician and mother agree that the immunization should be delayed. The patient's mother plans to discuss the decision with the child and return on a later date. Documentation includes the total immunization counseling time of 15 minutes. A follow-up appointment is scheduled.

ICD-10-CM	*CPT*
Z00.129 **Z28.21** (immunization not carried out because of patient refusal)	**99384 25** **90483**

Teaching Point: Because no vaccine was administered, no charge for the product or the administration would be reported. Written procedures for documentation and reporting of expired and wasted vaccine doses may be required for vaccines provided under the VFC program.

When the patient returns for follow-up, the codes reported will depend on the outcome of the encounter. If the vaccine is administered after additional physician counseling at the same encounter, **90460** will be reported in addition to the appropriate vaccine product code. If the patient returns for administration by clinical staff without additional counseling by a physician or QHP, **90471** will be reported in addition to the appropriate vaccine product code.

Additional counseling at the follow-up physician visit that does not result in immunization may be reported with **90482–90484** based on the physician's time spent in immunization counseling.

Note that modifier **JW** (drug amount discarded/not administered to any patient) is typically inappropriate when no vaccine is administered to the patient. Modifier **JW** is used to report waste from a single-dose vial/package when the required patient dose is less than the available single-dose amount. Two claim lines report the amounts administered and wasted. Follow payer instructions for reporting wasted vaccines and use of modifier **JW**.

Screening Tests and Procedures

Recommendations for age-appropriate screening services are outlined in the AAP/Bright Futures periodicity schedule, "Recommendations for Preventive Pediatric Health Care" (www.aap.org/en/practice-management/care-delivery-approaches/periodicity-schedule), or in your state's Early and Periodic Screening, Diagnostic, and Treatment plan.

When routine vision and/or hearing screening services are performed in conjunction with a preventive medicine visit, the diagnosis code for a routine infant or child health checkup should be linked to the appropriate screening service. The services/codes listed are examples of services that could be used to screen a patient. Some payers have specific policies that outline covered screening tools based on age; know your payer policies. For example, past a certain age, **92567** (tympanometry) may not be covered under preventive services.

Some payer policies bundle certain screening services (eg, vision screening) into the preventive medicine E/M service. This bundling does not align with *CPT* instruction or NCCI edits. But some payers allow separate payment for screening services. When billing is based on the most restrictive payer policy (or unsupported assumptions of noncoverage), earned revenue may be left unbilled.

Hearing Screening

92551 Screening test, pure tone, air only
92552 Pure tone audiometry (threshold); air only (full assessment)
92558 Evoked otoacoustic emissions, screening (qualitative measurement of distortion product or transient evoked otoacoustic emissions), automated analysis
92567 Tympanometry (impedance testing)
92568 Acoustic reflex testing, threshold portion
92583 Select picture audiometry

Audiometric tests require the use of calibrated electronic equipment, recording of results, and a written report with interpretation (eg, chart of hertz and decibels with pass/fail result for each ear tested and overall pass/fail result). Services include testing of both ears. If the test is applied to only 1 ear, modifier 52 (reduced services) must be appended to the code.

When hearing screening is performed in the physician office because of a failed screening in another setting (eg, school), report *ICD-10-CM* codes from category Z01.11-.

Z01.110 Encounter for hearing examination following failed hearing screening
Z01.118 Encounter for examination of ears and hearing with other abnormal findings (Use additional code to identify abnormal findings)

Code Z01.110 is reported for a normal screening result following a failed screening. Code Z01.118 indicates a failed repeat screening. An additional code is reported to identify the abnormality found following the failed repeat screening.

When addressing an abnormal result of newborn hearing screening, P09.6 (abnormal findings on neonatal screening for neonatal hearing loss) is reported. Codes in category Z01.11- may be reported in addition to P09.6, when appropriate.

Medicaid plans may provide specific hearing screening/testing coverage information and documentation forms/requirements. Follow the individual plan's guidance for reporting these services and any failed attempts to screen (eg, an attempt to screen an uncooperative child).

- Code 92551 (screening test, pure tone, air only) is used when the patient wears earphones and is asked to respond to tones of different pitches and intensities. This is a limited study.
- Code 92552 (full pure tone audiometric assessment; air only) is used when the patient wears earphones and is asked to respond to tones of different pitches and intensities. The threshold (lowest intensity of the tone heard by the patient 50% of the time) is recorded for multiple frequencies.
- Code 92558 (evoked otoacoustic emissions screening) is used when a probe tip is placed into the ear canal to screen for normal hearing function. Sounds that bounce back in low-intensity sound waves (ie, evoked otoacoustic emissions) are recorded and analyzed by computerized equipment and the results are automated.
- Code 92583 (select picture audiometry) is typically used for younger children. The patient is asked to identify different pictures with the instructions given at different sound intensity levels.
- Other commonly performed procedures include codes 92567 (tympanometry [impedance testing]) and 92568 (acoustic reflex testing, threshold portion). Both codes may, however, have limited coverage; check with payers.
- Automated audiometry testing is reported with Category III codes 0208T–0212T. Verify individual payer payment policy before providing these services.

Examples

➤ **A 16-year-old established patient presents for a preventive service and clearance to participate in school sports.** A complete preventive E/M service (99394) is provided. The patient has not undergone a hearing screening in the past 3 years, so pure tone, air-only screening audiometry is indicated (based on Bright Futures guidelines) and performed (92551). No abnormalities are found. Clearance to participate in sports is provided.

The *ICD-10-CM* code reported for each of the services is Z00.129 (encounter for routine child health examination without abnormal findings). Code Z02.5 (encounter for examination for participation in sports) is not reported in conjunction with codes for a routine child health examination per an *ICD-10-CM* Excludes1 note at category Z00. Clearance for sports is not separately reported when provided in conjunction with a preventive E/M service.

➤ **A 6-year-old who experienced a failed hearing screening at school is referred to a pediatrician for additional evaluation.** The child's parents indicate no prior concerns about hearing, and risk factor assessment is negative. The pediatrician chooses to perform screening audiometry (92551), which produces typical results.

The *ICD-10-CM* code reported is **Z01.110** (encounter for hearing examination following failed hearing screening). If the MDM or total physician time (not including time of testing) supports a separate office or other outpatient E/M service, an E/M code is separately reported (eg, **99212**).

Vision Screening

99173 Screening test of visual acuity, quantitative, bilateral

99174 Instrument-based ocular screening (eg, photoscreening, automated-refraction), bilateral; with remote analysis and report

99177 with on-site analysis

0333T Visual evoked potential, screening of visual acuity, automated, with report

0469T Retinal polarization scan, ocular screening with on-site automated results, bilateral

- Screening test of visual acuity (**99173**) must use graduated visual stimuli that allow a quantitative estimate of visual acuity (eg, Snellen or LEA Symbols chart).
  - Code **99173** is reported only when vision screening is performed in association with a preventive medicine visit.
  - Medical record documentation must include a measurement of acuity for both eyes, not just a pass or fail score.

Do not report 99173 when it is performed as part of an evaluation for an eye problem or condition (eg, examination to rule out vision problems in a patient presenting with problems with schoolwork) because the assessment of visual acuity is considered an integral part of the eye examination.

- Instrument-based ocular screening (**99174**, **99177**) is used to report screening for a variety of conditions, including esotropia, exotropia, isometropia, cataracts, ptosis, hyperopia, myopia, and others, that affect or have the potential to affect vision. These tests are especially useful for screening infants, preschool patients, and older patients whose ability to participate in traditional acuity screening is limited or very time intensive.
  - Code **99177** specifies screening with an instrument that provides an on-site (ie, in-office) pass or fail result. The result should be documented.
  - Code **99174** specifies the use of a screening instrument that incorporates remote analysis and report (by a physician located elsewhere). The result received from the external physician should be entered into the patient record.
  - These screenings cannot be reported in conjunction with codes **92002–92700** (general ophthalmologic services), **99172** (visual function screening), or **99173** (screening test of visual acuity, quantitative) because ocular screening is inherent to these services. An AAP policy statement on instrument-based pediatric vision screening is available at https://doi.org/10.1542/peds.2012-2548.
- Vision screening performed with an automated visual evoked potential system is reported with **0333T**. This code applies to automated screening via an instrument-based algorithm with a pass or fail result. A report of the result must be documented. Report **95930** only for comprehensive visual evoked potential testing with physician interpretation and report.
- Retinal polarization scanning (**0469T**) is used to detect amblyopia caused by strabismus and defocus. As with **99177**, results of each scan are generated on-site.

Codes 0333T and 0469T are *CPT* Category III codes for emerging services or technology. Verify payer policy for coverage and payment before providing these services.

Developmental Screening and Health Assessment

Standardized screening instruments (ie, validated tests that are administered and scored in a consistent or "standard" manner consistent with their validation) are used for screening and assessment purposes as reported by **96110** and **96127**.

Health risk assessments that are patient focused (**96160**) are differentiated from those such as maternal depression screening that are caregiver focused (**96161**) for the benefit of the patient.

Each of the screening and assessment codes discussed in this section represents the practice expense of administering, scoring, and documenting each standardized instrument. No physician work value is included. Physician interpretation is included in a related E/M service.

Chapter 8

Preventive Services

Developmental Screening

96110 Developmental screening, with scoring and documentation, per standardized instrument

Structured screening for developmental delay is a universal recommendation of the "Recommendations for Preventive Pediatric Health Care." At 18- and 24-month visits, specifically screen for autism spectrum disorder. Global developmental screening is recommended at 9-, 18-, and 30-month visits. When reporting these screenings, **96110** represents developmental screening with scoring and documentation per standardized instrument. (*Note:* Screening results should be documented in the patient medical record.)

ICD-10-CM codes **Z13.41** (encounter for autism screening) and **Z13.42** (encounter for screening for global developmental delays [milestones]) may be used to track developmental screening measures of the Child Core Set for patients receiving benefits through their Medicaid and Children's Health Insurance Program. Use of the Child Core Set is optional for state programs and physicians. Codes **Z13.41** and **Z13.42** may be reported at any encounter at which screening is performed (eg, with or without a preventive E/M service).

Code **96110**

- Is reported only for standardized developmental screening instruments. It is not reported when the pediatrician conducts an informal survey or surveillance of development as part of a comprehensive preventive medicine service (which is considered part of the history and is not separately billed).
- ✖ Does not require interpretation and report (ie, includes scoring and documentation only). The physician's or QHP's use of the score in determining the presence or absence of concern for developmental delay is included in the E/M service provided on that date.
- ✖ Is *not* reported for brief emotional or behavioral assessment (eg, depression screening); refer to **96127**.
- May be reported for each standardized developmental screening instrument administered. Medicaid Medically Unlikely Edits (MUEs) allow reporting of 3 screening instruments per DOS. If use of more than 3 instruments is clinically indicated and performed, report **96110** with 3 units billed on the first claim line and use modifier **59** (distinct procedural service) with 1 unit for each additional instrument reported on a separate claim line (ie, **96110 59**).

Example

➤ **An 18-month-old patient presents to a primary care physician for an established patient well-child examination.** The mother is given standardized screening instruments for developmental status and autism spectrum disorder by clinical staff, who explain their purpose and how they should be completed. The parent completes 2 standardized, validated questionnaires on a tablet device, and software scores the screening instruments and merges the scores into the patient's electronic health record. The physician reviews and interprets the scores and responses for each standardized instrument, which are normal in this example. The physician provides the recommended 18-month preventive E/M service (**99392**). The child will return for a scheduled 2-year-old preventive service.

ICD-10-CM	*CPT*
Z00.129 (routine child health examination [≥29 days] without abnormal findings)	**99392**
Z13.42 (screening for delayed milestones) **Z13.41** (autism screening)	**96110** × 2

Teaching Point: Code **96110** is reported with 2 units of service linked to *ICD-10-CM* codes **Z13.41** (autism screening) and **Z13.42** (screening for delayed milestones) to identify the reason for 2 units of service. Or, if required by a health plan, **96110** linked to **Z13.41** and **96110 59** linked to **Z13.42** are reported on 2 separate claim lines (1 unit per claim line). (For an illustration of how codes are linked on a claim form, refer to **Figure 1-1**.)

Emotional/Behavioral Assessment

96127 Brief emotional/behavioral assessment (eg, depression inventory, attention-deficit/hyperactivity disorder scale), with scoring and documentation, per standardized instrument

Code **96127**

- Is reported for documentation and scoring of standardized emotional/behavioral assessment instruments. For further discussion of **96127** for reporting use of standardized instruments in the diagnosis or management of an emotional/behavioral condition, refer to **Chapter 10**.

- Can involve 2 or more separately reported instruments (eg, screening instruments for anxiety and depression). Note that MUEs limit reporting to 3 units per claim line. When reporting to payers adopting MUEs, additional units beyond the first 3 must be reported on a separate claim line with an NCCI modifier (eg, 59, distinct procedural service). As always, documentation should support the appropriateness of the additional units of service.
- Can be reported for standardized depression and anxiety instruments that are required under US Preventive Services Task Force (USPSTF) and Bright Futures recommendations (refer to the AAP/Bright Futures "Recommendations for Preventive Pediatric Health Care" [periodicity schedule] insert).

Alternatively, there is a Healthcare Common Procedure Coding System code for depression screening that some payers (particularly Medicaid or managed Medicaid plans) prefer in lieu of 96127 for annual depression screenings. If required, report G0444 (annual depression screening, 5–15 minutes) to those payers.

The code descriptor for G0444 includes "5–15 minutes." Verify the payment policies of Medicaid plans that require G0444, specifically noting any requirement to document time spent providing the depression screening service.

✖ Is *not* reported in conjunction with preventive medicine counseling/risk factor reduction intervention (**99401–99404**) or psychiatric or neurological testing (**96130–96139** or **96146**).

Example

➤ **A 12-year-old is seen for an established patient preventive visit.** In addition to the preventive medicine E/M service, the physician's staff administers and scores 2 standardized instruments to screen for depression and anxiety. The physician reviews the scores, documents that the screening results are negative for symptoms of depression or anxiety, and completes the preventive medicine service.

ICD-10-CM	*CPT*
Z00.129	**99394**
Z13.31 (encounter for screening for depression) **Z13.39** (encounter for screening examination for other mental health and behavioral disorders)	**96127** × 2

Teaching Point: Codes **Z13.31** and **Z13.39** indicate that 2 screening instruments were used to screen for different conditions and may support quality measurement (eg, percentage of patients aged ≥12 years who were screened for depression).

When a positive screening results in a diagnosed condition, report the preventive service with abnormal findings (**Z00.121**) followed by the appropriate code for the diagnosed condition (eg, **F32.0**, major depressive disorder, single episode, mild). When appropriate, a significant and separately identifiable E/M service to evaluate and manage the condition may be reported by appending modifier **25** to an office or other outpatient E/M code (eg, **99214 25**). Documentation should clearly support the MDM of the separate service or, if billing according to time, the physician's total time (not including the time spent providing the separately reported preventive medicine service and screening) and a summary of the service provided (eg, education on the condition, questions answered, patient and/or caregiver concerns, management options discussed, plan of care). Link the diagnosis code for depression to the office or other outpatient E/M code.

When reporting an E/M service that addresses a positive screening, the physician's review and analysis of the score of each distinct instrument contributes to the amount and/or complexity of data to be reviewed and analyzed at the visit.

Health Risk Assessment

96160 Administration of patient-focused health risk assessment (eg, health hazard appraisal) with scoring and documentation, per standardized instrument

96161 Administration of caregiver-focused health risk assessment (eg, depression inventory) for the benefit of the patient, with scoring and documentation, per standardized instrument

Codes 96160 and 96161 are reported with 1 unit for each standardized instrument administered. Payer edits may limit the number of times 96160 and 96161 may be reported for an individual patient and/or on the same DOS. MUEs are set to 3 units for 96160 and 1 unit for 96161 per claim line. Append modifier 59 to the code for additional units on a second claim line.

Code 96160 is reported for administration of a patient-focused health risk assessment with scoring and documentation (eg, Hunger Vital Sign, Oral Health Risk Assessment Tool). This is differentiated from 96161, which is used to report a health risk assessment focused on a caregiver for the benefit of the patient (eg, maternal depression screening).

- Code 96160 cannot be used in conjunction with assessment and brief intervention for alcohol/substance abuse (99408, 99409).
- Check individual payer guidance to determine if and for what purposes 96160 is included as a covered and payable service under the payer's policies (eg, some Medicaid plans pay for adolescent health questionnaires reported with 96160).

Code 96161 is reported for administration and scoring of a health risk assessment to a patient's caregiver. Examples are a postpartum depression inventory administered to the mother of a newborn and administration of a standardized caregiver strain instrument to parents of a child who is seriously injured or ill.

- Screening for postpartum depression is caregiver focused (sign/symptoms of depression in mother) but performed in this setting for the benefit of the infant. This service is reported as a service provided to the infant with 96161 and the appropriate *ICD-10-CM* code for the infant's routine child health examination (eg, Z00.129).

Never report *ICD-10-CM* code Z13.32 (encounter for maternal depression screen) or Z13.31 (screening for depression) on the baby's medical record/bill.

- Check payer policy on adoption of 96161 versus a requirement to report as a service to the mother (ie, to mother's health plan) with 96127 (brief emotional/behavioral assessment [eg, depression inventory, attention-deficit/hyperactivity disorder scale], with scoring and documentation, per standardized instrument). Many Medicaid plans provide separate payment for maternal depression screening at well-child visits, but specific reporting instructions may apply. Vaccines and administration services would also be reported.

Prevent denials! NCCI edits bundle 96160 and 96161 with 96110, 96127, and IA (90460–90474) services, but a modifier is allowed when each code represents a distinct service and is clinically appropriate. Append modifier 59 (distinct procedure) to the bundled code (second column of NCCI edits) when these services are reported on the same date to a payer that has adopted NCCI edits.

Example

➤ **As part of a health supervision visit for a 9-month-old established patient, the physician directs clinical staff to administer a screening for postpartum depression that was not performed at the infant's 6-month visit.** After the mother has completed the screening instrument, clinical staff score and document the result in the patient record. The mother is also asked to complete a developmental screening instrument and a screening for social determinants of health (SDoH), which are scored and documented. The physician completes the preventive medicine service, including reviewing the score of the developmental screening and SDoH screening, with no abnormal findings and then counsels the patient's mother about influenza immunization. With the mother's consent, clinical staff administer a preservative-free split-virus vaccine. Anticipatory guidance that advises the mother that her screening indicates no current signs of postpartum depression is included, along with a list of symptoms that should prompt a call to her physician. The patient is scheduled to return for a second dose of influenza vaccine in 1 month.

ICD-10-CM	*CPT*
Z00.129 (encounter for routine child health examination without abnormal findings)	99391 25 (preventive medicine visit) 96161 59 (administration of caregiver-focused health risk assessment [eg, depression inventory] for the benefit of the patient, with scoring and documentation, per standardized instrument) 96160 59 (administration of patient-focused health risk assessment instrument [eg, health hazard appraisal] with scoring and documentation, per standardized instrument)
Z13.42 (screening for delayed milestones)	96110 (developmental screening)

Z00.129 (encounter for routine child health examination without abnormal findings) Z23 (encounter for immunization)	90460 (IA with physician counseling) Appropriate code for influenza vaccine administered

Teaching Point: NCCI edits bundle code pairs 99391 and 90460, 96110 and 96161, 96110 and 96160, 90460 and 96161, and 90460 and 96160. For each of the bundled code pairs, a modifier is allowed to override the edit when both services are provided and clinically appropriate. Electronic claim scrubbers are useful for identifying and addressing NCCI edit pairs before claim submission. Refer to **Chapter 2** for more on NCCI edits.

Prevention of Dental Caries

Application of Fluoride Varnish

99188 Application of topical fluoride varnish by a physician or other QHP

- Topical fluoride application by primary care physicians is a recommended preventive service for children from the age of primary tooth eruption up to 5 years (Grade B rating by the USPSTF). This service may be covered when provided alone or in conjunction with other services. Coverage varies by payer, typically limited to once every 6 months.
- *ICD-10-CM* code Z29.3 is reported to identify an encounter for prophylactic fluoride administration. When applicable, diagnosis of dental caries may be reported as a secondary diagnosis with codes in category K02. Encounter for prophylactic fluoride administration is reported separately from the encounter for routine child health examination (Z00.121 or Z00.129) when both services are provided at the same encounter.
- The percentage of members 1 to 4 years of age who received at least 2 fluoride varnish applications (on different dates) during the measurement year is a quality measure. Code 99188 (reported on 2 different dates for the same patient) indicates that this measure was met.

Example

➤ **A 4-year-old established patient undergoes a routine preventive medicine service without abnormal findings.** In addition, a medical assistant who has been qualified by a required online training and assessment program applies fluoride varnish to the child's teeth under supervision of the pediatrician, who remains in the office suite.

The pediatrician reports diagnosis code Z00.129 (routine child health examination without abnormal findings) linked to 99392 (established patient routine child health examination, age 1–4) and diagnosis code Z29.3 linked to 99188 (application of fluoride varnish).

Teaching Point: Although 99188 specifies application by a physician or QHP, payers may allow billing of services by trained clinical staff under direct physician supervision (incident to). Some Medicaid plans require training of clinical staff through specific programs and documentation of training and/or certification. It is important to identify the requirements of individual payers before providing this service and maintain documentation demonstrating that all coverage requirements were met.

Report 0792T (application of silver diamine fluoride 38%, by a physician or QHP) when silver diamine fluoride is applied to cavity lesions. Refer to individual payer policies to verify coverage and requirements for payment for this service.

Counseling to Prevent Dental Caries

Some payers will provide coverage for oral evaluation and health risk assessment or other dental preventive services when provided on the same day as a preventive medicine visit; other payers will allow services only when they are provided at an encounter separate from a preventive medicine visit. It is important to know payer requirements for reporting.

- Preventive counseling for oral health may be included as part of the preventive medicine service (99381–99395) or, if performed at a separate encounter, reported under the individual preventive medicine counseling service codes (99401–99404) or with an office or outpatient E/M service code (99202–99215). *ICD-10-CM* code Z13.84 may be reported for an encounter for screening for dental disorders.

Other Codes for Prevention of Dental Caries

- *Code on Dental Procedures and Nomenclature* codes also exist for topical application of fluoride varnish and fluoride. In addition, *Code on Dental Procedures and Nomenclature* codes exist for nutrition counseling to prevent dental disease, oral hygiene instruction, and oral evaluations. But acceptance of these codes by health plans may be limited to Medicaid plans.
- For those carriers (particularly Medicaid plans under Early and Periodic Screening, Diagnostic, and Treatment) that cover oral health care, some will require a modifier. These modifiers are payer specific and should be used only as directed by your Medicaid agency or other private payer.

  SC Medically necessary service or supply
  EP Services provided as part of Medicaid Early and Periodic Screening, Diagnostic, and Treatment program
  U5 Medicaid Level of Care 5, as defined by each state

Learn more about coding for services that support a child's oral health in the May 2023 *AAP Pediatric Coding Newsletter* article "Connecting Coding and Clinical Reports: Oral Health Care" (https://doi.org/10.1542/pcco_book229_document001).

Screening Laboratory Tests

- A test performed in the office laboratory should be billed with the appropriate laboratory code and, if performed, the appropriate blood collection code (36400–36416). Refer to the Blood Sampling for Laboratory Testing section in **Chapter 11**.
- Laboratories and physician offices performing waived tests should append modifier **QW** to the *CPT* code for Clinical Laboratory Improvement Amendments (CLIA)–waived procedures. To determine if a test is a CLIA-waived procedure, go to www.accessdata.fda.gov/scripts/cdrh/cfdocs/cfCLIA/search.cfm.
- *ICD-10-CM* allows separate reporting of special screening examinations (codes in categories **Z11–Z13**) in addition to the codes for routine child health examinations when these codes provide additional information. A screening code is not necessary if the screening is inherent to a routine examination. Payer guidelines for reporting screening examinations may vary. When specific *ICD-10-CM* codes are required to support payment for a screening service, be sure to link the appropriate *ICD-10-CM* code to the claim line for the screening service.

A positive finding on a screening test does not change the test to a diagnostic test. When a screening test results in an abnormal finding that has been identified at the time of code assignment, list first the code for the screening or preventive service followed by a code for the abnormal finding. Failure to list the screening code first may affect the patient's out-of-pocket costs for preventive services. Refer to Chapter 11 for information on coding for diagnostic tests in non-facility settings.

- To meet the HEDIS measure for percentage of children who turned 2 years of age in a measurement year and who had one or more capillary or venous lead blood test(s) for lead poisoning by their second birthday, a laboratory report of the lead screening test result or a note indicating the date the test was performed and the result or finding must be documented. Refer to **Chapter 3** for more information on HEDIS measures.

Follow payer instructions for reporting that patients were referred to an outside laboratory for lead screening (eg, report a code for the appropriate lead screening test with modifier 90, reference [outside] laboratory, and no charge).

- A table of common pediatric screening laboratory tests and codes is included at www.aap.org/cfp2026 ("Screening Laboratory Tests and Codes").

Preventive Care Provided Outside the Preventive Visit

Counseling and/or Risk Factor Reduction

Codes **99401–99404**, **99411**, and **99412** are used to report risk factor reduction services provided for the purposes of promoting health and preventing illness or injury in people without a specific illness.

Preventive medicine service codes (**99381–99395**) include counseling, anticipatory guidance, and/or risk factor reduction interventions that are provided at the time of the periodic comprehensive preventive medicine examination. *CPT* states to "refer to codes **99401–99404**, and **99411–99412** for reporting those counseling/anticipatory guidance/risk-factor reduction interventions that are provided at an encounter separate from the preventive medicine examination." Therefore, according to *CPT,* do not report **99401–99404** or **99411** or **99412** in addition to **99381–99397**.

- Risk factor reduction services will vary with age and address issues such as diet, exercise, sexual activity, dental health, injury prevention, travel safety, and family problems.
- Services are reported according to time, and time should be distinctly documented (eg, 15 minutes spent in counseling about diet and exercise to reduce risk for diabetes).
- Counseling, anticipatory guidance, and risk factor reduction interventions provided at the time of an initial or periodic comprehensive preventive medicine examination are components of the periodic service and not separately reported.
- Risk factor reduction may be reported separately with other E/M services.
  - E/M services (other than preventive medicine E/M services) reported on the same day must be separate and distinct.
  - Time spent in the provision of risk factor reduction may not be used as a basis for the selection of the other E/M code.
- When reporting a distinct E/M service, append modifier **25** to the code for the distinct E/M service.
- See the Coding for Counseling Without Same-Date Immunization section earlier in this chapter for discussion of codes for preventive counseling focused on the need for immunization.

Payment policies for preventive medicine counseling may vary by health plan. Ideally, recommended preventive medicine counseling provided outside a preventive E/M service (99381–99385, 99391–99395) is a covered preventive service paid with no out-of-pocket cost to the patient/caregiver. It is important to know if a payer considers preventive medicine counseling bundled to a problem-oriented E/M service when provided on the same DOS. Plans may require that the preventive counseling be included in the level of problem-oriented E/M service reported in lieu of reporting the appropriate preventive counseling code. Written copies of payment policies should be documented to support billing for preventive medicine counseling as part of a problem-oriented E/M service instead of reporting separately as directed by *CPT*.

Chapter 8

Preventive Services

Preventive Medicine, Individual Counseling Codes

Codes **99401–99404** are time-based codes, as shown by the following code descriptors. Each code descriptor is followed by the 2025 total non-facility RVUs and work RVUs (unadjusted for geographic locality). (The 2026 RVUs were not available at the time of this publication.)

Preventive medicine counseling and/or risk factor reduction intervention(s) provided to an individual (separate procedure)

99401 approximately 15 min (8–22 min, RVUs: total non-facility, 1.15; work, 0.48)
99402 approximately 30 min (23–37 min, RVUs: total non-facility, 1.87; work, 0.98)
99403 approximately 45 min (38–52 min, RVUs: total non-facility, 2.58; work, 1.46)
99404 approximately 60 min (≥53 min, RVUs: total non-facility, 3.30; work, 1.95)

Report codes **99401–99404**

- According to a physician's or other QHP's face-to-face time spent providing counseling
- For a new or an established patient
- When the medical record includes documentation of the total counseling time and a summary of the issues discussed

Time for codes 99401–99404 is met when the midpoint is passed (eg, 8 minutes of service required to report a 15-minute service).

Codes **99401–99404** may be reported when expectant parents request a consultation with a pediatric physician regarding risk reduction for the fetus. But consultation or office and other outpatient E/M services are reported when the service is requested by another physician, another QHP, or an appropriate source (eg, genetic counselor). Refer to the Consultations section in **Chapter 15** for information on reporting *ICD-10-CM* and *CPT* codes for expectant parent consultation services to the mother's health insurance.

Preventive Medicine E/M for Contraceptive Counseling

Counseling for contraception is included in comprehensive preventive medicine services (eg, **99384**, **99394**) when provided. Other E/M services provided for the purpose of contraceptive counseling may be reported with **99401–99404** or, when required by payer policy, office or other outpatient E/M codes (**99202–99215**, **99211–99215**).

Verify specific payer policies for contraceptive/family planning services that may specify codes and/or modifiers (eg, 99401–99404, 99213 FP). These codes may be necessary to support payment as a preventive service without out-of-pocket expense to the patient.

- Diagnosis codes in category Z30 for contraceptive counseling or surveillance should be linked to the procedure code for contraceptive services. For specific codes, refer to the "Contraception: Diagnosis Codes for Counseling, Initiation, and Surveillance by Method" at www.aap.org/cfp2026.
- Per *CPT* instruction, when preventive counseling is provided in conjunction with significant E/M of a problem, report office or other outpatient codes (99202–99215, 99211–99215) with modifier 25 and codes 99401–99404. Code selection for each service must be based on distinctly documented time (eg, 15 minutes spent in contraceptive counseling separate from 20 minutes' total time for E/M of nausea and vomiting).
- A urine pregnancy test performed at the visit for contraception is separately reported (eg, 81025, urine pregnancy test by visual color comparison method) and a diagnosis code to indicate the result (when negative, Z32.02).

Contraceptive supplies and medications are separately reported when purchased by the practice. Supply codes may include condoms (A4267, A4268), diaphragms (A4266), and hormone-containing patches (J7304).

Chapter 8

Preventive Services

Example

➤ **An adolescent presents to a pediatrician for a follow-up visit for moderate persistent asthma.** The patient completes an asthma symptom assessment tool that indicates no to minimal symptoms with current management, and medication refills are ordered. The patient also requests counseling about contraception. The adolescent expresses interest in intrauterine device implantation that may also alleviate heavy periods. A referral to a gynecologist for long-acting reversible contraception is provided. The physician documents 20 minutes of time spent on contraceptive counseling, distinct from and beyond the management of asthma.

ICD-10-CM	*CPT*
J45.40 (moderate persistent asthma, uncomplicated)	Office E/M code with modifier 25 (eg, 99214 25) 96160 (administration of patient-focused health risk assessment instrument [eg, health hazard appraisal] with scoring and documentation, per standardized instrument)
Z30.09 (encounter for other general counseling and advice on contraception)	99401

Teaching Point: The pediatrician's time of 20 minutes spent in preventive counseling supports reporting 99401 because the midpoint between 99401 and 99402 (23 minutes) was not passed. Distinct documentation of the time and work of the preventive counseling is important to support payment for both services provided. Time of the preventive counseling is distinctly documented and nonoverlapping with time spent reevaluating the patient's asthma symptoms. Code 96160 is reported for use of a standardized instrument in evaluation of asthma symptoms.

Refer to **Chapter 13** for discussion of codes for reporting contraceptive procedures, including injection, insertion, or implantation of a contraceptive product.

For additional information, refer to the September 2023 *AAP Pediatric Coding Newsletter* article "Connecting Coding to Clinical Policy: Contraception" (https://doi.org/10.1542/pcco_book233_document001).

Preventive Medicine, Group Counseling Codes

99411 Preventive medicine counseling and/or risk factor reduction intervention(s) provided to individuals in a group setting (separate procedure); approximately 30 minutes (16–45 min, RVUs: total non-facility, 0.59; work, 0.15)

99412 approximately 60 minutes (≥46 min, RVUs: total non-facility, 0.74; work, 0.25)

- Risk factor reduction services provided to a group are reported according to time. Time is met when the midpoint between the 2 codes is passed.

Refer to 99078 for reporting physician counseling to groups of patients with symptoms or an established illness. This service is reported for each participating child.

Example

➤ **A group of 10 patients aged 14 to 16 years attend a 60-minute session in the physician's office to discuss health habits to reduce risks related to family history of diabetes, type 2, and cardiovascular disease.** The physician conducts the session. (The session includes a 10-minute break that is not included in the time of service.) Services are documented in each patient's medical record and are reported for each child.

ICD-10-CM	*CPT*
Z71.3 (dietary counseling and surveillance) Z71.82 (exercise counseling) Z83.3 (family history of diabetes mellitus) Z82.49 (family history of ischemic heart disease and other diseases of the circulatory system)	99412 (risk-factor reduction counseling, group, 60 minutes)

Teaching Point: Although 10 minutes of break time is not included in the time of the counseling service, the 50 minutes of counseling support 99412 because the midpoint between the 30 minutes assigned to 99411 and the 60 minutes assigned to 99412 is passed. Services provided to a group of patients may not be reported as individual office E/M visits (99202–99215) except as specifically designated in payer policy and may be limited to time spent counseling each patient individually. Additional diagnosis codes may be appropriate to further specify the health concerns of individual patients (eg, obesity and BMI percentile).

Behavior Change Intervention

Behavior change interventions are for people who have a behavior that is often considered an illness, such as tobacco use and addiction or substance use or misuse. Behavior change services may be reported when performed as part of the treatment of conditions related to or potentially exacerbated by the behavior or when performed to change the harmful behavior that has not yet resulted in illness. Following are the codes and 2025 total non-facility and work RVUs (unadjusted for geographic locality) assigned to behavior change intervention codes:

99406 Smoking and tobacco use cessation counseling visit; intermediate, >3 min up to 10 min (RVUs: total non-facility, 0.43; work, 0.24)

99407 intensive, >10 min (RVUs: total non-facility, 0.82; work, 0.50)

99408 Alcohol and/or substance (other than tobacco) abuse structured screening (eg, Alcohol Use Disorders Identification Test, Drug Abuse Screening Test), and brief intervention services; 15–30 min (RVUs: total non-facility, 1.02; work, 0.65)

99409 >30 min (RVUs: total non-facility, 1.97; work, 1.30)

Codes 99406–99409 include specific time requirements that must be met (eg, at least 15 minutes must be spent in counseling to report 99408). The *CPT* midpoint rule does not apply to 99406–99409.

Behavior change interventions involve validated interventions, shown in **Figure 8-1**.

Behavior change intervention codes 99406–99409 are reported when

- Services are provided by a physician or QHP to patients to address a behavior that is often considered an illness (eg, tobacco use and addiction, substance use or misuse).
- Services involve specific validated interventions, including assessing readiness for and barriers to change, advising change in behavior, providing specific suggested actions and motivational counseling, and arranging for services and follow-up care.
  - ✖ Do not separately report 96160 for screening instruments used in conjunction with 99408 and 99409.
- Medical record documentation supports the total time spent in the performance of the service, and a detail of the behavior change intervention is provided.

Behavior change intervention services cannot be performed to a parent or guardian of a patient and reported under the patient's name.

Chapter 8 Preventive Services

Figure 8-1. Behavior Change Interventions

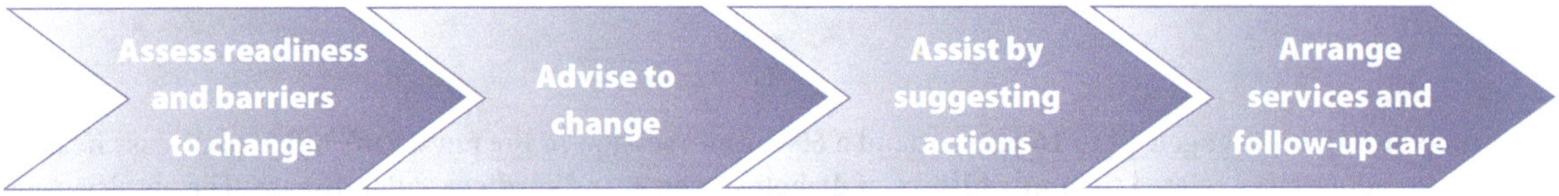

- Behavior change interventions may be reported separately with preventive medicine or other E/M services.
  - E/M services reported on the same day must be separate and distinct.
  - Time spent in the provision of behavior change intervention may not be used as a basis for the selection of the other E/M code.
- When reporting a distinct E/M service, append modifier **25** to the code for the distinct E/M service (eg, **99213 25**).

Refer to the Physician Group Education Services section in Chapter 11 for an example of how 99078 (physician educational services in a group) is used.

Examples

➤ **During an office visit for a 17-year-old new patient for an unrelated problem, it is learned the patient has been smoking for 2 years but would like to quit.** The physician spends 15 minutes applying motivational interviewing and discussing specific methods to overcome barriers, pharmacologic options, behavioral techniques, and nicotine replacement. The patient is referred to a community support group, and a follow-up visit is scheduled in 2 weeks to provide additional encouragement and counseling as needed. Diagnosis is tobacco use. The physician documents the time spent specific to tobacco use.

ICD-10-CM	*CPT*
Use the code appropriate for the problem addressed.	**99202–99205 25** (based on service performed and documented)
Z72.0 (tobacco use) **Z71.6** (tobacco abuse counseling)	**99407**

Teaching Point: If only general advice and encouragement to stop smoking was provided, it would be considered part of the new patient office visit. Counseling time must be documented. *ICD-10-CM* does not include a code for use of vaping products without a diagnosis of abuse or a vaping-related illness. Report **Z71.89** (other specified counseling) when counseling is focused on risks associated with vaping. Refer to **F17.29-** for codes for nicotine dependence and vaping.

➤ **A 14-year-old established patient with primarily hyperactive attention-deficit/hyperactivity disorder (ADHD) presents for a preventive E/M service.** The patient and parents report no problems in school and no concerns with current ADHD management. During time alone with the patient, the physician uses a structured screening tool to interview the patient about substance use. The result is positive, and the physician spends a total of 15 minutes interviewing the patient about substance use history and counseling the patient about risks associated with alcohol and drug use, not driving or riding with someone under the influence, and seeking an agreement to avoid future use. The physician documents 15 minutes of time spent on substance use, separate and distinct from the preventive visit.

ICD-10-CM	*CPT*
Z00.129 (routine child health examination without abnormal findings) **F90.1** (ADHD, predominantly hyperactive type)	**99394 25** (preventive medicine visit)
Z71.89 (other specified counseling)	**99408**

Time of counseling should be specifically documented as beginning after conclusion of the preventive medicine service. For example, "In addition to providing the routine child health examination, I spent 15 minutes in counseling against alcohol and drug use and seeking the patient's agreement to avoid associated health risk behaviors."

ICD-10-CM **guidelines state that substance use codes (eg, F10.99, alcohol use, unspecified with unspecified alcohol-induced disorder) should be assigned only when the use is associated with a mental or behavioral disorder and such a relationship is documented by the provider.**

Preventive Medicine Services Modifier

33 Preventive services

Modifier 33 is used to differentiate services provided as recommended preventive care when the service might also be provided for diagnostic indications. Some payers provide a listing of services for which modifier 33 is required when provided as a preventive service. Other payers, however, consider modifier 33 informational only and base benefit payment on the reported diagnosis and procedure codes.

- The appropriate use of modifier 33 will reduce claim adjustments related to preventive services and corresponding payments to members.
- Modifier 33 should be appended only to codes represented in one or more of the following categories:
  - Services rated A or B by the USPSTF
  - Immunizations for routine use in children, adolescents, and adults as recommended by the Advisory Committee on Immunization Practices
  - Preventive care and screenings for children as recommended by Bright Futures (AAP) and newborn testing (American College of Medical Genetics and Genomics)
  - Preventive care and screenings provided for women supported by the Health Resources and Services Administration

The USPSTF grades A and B are defined as follows:

- **Grade A: The USPSTF recommends the service. There is high certainty that the net benefit is substantial.**
- **Grade B: The USPSTF recommends the service. There is high certainty that the net benefit is moderate or there is moderate certainty that the net benefit is moderate to substantial.**

Most health plans cover preventive services with grade A or B without cost to the patient (ie, no deductible, co-payment, or coinsurance).

- **DO *NOT* USE MODIFIER 33**
  - ✖ **When the *CPT* code(s) is identified as inherently preventive (eg, preventive medicine counseling)**
  - ✖ **When the service(s) is not indicated in the categories noted previously**
  - ✖ **With an insurance plan that continues to implement the cost-sharing policy on preventive medicine services (legacy health plan)**
- Check with your payers before fully implementing the use of modifier 33 to verify reporting requirements. Modifier 33 *is not used for benefit determination by some payers* and may be required by others only for services that may be either diagnostic/therapeutic or preventive.

Example

➤ **An 8-year-old is seen for an established patient preventive visit.** In addition to providing the preventive medicine E/M service, the physician's staff administers and scores a standardized instrument to screen for anxiety. The physician reviews the scores, documents that the screening results are negative for symptoms of anxiety, and completes the preventive medicine service.

ICD-10-CM	*CPT*
Z00.129	99393
Z13.39 (encounter for screening examination for other mental health and behavioral disorders)	96127 33

Teaching Point: Code Z13.39 is used to report screening for anxiety. Modifier 33 indicates that use of the screening instrument was for preventive screening purposes.

Other Preventive Medicine Services

99429 Unlisted preventive medicine service

Code **99429** may be reported if these options are not suitable. If the unlisted code is used, most payers will require a copy of the progress notes filed with the claim.

Reporting a Preventive Medicine Visit With a Problem-Oriented Visit

When a problem or an abnormality is addressed (eg, symptomatic atopic dermatitis, exercise-induced asthma, migraine headache, scoliosis), *requires significant additional work*, and is medically necessary, it may be reported with the office or other outpatient services codes (**99202–99205**, **99212–99215**, and modifier **25**) in addition to the preventive medicine services code.

Know Payer Policies for Same-Day Preventive and Problem-Oriented Evaluation and Management Services

Some payers have adopted a policy that problem-oriented E/M services provided on the same date as a preventive medicine E/M service be paid at 50% of the contractual amount agreed on under the health plan contract. When reporting to these payers, be sure to include all work related to the problem-oriented encounter in determining the level of service provided. Physicians should not reduce the level of service reported.

- The presence of a chronic condition(s) in and of itself neither changes a preventive medicine visit to a problem-oriented visit nor unilaterally supports a separate problem-oriented E/M service (**99202–99205**, **99212–99215**) with the well-care visit, unless it has been separately addressed with a significant problem-oriented service.
- Although a separate E/M service is not reported when a minor problem or chronic condition requires less than significant additional work, the diagnosis code for the problem or chronic condition may be reported in addition to **Z00.121–Z00.129** (routine child health examination).
- It is important to make parents aware of any additional charges that may occur at the preventive medicine encounter. This includes, but is not limited to, a significant, separately identifiable E/M service.
  - Some patients will be required to provide a co-payment for the non–preventive medicine visit code under the terms of their plan benefit even when there is no co-payment required for the preventive medicine visit. Legally, this co-payment cannot routinely be written off.

Do not separately report an E/M service when

- ✖ An insignificant problem or condition is addressed (eg, minor diaper rash, stable chronic problem not evaluated at this visit).
- ✖ A prescription medication is renewed without reevaluation of the problem for which the medication is prescribed (eg, order for refill of as-needed short-acting β2-agonist that is nearing its expiration date).

When reporting both E/M services,

- The documentation of the problem-oriented service must be distinct from that of the preventive service (even if included in the same encounter note) and clearly support the level of service reported.
- When the level of service for the problem-oriented E/M service is selected according to the physician's total time on the date of the encounter, the physician's total time spent addressing the problem must be distinctly documented (not including any time spent providing and documenting the preventive service) in addition to documentation of the problem workup (eg, history of present illness, examination, records or test results reviewed), assessment, and plan. The total time of the problem-oriented E/M service does not include any time spent providing and documenting the preventive service.

Documentation of time spent managing a problem on the same date as a preventive medicine service might indicate "My total time of XX minutes was directed to activities of evaluating and managing X condition separate from the preventive service."

- Modifier 25 (significant, separately identifiable E/M service by the same physician on the same day of the procedure or other service) should be appended to the problem-oriented service code (eg, 99212 25). If vaccines are given at the same encounter, append modifier 25 to the problem-oriented E/M service code and to the preventive medicine service code to prevent payer bundling edits that may allow payment only for IA.
- *ICD-10-CM* well-care diagnosis codes (for the code list, refer to the *ICD-10-CM* Codes for Preventive Care Visits section earlier in this chapter) should be linked to the appropriate preventive medicine service code (99381–99395) and the code for problems or findings addressed that is linked to the problem-oriented service code (99202–99205, 99212–99215).

Examples

➤ **A 10-year-old patient receives health supervision at a well-child visit.** This established patient was previously diagnosed with gastroesophageal reflux disease (GERD). The patient notes an increase in symptoms and asks about a change in medication. After providing the preventive E/M service, the physician reevaluates the child's symptoms of GERD, medication adherence, and eating habits. A new medication is prescribed.

ICD-10-CM	*CPT*
Z00.121 (well-child check with abnormal findings) K21.9 (gastro-esophageal reflux disease without esophagitis)	99393 (preventive medicine visit)
K21.9 (gastro-esophageal reflux disease without esophagitis)	99214 25 (office E/M service, moderate level MDM)

Teaching Point: Documentation should clearly support the separate E/M of the GERD, discussion topics, and plan of care for the problem.

➤ **A 10-year-old patient with previously diagnosed GERD is seen for a preventive medicine visit.** The patient's mother requests a refill of a prescription medication that has helped alleviate the patient's GERD symptoms. There are no new abnormal findings at the encounter. An order for the medication refill is placed in addition to provision of the preventive E/M service.

ICD-10-CM	*CPT*
Z00.129 (routine child health examination without abnormal findings) K21.9 (gastro-esophageal reflux disease without esophagitis)	99393

Teaching Point: Because there was no significant evaluation of the GERD at the encounter, only the preventive E/M code is reported. The diagnosis code for GERD may be reported as an additional diagnosis to the code for the well-child checkup but is not a finding of the well-child checkup because the condition was not new or exacerbated.

Refer to the "Preventive and Problem-Oriented Services: Coding Continuum" box that follows for additional examples of coding for problems addressed at a preventive encounter.

To test your knowledge of coding for preventive services, complete the quiz found at the end of this chapter, after the continuum and resources. Answers to each quiz are found in **Appendix II**.

Preventive and Problem-Oriented Services: Coding Continuum

Continuum Model for Problem-Oriented and Preventive Evaluation and Management on the Same Date			
Code selection may be based on the level of MDM or the total time[a] spent by the physician or QHP devoted to the problem-oriented E/M on the date of the encounter.			
	Medical Decision-Making (2 of 3 Elements Required)		
***CPT* Code With Time and Vignette (Appropriate preventive E/M service codes are also reported)**	**No. and Complexity of Problems Addressed**	**Amount and/or Complexity of Data Reviewed and Analyzed**	**Risk of Complications and/or Morbidity or Mortality of Patient Management**
99212 25 (10–19 minutes) A 10-year-old patient presents with a stuck earring that requires removal without incision.	**Minimal:** Minor problem	**Limited:** Assessment requiring an independent historian(s)	**Minimal**
99213 25 (20–29 minutes) A 14-year-old presents today for a rash on their forearms after a recent camping trip. Diagnosis is poison ivy.	**Low:** 1 acute, uncomplicated illness or injury	**Minimal or none**	**Low:** Home management with over-the-counter products
99214 25 (30–39 minutes)[b] A 6-year-old child presents with a new-onset rash and history of fever and sore throat in the past week as well as abdominal pain, nausea, and decreased appetite.	**Moderate:** Acute illness with systemic symptoms and high risk of morbidity without treatment	**Moderate:** Rapid streptococcal test and viral swab performed. Assessment requiring an independent historian(s).	**Moderate:** Prescription of antibiotic for treatment of streptococcal sore throat
99215 25 (40–54 minutes)[b] A 14-year-old presents with concern of recent-onset anxiety with palpitations and depression for which they are seeing a therapist. Patient describes suicidal ideation without plan or intent. Mother provides family history, which is negative for bipolar disorder and positive for anxiety disorders.	**High:** 1 acute or chronic illness or injury that poses a threat to life or bodily function	**High:** Independent historian. Tests ordered are CBC, thyroid function tests, comprehensive metabolic panel, and electrocardiography. Phone discussion with therapist regarding prescription of SSRI and other options for management.	**High:** Discussion regarding hospitalization and advice to go to the ED if suicidal ideation includes intent

Abbreviations: CBC, complete blood cell count; *CPT, Current Procedural Terminology;* ED, emergency department; E/M, evaluation and management; MDM, medical decision-making; QHP, qualified health care professional; SSRI, selective serotonin reuptake inhibitor.

[a] Time-based E/M: Time is the total time spent in activities related to the problem-oriented E/M service by the physician or QHP on the date of the encounter. Do not include time of the preventive medicine service or time of other separately reported services.

[b] In some cases, a problem that requires higher levels of E/M service (ie, 99214 or 99215) may warrant delay of the preventive E/M service.

Chapter Takeaways

In this chapter, common pediatric preventive services and reporting for a combination of preventive and problem-oriented services were discussed. Following are takeaways from this chapter:

- Well-child or preventive medicine services are a type of E/M service and are reported with codes **99381–99395** according to the patient's age and status as a new or established patient.
- Appropriate diagnosis coding for preventive medicine is based on the patient's age and, except for newborn services, on whether an abnormality is identified during the service.
- Immunization services are reported with 2 families of procedure codes: one for the product (vaccine, toxoid, or immunoglobulin) and one for the services associated with the IA (eg, intramuscular injection, intranasal administration).
- IA is reported according to the type of product administered and, in most cases, the age of the patient and inclusion of counseling by a physician or QHP. IA codes for vaccines and toxoids are distinct from IA of an immunoglobulin for passive immunization (ie, seasonal RSV-mAb).
- New codes **90482–90484** are time-based codes reported for immunization counseling of 3 or more minutes without same-date administration of one or more recommended immunizations.
- Codes **99401–99404**, **99411**, and **99412** are used to report risk factor reduction services provided for the purposes of promoting health and preventing illness or injury in people without a specific illness. Codes **99406–99408** are reported for behavior change intervention services.
- When a provider manages a condition at a preventive visit, an office E/M service may be reported when the service is separate and significantly beyond the preventive service.
- An insignificant problem or condition that does not require significant MDM or time cannot be reported as a separate E/M service in addition to a preventive service.

Resources

AAP Coding Assistance and Education

AAP *Bright Futures: Guidelines for Health Supervision of Infants, Children, and Adolescents,* 4th Edition (www.aap.org/en/practice-management/bright-futures)

AAP/Bright Futures periodicity schedule, "Recommendations for Preventive Pediatric Health Care" (refer also to the insert) (www.aap.org/en/practice-management/care-delivery-approaches/periodicity-schedule)

AAP Section on Ophthalmology and Committee on Practice and Ambulatory Medicine, American Academy of Ophthalmology, American Association for Pediatric Ophthalmology and Strabismus, and American Association of Certified Orthoptists "Instrument-Based Pediatric Vision Screening Policy Statement," *Pediatrics* (https://doi.org/10.1542/peds.2012-2548)

"Payment for Oral Health Services" (www.aap.org/en/patient-care/oral-health/payment-for-oral-health-services)

Pediatric Immunizations: Coding Quick Reference Card 2026 (www.aap.org/Pediatric-Immunizations-Coding-Quick-Reference-Card-2026)

"Refusal to Vaccinate," including an immunization refusal form and template (www.aap.org/en/patient-care/immunizations/implementing-immunization-administration-in-your-practice/refusal-to-vaccinate)

"Respiratory Syncytial Virus (RSV) Prevention" (www.aap.org/en/patient-care/respiratory-syncytial-virus-rsv-prevention)

"7 Rights of Vaccine Administration" (www.aap.org/en/patient-care/immunizations/implementing-immunization-administration-in-your-practice/vaccine-administration)

"Vaccine Financing and Coding" (www.aap.org/en/practice-management/child-health-finance-payment-strategy/coding-and-valuation/vaccine-financing-and-coding/)

AAP Pediatric Coding Newsletter

"2024 *Current Procedural Terminology* Updates: Female Pelvic Examination," December 2023 (https://doi.org/10.1542/pcco_book236_document002)

"Connecting Coding and Clinical Reports: Oral Health Care," May 2023 (https://doi.org/10.1542/pcco_book229_document001)

"Connecting Coding and Policy: Getting Paid for Tobacco and Substance Use Screening and Intervention," June 2023 (https://doi.org/10.1542/pcco_book230_document001)

"Connecting Coding to Clinical Policy: Contraception," September 2023 (https://doi.org/10.1542/pcco_book233_document001)

"Important *ICD-10-CM* Changes to Reporting Obesity and Pediatric Body Mass Index," September 2024 (https://doi.org/10.1542/pcco_book245_document003)

"Refresh Your Knowledge: Reporting National Drug Codes," September 2025 (https://doi.org/10.1542/pcco_book257_document003)

Immunization and Vaccines

AMA Category I vaccine codes (www.ama-assn.org/practice-management/cpt/category-i-immunization-codes)

CDC VFC program (www.cdc.gov/vaccines/programs/vfc/index.html)

Laboratory Testing

FDA CLIA test category database (www.accessdata.fda.gov/scripts/cdrh/cfdocs/cfCLIA/search.cfm)

National Drug Codes

FDA National Drug Code Directory (www.fda.gov/drugs/drug-approvals-and-databases/national-drug-code-directory)

Online-Exclusive Content at www.aap.org/cfp2026

"FAQ: Immunization Administration"

"Preventive Medicine Encounters: What's Included? (Letter Template)"

"Screening Laboratory Tests and Codes"

Quality Measurement Information

Agency for Healthcare Research and Quality, US Department of Health and Human Services, National Guideline Clearinghouse (www.ahrq.gov/gam/index.html)

CPT Category II codes (www.ama-assn.org/practice-management/cpt/category-ii-codes)

Vaccines for Children

Vaccines for Children eligibility criteria (www.cdc.gov/vaccines-for-children/about/index.html)

Test Your Knowledge!

1. **What is true for IA codes 90460–90461 and 96380 but not 90471–90474 or 90480?**
   a. Codes 90460–90461 and 96380 are reported per injection.
   b. Codes 90460–90461 and 96380 require same-date counseling by a physician or other QHP.
   c. Codes 90460–90461 may be reported on the same date as 96380 but not on the same date as 90471–90474 or 90480.
   d. Codes 90460–90461 and 96380 are never reported with more than 1 unit.
2. **What is the minimum time required to report immunization counseling without same-date IA (code 90482)?**
   a. 10 minutes
   b. 6 minutes (based on the midpoint rule)
   c. 11 minutes
   d. 3 minutes
3. **True or false? Codes 90482–90484 cannot be reported on a date when any IA service is provided.**
   a. True
   b. False
4. **Which is the appropriate diagnosis code linked to 96161 for administration and scoring of a maternal depression screening instrument when billed to an infant's health plan?**
   a. Z00.121 or Z00.129
   b. Z13.32 (encounter for maternal depression screen)
   c. Z13.31 (screening for depression)
   d. Z00.00 or Z00.01
5. **Which differentiates behavior change intervention codes 99406–99409 from preventive medicine counseling codes 99401–99404?**
   a. Behavior change interventions involve validated interventions provided to a patient who has a behavior that is often considered an illness itself.
   b. The *CPT* midpoint rule applies to 99406–99409.
   c. Codes 99406–99409 are not selected according to time.
   d. Codes 99406–99409 are reported only for services provided to a new patient.

CHAPTER 9

Indirect Management of Chronic and Complex Conditions

Contents

Chapter Highlights

- Options for reporting evaluation and management (E/M) services provided without direct patient contact
- Tracking time of services provided within a 30-day or calendar-month period
- Differentiating types of care management services provided to improve care for chronic conditions
- Providing and reporting care management services during a patient's transition from a facility stay to the community setting
- Related but separately reported indirect management services

In addition to codes for services provided on a single date of service, *Current Procedural Terminology* (*CPT*®) includes categories of codes created to recognize episodes of care for complex health care needs that go beyond the work included in preservice, intraservice, and postservice values of the traditional E/M service provided directly (in person or by telecommunications technology) by a physician or other qualified health care professional (QHP) whose scope of practice includes E/M services (eg, nurse practitioner, physician associate). Several code categories include codes for reporting care management services performed by clinical staff under the supervision of a physician or QHP and for reporting a combination of physician or QHP and clinical staff services.

The American Academy of Pediatrics (AAP) *Pediatric Care Management: Coding Quick Reference Card 2026* outlines these codes and includes decision trees to help guide users to the correct codes (www.aap.org/Pediatric-Care-Management-Coding-Quick-Reference-Card-2026).

Indirect Management of Chronic and Complex Conditions

Management of complex medical conditions may be reported with multiple codes for individual services and/or single codes that describe a combination of direct and indirect services or a period of indirect services reported with one or more codes based on time of service.

Four of 5 key categories of E/M services that include indirect services are discussed in this chapter.

1. Principal care management (PCM) (**99424–99427**) is a monthly service provided by a physician with a focus on the medical and/or psychological needs manifested by a single complex chronic condition (eg, poorly controlled diabetes). PCM services do not require management and coordination of services for all of a patient's health care needs.
2. Chronic care management (CCM) (**99490**, **99439**, **99491**, **99437**) and complex CCM (**99487**, **99489**) are monthly services provided by a single physician to manage or coordinate services for patients with 2 or more complex chronic conditions. The reporting individual provides or oversees the management and/or coordination of services, as needed, for all the patient's health care needs. Direct services are separately reported.
3. Care plan oversight (CPO) (**99374**, **99375**; **99377**, **99378**; **99379**, **99380**) is another monthly service provided by a single physician in supervision of health care services typically delivered by nonphysician qualified health care professionals (NQHCPs) (eg, therapists), home health, or hospice services. CPO is reported by only 1 individual who has the sole or predominant supervisory role with a particular patient.
4. Transitional care management (TCM) (**99495**, **99496**) services support patient transition from a stay in a facility to their home environment without gaps in their care management. The reporting physician or QHP provides or oversees the management and/or coordination of services, as needed, for all the patient's health care needs. TCM includes a combination of 1 direct service and indirect services over a 30-day period, as needed.

A fifth category of indirect services, psychiatric collaborative (**99492–99494**) and general behavioral health integration (**99484**) care management services, is discussed in **Chapter 10**.

Each of these categories of service is reported according to time and/or specified levels of service devoted to care of the individual patient in a specified period. *CPT* instructions for each category of services specify the service requirements, eligible service providers, required time (when applicable), and whether certain other services may be separately reported within the period of each service. A table comparing requirements for reporting PCM, CCM, and CPO services is included at www.aap.org/cfp2026 ("Monthly Care Management and Care Plan Oversight Services: A Comparison").

Care management services cannot be reported when provided during a postoperative portion of the global period of a service reported by the same physician or other physician of the same specialty and same group practice. For example, a surgeon would not report TCM during a postoperative period, but a primary care pediatrician may report TCM when coordinating care for all the patient's medical conditions following hospital discharge. Care management services are not reported for postoperative care alone (eg, when reporting a surgical service code with modifier 55 only for postoperative management).

- Review the codes for these services and the related coding instructions to take advantage of opportunities to be paid for providing and/or coordinating care between visits for children with complex health care needs.
- Identify the services that practice capabilities will support to take advantage of opportunities to be paid for providing and reporting services related to managing chronic conditions and complex health care needs. For instance, provision of TCM services requires timely identification of patients discharged from an inpatient or observation stay so contact may be made with the patient or caregiver within 2 business days of facility discharge.
- Payers may require specific electronic capabilities (eg, an electronic health record [EHR] that meets specific certification and/or standards for interoperability).
- Codes and payment policy for many of these services continue to evolve. Be sure to review reporting instructions for any changes that will take place on January 1 of each year.
- Report these services and the diagnosis codes representing the patient's chronic and complex conditions to demonstrate the higher-quality, lower-cost care that is a key element of emerging payment methodologies.

Refer to Chapter 4 for information on emerging payment methodologies such as value-based payment incentives. Some health plans cover care management services only as part of a value-based payment program (ie, not fee-for-service [FFS]).

- Payers that have adopted value-based or enhanced payment initiatives, such as per-member-per-month payment models, may consider certain care management services bundled into the services for which the enhanced payment is made. Practices may, however, choose to assign codes for use in internal calculations of the cost to provide enhanced care in comparison to any enhanced payments.

For more information on preparing your practice to care for patients with complex health care needs, refer to the AAP policy statement "Patient- and Family-Centered Care Coordination: A Framework for Integrating Care for Children and Youth Across Multiple Systems" (https://doi.org/10.1542/peds.2014-0318).

- This policy statement, coauthored by the AAP Council on Children With Disabilities and the Medical Home Implementation Project Advisory Committee, outlines the essential partnerships that are critical to this framework.

Services such as CCM do not prevent separate reporting of preventive services when provided to children with complex health care needs. Refer to Chapter 8 for more information on reporting preventive E/M services and separately reportable services on the same date.

Tracking Time of Periodic Services

Care management services, other than TCM, are reported only when a specific amount of time is spent providing the service during 1 calendar month. CPO also requires specified amounts of time spent within a calendar month. Services typically occur on multiple days within the month. *Each segment of time must be documented.*

In 2025, Healthcare Common Procedure Coding System (HCPCS) codes **G0556–G0558** (for full descriptors, refer to your HCPCS reference) were introduced for reporting advanced primary care management services provided to patients with Medicare coverage. In recognition of the burden associated with tracking and documenting the clinical staff minutes spent on each activity of a care management service, the services reported with **G0556–G0558** are not time based. Payment for services reported with **G0556–G0558** may vary by Medicaid and private health plan, and benefits should be verified prior to provision of services. These codes may also be included in a payer's incentive program (eg, primary care incentive program) that provides incentive payments in addition to or in lieu of a FFS contract. Refer to the Resources at the end of this chapter for an article providing additional details.

Documentation and tracking of time for services that are reported periodically, such as time spent in CCM activities in a calendar month, require establishing routine processes to capture all billable services. Failure to track the time and activities may result in practice expense that does not yield revenue.

Practice and system capabilities vary. Potential tracking mechanisms include

- EHR flowcharts designed to capture each activity and the related time throughout a period of service and prompt code assignment when required service time is met.
- Stand-alone time-tracking software, which may also offer a solution for documenting time of service.
- Manual systems, such as spreadsheets, that are updated at the time of each activity.
- Work-arounds in existing electronic systems, such as EHR templates for clinical staff appointments that are assigned pseudocodes to track time (refer to the example that follows). Pseudocodes are never used on claims; instead, they provide a basis for tracking time-based services.

Collaboration with system vendors, professional colleagues, and practice management consultants may be invaluable to successful delivery, documentation, and reporting of time-based services.

The following example illustrates one semiautomated method of using pseudocodes:

Example

➤ **Clinical staff members of a physician who is providing PCM services to a child with a single high-risk disease spend 35 minutes over 1 month in PCM activities in support of the patient's plan of care.** On the date of each activity, clinical staff document the nature of the activity as well as the time spent. They also select a pseudocode (eg, COORD or PCMAN) and 1 unit of service for each minute spent providing a service. No charge is generated by entry of the pseudocode. Billing staff, however, will generate a report of the patients for whom the pseudocode was entered during a calendar month and bill for services that meet the time requirements of the service.

Because 35 minutes of clinical staff time was spent providing the PCM service to this child, the pediatrician reports **99426** (PCM, first 30 minutes of clinical staff time directed by physician or QHP, per calendar month).

Chapter 9

Indirect Management of Chronic and Complex Conditions

Monthly Care Management Services

Monthly care management services are management and support services that are not limited to the period following discharge from a facility stay. These services are provided by physicians or QHPs or by clinical staff under the direction of a physician or QHP to individuals who reside at home or in a domiciliary, rest home, or assisted living facility. The goals of care management services are to improve care coordination, reduce avoidable hospital services, improve patient engagement, and decrease care fragmentation.

CPT includes 3 types of continuous care management services. Details of patient eligibility, providers of service, and time requirements vary for these services, as discussed in detail in the Principal Care Management Services section earlier in this chapter and the Chronic Care Management and Complex CCM section later in this chapter.

- *PCM services:* provision or supervision of the management and/or coordination of services, as needed, for a patient's single complex chronic condition
- *CCM services:* provision or supervision of the management and/or coordination of services, as needed, *for all the patient's medical conditions, psychosocial needs, and activities of daily living*
- *Complex CCM services:* CCM *services* that require at least 60 minutes of clinical staff time under the direction of a physician or QHP and moderate or high medical decision-making (MDM)

Time, activities (eg, patient education), and identification of the individual conducting each activity must be documented. An example of a worksheet for tracking care management activities and service times is included at www.aap.org/cfp2026 ("Care Management Tracking Worksheet Template").

- Each minute of time is counted only once and only for 1 service.
- In-person or telemedicine E/M services are separately reported, when provided. A physician or QHP may separately provide and report a distinct time-based service (eg, time-based office E/M service) when *other distinct time* is used to report care management services provided to the same patient during the same calendar month.
- Only time spent by clinical staff employed directly by or under contract and clinically integrated with the reporting professional's practice is included in the time of care management services.

The midpoint rule applied for some time-based coding does not apply to care management services (99424–99427, 99437, 99439, 99487, 99489, 99490, 99491). Times specified in code descriptors for care management services must be met or exceeded.

- When provided during the same calendar month as care management services, behavioral or psychiatric collaborative care management services (**99484**, **99492–99494**) may be separately reported. Do not count the same minutes (eg, 1:00–1:15 pm) toward care management and behavioral or psychiatric collaborative care management services.
- ✖ Care management services are not reported by the same individual for services to the same patient in the same calendar month as end-stage renal disease services (**90951–90970**), CPO (**99374–99380**), or other care management services (eg, do not report both CCM and complex CCM).

Required Practice Capabilities

A practice providing PCM, CCM, or complex CCM services must have all the following specific capabilities:

- Use of an EHR system that supports timely access to clinical information.
- Provide patients and caregivers with a means to contact health care professionals in the practice to address urgent needs, regardless of the time of day or day of the week.
- Provide continuity of care through scheduling of the patient's successive routine appointments with a designated member of the care team.
- Provide timely access and management for necessary follow-up when a patient is discharged from the emergency department or hospital.
- Patient and caregiver engagement, education, and integration of care among all service professionals, as appropriate for each patient.
- The individual reporting care management services oversees activities of the care team.
- All care team members providing services are clinically integrated.

CPT no longer requires use of a standardized methodology to identify patients who may qualify for care management services. Yet such processes may be beneficial in identifying and offering care management services to patients. Processes may involve developing checklists or processes for identifying characteristics of patients with complex health care needs (eg, any patient with chronic or episodic conditions that are expected to last at least 12 months and increase the risk of morbidity and mortality, acute exacerbation or decompensation, or functional decline may require CCM services). Examples of such characteristics (*examples only, not a practice guideline*) include

- Number of chronic conditions
- Number of visits for nonroutine care in the past year
- Emergency department visits or hospitalizations in the past 6 months
- Number of current medications or medications prescribed or revised in the past 6 months
- Number of physicians and other providers (eg, home health care provider, nutritionist)
- Lack of resources (eg, housing, health plan coverage, access to care in community)
- Assistance required for activities of daily living
- Other psychosocial considerations (eg, language barriers, multiple family members with complex care needs)

Activities of Care Management Services

Services include all clinical staff time spent in face-to-face and non–face-to-face services or a physician's time personally spent in care management activities. Time spent in other reported services (eg, time of prolonged clinical staff service [**99415**, **99416**] or time of collection and interpretation of physiologic data [**99091**]) may not be included to meet requirements for reporting care management services.

Care management activities include

- Face-to-face and non–face-to-face time spent communicating with and engaging the patient and/or family, caregivers, other professionals, community services, and agencies
- Developing, revising, documenting, communicating, and implementing a disease-specific care plan (PCM) or comprehensive care plan (CCM, complex CCM)
- Collecting health outcomes data and registry documentation
- Teaching the patient and/or family/caregiver to support patient self-management, independent living, and activities of daily living
- Identifying community and health resources
- Facilitating access to care and other services needed by the patient and/or family
- Management of care transitions not reported as part of TCM (**99495**, **99496**)
- Ongoing review of patient status, including review of laboratory and other studies not reported as part of an E/M service
- Assessment and support for adherence to the care plan

Development of a Plan of Care

A plan of care (also referred to as a *care plan*) must be developed, monitored, or revised *and a copy provided to each patient* receiving care management services. For PCM, the plan of care is focused on management of the patient's single complex chronic health condition. For CCM and complex CCM services, the plan of care addresses all the patient's health care needs.

- A plan of care for health problems is based on a physical, mental, cognitive, social, functional, and environmental evaluation. It is intended to provide a simple and concise overview of the patient and the patient's medical conditions and to be a useful resource for patients, caregivers, and providers. Refer to **Figure 9-1** for an example of a plan of care.
- Creation, monitoring, or revision of a plan of care must be documented. Plans created by other entities (eg, home health agencies) cannot be substituted for a care plan established by the individual reporting PCM or CCM services.
  - The entire plan of care should be reviewed and revised (as needed) at least annually. Updates to the plan of care may occur periodically based on changes in status or goal.

CPT defines a *care plan* or *plan of care* as required for care management services (ie, PCM, CCM, and complex CCM) as

- Based on a physical, mental, cognitive, social, functional, and environmental assessment
- Comprehensive for a single complex chronic health problem or for all health problems, as applicable
- Typically not limited to but possibly including
  - Problem list
  - Expected outcome and prognosis
  - Measurable treatment goals
  - Cognitive assessment
  - Functional assessment
  - Caregiver assessment
  - Environmental evaluation
  - Symptom management
  - Medical management
  - Planned interventions
  - Interaction and coordination with outside resources and other health care professionals and providers
  - Summary of advance directives

These elements are intended to be a guide for creating a meaningful plan of care rather than a strict set of requirements. They should be used only as appropriate for the individual.

The plan should be updated periodically to account for status or goal changes. The entire care plan should be reviewed at least annually.

To help illustrate the use of codes for management of complex medical conditions, most examples in this chapter focus on Patient A, an adolescent who was recently diagnosed with major depression resulting from distress caused by hemoglobin SS disease and mild persistent asthma.

Principal Care Management Services

PCM services are focused on the medical and/or psychological needs manifested by a single complex chronic condition with all the following characteristics:

- Is expected to last at least 3 months
- Requires frequent adjustments in the medication regimen, and/or the management of the condition is unusually complex because of coexisting conditions
- Places the patient at significant risk of hospitalization, acute exacerbation/decompensation, functional decline, or death
- Requires development, monitoring, or revision of disease-specific care plan

Refer to **Box 9-1** for codes and work descriptions for PCM services.

The patient may have multiple chronic conditions that may warrant provision of CCM or complex CCM services, but the focus on the single condition differentiates PCM from these services (eg, a patient may require ongoing CCM by a pediatrician as well as a period of PCM by a pulmonologist or hematologist focused solely on a single condition). Individual(s) of the same group practice *and same specialty* cannot report PCM in conjunction with CCM or complex CCM.

A patient's primary care pediatrician may provide PCM services to a patient who does not have the 2 or more chronic or episodic health conditions required to report CCM services. For example, a pediatrician may provide PCM to a patient with asthma who has had severe exacerbation until the patient's condition stabilizes. PCM does not, however, require the reporting individual to address, as needed, all medical conditions, psychosocial needs, and activities of daily living, as required for CCM and complex CCM.

Figure 9-1. Example Plan of Care

This plan of care has been written by A Great Pediatric Practice to help us work with you to be as healthy as possible. This plan will allow you to share with us what is important to you and will let you know what to expect from us.

We will keep a copy of this plan and make changes as necessary. We will share this with other people who care for you (like other doctors or therapists), as needed, to help them care for you. You can also share this with others (like family members) who help you care for yourself.

Date	01/15/2026	Primary physician	Dr J	Page 1 of 2

About Me

Name	Patient A	I like to be called	Patient A	Date of birth	12/25/2008

Primary caregivers	Mother and maternal grandmother		
Preferred contact information	123 Home St Anywhere, US 98765 555-999-6655		
Secondary contact information	555-999-8877		
Preferred pharmacy	Family Drug Store	Preferred hospital	Children's Hospital-Main

Who to Call When I Need Care or Have Questions?

My care coordinator	Nurse B

Important Health Information

I am allergic to	No known allergies
I have difficulty with	Pain episodes, asthma symptoms in late summer/fall, missing school for medical appointments
Equipment I need (like a wheelchair)	Nebulizer, inhaler
Community assistance	No food or housing insecurity (as described by mother)

My Health Concerns (Include concerns from patient and caregiver perspectives.)

Concerns	What I can expect for each concern
Asthma	Coordinated care with pulmonologist
Sickle cell disease	• Coordinated care with team at Children's Hospital for hematology, pulmonary, pain management, and behavioral health • Assistance with obtaining prompt and appropriate care in the emergency department, when needed
Depression	Coordination with behavioral health team of Children's Hospital

My Health Care Plans

Concerns	Plans
Asthma	• Maintain symptom control through consistent use of daily control medication. • Follow asthma action plan when symptomatic. • Go to emergency department if asthma is unresponsive to 4 puffs of rescue inhaler (albuterol).
Sickle cell disease	• Continue current medications for control and pain management. • Maintain hydration daily. • Alert Dr J of any fever or increased fatigue, pain, or other symptoms. • Get annual transcranial Doppler ultrasonography. • Go to emergency department if there are signs of stroke, uncontrolled pain, or other symptoms that are unresponsive to home treatment.
Depression	• Continue medication and telemedicine appointments with behavioral health team at Children's Hospital. • Call Dr J for any side effects of management or mild to moderate escalation of symptoms. • Call 988 and go to the emergency department if thoughts of hurting yourself or others.

Figure 9-1 (*continued*)

My Planned Care

Specialty care	Children's Hospital Sickle Cell Program for periodic hematology, pulmonary, pain medicine, and behavioral health care
Preventive care	• Next preventive visit on 04/14/2025 at 4:00 pm • Annual transcranial Doppler ultrasonography due 06/2025 (Children's Hospital will schedule for same date as visit with hematologist.)
Scheduled follow-up visit	On 02/20/2025 at 4:00 pm—Call for urgent appointment as needed.
School counselor	Coordinates IEP (individualized education program) changes, available at 555/555-1234
Other: School nurse is available only 2 days per week. School plan addresses physical limitations with accommodations for medication, hydration, frequent restroom trips, and rest. School requires physician signature annually on chronic illness form because of potential for missed school.	
Additional notes	
Patient signature	
Parent signature	
Care coordinator signature	

Box 9-1. Principal Care Management Services

A care plan specific to the single disease must be developed, revised, or monitored and shared with the patient/caregivers for each type of PCM service. Ongoing communication and care coordination with relevant practitioners furnishing care is also required. PCM services of <30 minutes in a calendar month are not reported separately.

Patient Population for All PCM Services

Patients have a single complex chronic condition expected to last ≥3 months that presents significant risk of death, acute exacerbation/decompensation, or functional decline. The condition requires frequent adjustments in the medication regimen, and/or the management of the condition is unusually complex because of coexisting conditions.

Required Time and RVUs: PCM by Physician or QHP Time

#99424 PCM services ≥30 minutes of physician or QHP time, per calendar month

Total non-facility RVUs: 2.50; work RVUs: 1.45.[a]

#✚99425 *each* additional 30 minutes of physician or QHP time, per calendar month (List separately in addition to **99424** for each full 30 minutes beyond the first 30 minutes)

Total non-facility RVUs: 1.82; work RVUs: 1.00.[a]

Required Time and RVUs: PCM by Clinical Staff Time

#99426 PCM services ≥30 minutes of clinical staff activity directed by a physician or other QHP, per calendar month (may include time spent personally by a physician or other QHP)

Total non-facility RVUs: 1.91; work RVUs: 1.00.[a]

#✚99427 each additional 30 minutes per calendar month (List up to 2 units separately in addition to **99426**)

Total non-facility RVUs: 1.56; work RVUs: 0.71.[a]

Abbreviations: PCM, principal care management; QHP, qualified health care professional; RVU, relative value unit.

[a] 2025 National Physician Fee Schedule Relative Value File, total non-facility and work RVUs, not geographically adjusted. 2026 RVUs were not available at the time of this publication. Individual payers may use different relative value files (eg, from previous years).

● indicates a new code; ▲, revised; #, re-sequenced; ✚, add-on; ★, audiovisual technology; and ◀, synchronous interactive audio.

PCM services include

- Establishing, implementing, revising, or monitoring a care plan specific to a single disease
- Thirty minutes or longer of time personally spent by a physician or QHP (99424, 99425) or by clinical staff under the supervision of an employing (direct or contractual) physician or QHP (99426, 99427)

If a physician or QHP spends less than 30 minutes in a calendar month providing PCM services, 99426 and 99427 may be reported for 30 or more minutes of combined time of the physician and clinical staff.

- Ongoing communication and care coordination between relevant practitioners furnishing care

Unlike CCM or complex CCM services, PCM services may be provided by more than one physician or QHP in the same calendar month for the same patient. Documentation in the patient's medical record should reflect coordination among relevant managing clinicians.

Table 9-1 includes examples of PCM services.

Table 9-1. Principal Care Management Coding Examples

The patient in each example is Patient A, with hemoglobin SS disease, asthma, and new-onset depression with suicidal thoughts, and they just completed a 30-day period of TCM. *ICD-10-CM* diagnosis codes may include, when addressed, F32.2 (major depressive disorder, single episode, severe without psychotic features), J45.30 (mild persistent asthma, uncomplicated), and D57.1 (sickle-cell disease without crisis), in addition to codes for any other conditions addressed.

Example	Code Assignment
Patient A is receiving PCM services. A hematologist spends 35 minutes in the calendar month implementing a care plan focused on managing hemoglobin SS disease in coordination with the other physicians and caregivers.	99424 (PCM of ≥30 minutes by a physician or QHP) is reported by the hematologist. If time in the calendar month exceeds 59 minutes, 99425 is reported for each additional period of ≥30 minutes in addition to 99424.
Patient A is receiving PCM services. A hematologist spends 35 minutes in the calendar month implementing a care plan focused on managing hemoglobin SS disease in coordination with the other physicians and caregivers. An NP in the same hematology practice spends 30 minutes coordinating care with the behavioral health team and student's school nurse with regard to the sickle cell disease.	The hematologist reports 99424 (PCM of ≥30 minutes by a physician or QHP) and 99425 (each additional 30 minutes) for the combined time of 65 minutes spent by the physician and QHP during the calendar month. No overlapping time is counted. If the hematologist and NP meet to discuss the patient's care, only 1 person counts the time spent in the meeting.
Patient A is also receiving PCM services focused on pain management. During the calendar month, clinical staff of a pain management specialist spend 25 minutes in PCM activities. The pain management physician also spends 20 minutes in the same calendar month in PCM activities.	The pain management physician reports 99426 for combined clinical staff and physician time (45 minutes). If the combined time were 60–89 minutes in a calendar month, 99427 would also be reported with 1 unit. For any time ≥90 minutes, 2 units of service may be reported with 99427.

Abbreviations: *ICD-10-CM, International Classification of Diseases, 10th Revision, Clinical Modification;* NP, nurse practitioner; PCM, principal care management; QHP, qualified health care professional; TCM, transitional care management.

Chronic Care Management and Complex CCM

The appropriate CCM or complex CCM code(s) is (are) reported once per calendar month by only 1 individual who has assumed the management role for all the patient's care. This may be a primary care pediatrician or a subspecialist, but only the 1 individual may report CCM or complex CCM services in a calendar month. Face-to-face E/M services may be separately reported by the same individual during the same calendar month.

Time spent by physicians and other QHPs of the same specialty in the same group practice (eg, covering physician) may be combined to meet the time requirements for care management services, but the service must be reported by the individual who is overseeing the patient's care.

CCM services are performed personally by a physician or QHP (99491, 99437) or by clinical staff under supervision by an employing (direct or contractual) physician or QHP (99490, 99439, or complex CCM [99487, 99489]). Refer to **Box 9-2**, which provides requirements for CCM and complex CCM services.

Box 9-2. Chronic Care Management Services

A comprehensive care plan for all the patient's medical conditions, psychosocial needs, and activities of daily living must be developed, revised, or monitored and shared with the patient/caregivers for each type of CCM service.

Patient Population for All CCM Services

Patients have multiple (≥2) chronic or episodic conditions expected to last ≥12 months, or until the death of the patient, that present significant risk of death, acute exacerbation/decompensation, or functional decline.

Time Required and RVUs: CCM by Clinical Staff Time

#99490 CCM services ≥20 minutes of clinical staff activity directed by a physician/QHP, per calendar month
Total non-facility RVUs: 1.87; work RVUs: 1.00.[a]

#+99439 each additional 20 minutes of clinical staff time directed by a physician or QHP, per calendar month (List up to 2 units separately in addition to 99490)
Total non-facility RVUs: 1.42; work RVUs: 0.70.[a]

May combine physician or QHP time of <30 minutes personally spent in CCM services with clinical staff time as long as ≥20 minutes is spent within a calendar month

Time Required and RVUs: CCM by Physician or QHP Time

#99491 CCM services by physician/QHP, first 30 minutes (≥30–59 minutes), per calendar month
Total non-facility RVUs: 2.54; work RVUs: 1.50.[a]

+99437 each additional full 30-minute period (eg, 60–89 minutes equals 1 unit)
Total non-facility RVUs: 1.78; work RVUs: 1.00.[a]

Time Required and RVUs: Complex CCM

Moderate- or high-level MDM required in addition to time requirements.

99487 Complex CCM services ≥60 minutes of clinical staff activity directed by a physician/QHP, per calendar month (may include time spent personally by a physician or QHP)
Total non-facility RVUs: 4.07; work RVUs: 1.81.[a]

+99489 each additional 30 minutes per calendar month (List separately in addition to 99487)
Total non-facility RVUs: 2.18; work RVUs: 1.00.[a]

Abbreviations: CCM, chronic care management; MDM, medical decision-making; QHP, qualified health care professional; RVU, relative value unit.

[a] 2025 National Physician Fee Schedule Relative Value File, total non-facility and work RVUs, not geographically adjusted. 2026 RVUs were not available at the time of this publication. Individual payers may use different relative value files (eg, from previous years).

CCM

- Is provided to patients with 2 or more chronic continuous or episodic health conditions expected to last 12 months or longer, or until the death of the patient, and that place the patient at significant risk of death, acute exacerbation/decompensation, or functional decline.
- Addresses *all* the patient's medical conditions, psychosocial needs, and activities of daily living.
- Requires creation, implementation, monitoring, and revision (as needed) of a comprehensive care plan for all the patient's health-related problems.
- Codes 99491 and 99437 are not reported for time spent by a physician or QHP on the date of a face-to-face E/M visit.

In addition to requirements for CCM, complex CCM (99487, 99489) requires

- Moderate- or high-level MDM during the calendar month
- At least 60 minutes of clinical staff time, under the direction of a physician or other QHP (may include time spent by the physician or QHP)

Reporting CCM and Complex CCM

There are significant differences in work and practice expense required for each type of CCM and complex CCM service. It is important to consider the amount and type of time (clinical staff and/or physician/QHP) and type of MDM required to determine the most appropriate code for each calendar month. A patient who requires CCM in January may require complex CCM in February, or vice versa, as clinical circumstances change.

- Only 1 type of CCM or complex CCM service is reported per calendar month.
  - No combination of codes 99487 and 99490 or 99491 may be reported for the same month.
  - One of these codes is reported in any calendar month when the requirements of the code descriptor are met.

- For 99491 and 99437, count only the time personally performed by the physician or other QHP. Time spent by clinical staff is not counted toward the time to support 99491 or 99437.
- More than one clinical staff member may spend time in CCM activities on a single date. Count all time that is not overlapping, but do not count the same period more than once.
- If multiple clinical staff members meet about 1 patient, count the time for only 1 staff member (eg, 3 staff members spend 5 minutes discussing a patient; the total time of the CCM activity is 5 minutes).
- ✖ Do not count any time of the clinical staff spent as part of a separately reported service (eg, providing patient and caregiver education on the date of a physician or QHP visit).
- If the physician personally performs clinical staff activities of care management, their time may be counted toward the required clinical staff time supporting 99487, 99489, 99490, and 99439. If a physician or QHP personally performs at least 30 minutes of CCM services, refer to 99491 and 99437.

Refer to examples for each level of CCM in **Table 9-2**.

Table 9-2. Chronic Care Management Coding Examples

The patient in each example is Patient A, who has hemoglobin SS disease, asthma, and new-onset depression with suicidal thoughts. *ICD-10-CM* diagnosis codes may include F32.2 (major depressive disorder, single episode, severe without psychotic features), J45.30 (mild persistent asthma, uncomplicated), and D57.1 (sickle-cell disease without crisis), in addition to codes for any other conditions addressed.
Each activity included in the CCM service must be documented in the patient record with the date and description of the activity and authenticated with the performing clinician's signature, electronic or written, and date completed.

Example	Code Assignment
Patient A is receiving CCM services. Time begins the day after the 30-day period of TCM was completed. Clinical staff spend 65 minutes in the remainder of the calendar month implementing the care plan and responding to questions and concerns. MDM is moderate.	99487 (complex CCM of at least 60 minutes with moderate to high MDM) is reported by supervising physician Dr J. *Tip:* No time spent during the TCM period is counted toward the time of CCM or complex CCM.
Patient A is receiving continued CCM services. During the calendar month, MDM includes management of increased asthma symptoms and a decision to prescribe a new asthma control medication. A total of 95 minutes of combined physician and clinical staff time is spent in CCM activities in the calendar month.	Dr J reports 99487 for the first 60 minutes and 99489 (complex CCM, each additional 30 minutes) for the additional 35 minutes. One unit of 99489 is reported for each full 30 minutes after the first 60 minutes of CCM in a calendar month.
Patient A is receiving continuing CCM services. Dr J spends 40 minutes revising the plan of care following review of records from a visit with specialists at the Children's Hospital Sickle Cell Program. Clinical staff also spend 15 minutes in CCM activities during the calendar month.	Dr J reports 99491 (CCM, personally performed by a physician or QHP, at least 30 minutes in the calendar month). Only Dr J's time is counted toward 99491. If Dr J's total time in the month is at least 60 minutes, 99491 and 99437 are reported.
Patient A is receiving CCM services for symptom monitoring and management. Dr J's clinical staff spend 15 minutes in CCM activities. Dr J also personally spends 10 minutes in CCM activities.	Dr J reports 99490 (CCM with at least 20 minutes of clinical staff time). Dr J and the clinical staff's combined time is counted toward 99490. *Tip:* Dr J did not personally spend 30 minutes in CCM activities to support 99491.
Patient A is receiving continued CCM services. Dr J personally spends 10 minutes in CCM activities in addition to 30 minutes spent by clinical staff.	99490 and 99439 × 1 (CCM of at least 20 minutes and at least 20 minutes beyond the first 20 minutes in a calendar month) are reported for 40 minutes' combined time of Dr J and clinical staff.

Abbreviations: CCM, chronic care management; *ICD-10-CM, International Classification of Diseases, 10th Revision, Clinical Modification;* MDM, medical decision-making; QHP, qualified health care professional; TCM, transitional care management.

Care Plan Oversight Services

CPO is recurrent physician or QHP supervision of a patient who has complex health care needs or a patient who requires multidisciplinary care and ongoing physician or QHP involvement. CPO services are not provided face-to-face and reflect the complexity and time required to supervise the care of the patient who is receiving home health, hospice, or nursing facility services. The codes are reported separately from E/M office visits.

Box 9-3 compares CPO services, including patient population served, work included, and services not separately reported. (Work included and services not separately reported are the same for all CPO services.)

Box 9-3. Care Plan Oversight Service Codes at a Glance

Time of CPO service is a physician's or QHP's time spent in a calendar month. Activity by clinical staff is not included in the time of CPO service.

All patients receiving CPO require complex and multidisciplinary care modalities involving regular development and/or revision of care plans by the physician. The patient is not present at the time of service.

Codes by Patient Population

Supervision of a *patient under care of home health agency* (not in hospice or nursing facility)	Supervision of a *hospice patient*	Supervision of a *nursing facility patient*
99374 15–29 min Total non-facility RVUs: 2.04; work RVUs: 1.10.[a] 99375 ≥30 min Total non-facility RVUs: 3.07; work RVUs: 1.73.[a]	99377 15–29 min Total non-facility RVUs: 2.04; work RVUs: 1.10.[a] 99378 ≥30 min Total non-facility RVUs: 3.07; work RVUs: 1.73.[a]	99379 15–29 min Total non-facility RVUs: 2.04; work RVUs: 1.10.[a] 99380 ≥30 min Total non-facility RVUs: 3.07; work RVUs: 1.73.[a]

Work Included in CPO Services

- At least 15 minutes by the physician in regular development and/or revision of care plans
- Review of subsequent reports of the patient's status and related laboratory or other diagnostic studies
- Communication, including telephone calls, for assessment or care decisions with individuals (eg, family, caregivers, health care professionals) involved in the patient's care
- Integration of new information into the medical treatment plan or adjustment of medical therapy

May Be Separately Reported When Each Service Time Is Distinct and Nonoverlapping

98012–98015 Synchronous audio-only visit
98016 Brief communication technology-based service (eg, virtual check-in)
98966–98968 Telephone services by QHPs who cannot provide/report E/M services
98970–98972, 99421–99423 Online digital services
99358, 99359 Prolonged non-face-to-face E/M service not on the date of a visit

May Not Be Reported in the Same Calendar Month as CPO

94005 Home ventilator management CPO
99091 Collection and interpretation of physiologic data
99424–99427 PCM services
99487, 99490, 99491 Complex and CCM services

Abbreviations: CCM, chronic care management; CPO, care plan oversight; E/M, evaluation and management; PCM, principal care management; QHP, qualified health care professional; RVU, relative value unit.

[a] 2025 National Physician Fee Schedule Relative Value File, total non-facility and work RVUs, not geographically adjusted. 2026 RVUs were not available at the time of this publication. Individual payers may use different relative value files (eg, from previous years).

Medicare requires the use of Level II HCPCS codes for CPO services provided to patients under the care of a home health agency (G0181) or hospice (G0182). To report these G codes, Medicare requires a minimum of 30 minutes of physician supervision per calendar month. Because some Medicaid programs may follow suit, check with your payer to learn its requirements for reporting these services.

CPO services

- Are reported only by the individual (ie, physician/QHP) who has the predominant supervisory role in the care of the patient or is the sole provider of the services.
- The Centers for Medicare & Medicaid Services (CMS) requires a face-to-face visit within 6 months before CPO services. Verify individual payer policies for similar requirements and possible inclusion of telemedicine services in support of a face-to-face visit requirement.
- Include
  - Regular development and/or revision of care plans
  - Review of subsequent reports of the patient's status
  - Review of related laboratory or other diagnostic studies
  - Communication, including telephone calls, for the purpose of assessment or care decisions with health care professionals, family members, surrogate decision-makers (eg, legal guardians), and/or key caregivers involved in the patient's care

- Integration of new information into the medical treatment plan or adjustment of medical therapy
- Team conferences
- Prolonged E/M service before and/or after direct patient care when the same time is attributed to CPO (Count the time toward either prolonged service or CPO.)

- Are reported once per month according to the amount of time spent by the physician during that calendar month.

Unlike with care management services, time included in CPO is only that of the physician or other QHP and not that of clinical staff.

- Include all cumulative time within the same calendar month.
- Are reported according to the patient's location or status (eg, nursing facility, hospice) and the total time spent by the physician within a calendar month. Less than 15 minutes' cumulative time within a calendar month cannot be reported.
- Are reported separately from other office or other outpatient, hospital, home, or nursing facility E/M services.
- Require recurrent supervision of therapy.
- ✖ Do not require specific practice capabilities as are defined for CCM services.
- ✖ Are not reported in conjunction with PCM/CCM/complex CCM and TCM services.

CCM or PCM services personally performed by a physician or other QHP (99491, 99424, 99425, 99437) are similar to CPO for patients under the care of home health (99374, 99375) or hospice (99377, 99378). Practices reporting CCM/PCM, however, must meet certain qualifications as discussed in the Required Practice Capabilities section earlier in this chapter. Specific practice qualifications are not required for CPO. Compare requirements for reporting PCM, CCM, and CPO services in the "Monthly Care Management and Care Plan Oversight Services: A Comparison" table included at www.aap.org/cfp2026.

Time spent on the following activities may not be considered CPO:

- ✖ Travel time to or from the facility or place of domicile
- ✖ Services furnished by clinical staff (ancillary or incident-to staff)
- ✖ Interpretation of laboratory or other diagnostic studies associated with a face-to-face E/M service
- ✖ Informal consultations with health professionals not involved in the patient's care
- ✖ Routine postoperative care provided during the global surgery period of a procedure
- ✖ Time spent on online digital E/M or in medical team conferences if they are separately reported with 99421–99423 or 99367
- ✖ Very low-intensity or infrequent supervision services included in the pre- and post-encounter work for an E/M service

Example

➤ **A physician reviews a final report from a home health nurse on a patient who no longer requires home health after the first week of the calendar month.** These low-intensity services are considered part of the pre- and post-encounter work of related E/M services and are not reported as CPO services.

A CPO billing worksheet can be used to track time of CPO services based on documentation in the patient's medical record and used to support billing when time in a calendar month supports reporting a CPO service. A template is included at www.aap.org/cfp2026 ("Care Plan Oversight Billing Worksheet Template"). An example of a completed CPO log follows. Electronic time-tracking software may be used in lieu of a worksheet.

Home Ventilator Management

94005 Home ventilator management CPO of a patient (patient not present) in home, domiciliary or rest home (eg, assisted living) requiring review of status, review of laboratories and other studies and revision of orders and respiratory care plan (as appropriate), within a calendar month, 30 minutes or more

Services include determining ventilator settings, establishing a plan of care, and providing ongoing monitoring. Code **94005** is used to report home ventilator management CPO. It may be reported only when 30 or more minutes of CPO is provided within a calendar month.

Home ventilator management CPO is distinct from CPO to patients under care of a home health care or hospice agency (**99374–99378**) when provided and reported by a separate physician or QHP (eg, pulmonologist reports **94005** and primary care physician reports **99374**).

Care Plan Oversight Billing Worksheet Template[a]			
Physician: Dr J Patient Name: Patient A Month: February 2026 *Supporting documentation is found in patient's medical record. Patient A is receiving home health care at home under a wound care plan approved by Dr J.*			
Date of Service	**Documented Service**	**Total Minutes**	**Monthly Subtotal**
02/04/2025	Development of wound care plan and order for home health	20	20
02/04/2025	Discussion with wound care nurse concerned about drainage from wound	6	26
02/15/2025	Discussion with pain management physician	10	36
02/16/2025	Review of report from wound care nurse	5	41
Total time in the calendar month			41
Time Requirements (min) per Calendar Month	**Patient Under the Care of a Home Health Care Agency**	**Hospice Patient**	
15–29	99374	99377	
≥30	99375	99378	
≥30 Medicare code	G0181	G0182	
Code Supported: **99375** or **G0181**, depending on payer			

Abbreviation: CPO, care plan oversight.

[a]Follow individual payer guidelines for reporting CPO for a pediatric-prescribed extended care facility. Codes 99374 and 99375 (home health CPO) are required by some plans.

Chapter 9

Indirect Management of Chronic and Complex Conditions

Coding for Episodes of Care

CPT instructions explain requirements and guide which activities are included in each service and which are separately reported. Many inclusion and exclusion rules are applied to the services discussed in this chapter.

- Certain niche services (eg, management of end-stage renal disease) may be considered components of or an alternative to PCM or CCM.
- The same time and activity are never used to support multiple codes (eg, time used to support reporting of an online digital E/M service code is not included in time of CCM).

Transitional Care Management Services

TCM (99495 and 99496) includes services provided to a new or established patient whose medical and/or psychosocial problems require moderate- or high-level MDM during the transition to the patient's community setting (eg, home, domiciliary, rest home, or assisted living facility) from the following settings:

- Inpatient hospital including partial, acute, rehabilitation, and long-term acute stays
- Observation care
- Skilled nursing or nursing facility

Box 9-4 includes code descriptors for TCM services. TCM commences on the date of discharge and continues for the next 29 days. *There are no specific requirements for time spent in TCM services,* but TCM activities still should be documented on the dates provided. Refer to **Table 6-4** to determine the level of MDM.

TCM services are valued significantly higher than other care management services. If the dates and/or time for TCM and other care management services overlap, it is advantageous to report TCM, provided all required elements of service have been met. Total non-facility and work RVUs for TCM are included in **Box 9-4**. Using a hypothetical conversion factor of $40 per RVU, an average allowed amount for TCM services would be approximately $248.80 for 99495 (total non-facility RVUs: 6.22 × 40) and $337.20 for 99496 (total non-facility RVUs: 8.43 × 40). Payment allowance will vary by contracted conversion factors and the fee schedule used by a payer (eg, prior year's Medicare Physician Fee Schedule).

Box 9-4. Transitional Care Management at a Glance

Patient Population New or established patients whose medical and/or psychosocial problems require moderate- or high-level MDM during a 30-day transition period beginning with the date of discharge from a facility setting to the patient's home, domiciliary, rest home, or assisted living facility	
★**99495** TCM services with the following required elements: • Communication (direct contact, telephone, electronic) with the patient and/or caregiver within 2 business days after the date of discharge • At least moderate level of MDM during the service period • Face-to-face or telemedicine visit within 14 calendar days, starting on the date of discharge[a]	★**99496** TCM services with the following required elements: • Communication (direct contact, telephone, electronic) with the patient and/or caregiver within 2 business days after the date of discharge • High level of MDM during the service period • Face-to-face or telemedicine visit within 7 calendar days, starting on the date of discharge[a]
Total non-facility RVUs: 6.22.[b] Work RVUs: 2.78.[b]	Total non-facility RVUs: 8.43.[b] Work RVUs: 3.79.[b]

Abbreviations: MDM, medical decision-making; RVUs, relative value units; TCM, transitional care management.

[a] Medication reconciliation and management must occur no later than the date of the face-to-face visit.

[b] 2025 National Physician Fee Schedule Relative Value File, total non-facility and work RVUs, not geographically adjusted. 2026 RVUs were not available at the time of this publication. Individual payers may use different relative value files (eg, from previous years).

One face-to-face visit (in person or by telemedicine) with the reporting physician or QHP is included in addition to indirect services performed by the physician/QHP and/or licensed clinical staff under the direction of the physician/QHP. Any additional face-to-face visits during the service period are separately reported.

Moderate to high MDM (as defined in the E/M service guidelines) is a requirement for TCM. Follow-up care that includes low-intensity services such as discussion of improvement or normal laboratory results, which require only straightforward or low MDM, are not reported with codes for TCM.

A combination of patient care activities by a physician or other QHP and clinical staff working under supervision of a physician or QHP are included in TCM.

Non–face-to-face services provided by the physician or other QHP may include

- Obtaining and reviewing the discharge information
- Reviewing, ordering, or following up on pending diagnostic tests and treatments
- Communicating with or educating the family and/or other caregivers
- Interacting with other QHPs who will assume/reassume care of the patient's system-specific problems
- Scheduling assistance for necessary follow-up services
- Arranging referrals and community resources as necessary

Licensed clinical staff time (under the direction of the physician or other QHP) may include face-to-face and non–face-to-face time spent

- Communicating with the patient and/or family or other caregivers about aspects of care and with other agencies and community services used by the patient
- Educating the patient and/or family or other caregivers to support self-management, independent living, and activities of daily living
- Assessing and supporting adherence to the treatment plan and medication management
- Facilitating access to care and other services needed by the patient and/or family, including identifying community and health resources

TCM services are not limited to the attending provider of the related facility stay (eg, hospitalist) or to physicians of any specific specialty.

- The individual reporting TCM provides or oversees the management and/or coordination of services necessary *for all* the patient's medical conditions, psychosocial needs, and activities of daily living.
- Only 1 individual may report TCM for each qualifying patient within 30 days of discharge. Another TCM service may not be reported by the same individual or group for any subsequent discharge(s) within those 30 days.

Other physicians and QHPs (eg, covering physician) may contribute to the TCM service, but only the physician who provides the initial face-to-face service after discharge reports the service.

- Hospital or observation discharge services (eg, **99238**, **99239**) may be reported by the same individual reporting TCM services. Discharge services do not qualify as the required face-to-face visit for TCM.

Codes 99495 and 99496

- Require initial patient contact, a face-to-face visit with the reporting physician or QHP, and medication reconciliation *within specified time frames.*

To provide direct patient contact within 2 business days after the date of discharge and to schedule appointments within 7 or 14 calendar days (counting the date of discharge as day 1), practices must have a process for receiving notification of observation and inpatient hospital discharges. Failure to make contact within 2 business days or to provide a face-to-face visit within 14 calendar days eliminates the possibility of reporting TCM services.

- Initial patient contact must occur with 2 business days after the date of discharge (eg, by close of the business day on Tuesday when the patient is discharged on Saturday).
- The included face-to-face visit must occur within 7 or 14 days of discharge, counting the day of discharge as day 1.
- Medication management must occur *no later than* the date of the face-to-face visit.
  - *Medication reconciliation* refers to the process of avoiding inadvertent inconsistencies across transitions in care by reviewing the patient's complete medication regimen at the time of admission, transfer, and discharge and comparing it with the regimen being considered for the new setting of care.
  - Clinical staff may perform and document medication reconciliation under general supervision of the physician or QHP.

When medication management occurs in conjunction with a face-to-face visit, 1111F (discharge medications reconciled with the current medication list in outpatient medical record) may be reported in addition to the code for the service provided. Code 1111F is a Category II *CPT* code used for performance measurement in some quality initiatives and is not associated with FFS payment. Learn more about Category II codes in Chapter 3.

- Follow payer guidelines for reporting. The CMS allows reporting of TCM services following completion of the required face-to-face visit (ie, before the end of the service period). Other payers may not allow billing until the complete service period has elapsed.
- Code selection is based on the level of MDM and the date of the first face-to-face visit, as shown in **Table 9-3**. Note that all 4 components (communication within 2 business days, medication reconciliation, type of MDM, and timing of face-to-face visit) must be met and supported in the documentation to report TCM services, although only the MDM and timing of the face-to-face visit differentiate code selection.
  - **Figure 9-2** shows the required elements of the TCM service.

Figure 9-2. Required Elements of Transitional Care Management

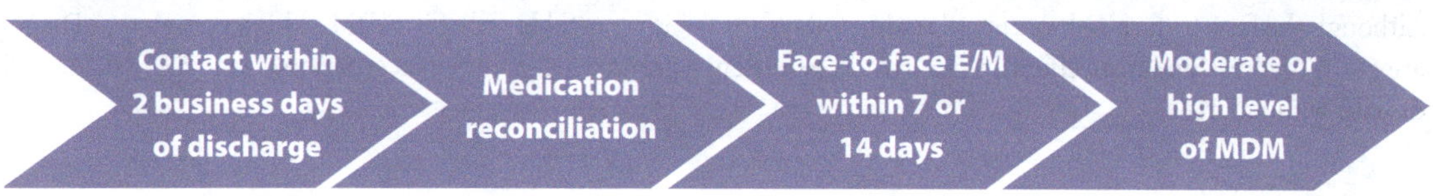

E/M indicates evaluation and management; MDM, medical decision-making.

Table 9-3. Levels of Transitional Care Management

Documentation must support that interactive communication with the patient/caregiver took place within 2 business days of discharge for either level of service, the date and level of MDM of the initial face-to-face visit, and medication reconciliation. Unlike other care management services, time is not a factor in code selection for TCM.

Level of Medical Decision-Making	Face-to-Face Visit Within 7 Days	Face-to-Face Visit Within 8 to 14 Days
Moderate	99495	99495
High	99496	99495

Abbreviations: MDM, medical decision-making; TCM, transitional care management.

Examples

➤ **A patient with hemoglobin SS disease and asthma is discharged from the hospital after a 3-day admission for asthma symptoms and concern for acute chest syndrome.** The patient is discharged on Sunday morning. On Tuesday morning, the patient's primary care pediatrician reviews records from the hospital stay and notes concerning issues with mental health. The pediatrician telephones the parent, who shares a concern about a new diagnosis of depression because the first available follow-up appointment with a psychologist is more than 3 weeks from discharge. The patient is seen by the pediatrician later that day. Asthma symptoms improve, and pain is currently controlled. The depression is reassessed, and the patient is determined to have suicidal thoughts, although there is no current intent. The pediatrician telephones the sickle cell program at the children's hospital 130 miles away, where the patient has received behavioral health care in the past. After speaking with a psychiatrist specializing in caring for children with chronic illness, it is agreed that the patient will receive care from the clinic rather than wait to meet with the local psychologist. Although admission for psychiatric care is discussed as an option, intensive telemedicine treatment is scheduled. The patient is also advised to keep an in-person follow-up appointment with the pulmonologist the following week. The pediatrician and clinical staff closely monitor and coordinate ongoing treatment for the duration of the 30-day period that began on the date of discharge. The MDM is considered to be high complexity, given the management of depression with suicidal ideation and a decision regarding hospitalization.

Code **99496** is reported given the high-complexity MDM, a face-to-face visit within 7 calendar days of the date of discharge, and other requirements, including interactive contact within 2 business days after the date of discharge. Diagnosis codes may include **R45.851** (suicidal ideations), **F32.2** (major depressive disorder, single episode, severe without psychotic features), **J45.31** (mild persistent asthma with [acute] exacerbation), and **D57.1** (sickle-cell disease without crisis).

➤ **Patient A has hemoglobin SS disease and mild persistent asthma and is discharged Sunday from the hospital after an admission for asthma symptoms and concern for acute chest syndrome.** On the following Tuesday, a member of the pediatrician's clinical staff telephones the patient's mother, who shares concerns about the child's depression because the first available follow-up appointment with a psychologist is 3 weeks from today. Following consultation with the pediatrician, clinical staff assist with arranging an earlier follow-up appointment via telemedicine with a psychiatrist who specializes in caring for children with chronic medical conditions instead of the local psychologist. Patient A is seen by the pediatrician in follow-up on the sixth calendar day after discharge. At the visit, the pediatrician reassesses the patient's asthma, hemoglobin SS disease, and depression; reconciles medications and enters related orders; and revises the patient's plan of care, adding a plan for depression management. The pediatrician and clinical staff monitor and coordinate the child's ongoing treatment through the conclusion of the 29th day following discharge. The MDM meets the requirements of moderate complexity for management of depression, asthma, and hemoglobin SS disease with prescription drug management.

Code **99495** is reported because the MDM was moderate and other requirements for TCM services were met. Although the face-to-face visit occurred within 7 days, **99496** is reportable only for MDM of high complexity. Diagnoses are **F32.A** (depression, unspecified), **J45.31** (mild persistent asthma with [acute] exacerbation), and **D57.1** (sickle-cell disease without crisis).

Care Management After TCM

A patient may require ongoing care management services after the 30-day TCM service period has ended. When a TCM service period begins or ends in the same month that other care management services are provided, each service may be reported by the same physician or QHP as long as the same period is not attributed to more than one service (ie, time during the TCM service period cannot be attributed to another care management service).

Example

➤ **Patient A is discharged on January 14, 2026. TCM is provided through a period ending on February 12, 2026.** The pediatrician provides CCM services for the remainder of the month of February. Only the time spent in CCM services provided from February 13, 2026, through February 28, 2026, may be considered for that calendar month per *CPT*.

Interprofessional Telephone/Internet/Electronic Health Record Consultations

Remote interprofessional consultations include a request by a patient's treating physician or other QHP for an opinion and/or treatment advice by telephone, internet, or EHR from a physician or other QHP with specialty expertise (ie, consultant). This consultation does not require face-to-face contact with the patient by the consultant. The patient may be in the inpatient or outpatient setting.

- ✖ When the purpose of communication is to arrange a transfer of care or face-to-face patient encounter, interprofessional consultation codes are not reported.
- As with all consultations, the request for advice or an opinion, including what advice or opinion was sought, should be documented in the patient record. For a new patient with no record, the consultant should create a record to document this service.

Interprofessional consultations have been identified by the CMS as a means of increasing access to specialty care that might otherwise be inaccessible to a patient. The CMS has encouraged state Medicaid programs to include payment for interprofessional consultation services in Medicaid benefits.

Interprofessional Consultation Reporting by a Treating/Requesting Physician

The physician or QHP who is treating the patient and requesting the interprofessional consultation should document the request for information and time spent preparing for and communicating during the consultation. This work is a referral service with code selection based on whether another E/M service is provided by the requesting physician or QHP to the same patient on the same date.

On a date when no other E/M service is furnished to the patient, the treating/requesting physician or QHP who spends 16 to 30 minutes preparing for the referral and/or communicating with the consultant may report the service with **99452**.

#99452 Interprofessional telephone/Internet/EHR referral service(s) provided by a treating/requesting physician or QHP, 30 minutes

Do not report **99452**

- ✖ On the same date an E/M service is reported by the same individual or other individuals of the same exact specialty and same group practice
- ✖ When less than 16 minutes is spent on the date of the consultation preparing for the referral and/or communicating with the consultant
- ✖ More than once in a 14-day period

When the referral service and another E/M service are performed on the same day by the same physician or QHP, the combined services are reported with the code for the other E/M service (eg, **99214**, established patient office visit). The code for the combined services may be selected according to either the physician's or QHP's total time or MDM.

- When selecting a code based on the total time, the time spent providing the referral service is included in the total time of the E/M service provided on the same date.
- When MDM is used to select the level of E/M service, the work of performing the referral service is considered part of the MDM (eg, discussion of management with an external physician or QHP).

Interprofessional Consultation Reporting by a Consultant

A physician with specialty expertise (consultant) who provides opinion or treatment advice *by telephone, internet, or EHR* at the request of and to a patient's treating physician or QHP reports the service with interprofessional consultation codes **99446–99449** or **99451**. These consultations do not require face-to-face contact with the new or established patient by the consultant.

99446 Interprofessional telephone/Internet/EHR assessment and management service provided by a consultative physician or other QHP including a verbal and written report to the patient's treating/requesting physician/QHP; 5–10 minutes of medical consultative discussion and review

99447 11–20 minutes of medical consultative discussion and review

99448 21–30 minutes of medical consultative discussion and review

99449 31 minutes or more of medical consultative discussion and review

#99451 Interprofessional telephone/Internet/EHR assessment and management service provided by a consultative physician or QHP including a written report to the patient's treating/requesting physician or other QHP, 5 or more minutes of medical consultative time

Guidelines for the consultant reporting interprofessional telephone/internet/EHR consultations include

- For a new patient with no record, create a record to document this service.
- As with all consultations, the request for opinion or treatment advice should be documented in the patient record.
- For **99446–99449**, *more than 50% of the time* reported as interprofessional consultation must have been spent in medical consultative verbal or internet discussion rather than review of data (eg, medical records, test results).
- Code **99451** is reported according to the total time of review and interprofessional consultation.
- Both verbal and written reports are required for completion of the services represented by **99446–99449**. Only a written report is required for **99451**.
- A single interprofessional consultation code is reported for the cumulative time spent in discussion and information review regardless of the number of contacts necessary to complete the service.

Do not report **99446–99451**

- ✖ When the consultant has provided a face-to-face service to the patient within the past 14 days or when the consultation results in scheduling of a face-to-face service within the next 14 days or at the consultant's next available appointment date
- ✖ For less than 5 minutes of medical consultative time
- ✖ More than once in a 7-day interval
- *Less than 50% of the time* reported as interprofessional consultation must have been spent in medical consultative verbal or internet discussion rather than review of data (eg, medical records, test results).
- Consultation services provided directly to the patient and/or family may be reported with **98000–98007** (synchronous audio-video visit), **98008–98015** (synchronous audio-only visit), or **99421–99423** (online digital E/M), and the time related to these services is not included in the time attributed to interprofessional consultation services. Nonphysician qualified health care professionals (eg, therapists) report **98966–98968** or **98970–98972** for these services.
- Time spent by the consultant reviewing pertinent medical records, studies, or other data is included in the time of the interprofessional consultation and not separately reported.
- ✖ Do not report prolonged E/M service before and/or after direct patient care (**99358**, **99359**) for any time within the service period if reporting **99446–99451**.

Example

➤ **A 15-year-old is seen by a primary care pediatrician for follow-up of Crohn disease.** The patient reports increased symptoms, including rectal bleeding. The patient's gastroenterologist is located 250 miles away, so the pediatrician arranges an interprofessional consultation to discuss a potential change in treatment. The pediatrician's total time on the date of the visit is 30 minutes, including time spent arranging for a telephone consultation with the patient's gastroenterologist to discuss management options for the patient's poorly controlled Crohn disease of the small intestine with rectal bleeding.

The next day, the gastroenterologist spends 5 minutes reviewing the pediatrician's documentation of the patient's evaluation. Later that day, the pediatrician and gastroenterologist spend a total of 21 minutes discussing the pediatrician's findings, diagnosis, and appropriate treatment options. The gastroenterologist provides the pediatrician with a written report of the recommendations discussed. The diagnosis is poorly controlled Crohn disease with rectal bleeding. The pediatrician calls the patient and parents to inform them that the gastroenterologist recommended a new medication that requires prior authorization by the patient's health plan. The patient is to continue current medications for now. The pediatrician's nurse will call when the health plan's determination of coverage is received.

Service	*ICD-10-CM*	*CPT*
First date of service (pediatric E/M visit)	**K50.011** (Crohn's disease of small intestine with rectal bleeding)	**99214** (established patient office or other outpatient visit E/M, 30–39 minutes of total time)
Second date (interprofessional consultation)	The pediatrician and gastroenterologist each report **K50.011**.	The pediatrician reports **99452** for the 21 minutes spent in interprofessional referral service. The gastroenterologist reports **99448** (21–30 minutes of medical discussion and review).

Teaching Points: In this vignette, the patient and parents are not present for the interprofessional consultation. The consultation service by the gastroenterologist included 5 minutes of record review and 21 minutes of conversation with the pediatrician. If less than 50% of the gastroenterologist's time was devoted to the medical consultative verbal or internet discussion, an interprofessional consultation would not be reported. The pediatrician may report **99452**

for 16 to 30 minutes of interprofessional consultation, not including the time spent in telephone conversation with the patient and parents. Only time spent preparing for the referral and communicating with the gastroenterologist is included in the time of 99452. The pediatrician's time spent communicating with the patient or parent after the date of the visit may contribute to the time of a monthly care management service, when performed.

Medical Team Conferences

Medical team conference codes 99366–99368 are used to coordinate or manage care and services for established patients with chronic or multiple health conditions (eg, child who experienced a stroke caused by sickle cell disease and requires physical and occupational therapy, speech therapy, pain management, and scheduled transfusions).

Codes differentiate reporting provider (physician or other QHP who may provide and independently report E/M services vs other NQHCP) and face-to-face versus non–face-to-face (patient and/or family is or is not present) team conference services.

Code 99367 is the only code that may be reported by a physician or other QHP who may report E/M services, and it can be reported only when the patient and/or family is not present at the team conference.

Codes 99366 and 99368 are reported only for services provided by NQHCPs who do not independently provide and report E/M services. For discussion of codes 99366 and 99368, refer to **Chapter 12**.

Box 9-5 provides an overview of the patient population, code descriptor, and services not separately reported with medical team conference services.

Box 9-5. Medical Team Conference Services

Patient Population

Established patients with chronic and multiple health conditions or with congenital anomalies (eg, cleft lip and palate, craniofacial abnormality)

Physician or QHP Service

99367 Medical team conference with interdisciplinary team of health care professionals, patient and/or family not present, 30 minutes or more; participation by physician

(When patient or caregivers attend conference, report other E/M codes.)

Total RVUs (facility or non-facility): 1.59; work RVUs: 1.10.[a]

Work Required

At least 30 minutes of face-to-face services from different specialties or disciplines

Face-to-face evaluations or treatments of the patient performed, independent of any team conference, within the previous 60 days

Presentation of findings and recommendations

Formulation of a care plan and subsequent review/proofing of the plan

Services Not Separately Reported

Do not report 99367 during the same month as 99437, 99439, 99487, 99489, 99490, 99491 CCM and complex CCM services.[b]

Abbreviations: CCM, chronic care management; E/M, evaluation and management; PCM, principal care management; RVU, relative value unit; QHP, qualified health care professional.

[a] 2025 National Physician Fee Schedule Relative Value File, total non-facility and work RVUs, not geographically adjusted. 2026 RVUs were not available at the time of this publication. Individual payers may use different relative value files (eg, from previous years).

[b] When not reporting 99367, time spent in the medical team conference may contribute to either the total time of an E/M service provided on the same date as the medical team conference or the time of PCM or CCM service code(s).

Medical team conferences require

- *Face-to-face participation* by a minimum of 3 care team members, such as physicians and/or QHPs from different subspecialties and/or NQHCPs from different disciplines (eg, speech pathologists, dietitians, social workers), with or without the presence of the patient, family member(s), community agencies, surrogate decision-maker(s) (eg, legal guardian), and/or caregiver(s).
  - Participation by telephone is not reported.
  - Verify payer policies for participation via interactive audiovisual communication (telemedicine). Participation in team conferences via telemedicine *has not yet been added* to the lists of services reported with modifier 95 or the Medicare list of services approved for provision via telehealth.
- Active involvement in the development, revision, coordination, and implementation of health care services needed by the patient by each participant.
- Face-to-face evaluations and/or treatments within the previous 60 days, by the participating physician or QHP, that are separate from any team conference.

Chapter 9 Indirect Management of Chronic and Complex Conditions

Only 1 individual from the same specialty reports 99367 for the same encounter. Physicians and other QHPs of different specialties, however, may each report their participation in a team conference.

- Medical record documentation should include the reporting physician's or QHP's contributed information and subsequent treatment recommendations and the time spent from the beginning of the review of an individual patient until the conclusion of the review.
- Medical team conferences may not be reported if the facility or organization is contractually obligated to provide the service, they are informal meetings or simple conversations between physicians and other QHPs and NQHCPs, or less than 30 minutes of conference time is spent in the team conferences.
- *CPT* instructs that physicians *or other QHPs* report their participation in a team conference with the patient and/or family present using E/M codes for the place of service (POS) based on the instructions for the E/M service provided.

Examples

➤ **A primary care pediatrician, a neurologist, a urologist, a physical therapist, and an occupational therapist participate in discussion and planning for transitioning a patient from pediatric to adult care.** The conference lasts 60 minutes and neither patient nor parents attend. Each participant in the conference has completed their evaluation of the patient within 60 days before the conference.

CPT	
99367	Each participating physician from different specialties
99368	Each NQHCP (eg, physical and occupational therapists)

Physicians who provide a face-to-face visit (eg, consultation, 99242–99245) on the same date as a *medical team conference without the patient/family present* should report codes for the individual services provided. A payer may require modifier 25 (significant, separately identifiable E/M service) on the code for the face-to-face visit. If 99367 will not be paid because of payer policy, the physician's time participating in the conference may be included in the total time of another E/M service provided on the same date, when applicable.

➤ **A primary care pediatrician, hematologist, pulmonologist, and licensed clinical social worker (LCSW) participate in discussion and planning with Patient A and the patient's parents present.** The conference lasts 60 minutes. No other E/M services are provided by the physicians on this date.

CPT	
99366	Each nonphysician QHCP (eg, LCSW)
99202–99499	Each participating physician, if they are from different specialties and/or from different practices (ie, separate tax ID numbers) reports an E/M service based on the POS and applicable time-based coding instructions.

Physicians who provide a face-to-face visit on the same date as a medical team conference *with the patient/family present* should report the appropriate E/M code for the site of the visit and may also report an appropriate prolonged service code (eg, 99418 for inpatient or observation services or, for E/M services in office or outpatient settings, 99417) for time extending beyond the parameters designated by the E/M code and to the minimum time of the appropriate prolonged service code.

Advance Care Planning

★99497 Advance care planning including the explanation and discussion of advance directives such as standard forms (with completion of such forms, when performed), by the physician or other QHP; first 30 minutes, face-to-face with the patient, family member(s) and/or surrogate

★✚99498 each additional 30 minutes (List separately in addition to code for primary procedure)

Advance care planning includes

- A face-to-face service by a physician or QHP, including telemedicine services, to a patient, family member, or surrogate spent in counseling and discussion of advance directives
- Completion of forms, when applicable (eg, Health Care Proxy, Durable Power of Attorney for Health Care, Living Will, and Medical Orders for Life-Sustaining Treatment)

● indicates a new code; ▲, revised; #, re-sequenced; ✚, add-on; ★, audiovisual technology; and ◀, synchronous interactive audio.

Active management of problems is not included in advance care planning. Other E/M services provided on the same date as advance care planning may be separately reported *except for* hourly critical care services (99291, 99292), inpatient neonatal and pediatric critical care (99468, 99469; 99471–99476), and initial and continuing intensive care services (99477–99480). Append modifier 25 to the E/M code for active management of problems.

Because the *CPT* prefatory language and code descriptors for advance care planning do not include other instruction on the time required for reporting, these services may be reported according to general *CPT* instruction to report when the midpoint is passed (eg, 1 unit of 99498 may be reported for services of 46–75 minutes).

Do not report 99497 for less than 16 minutes of physician face-to-face time.

Exceptions may apply for payers with policy requiring that the time included in the code descriptor be met or exceeded.

Advance care planning services may be considered bundled to enhanced payment methodologies (eg, patient-centered medical home receiving per-member-per-month care coordination fees) and not separately paid. But *CPT* requires reporting of the code that is specific to the service provided regardless of payment policy. Advance care planning services should not be reported as another service (eg, office visit) in an effort to prevent denial as a bundled service or because another service has higher RVUs and payment values.

RVUs assigned for a non-facility site of service are 2.46 for 99497 and 2.13 for 99498 ($98.40 and $85.20, respectively, if paid at $40 per RVU).

However, when a payer does not recognize advance care planning codes or the main reason for an encounter is other than advance care planning, consultation codes 99242–99245 or other E/M service codes (eg, 99212–99215) may be appropriately reported.

Chapter 9

Indirect Management of Chronic and Complex Conditions

Examples

➤ **A child and their parents, who have learned at a recent visit that the child's prognosis is poor, return for advance care planning.** The physician spends 50 minutes face-to-face with the patient and parents, assesses their understanding of the diagnosis, and confirms and documents decisions about palliative care and the desire to limit lifesaving measures. A plan of care is developed and documented, and an appointment with the palliative care team at the hospital is scheduled.

CPT
99497 (advance care planning, initial 30 minutes) 99498 × 1 (each additional 30 minutes)

The physician's face-to-face time of 50 minutes spent providing the advance care planning supports reporting 99497 with 1 unit of 99498 for the final 20 minutes of service.

➤ **An adolescent with cystic fibrosis wishes to discuss and be involved in planning her care after learning she will require a lung transplant.** The pulmonologist spends 80 minutes face-to-face with the patient and her parents, assessing their understanding of the diagnosis and prognosis, their continued hope that treatment is successful, and the patient's wishes to be included in decisions about her care. A plan of care is developed and documented, and an appointment with the palliative care team at the hospital is scheduled to provide additional counseling and support services to the patient and family.

The physician may report codes 99497 and 99498 × 2 for the 80 minutes of face-to-face time spent providing the advance care planning. Per *CPT* instruction, an additional unit of 99498 is reported because the midpoint (16 minutes) between the time reported with the first unit (31–60 minutes) and the second unit (61–90 minutes) was passed.

Indirect Prolonged Service on Date Other Than the Face-to-Face E/M Service

Prolonged services without direct patient contact (99358, 99359) are reported when a physician or QHP provides prolonged service *on a date other than* the date of a face-to-face E/M service.

Indirect prolonged services may be reported in relation to any level or category of E/M service that was or will be provided on another date of service regardless of whether time was used to select the level of the face-to-face service. The POS does not affect reporting.

Refer to discussion of 99417 in **Chapter 7** and 99418 in **Chapter 16** for prolonged service on the date of a face-to-face E/M service.

Guidelines for reporting non-direct prolonged services include

- Only time spent on a single date of service is reported with 99358 and 99359. Do not add segments of time from more than one date of service.
- Time is met when the midpoint is passed.
  - Less than 30 minutes' total duration on a given date cannot be reported.
  - Less than 15 minutes beyond the first hour or beyond the final 30 minutes is not reported separately. Use 99359 to report the final 15 to 30 minutes beyond the time reported with 99358 on a given date. **Table 9-4** breaks down the time requirements.
- Must be reported on a different date than the related primary service within a time frame to contribute to ongoing patient management. *CPT* does not specify a time frame (eg, within 1 week of related service) for provision of prolonged service before and/or after direct patient care.

Table 9-4. Non–Face-to-Face Prolonged Services at a Glance

99358 Prolonged E/M service before and/or after direct patient care; first hour
+99359 each additional 30 minutes (Use in conjunction with 99358.)

Prolonged service must be related to another service provided by the same individual.

Total Duration (min) of Prolonged Service Without Direct Face-to-Face Contact	Code(s) and Unit(s) of Service Reported
<30	Not separately reported
30–74	99358 × 1
75–104	99358 × 1 and 99359 × 1
≥105	99358 × 1 and 99359 × 2

Abbreviation: E/M, evaluation and management.

Prolonged service before and/or after direct patient care

- ✖ Does not include time spent by clinical staff
- ✖ Cannot be reported for time spent in provision of and reported with codes for
  - CPO services (99374–99380)
  - CCM (99491, 99437)
  - PCM (99424, 99425)
  - Medical team conferences (99366–99368)
  - Online medical evaluations (99421–99423)
  - Interprofessional telephone/Internet/EHR consultations (99446–99452)
  - Anticoagulant management for a patient taking warfarin (93792, 93793)
- ✖ Is not reported when any other E/M service is provided on the same date

Example

➤ **A physician requested and received medical records from multiple sources for a child with hemoglobin SS disease who was placed into foster care and had multiple hospitalizations and inconsistent care over the past 3 years.** On a day before the date of the initial consultation service, the physician spends 35 minutes reviewing and summarizing the medical records and documents the time spent in the medical record. The physician reports

CPT	*ICD-10-CM*
99358 (prolonged physician services without direct patient contact; 30–74 minutes)	D57.1 (sickle-cell disease without crisis)

The prolonged service without direct patient contact could also have taken place between the first and subsequent patient visits but not on the date of an E/M visit.

Related Services Discussed in Other Chapters

From Chapter 7

After-Hours and Special Services

Codes **99050–99060** are used to report services provided after hours or on an emergency basis and are an adjunct to the basic E/M service provided.

From Chapter 20

Brief Communication Technology-Based Service

A brief communication technology-based service (virtual check-in [**98016**]) is reported by a physician or other QHP who can independently provide and report E/M services *at the request of an established patient* to evaluate whether a more extensive type of service (eg, office visit) is required to address the patient's concern. At least 5 minutes of medical discussion between the patient and reporting physician or QHP is required to report **98016**. This service is not reported when the virtual check-in leads to an E/M service on the same date, but the time of the virtual check-in is included in the total time of the other E/M service provided.

Medical discussion of longer than 10 minutes may support reporting a more extensive E/M service (eg, **98012**, synchronous audio-only established patient visit with more than 10 minutes of medical discussion).

Online Digital E/M Services

An online digital medical evaluation (**99421–99423**) is a non–face-to-face E/M service by a physician or other QHP who may report E/M services to a patient by using internet communication (eg, patient portal messaging) in response to a patient's online inquiry.

This is in contrast with telemedicine services, which represent interactive audio and/or video telecommunications systems that permit real-time communication between the physician, at the distant site, and the patient, at the originating site.

Codes **98970–98972** are used to report an online assessment and management service by an NQHCP (eg, occupational therapist, speech pathologist) who cannot report E/M codes. The reporting guidelines for codes **98970–98972** are the same as those for online services provided by the physician or QHP.

Telemedicine Services

Synchronous office E/M services provided via audio-video (**98000–98007**) or audio-only (**98008–98015**) communications technology are reported similarly to outpatient office E/M services (**99202–99205**, **99212–99215**) based on total time or MDM. More than 10 minutes of medical discussion is required to report **98008–98015**.

Codes **98966–98968** are used to report telephone assessment and management services by NQHCPs who may not report E/M services.

From Chapter 21

Remote Physiologic Monitoring

#●99470 Remote physiologic monitoring treatment management services, clinical staff/physician/other QHP time in a calendar month requiring interactive communication with the patient/caregiver during the month; first 10 minutes

#▲99457 first 20 minutes

#✚▲99458 each additional 20 minutes

Code **99457** is reported for time spent managing care when the results from a monitoring device(s) are used for treatment management services. This code requires 20 or more minutes of time spent using the results of physiologic monitoring (eg, transmitted glucose monitor results) to treat a patient under a specific treatment plan. When the time of service extends a full 20 minutes beyond the first 20 minutes (ie, at least 40 minutes total), report **99458** in addition to **99457**.

Reporting a Combination of Complex Medical Management Services

Services such as CCM and TCM offer a means of reporting many activities of care management with 1 or 2 codes that describe the complexity and period of care. But when these codes do not apply (eg, patient does not meet criteria) or a payer does not provide benefits for care management services, it may be necessary to report a combination of codes for non–face-to-face services provided to a child with complex health care needs. These may include CPO, online or telemedicine E/M services, prolonged services, and team conference services. Some of these services may also be reported in addition to care management services when the time of each service is distinct.

To test your knowledge of the information presented in this chapter, complete the quiz found at the end of it, after the resources. Answers to each quiz are found in **Appendix II**.

Chapter Takeaways

- CCM and complex CCM services are reported for services provided to a patient with 2 or more chronic conditions that are expected to last at least 1 year. They include ongoing coordination of care for all the patient's health care needs.
- PCM is a service provided to a patient with a single serious chronic condition that is expected to last at least 3 months. PCM does not require management of all the patient's health care needs, and more than one physician may provide PCM services when provided for distinct conditions.
- CPO is similar to other care management services but includes only time spent by a physician or QHP and does not require the practice capabilities of CCM or PCM.
- Practices with the capabilities required for reporting CCM services in lieu of CPO may still report CPO codes when the service provided and nature of the patient presentation support reporting CPO. Physicians must determine the appropriate code selection according to the practice capabilities, services rendered, and nature of the patient presentation.
- TCM is reported by a single physician or QHP who assumes management of all the patient's health care needs following discharge from a facility stay during a 30-day period.
- Although other services may be provided and separately reported during the service period of an indirect care management service, times of service cannot be overlapping.
- Be sure to review payer guidance on reporting these services, as National Correct Coding Initiative edits or other payment policy may require appending modifiers to indicate that distinct periods were spent in the provision of each service. For instance, prolonged E/M service is bundled to CPO, but a modifier may be appended to indicate distinct services within the same reporting period. Guidance for reporting and coverage may vary.

Resources

AAP Coding Assistance and Education

AAP policy statement, "Patient- and Family-Centered Care Coordination: A Framework for Integrating Care for Children and Youth Across Multiple Systems" (https://doi.org/10.1542/peds.2014-0318)

Pediatric Care Management: Coding Quick Reference Card 2026 (www.aap.org/Pediatric-Care-Management-Coding-Quick-Reference-Card-2026)

AAP Pediatric Coding Newsletter™

"Advanced Primary Care Management Services: A Step Toward Value-based Care?" April 2025 (https://doi.org/10.1542/pcco_book252_document001)

"Care Management Services by Specialists and by Primary Care," January 2022 (https://doi.org/10.1542/pcco_book213_document002)

"Coding Hotline," July 2023 (https://doi.org/10.1542/pcco_book231_document004)

"Connecting Coding and Clinical Practice Guidelines: Obesity," May 2024 (https://doi.org/10.1542/pcco_book241_document003)

"Revisiting Transitional Care Management Services," August 2024 (https://doi.org/10.1542/pcco_book244_document003)

Online-Exclusive Content at www.aap.org/cfp2026

"Care Management Tracking Worksheet Template"

"Care Plan Oversight Billing Worksheet Template"

"Monthly Care Management and Care Plan Oversight Services: A Comparison"

Test Your Knowledge!

1. **Which service is only reported by a physician or QHP who provides or oversees the management and/or coordination of services, as needed, for all the patient's health care needs?**
   a. Advance care planning
   b. CCM
   c. CPO
   d. PCM
2. **Which is true of PCM services?**
   a. The patient receiving the service has a serious chronic condition expected to last a minimum of 12 months.
   b. PCM services are never reported by a physician or QHP providing primary care.
   c. PCM addresses all of a patient's health care needs.
   d. PCM services require development, monitoring, or revision of disease-specific care plan.
3. **How are complex CCM services (99487) different from CCM services reported with 99490 or 99491?**
   a. Complex CCM requires at least 60 minutes of clinical staff time and moderate or high MDM.
   b. Complex CCM requires at least 60 minutes of physician or QHP time.
   c. CCM reported with 99490 or 99491 requires moderate medical decision-making.
   d. Complex CCM and CCM are differentiated only by the required time of service.
4. **Which of the following is accurate for reporting a treating physician's or QHP's time spent preparing for and participating in an interprofessional consultation?**
   a. The treating physician or QHP always reports 99452 for time spent in interprofessional consultation referral service.
   b. The treating physician or QHP reports 99452 for time spent in interprofessional consultation only when no other E/M service is provided to the patient on the same date.
   c. The treating physician or QHP reports 99452 only when at least 30 minutes is spent in an interprofessional consultation referral service.
   d. The treating physician or QHP always reports an E/M code for the appropriate site of service for time spent preparing for and participating in an interprofessional consultation.
5. **True or false? Prolonged service without direct patient contact on a date other than the face-to-face E/M service is only reported in conjunction with another E/M service for which the code was selected on the basis of time.**
   a. True
   b. False

CHAPTER 10

Mental and Behavioral Health Services

Contents

Chapter Highlights

- Who may provide mental and behavioral health services
- Important payment considerations
- Diagnosis coding guidelines for mental and behavioral health services
- Integration of behavioral health into primary care practice
- Codes for evaluation and treatment of alcohol and substance use
- Differentiation of codes for testing for neuropsychological and psychological conditions
- Coding for psychiatric evaluation, psychotherapy, and other psychiatric services

Mental and Behavioral Health Services

This chapter focuses on services that are provided to diagnose, manage, or treat mental and behavioral health conditions. Mental and behavioral health services are an important part of pediatric medicine. In recent years, strategies to address issues with access to mental and behavioral health care have included integration of mental health and substance use treatment into primary care settings and expansion of access to care through telephone and digital platforms. Yet obtaining/providing mental and behavioral health services for/to children still involves complexities that physicians must understand to help their patients access needed services.

Pediatric mental and behavioral health conditions may be recognized through preventive screening for anxiety or depression or evaluation of signs and symptoms. Screening and/or assessment for mental and behavioral conditions (96127) and screening for social determinants of health (health risk assessment, 96160–96161) that may influence diagnosis and treatment are discussed in **Chapter 8**. Standardized instruments may also be used for diagnosis and follow-up of mental and behavioral health conditions and reported in addition to office visits and/or psychotherapy, when performed. Use of standardized instruments is included in behavioral health integration services (ie, not separately reported).

Chapter 10

Mental and Behavioral Health Services

Physicians and Other Mental/Behavioral Health Professionals

Services included in this chapter may be provided by

- Physicians, other qualified health care professionals (QHPs, whose scope of practice includes evaluation and management [E/M] services). State regulations and payment policies are often least restrictive for these professionals.
- Nonphysician qualified health care professionals (NQHCPs), who are licensed clinical psychologists (LCPs) and licensed clinical social workers (LCSWs) and may include licensed therapists (eg, licensed marriage and family therapists) and counselors. State regulations and payment policies may vary, but often these professionals may provide and independently report services other than E/M services.
- Allied health care professionals, such as registered behavior technicians and licensed master social workers who provide services ordered by and under the general supervision of physicians, QHPs, and NQHCPs. State regulations and payment policies are often somewhat restrictive for these professionals.
- Clinical staff (eg, registered nurse, medical assistant, behavioral health care manager [BHCM]) working under direct (immediately available in the office or, when allowed, by real-time audio-video communication) supervision of a physician, QHP, or NQHCP. State regulations and payment policies are typically most restrictive for these professionals.

Including Nonphysician Professionals in Your Practice

Services such as behavioral health assessment by an LCSW or licensed psychologist may be provided within a general pediatric group practice and can be an integral part of providing a full scope of care in the medical home. Billing and coding of these services, however, must align not only with coding guidelines but also state scope of practice and individual payer policies on credentialing, contracting, and billing for services of the specific NQHCP. Know your state regulations and payer policies when integrating mental/behavioral health professionals into your practice.

Payment and Coverage Issues for Mental/Behavioral Health Services

Behavioral health services may be covered through a plan and provider network separate from other health care services. When arranging for or providing behavioral health services, it is very important to explore the patient's health plan policy options.

- Failure to credential and, when applicable, contract with behavioral health plans may lead to unpaid or underpaid charges or unanticipated takebacks of previously paid amounts.
- Payer policies may allow specific licensed professionals, such as LCPs and LCSWs, to directly provide and report certain services. Other NQHCPs (eg, licensed master social workers) may be limited to providing services under direct supervision and reporting in the name of the participating health care professional (eg, LCP or psychiatrist).
- General pediatricians and other QHPs may be ineligible to participate in the behavioral health plan network and limited to reporting E/M (eg, **99214**) services to the health plan. Likewise, psychiatrists and QHPs specializing in mental health but able to provide other medical services may participate in both medical and behavioral health networks.

The American Academy of Pediatrics (AAP) Council on Early Childhood, Committee on Psychosocial Aspects of Child and Family Health, and Section on Developmental and Behavioral Pediatrics included the following information about treatment coverage for emotional and behavioral health problems in the policy statement "Addressing Early Childhood Emotional and Behavioral Problems" (https://doi.org/10.1542/peds.2016-3023).

American Academy of Pediatrics Policy Statement

"Without adequate payment for screening and assessment by primary care providers and management by specialty providers with expertise in early childhood mental health, treatment of very young children with emotional and behavioral problems will likely remain inaccessible for many children. Given existing knowledge regarding the importance of early childhood brain development on lifelong health, adequate payment for early childhood preventive services will benefit not only the patients but society as well and should be supported. Mental health carve-outs should be eliminated because they provide a significant barrier to access to mental health care for children. Additional steps toward equal access to mental health and physical health care include efficient prior authorization processes; adequate panels of early childhood mental health providers; payment to all providers, including primary care providers, for mental health diagnoses; sustainable payment for co-located mental health providers and care coordination; payment for evidence-based approaches focused on parents; and payment for the necessary collection of information from children's many caregivers and for same-day services. Advocacy for true mental health parity must continue."

Integration of psychiatric/behavioral health care professionals into the primary care practice may also require an understanding of health plan payment policies. Payer edits may not allow separate payment for mental and behavioral health services when E/M services are provided in the same practice on the same date. Verify coverage and billing options before provision of services.

To learn more about payer edits, refer to Chapter 2. To learn more about AAP payer advocacy, refer to Chapter 4.

- Payers often place limitations on the diagnoses that may be paid under a patient's health benefits versus a separate behavioral health benefit.
  - Pediatricians may be required to report codes for symptoms rather than diagnosed conditions (eg, sadness in lieu of depression). This conflicts with *International Classification of Diseases, 10th Revision, Clinical Modification* (*ICD-10-CM*) guidelines, which instruct, "Codes that describe symptoms and signs, as opposed to diagnoses, are acceptable for reporting purposes *when a related definitive diagnosis has not been established (confirmed) by the provider*."
  - Adherence to *ICD-10-CM* guidelines when assigning diagnosis codes is required under the Health Insurance Portability and Accountability Act (HIPAA) of 1996. Payers are required to accept codes reported in compliance with the official guidelines for code selection and reporting.
  - When payers deny claims appropriately reported with codes **F01–F99** (mental, behavioral, and neurodevelopmental disorders), pediatricians may report the issue through the AAP Coding and Payment Hotline (www.aap.org/en/practice-management/child-health-finance-payment-strategy/coding-payment-hotline) or seek the assistance of an AAP pediatric council (www.aap.org/en/practice-management/child-health-finance-payment-strategy/payment-and-finance-advocacy/aap-pediatric-councils). HIPAA code set violations may also be reported with the Centers for Medicare & Medicaid Services complaint form at https://asett.cms.gov/ASETT_ST_CMP_HomePage.

Healthcare Common Procedure Coding System (HCPCS) modifiers identifying the type of health care professional (eg, **AJ**, clinical social worker) may be necessary to override edits that bundle E/M services provided by a physician/QHP and mental/behavioral health services provided by an NQHCP on the same date.

Relevant HCPCS modifiers include

AH	Clinical psychologist
AJ	Clinical social worker
AM	Physician, team member service
FQ	Furnished using audio-only communication technology

GT	Via interactive audio and video telecommunication systems
HA	Child/adolescent program
HN	Bachelor's degree level
HO	Master's degree level
HP	Doctoral level
HQ	Group setting
TL	Early intervention/individualized family service plan (IFSP)
UN	Two patients served
UP	Three patients served
UQ	Four patients served
UR	Five patients served
US	Six or more patients served

Telemedicine for Mental Health Services

In 2025, codes for office or other outpatient E/M visits via synchronous audio-visual (98000–98006) or audio-only (98008–98015) communications technology were added to *CPT*®. However, the Medicare program elected to continue paying for telemedicine office/outpatient E/M visits reported with E/M office visit codes (99202–99215) appended with telemedicine modifiers. Payer policies for telemedicine services may influence reporting of an E/M service performed in conjunction with psychotherapy. Verification of payer policy is advised prior to claim submission. Another code, 98016, is reported for a brief communication technology-based service (eg, telephone call) of 5 to 10 minutes' duration to determine if a more extensive service is indicated.

Access to health care services via electronic communication technology has advanced significantly since the COVID-19 public health emergency. Although many advances were short-term amendments to payer policies, payment policies for services provided for mental health and substance use diagnoses have changed permanently in many areas. It is important for physicians and other providers of these services to be aware of changing regulations and payment policies that may support greater use of telemedicine.

Refer to **Chapter 2** for more information on use of modifiers and **Chapters 19** and **20** for discussion of coding and documentation for telemedicine services.

Reporting Codes F01–F99

Diagnosis of behavioral and mental health conditions is typically based on the criteria set forth in the *Diagnostic and Statistical Manual of Mental Disorders, 5th Edition, Text Revision* (*DSM-5-TR*) classification system.

- Often, a simple crosswalk from the *DSM-5-TR* diagnosis to the *ICD-10-CM* code supporting the diagnosis can be made. However, the classifications are not always equivalent.
- It is important that documentation clearly reflects a diagnostic statement separate from the assignment of an *ICD-10-CM* code as required by official guidance for *ICD-10-CM*.
  - Documentation should include the findings supporting the diagnosis (eg, observations made during the appointment, history, standardized rating scale results, pertinent physical examination findings).
  - Failure to document the information supporting the diagnostic statement could affect the patient's access to care and the physician's payment for services provided.
- *ICD-10-CM* includes codes for specifying how an accident or injury happened (eg, unintentional or accidental; intentional, such as suicide or assault).
  - Treatment of patients who have sustained injury or illness (eg, poisoning) resulting from intentional self-harm are reported with codes signifying the intent—for example, **T52.92XA** (toxic effect of unspecified organic solvent, intentional self-harm, initial encounter) or **R45.88** (nonsuicidal self-harm).
  - If the intent of the cause of an injury or another condition is unknown or unspecified, code the intent as accidental intent. All transport accident categories assume accidental intent.
  - Codes for events of undetermined intent are for use only if the documentation in the record specifies that the intent cannot be determined at the encounter (eg, suspected abuse under investigation).

To fully report conditions such as poisoning, follow *ICD-10-CM* instructions in the tabular list. For example, instructions for T52.92XA include "Use additional code(s) for all associated manifestations of toxic effect, such as: respiratory conditions due to external agents (J60–J70)."

Current Procedural Terminology Add-On Codes

Many mental and behavioral health services are described by a combination of a base code with add-on codes (AOCs) representing extended services. AOCs (marked with a + before the code) are always performed in addition to a primary procedure and are never reported as a stand-alone service. Like most other codes, AOCs describe additional intraservice work and are not valued to include preservice and postservice work.

Behavioral Health Integration

Integration of mental/behavioral health care into primary care pediatrics has been identified as a means of providing early and ongoing access to behavioral health services. Integration of medical and behavioral health services does not always mean inclusion and/or colocation of behavioral health professionals in a medical practice. Integration may include care management services provided under the supervision of a physician or QHP to initiate a plan of care, coordinate care, and monitor and/or respond to changes in the status of mental/behavioral health conditions.

Following are 2 sets of codes that describe integrated behavioral health services:

1. Psychiatric collaborative care management services (99492–99494) include a defined team of health care professionals providing care through a specific method.
2. General behavioral health integration (99484) services do not include specific types of professionals or a specified method of delivery.

These behavioral health integration services are differentiated by the required elements of service.

Psychiatric Collaborative Care Management Services

Psychiatric collaborative care management services are reported by a physician or QHP who supervises a BHCM who delivers the services in collaboration with a psychologist or other mental health professional (QHP) who can prescribe a full range of medications. Psychiatric collaborative care management services are provided to patients who have a new or existing psychiatric disorder that requires a behavioral health assessment; care plan implementation, revision, or monitoring; and provision of brief interventions. The treating physician or QHP reports codes 99492–99494 when all requirements for reporting are met. E/M and other services may be reported separately by the same physician or QHP during the same calendar month.

99492 Initial psychiatric collaborative care management, first 70 minutes in the first calendar month of BHCM activities, in consultation with a psychiatric consultant, and directed by the treating physician or other QHP, with the following required elements:

- outreach to and engagement in treatment of a patient directed by the treating physician or other QHP,
- initial assessment of the patient, including administration of validated rating scales, with the development of an individualized treatment plan,
- review by the psychiatric consultant with modifications of the plan if recommended,
- entering patient in a registry and tracking patient follow-up and progress using the registry, with appropriate documentation, and participation in weekly caseload consultation with the psychiatric consultant, and
- provision of brief interventions using evidence-based techniques such as behavioral activation, motivational interviewing, and other focused treatment strategies.

Payer policies vary in coverage of psychiatric collaborative care management. For instance, some programs allow one unit of 99492 per year rather than once per lifetime per physician or other QHP. Billing staff should regularly review payer policies to inform correct coding.

99493 Subsequent psychiatric collaborative care management, first 60 minutes in a subsequent month of BHCM activities, in consultation with a psychiatric consultant, and directed by the treating physician or other QHP, with the following required elements:

- tracking patient follow-up and progress using the registry, with appropriate documentation,
- participation in weekly caseload consultation with the psychiatric consultant,
- ongoing collaboration with and coordination of the patient's mental health care with the treating physician or other QHP and any other treating mental health providers,
- additional review of progress and recommendations for changes in treatment, as indicated, including medications, based on recommendations provided by the psychiatric consultant,

- provision of brief interventions using evidence-based techniques such as behavioral activation, motivational interviewing, and other focused treatment strategies,
- monitoring of patient outcomes using validated rating scales, and
- relapse prevention planning with patients as they achieve remission of symptoms and/or other treatment goals and are prepared for discharge from active treatment.

+99494 Initial or subsequent psychiatric collaborative care management, each additional 30 minutes in a calendar month of BHCM activities, in consultation with a psychiatric consultant, and directed by the treating physician or other QHP (List separately in addition to code for primary procedure)
(Use **99494** in conjunction with **99492** or **99493**.)

Medicaid plans and other payers may also accept HCPCS code **G2214**, which requires less time within a calendar month than **99492** or **99493**. Report **G2214** for either initial or subsequent psychiatric collaborative care management.

G2214 Initial or subsequent psychiatric collaborative care management, first 30 minutes in a month of BHCM activities, in consultation with a psychiatric consultant, and directed by the treating physician or other QHP

Other payers that follow the *CPT* midpoint rule for time may allow reporting of **99492** for 36 minutes or more and **99493** for 31 minutes or more. Verify the policies and initiatives of plans in your area to determine the correct codes, payment policies, and fee schedules for these services.

As shown in **Figure 10-1**, codes **99492–99494** represent services provided by a team that includes 3 distinct roles.

Figure 10-1. Psychiatric Collaborative Care Team

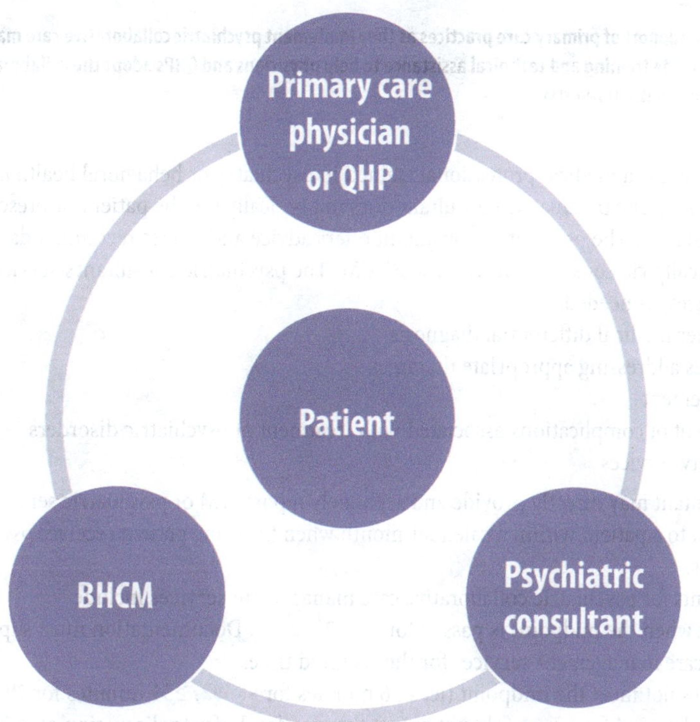

Abbreviations: BHCM, behavioral health care manager; QHP, qualified health care professional.

Each team member's role is defined in *CPT* as follows:

- The treating physician or QHP
  - Directs the BHCM and continues to oversee the patient's care, including prescribing medications, treating medical conditions, and making referrals for specialty care when needed.
  - Engages the services of the psychiatric consultant, who does not directly bill for psychiatric collaborative care management services (ie, the treating physician's or QHP's practice contracts with the psychiatric consultant for this component of the psychiatric collaborative care management service).

- Acts in a supervisory role to the BHCM (may be a direct employee or contractual employee but should represent a practice expense, as other clinical staff and NQHCPs do).
- May personally perform behavioral health care management activities. When those activities are not used to meet criteria for a separately reported service (eg, office E/M), their time may be counted toward the required time for psychiatric collaborative care management.
- Is ultimately responsible for delivery, documentation, and billing of psychiatric collaborative care management services in compliance with *CPT* and payer policies.

- The BHCM is an NQHCP or clinical staff member with master- or doctoral-level education *or* specialized training in behavioral health who provides behavioral health care management services under the treating physician's or QHP's supervision and in consultation with a psychiatric consultant. The BHCM provides the following services, as needed:
  - Assessment of needs, including the administration of validated rating scales.
  - Development of a care plan.
  - Provision of brief face-to-face and non–face-to-face interventions.
  - Ongoing collaboration with the treating physician or QHP.
  - Consultation with the psychiatric consultant at least weekly (typically non–face-to-face).
  - Maintenance of a registry.
  - Sometimes, provision and reporting of other services (within the BHCM's scope of practice) in the same calendar month as psychiatric collaborative care management. These may include psychiatric diagnosis, psychotherapy, smoking and tobacco use cessation counseling (**99406**, **99407**), and alcohol and/or substance use structured screening and brief intervention services (**99408**, **99409**).

Chapter 10

Mental and Behavioral Health Services

State initiatives may include support of primary care practices as they implement psychiatric collaborative care management. For instance, some Medicaid programs provide training and technical assistance to help physicians and QHPs adopt the collaborative care model, including access to and use of a patient registry.

- The psychiatric consultant is a medical professional trained in psychiatry or behavioral health *and qualified to prescribe a full range of medications.* The psychiatric consultant does not typically see the patient or prescribe medications, except in rare circumstances. The psychiatric consultant offers advice and makes recommendations to the treating physician or QHP, typically via consultation with the BHCM. The psychiatric consultant's services include recommending the following services, as needed:
  - Psychiatric and other medical differential diagnosis
  - Treatment strategies addressing appropriate therapies
  - Medication management
  - Medical management of complications associated with treatment of psychiatric disorders
  - Referral for specialty services

The psychiatric consultant may directly provide and separately report E/M or psychiatric services, such as psychiatric evaluation (**90791**, **90792**), to a patient within a calendar month when the same patient receives psychiatric collaborative care management services.

Reporting requirements for psychiatric collaborative care management services include

- Time of service is met when the midpoint is passed for **99492–99494**. Documentation must support provision of psychiatric collaborative care management services for the required time.
- ✖ When service time does not meet the midpoint (ie, ≥36 minutes for **99492**, ≥31 minutes for **99493**, ≥16 minutes beyond most recent full period for **99494**), do not report these codes. Refer to discussion of **G2214** earlier in this section for a potential alternative.
- Services are provided for an episode of care defined as beginning when the treating physician or QHP directs the patient to the BHCM and ending with
  - The attainment of targeted treatment goals, which typically results in the discontinuation of care management services and continuation of usual follow-up with the treating physician or other QHP
  - Failure to attain targeted treatment goals, culminating in referral to a psychiatric care provider for ongoing treatment
  - Lack of continued engagement, with no psychiatric collaborative care management services provided over a consecutive 6-month calendar period (break in episode of care)
- A new episode of care starts after a break in an episode of care of 6 calendar months or more.

- Following are typical indications of medical necessity for psychiatric collaborative care management services, when documented. Other reasons for services may support medical necessity.
  - A newly diagnosed condition
  - A patient's need for help engaging in treatment
  - A patient who has not responded to standard care delivered in a nonpsychiatric setting or who requires further assessment and engagement before consideration of referral to a psychiatric care setting
  - Documentation of the patient's behavioral health conditions, psychosocial needs, and other factors influencing patient care may help support the necessity of services when health plans implement specific coverage criteria and/or prior authorization for psychiatric collaborative care management services

Psychiatric collaborative care management services do not require establishment of a care plan for *all* the patient's health care needs. The services are directed to behavioral health needs. Patients may or may not have coexisting conditions that affect treatment and management.

- Psychiatric collaborative care management services may be reported in the same month as chronic care management or principal care management services (**99439, 99487, 99489–99491, 99424–99427, 99437**) when the requirements for each service are met without overlap.
- Remote therapeutic monitoring treatment management services for cognitive behavioral therapy (**98980, 98981**) are separately reported when they are provided and the time is not overlapping with that of psychiatric collaborative care management.

Refer to Chapter 21 for discussion of 98980 and 98981.

- Provision of psychiatric collaborative care management services may support quality initiatives such as use of an electronic clinical data system to track care and administration of a validated rating scale (eg, depression screening instrument) during a 4-month period for patients diagnosed with major depression or dysthymia.
- Psychiatric collaborative care management includes use of validated rating scales in monitoring patient outcomes.
- ✖ Do not separately report use of standardized rating scales (eg, **96127**).
- ✖ Do not include any time spent in separately reported services in the time of psychiatric collaborative care management.
- ✖ Do not separately report interprofessional consultation (eg, **99446–99449, 99451**, or **G0546–G0551**) for consultations between the treating physician, BHCM, and consulting psychiatrist.

Chapter 10

Mental and Behavioral Health Services

Example

➤ **A pediatrician orders psychiatric collaborative care management services for a 15-year-old patient diagnosed with moderate depression, single episode.** An LCSW, as the BHCM, discusses psychiatric collaborative care management services with the patient and performs an initial assessment. Standardized assessment instruments are used in the assessment, and a treatment plan including psychotherapy is agreed on. Later, the LCSW enters the patient information into a registry that will be used to track medication adherence and progress. At a regularly scheduled conference call between the BHCM and a consulting psychiatrist, the patient's assessment is reviewed and the treatment plan approved. The supervising pediatrician is also consulted and approves the treatment plan. The LCSW documents the time and activities directed to the patient's care throughout the calendar month. The LCSW, whose scope of practice includes psychotherapy, provides 3 separately reported individual psychotherapy sessions within the calendar month in addition to psychiatric collaborative care management services. During the calendar month, the BHCM documents 60 minutes of time spent in psychiatric collaborative care management services.

Throughout the month, the treating physician or QHP directs the BHCM and continues to oversee the patient's care, including prescribing medications, treating medical conditions, and making referrals for specialty care when needed. When the treating physician or QHP personally performs activities of psychiatric collaborative care management that are not included in an E/M or other separately reported service, the physician's or QHP's time contributes to the psychiatric collaborative care management service time. The treating physician or QHP documents review of patient progress and approval of change in treatment, as indicated, based on recommendations of the psychiatric consultant.

ICD-10-CM	*CPT*
F32.1 (major depressive disorder, single episode, moderate)	The treating physician or QHP reports 99492 (initial month psychiatric collaborative care management service, first 70 minutes) The LCSW reports (when provided) 90832, 90834, or 90837 (psychotherapy without E/M based on time of service; 30, 45, or 60 minutes)

Teaching Point: Time of services for psychiatric collaborative care management is met when the midpoint is passed. In this example, the 60 minutes spent by the BHCM supports reporting 99492, which includes the first 70 minutes of psychiatric collaborative care management services in the initial month of service.

Psychotherapy services may be reported on a separate claim before fulfilling the time requirement for psychiatric collaborative care management. No time spent in providing separately reported psychotherapy may be attributed to the time of psychiatric collaborative care management services. If psychotherapy services were not within the scope of practice for the BHCM, the patient might be referred to another provider (eg, the consulting psychiatrist), who would report the services rendered.

General Behavioral Health Integration Care Management

General behavioral health integration care management (99484) is reported by a physician or QHP for supervision of clinical staff who provide at least 20 minutes of outpatient general behavioral health integration services within a calendar month to a patient with a behavioral health condition (including substance use). The individual reporting 99484 must be able to perform and report E/M services, including an initiating visit. A treatment plan must be documented and address the patient's behavioral health condition(s), but a comprehensive health care plan is not required. Code 99484 does not include requirements for a BHCM or collaboration with a psychiatrist.

#99484 Care management services for behavioral health conditions, at least 20 minutes of clinical staff time, directed by a physician or other QHP, per calendar month, with the following required elements:

- Initial assessment or follow-up monitoring, including the use of applicable validated rating scales,
- Behavioral health care planning in relation to behavioral/psychiatric health problems, including revision for patients who are not progressing or whose status changes,
- Facilitating and coordinating treatment such as psychotherapy, pharmacotherapy, counseling and/or psychiatric consultation, and
- Continuity of care with a designated member of the care team

Clinical staff providing general behavioral health integration services are not required to have qualifications that would permit them to separately report services (eg, psychotherapy), but if they are qualified and they perform such services, they may report such services separately. The time of the separately reported service is not used to support reporting 99484.

Services must be provided under general physician supervision and in accordance with the licensing and scope of practice requirements of the state where services are provided. The individual supervising and reporting general behavioral health integration care management services must be able to report E/M services.

All the required elements of service listed in the code descriptor must be provided and documented.

When psychologists and/or LCSWs are integrated into a medical practice, the NQHCPs may provide and report behavioral health care management services with G0323 (care management services for behavioral health conditions, at least 20 minutes of clinical psychologist or clinical social worker time, per calendar month). These services include coordination with and/or referral to physicians and QHPs whose scope of practice includes prescribing medications and furnishing E/M services; counseling; and/or psychiatric consultation in addition to the required elements of general behavioral health integration. Refer to individual payer policies for guidance on coverage, billing, and documentation. Codes 99484 and G0323 would not be reported for the same patient by health care professionals in the same group practice.

Example

➤ **A 15-year-old established patient presents to a primary care pediatrician with concerns of social anxiety and lack of interest in previously enjoyed activities.** In addition to obtaining the patient's history, the physician uses scores from 2 patient-completed standardized behavioral health assessment instruments (eg, depression and anxiety rating scales) and a standardized health risk assessment instrument to inform the diagnostic and treatment considerations. The primary care physician diagnoses the patient with a behavioral health disorder and prescribes medication. The physician also recommends that the patient receive behavioral health care management as part of the treatment plan. The physician reports the appropriate code for the E/M service (eg, 99214), 96127 × 2 (brief emotional/behavioral assessment [eg, depression inventory, attention-deficit/hyperactivity disorder (ADHD) scale], with scoring and documentation, per standardized instrument), and 96160 (administration of patient-focused health risk assessment instrument [eg, health hazard appraisal] with scoring and documentation, per standardized instrument) for the services provided on that date.

A few days later, clinical staff (eg, a nurse with specialized training in behavioral health services) meets with the patient and parents to develop a behavioral health plan of care based on the physician's orders. During the calendar month, clinical staff, working under the physician's supervision, provide coordination of care with a psychologist in another practice and with a school counselor. At least 20 minutes of clinical staff time is documented for activities of general behavioral health integration during the calendar month to assess adherence to the plan of care, assess progress through standardized rating scales, and coordinate care, including facilitating access to community resources, as needed.

Teaching Point: If clinical staff time of less than 20 minutes is documented in a calendar month, 99484 is not reported. Provision and scoring of standardized rating scales is not separately reported when performed in conjunction with behavioral health integration services. Physician services are separately reportable when the time and activities of those services are not included toward meeting the criteria of 99484.

Refer to individual payer policies for reporting general behavioral health integration services on the same date that a physician provides a significant and separately identifiable E/M service.

- Time may be face-to-face but more typically may be non–face-to-face. Clinical staff must be available to provide face-to-face services to the patient when requested.
- E/M and/or psychiatric services may be reported on the same date or in the same calendar month as general behavioral health integration services when performed, but the time of separately reported services is not counted toward the time of general behavioral health integration services.
- General behavioral health integration (99484) may be reported in the same month as chronic care management or principal care management services (99439, 99487, 99489–99491, 99424–99427, 99437) when the requirements for each service are met without overlap. Psychiatric collaborative care management (99492–99494, G2214) may not be reported by the same provider in the same month as general behavioral health integration.
- The reporting individual may personally provide elements of general behavioral health integration services and combine the time of service with that of clinical staff to support reporting 99484. However, the time of services that are separately reported (eg, 20 minutes' total time spent providing an E/M service reported with 99213) cannot be included in the time supporting 99484.
- Clinical staff time spent coordinating care with the emergency department (ED) may be reported with 99484, but time spent while the patient is an inpatient or is admitted to observation status may not be reported with 99484.
- ✖ *Use of validated rating scales is required and is not separately reported* (ie, do not report 96127 for rating scales administered during the period of behavioral health care management services).
- ✖ Do not include time spent in separately reported services in the time of general behavioral health integration services.

Evaluation and Treatment of Alcohol and Substance Use

The initial evaluation of a child for alcohol and/or substance use is often in the context of an E/M service (eg, office and other outpatient E/M 99202–99205 or 99212–99215). E/M codes may be selected according to the total time spent by the physician or QHP in care of the individual patient on the date of service (DOS).

Additionally, codes 99408 and 99409 are reported for screening and an initial brief assessment and intervention for alcohol or substance use *of at least 15 minutes* (known as screening, brief intervention, and referral for treatment, or SBIRT). This behavior change service involves specific validated interventions of assessing readiness for change and barriers to change, advising a change in behavior, assisting by specifically suggesting actions and motivational counseling, and arranging for services and follow-up. The AAP policy statement "Substance Use Screening, Brief Intervention, and Referral to Treatment" (https://doi.org/10.1542/peds.2016-1210) recommends that pediatricians become familiar with adolescent SBIRT practices and their potential to be incorporated into universal screening and comprehensive care of adolescents in the medical home.

★◀99408 Alcohol and/or substance (other than tobacco) abuse structured screening (eg, Alcohol Use Disorder Identification Test, Drug Abuse Screening Test), and brief intervention (SBI) services; 15 to 30 minutes

★◀99409 greater than 30 minutes

- Services are time based, so the time spent providing the service must be documented and may not overlap with any time spent providing other services on the same date.

● indicates a new code; ▲, revised; #, re-sequenced; ✚, add-on; ★, audiovisual technology; and ◀, synchronous interactive audio.

- Append modifier **25** (significant, separately identifiable E/M service) to codes for other E/M services (eg, **99214 25**) when a significant E/M service is provided on the same date as the service described by **99408** and **99409**.
- When performed, counseling regarding use of naloxone is included in the brief intervention service. Counseling about and prescription of naloxone may also be included in total time or medical decision-making (MDM) of other E/M services provided to address substance use.

Codes **99408** and **99409** are included in the lists of codes that may be reported with telemedicine modifiers **93** (audio-only telemedicine service) and **95** (synchronous audiovisual telemedicine service), when applicable.

> ***CPT* instruction allows reporting of behavior change intervention codes 99406–99409 when provided on the same date as a preventive E/M service. Append modifier 25 to codes 99381–99397 when reporting on the same date as 99406–99409. Behavior change interventions are preventive services that may be covered without out-of-pocket cost (eg, deductible or coinsurance) to the patient.**

ICD-10-CM Coding for Use, Abuse, and Dependence

The guidelines for *ICD-10-CM* offer specific guidance for reporting diagnoses of mental and behavioral disorders caused by psychoactive substance use.

- Code **Z71.41** is reported as the first-listed code when an encounter is primarily focused on alcohol abuse counseling and surveillance. A code for alcohol abuse or dependence (**F10.-**) is additionally reported.
- Code **Z71.51** is reported as the first-listed code when an encounter is primarily for counseling on drug abuse and surveillance of a person with drug abuse. Codes for drug abuse or dependence (**F11–F16**, **F18**, or **F19**) are reported in addition to **Z71.51**.
- When substance use is addressed and/or affects patient management during an encounter that is primarily for management or treatment of other conditions, report a code for management of the other condition(s) first, followed by a code for substance use.
- The codes for unspecified psychoactive substance *use* disorders (**F10.9-**, **F11.9-**, **F12.9-**, **F13.9-**, **F14.9-**, **F15.9-**, **F16.9-**) are to be used only when the psychoactive substance use is associated with a physical, mental, or behavioral disorder and such a relationship is documented by the provider. Note that codes for inhalant use (**F18.9-**) and polysubstance or indiscriminate drug use (**F19.9-**) are not included in this instruction.

> **For a diagnosis of nicotine vaping, assign a code from subcategory F17.29- (nicotine dependence, other tobacco products) that includes noncombustible electronic nicotine delivery systems.**

- Subcategories of codes for mental and behavioral disorders caused by psychoactive substance use indicate *use* and *abuse* of and *dependence* on various psychoactive substances. These categories do not include abuse of nonpsychoactive substances such as antacids, laxatives, or steroids that are reported with category **F55**. Each subcategory offers a spectrum of use, abuse, and dependence with extended information such as *with intoxication, with withdrawal,* and *with delusions.*
- For each encounter, only 1 code should be assigned to identify the pattern of use (use, abuse, or dependence) based on the hierarchy shown in **Figure 10-2**. Report a code for the condition farthest to the right in the figure.

Figure 10-2. Coding Hierarchy for Substance Use, Abuse, or Dependence

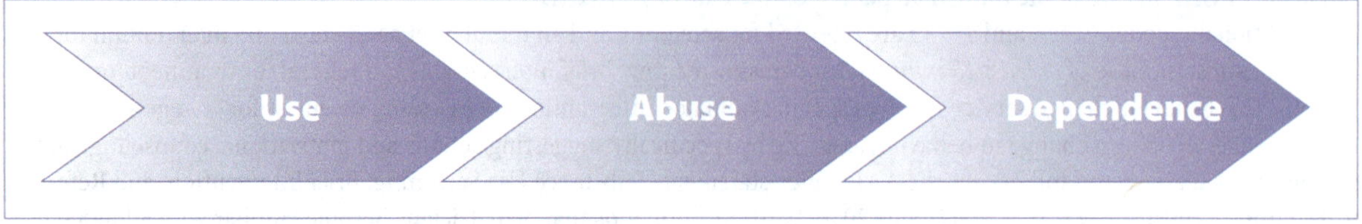

- Selection of codes for mental and behavioral disorders caused by psychoactive substance use for substance abuse or dependence in remission (categories **F10–F19** with **-.11**, **-.21**) requires the provider's clinical judgment. The appropriate codes for in remission are assigned only according to provider documentation unless otherwise instructed by the classification.

- Mild substance use disorders in early or sustained remission are classified to the appropriate codes for substance abuse in remission, and moderate or severe substance use disorders in early or sustained remission are classified to the appropriate codes for substance dependence in remission.

Management/Treatment of Alcohol and/or Substance Use Disorders

Treatment of alcohol and/or substance use disorders may be covered only when provided by physicians with certification in addiction medicine or by other licensed health care professionals whose scope of practice includes treating substance use disorders. Verify health plan benefits and eligible providers before beginning treatment services. Prior authorization of services is often required.

Coding for management/treatment of alcohol and/or substance use disorders is largely payer driven. Psychotherapy codes may be applicable, or E/M codes may be selected according to time of counseling and/or coordination for ongoing counseling on alcohol and/or substance use disorders. Yet many health plans and Medicaid programs require use of HCPCS codes and/or modifiers for reporting assessments and management/treatment of alcohol and/or substance use disorders.

Examples of HCPCS codes include

H0016 Alcohol and/or drug services; medical/somatic (medical intervention in ambulatory setting)

T1007 Alcohol and/or substance abuse services, treatment plan development and/or modification

Modifiers **HF–HI** provide details such as whether the program is an integrated mental health/substance abuse program. Refer to payer guidelines for use of these modifiers.

Opportunities may exist to treat alcohol and substance use through integrated behavioral health such as psychiatric collaborative care management services (for discussion of these, refer to the Psychiatric Collaborative Care Management Services section earlier in this chapter).

Central Nervous System Assessments/Tests

The following codes are used to report the services provided during testing of central nervous system functions. Central nervous system assessments include, but are not limited to, memory, language, visual/motor responses, and abstract reasoning/problem-solving abilities. The mode of completion can be by a person (eg, with paper and pencil) or via automated means. The administration of these tests will generate material that is interpreted and formulated into a report by a physician or other QHP or an automated result.

Standardized instruments are used in the performance of central nervous system assessment/testing services. Standardized instruments are validated tests administered and scored in the consistent or "standard" manner performed during their validation. Informal checklists created by a physician or an electronic health record developer are not considered standardized instruments.

Claims for testing are typically reported after the final date of testing services, with the appropriate codes for each DOS reported on the single claim. But payer instructions may vary, and some require reporting with only the date on which testing services are completed.

Payers may require prior authorization of tests. Practices should adopt procedures for verifying coverage and obtaining prior authorization, when required.

Central nervous system assessments and tests are not reported in conjunction with adaptive behavior treatment (**97151–97158**, **0362T**, **0373T**).

Neuropsychological and Psychological Testing

Mini–mental status examination performed by a physician is included as part of the central nervous system physical examination of an E/M service and is not separately reportable.

Neurobehavioral Status Examination

When reporting an assessment of fine and/or gross motor, language, cognitive level, social, memory, and/or executive functions via standardized developmental instruments, refer to codes 96112–96113 as discussed in Chapter 11.

The neurobehavioral status examination is a clinical interview and a collection of clinical information (eg, review of medical records, interview of family/caregivers). When it precedes neuropsychological or psychological evaluation services, the neurobehavioral status examination determines the types of tests to be administered. Neurobehavioral status examination does not require completion of a standardized instrument.

★◀96116 Neurobehavioral status examination (clinical assessment of thinking, reasoning and judgment [eg, acquired knowledge, attention, language, memory, planning and problem solving, and visual spatial abilities]), by physician or other QHP, both face-to-face time with the patient and time interpreting test results and preparing the report; first hour

✚96121 each additional hour

- Documentation of these services includes clinical assessment of the patient, collateral interviews (as appropriate), review of previous records, informal observation of behavior during examination, and interpretation and report. Include the reason for examination, date, and time spent, including examination, interpretation, and report of findings and recommendations.
- Report neurobehavioral status examination based on face-to-face time, and include time interpreting findings and preparing a report.
- The unit of time is 60 minutes, and time is met when the midpoint is passed (ie, at least 31 minutes of time is required for the first or last unit of service).
- These services may be provided via telemedicine; append modifier **95** to indicate a service provided via real-time audiovisual technology or modifier **93** to indicate a service provided via audio-only communication.
- A physician or a QHP who can independently provide and report E/M services may elect to report codes for E/M services and, when applicable, prolonged E/M service in lieu of codes **96116** and **96121**.

Chapter 10

Mental and Behavioral Health Services

Example

➤ **An 8-year-old boy, previously diagnosed with ADHD, predominantly inattentive type, is being evaluated for gradual problems with remembering directions, organizing his school materials and his room at home, and other behavior concerns.** The physician or QHP performs a neurobehavioral status examination, which involves clinical assessments and observations for impairments in acquired knowledge, attention, learning, and memory. The results indicate the need for further standardized language, memory, and intelligence testing. The total time for testing, scoring, and report writing is 3½ hours.

This service is reported with **96116** (neurobehavioral status examination) and **96121** with 2 units for the additional 2½ hours of examination and report writing. The diagnosis code would be *ICD-10-CM* **F90.0** (ADHD, predominantly inattentive type). Additional *ICD-10-CM* codes may be assigned for specific developmental disorders diagnosed following testing (eg, **F81.2**, mathematics disorder).

Psychological and Neuropsychological Testing Services

Codes for psychological and neuropsychological testing differentiate test administration by physicians, QHPs, and NQHCPs from that by technicians or automated systems. A combination of testing evaluation and test administration and scoring services is typically reported on a single claim.

The test selection, test administration, and method of testing and scoring are the same regardless of who performs testing.

Testing Evaluation Services by a Physician or Other QHP With Interpretation and Report

★◀96130 *Psychological* testing evaluation services by physician or other QHP, including integration of patient data, interpretation of standardized test results and clinical data, clinical decision-making, treatment planning and report, and interactive feedback to the patient, family member(s) or caregiver(s), when performed; first hour

★✚◀96131 each additional hour (List separately in addition to code for primary procedure)

★◀96132 *Neuropsychological* testing evaluation services by physician or other QHP, including integration of patient data, interpretation of standardized test results and clinical data, clinical decision making, treatment planning and report, and interactive feedback to the patient, family member(s) or caregiver(s), when performed; first hour

★✚◀96133 each additional hour (List separately in addition to code for primary procedure)

● indicates a new code; ▲, revised; #, re-sequenced; ✚, add-on; ★, audiovisual technology; and ◀, synchronous interactive audio.

- Report codes 96130–96133 according to the face-to-face time with the patient and the time spent integrating and interpreting data. The standard *CPT* time definitions apply (ie, midpoint rule, a minimum of 31 minutes must be provided to report a 1-hour unit of service).
- *Time spent in test administration and scoring is not included in time used to support codes 96130–96133.* Separately report psychological/neuropsychological test administration and scoring services (96136–96139) on the same or different days (ie, each service is separately reported on the same claim). Report the total time of evaluation and testing services at the completion of the entire episode of evaluation on a single claim, with each DOS listed separately.

Time of 30 minutes or less would not be reported with codes 96130–96133.

- Documentation of these services includes scoring, observation of behavior, and interpretation and report. It should include the date and time spent in testing and the time spent integrating and interpreting data, reason for the testing, and titles of all instruments used.

The time reported in 96130–96133 is a combination of the *documented* face-to-face time with the patient and the time spent integrating and interpreting data. An itemization of time for each activity is preferable.

Example

➤ **An adolescent patient with history of traumatic brain injury is referred for neuropsychological evaluation to assess difficulties with memory and reading.** A physician spends 2 hours reviewing the patient's medical records, interpreting data from tests administered and scored on an earlier date by a technician, and creating a report (copied to the referring physician) of the diagnosis and recommendations for treatment. Another 40 minutes was spent providing interactive feedback to the patient and caregivers.

Code 96132 and 2 units of 96133 are reported for 160 minutes spent in data interpretation, interactive feedback, and report writing. If the physician had also personally administered and scored tests, 96136 and 96137 would have also been reported according to the time of testing and scoring. Test administration and scoring by a technician would be reported separately with 96138 and 96139 according to the time of service (for discussion of 96138 and 96139, refer to the Technician-Administered Testing section later in this chapter).

Teaching Point: Report 96133 with 1 unit of service in addition to 96132 for time of 91 to 150 minutes. Time of 151 minutes or more supports additional units of service for 96133 (include 1 unit for 31–59 minutes beyond the last full hour).

Testing Administration Services

Test administration and scoring services are selected according to time of service. The midpoint rule applies. Separate codes are reported depending on whether testing and scoring are personally performed by a physician, QHP, or NQHCP or are performed by a technician.

At least 2 distinct tests must be administered and scored to report codes 96136–96139. Do not separately count subtests in a multifaceted test (eg, Wechsler Preschool and Primary Scale of Intelligence is 1 test with 14 subtests). Code 96127 (brief emotional/behavioral assessment, with scoring and documentation, per standardized instrument) may be reported for administration and scoring of a single standardized test.

Physician or QHP Administration and Scoring

★◀96136 Psychological or neuropsychological test administration and scoring by physician or other QHP, two or more tests, any method; first 30 minutes

★✚◀96137 each additional 30 minutes after first 30 minutes (List separately in addition to code for primary procedure)

Services include administration of a series of tests, recording of behavioral observations made during testing, scoring, and transcription of scores to a data summary sheet.

- Codes are selected according to time of testing and scoring. Time is met when the midpoint is passed (ie, a minimum of 16 minutes for 30-minute codes). Refer to **Table 10-1** for more details.

• indicates a new code; ▲, revised; #, re-sequenced; ✚, add-on; ★, audiovisual technology; and ◀, synchronous interactive audio.

Chapter 10

Mental and Behavioral Health Services

Table 10-1. Calculating Units of Service for Time of Test Administration and Scoring

Total Time (min) of Administration and Scoring Performed By	First 30 min (16–45 min)	First Additional 30 min (46–75 min)	Second Additional 30 min (76–105 min)	Each Additional 30 min or Last 16 min Beyond Final Full 30-min Period (>106 min)
Physician, QHP, or NQHCP	96136 (1 unit)	96136 and 96137 (1 unit each)	96136 (1 unit) and 96137 (2 units)	96136 (1 unit) and units of 96137 for each 30 min or last 16 min beyond final full 30-min period
Technician	96138 (1 unit)	96138 and 96139 (1 unit each)	96138 (1 unit) and 96139 (2 units)	96138 (1 unit) and units of 96139 for each 30 min or last 16 min beyond final full 30-min period

Abbreviations: NQHCP, nonphysician qualified health care professional; QHP, qualified health care professional.

- ✖ *Do not include* time spent in integration of patient data or interpretation of test results in the time reported with 96136 and 96137. This time is included with psychological and neuropsychological test evaluation services (96130–96133).
- Psychological or neuropsychological test administration *through a single test/instrument,* with interpretation and report, is reported with 96127 (brief emotional/behavioral assessment [eg, depression inventory, ADHD scale], with scoring and documentation, per standardized instrument).

Examples

➤ **A physician spends 80 minutes administering tests, recording observations, scoring, and transcribing results to a data summary sheet.** Codes 96136 × 1 unit and 96137 × 2 units are reported.

Teaching Point: Code 96136 is reported for the first 30 minutes. Two units of 96137 are also reported for the remaining 50 minutes (1 full period of 30 minutes and the final 20 minutes). If the final period of service were less than 16 minutes, only 1 unit of 96137 would be reported.

➤ **An adolescent is referred for psychological testing evaluation.** The patient undergoes physician-administered psychological testing to evaluate emotionality, intellectual abilities, personality, and psychopathology and to make a mental health diagnosis and treatment recommendations as applicable. The total time of face-to-face testing is 45 minutes. The physician's total time of evaluation and data integration and interpretation is 75 minutes. Codes 96136 and 96130 are reported.

Teaching Point: Test administration and scoring time of 45 minutes are reported with 96136. Seventy-five minutes of physician testing evaluation service is reported with 96130.

Technician-Administered Testing

Testing and administration services performed by a technician are reported with 96138 and 96139.

★◂96138 Psychological or neuropsychological test administration and scoring by technician, two or more tests, any method; first 30 minutes

★✚◂96139 each additional 30 minutes (List separately in addition to code for primary procedure)

Codes 96138 and 96139 do not include the work of a physician or QHP. These codes are valued only for practice expense and medical liability.

- Evaluation services by the physician, QHP, or NQHCP are reported with 96130–96133 whether provided on the same or a different date. Do not include time for evaluation services (eg, integration of patient data or interpretation of test results) in time of test administration and scoring.

Example

➤ **An adolescent patient is referred for neuropsychological testing.** A technician spends 40 minutes administering and scoring tests. The technician also notes any behavioral observations. Code **96138** is reported with 1 unit of service.

Teaching Point: When a physician, QHP, or NQHCP provides evaluation services, including integration and interpretation of data from tests administered by a technician, on the same or a different date, refer to **96132** and **96133** for those services.

Automated Testing and Result

When a single test instrument is completed by the patient via an electronic platform without administration and scoring by a clinician, report **96146**.

96146 Psychological or neuropsychological test administration, with single automated, standardized instrument via electronic platform, with automated result only

Code **96146** does not include scoring by a health care professional or interpretation and report. Results are generated via the electronic platform.

✖ If a test is administered by a clinician, do not report **96146**. For brief emotional/behavioral assessment using a standardized instrument with scoring by a clinician, refer to **96127**.

Example

➤ **A child who is recovering from a concussion is provided a single computerized test for postconcussion symptoms.** The patient completes the test, and the automated result is included in the patient's medical record.

Code **96146** is reported in addition to the code representing the physician's related E/M service (eg, **99213**). Append modifier **25** (significant, separately identifiable E/M service) if the services are provided on the same date and the payer uses National Correct Coding Initiative edits.

Behavior Management Services

★◀**96202** Multiple-family group behavior management/modification training for parent(s)/guardian(s)/caregiver(s) of patients with a mental or physical health diagnosis, administered by physician or other QHP (without the patient present), face-to-face with multiple sets of parent(s)/guardian(s)/caregiver(s); initial 60 minutes

★✚◀**96203** each additional 15 minutes

Behavior management/modification training is provided to a multiple-family group of parent(s)/guardian(s)/caregiver(s), without the patient present. The physician, QHP, or NQHCP provides a *face-to-face service* to train parent(s)/guardian(s)/caregiver(s) to use skills and strategies to address behaviors affecting the patient's mental or physical health diagnosis and to support adherence to the patient's treatment and the plan of care.

Training may include

- Verbal instruction
- Video and live demonstrations
- Feedback from a physician, QHP, or NQHCP or other parents in group sessions

The time of service is the reporting individual's face-to-face time with multiple sets of parent(s)/guardian(s)/caregiver(s). Code **96202** requires at least 31 minutes of service. No specific instruction for the required time to report **96203** is included in *CPT* instructions. Given the midpoint rule, time is met when the midpoint is passed (ie, at least 8 minutes for a service time of 15 minutes). *Time must be documented to support the service provided.*

The services reported with **96202** and **96203**

- Must take place without the patient present
- Are provided to a multiple-family group of parent(s)/guardian(s)/caregiver(s)
- Emphasize active engagement and involvement of the parent(s)/guardian(s)/caregiver(s) in the treatment of a patient with a mental or physical health diagnosis

Do not report **96202** and **96203**

✖ For preventive medicine counseling (**99401–99404**; **99410**, **99411**)

✖ For risk factor reduction interventions (**99406–99409**)

- ✖ For services to the patient and the parent(s)/guardian(s)/caregiver(s) during the same session (Report with appropriate E/M code[s] for site of service.)
- ✖ For educational services rendered to patients in a group setting (eg, prenatal, obesity, or diabetic instructions) (Report with 99078.)

Example

➤ **A psychiatric clinical nurse specialist provides behavior management services to a group of parents and caregivers whose children have diagnosed illnesses and behaviors that affect their illnesses and management or treatment.** The group participates in activities to learn interventions that participants can independently use to effectively manage their children's illnesses/diseases. The psychiatric clinical nurse specialist documents a total of 45 minutes spent face-to-face providing behavior management services to the group.

Codes reported to the health plan for each child include diagnosis codes for the child's illness/disease.

96202 Multiple-family group behavior management/modification training for parent(s)/guardian(s)/caregiver(s) of patients with a mental or physical health diagnosis, administered by physician or other QHP (without the patient present), face-to-face with multiple sets of parent(s)/guardian(s)/caregiver(s); initial 60 minutes

Teaching Point: The clinical nurse specialist reports 96202 for each patient whose parent(s)/guardian(s)/caregiver(s) participated in the service. If the time of service had exceeded the first 60 minutes by at least 8 minutes (the midway point between 60 minutes and 75 minutes), 96203 would have been reported in addition to 96202.

A psychiatric clinical nurse specialist, like other advanced practice registered nurses, may practice independently in some states but only under physician supervision in other states. Where independent practice is not within the psychiatric clinical nurse specialist scope of practice, a plan may require reporting under the name of the supervising physician or other QHP.

Health and Behavior Assessments/Interventions

Health and behavior assessment and intervention procedures (96156, 96158, 96159, and 96164–96171) are provided by NQHCPs who cannot report E/M services but can independently provide and report assessment and intervention procedures. These services are used to identify and address psychosocial, behavioral, emotional, cognitive, and interpersonal factors important to the assessment, treatment, or management *of physical health problems.*

The patient's primary diagnosis must be a medical (physical) issue, and the focus of the assessment and interventions is on factors complicating medical conditions and treatments. These codes describe assessments and interventions to improve the patient's health and well-being using psychological and/or psychosocial interventions designed to ameliorate specific disease-related problems.

These services do not represent preventive medicine counseling and risk factor reduction interventions.

- Physicians and QHPs who can provide and report E/M services do not report 96156, 96158, 96159, or 96164–96171. E/M codes including preventive medicine services are reported instead depending on the type of service provided.
- When an E/M service is provided by a physician or QHP on the same date that an NQHCP (eg, LCSW) provides health and behavior assessment/intervention, each service is separately reported by the individual providing the service. The same provider cannot report both services.
- May be reported by psychologists, clinical social workers, licensed therapists, and other NQHCPs within their scope of practice who have specialty or subspecialty training in health and behavior assessment or intervention procedures.
- Codes 96156, 96158, 96159, and 96164–96171 are reported with telemedicine modifier 93 (audio-only) or 95 (synchronous audiovisual), when applicable.
- ✖ Are not reported with psychiatric codes (90785–90899) when provided on the same day. Only the primary service is reported (ie, 96156, 96158, 96159, and 96164–96171 or 90785–90899).
- ✖ Are not reported with adaptive behavior assessment or treatment (97151–97158, 0362T, 0373T).
- ✖ Are not used in conjunction with a primary diagnosis of mental disorder. (Payers may deny claims when a diagnosis code indicating mental disorder is included for these services.)

When required by a payer, a health behavior assessment or reassessment may qualify as an initiating visit before performing care management services for behavioral health conditions by a clinical psychologist or clinical social worker (G0323).

Health Behavior Assessment

96156 Health behavior assessment, or re-assessment (ie, health-focused clinical interview, behavioral observations, clinical decision making)

Health behavior assessment includes evaluation of the patient's responses to disease, illness or injury, outlook, coping strategies, motivation, and adherence to medical treatment. Assessment is conducted through health-focused clinical interviews, observation, and clinical decision-making.

Code 96156 is not reported according to time. Report only 1 unit of service.

Example

➤ **A 13-year-old girl with multiple food allergies and newly increased anxiety is assessed for response to management of food allergies.** The patient notes feelings of social isolation at home and school resulting from restricted diet. She is fearful of having an allergic reaction in front of her peers. The patient is assessed with standardized questionnaires. The child's parents are also interviewed.

Code 96156 would be reported with, for example, *ICD-10-CM* code Z91.010 (allergy to peanuts). If the patient has been diagnosed with an anxiety disorder, report also a code for the anxiety disorder (eg, F41.9, anxiety disorder, unspecified). Codes for mental and behavioral health conditions, however, should not be reported as the first-listed or primary reason for health behavior assessment. The health behavior assessment is not primarily focused on behavioral health conditions.

When neuropsychological and/or psychological testing is performed at the same session as health behavior assessment or reassessment, payer edits may require modifier 59 to be appended to the code for the testing to indicate a distinct service.

Health Behavior Intervention

Codes 96158, 96159, and 96164–96171

- Are time-based services requiring documentation of the time spent face-to-face with the patient(s) and/or family.
- ✖ Do not report 96158, 96164, 96167, or 96170 for less than 16 minutes of service.
- Include promotion of functional improvement, minimizing psychological and/or psychosocial barriers to recovery, and management of and improved coping with medical conditions.
- Emphasize active patient/family engagement and involvement. These interventions may be provided individually, to a group (≥2 patients), and/or to the family, with or without the patient present.

Refer to **Table 10-2** for a breakdown of the health behavior intervention codes.

Table 10-2. Health Behavior Intervention Codes

Health Behavior Intervention Provided To	Initial Code	Add-On Code
Individual, face-to-face	◀96158 initial 16–30 min	◀✚96159 each additional 15 min (List separately in addition to code 96158)
Group (2 or more patients), face-to-face	◀#96164 initial 16–30 min	◀#✚96165 each additional 15 min (List separately in addition to code 96164)
Family (with the patient present), face-to-face	◀#96167 initial 16–30 min	◀#✚96168 each additional 15 min (List separately in addition to code 96167)
Family (without the patient present), face-to-face	◀#96170 initial 16–30 min	◀#✚96171 each additional 15 min (List separately in addition to code 96170)

● indicates a new code; ▲, revised; #, re-sequenced; ✚, add-on; ★, audiovisual technology; and ◀, synchronous interactive audio.

Examples

➤ **Health behavior intervention is provided to an adolescent who has morbid obesity (caused by excess intake of calories) with familial hypercholesterolemia and who does not adhere to the plan of care.** Results from a health behavior assessment are used to develop a plan to address health risk behaviors and factors impeding adherence to a plan of care developed through shared decision-making by the patient, his parents, and his physician. Thirty minutes is spent with the patient discussing the behavior and steps to help him adhere to the plan of care.

Code 96158 with 1 unit of service would be reported with diagnosis codes for the morbid obesity due to excess calories (E66.01) (and body mass index, if documented) and familial hypercholesterolemia (E78.01).

➤ **Three patients with type 1 diabetes and identified needs for better treatment adherence take part in a group intervention.** Using results of assessments conducted at previous encounters, the clinical psychologist works with the patients to gain understanding and acceptance of their physician's care plan, addresses barriers to adherence, and helps each patient develop goals for better adherence. A total of 55 minutes is spent face-to-face with the group of patients.

Codes 96164 (1 unit for first 30 minutes) and 96165 with 2 units of service (1 full 15-minute period and 1 unit for the last 10 minutes because the midpoint of 8 minutes beyond the last full period was passed) are reported. *ICD-10-CM* codes appropriate to each patient's condition (eg, appropriate codes from category E10, type 1 diabetes, and codes for any manifestations) are reported.

Psychiatric Services

Psychiatric services include diagnostic services, psychotherapy, and other services to an individual, a family, or a group. Comprehensive services may be provided by a multidisciplinary team (eg, psychiatrist, developmental-behavioral pediatrician, NP, psychologist, clinical social worker, and/or clinical counselor).

But in many parts of the country, children's mental and behavioral health professionals are unavailable. General pediatricians must often take on management of mental health problems and, when possible, consult with a mental/behavioral health professional at a distant location or arrange for telemedicine services. (Refer to the Payment and Coverage Issues for Mental/Behavioral Health Services section earlier in this chapter for important considerations for general pediatricians providing psychiatric services.)

Psychiatric services described by 90785, 90791 and 90792, 90832–90840, and 90845–90847 are included in Appendix T of the AMA *CPT* manual and preceded by the ◀, indicating that these services may be reported with modifier 93 (audio-only telemedicine service). Refer to Chapters 2 and 20 for additional information on reporting codes with modifier 93.

Interactive Complexity

★◀✚90785 Interactive complexity

Psychiatric services to children may include interactive complexity. According to *CPT*, psychiatric procedures may be reported "with interactive complexity" when at least 1 of the following circumstances is present:

- The need to manage maladaptive communication (eg, related to high anxiety, high reactivity, repeat questions, or disagreement) among participants that complicates delivery of care
- Caregiver emotions or behavior interfering with the caregiver's understanding and ability to assist in the implementation of the treatment plan
- Evidence or disclosure of a sentinel event and mandated report to third party (eg, abuse or neglect with report to state agency) with initiation of discussion of the sentinel event and/or report with the patient and other visit participants
- Use of play equipment or other physical devices to overcome barriers to therapeutic or diagnostic interaction between the physician or other QHP and a patient who has not developed or has lost either (a) expressive language communication skills to explain their symptoms and response to treatment or (b) receptive communication skills to understand the physician or other QHP if they were to use typical language for communication

AOC 90785 is reported when interactive complexity complicates delivery of psychiatric services, including diagnostic psychiatric evaluation (90791, 90792), psychotherapy (90832–90834, 90836–90838), and group psychotherapy (90853). Report 90785 in conjunction with 90853 for the specified patient when group psychotherapy includes interactive complexity.

- Interactive complexity indicates an *increased complexity of work* as opposed to an extended duration of services. The increased complexity of the psychiatric service arises from specific communication factors that can result in barriers to diagnostic or therapeutic interaction with the patient.
- Interactive complexity is not billed in conjunction with psychotherapy for crisis (**90839**, **90840**) or with psychiatric or neuropsychiatric testing (**96130–96134**, **96136–96139**, **96146**).
- *Interactive complexity applies only to the psychiatric portion of a service* including both psychiatric and E/M components.
- ✖ Code **90785** is never reported alone and is not reported in conjunction with E/M services alone. When provided in conjunction with time-based psychotherapy services, the time spent providing interactive complexity services is reflected in the time of the psychotherapy service and must relate only to the psychotherapy service.
- ✖ Do not report **90785** in conjunction with adaptive behavior assessment or treatment services (**97151–97158**, **0362T**, **0373T**).

Examples

➤ **A 10-year-old patient undergoes psychiatric evaluation.** The child is accompanied by separated parents who report that the child has recently demonstrated significant anxiety about abandonment and has new-onset tantrums. The child's teachers report that the child requires a plan for anxiety management during the school day and is easily influenced by peers. The parents are extremely anxious and repeatedly ask questions about the treatment process. Each parent continually challenges the other's observations of the patient.

Codes **90791** (psychiatric diagnostic evaluation) and **90785** (interactive complexity) are reported.

➤ **A 6-year-old girl is seen for psychotherapy.** The child was placed into foster care following hospitalization for injuries sustained from physical abuse and neglect by her mother 3 years before this evaluation. The service includes the psychologist's review of the child's medical record and telephone interviews with the child's social worker and teacher. The mother refuses a request for interview. The psychologist interviews current and former foster parents, who express concerns that the child is easily offended and retaliates against perceived offenses with violent outbursts. The psychologist uses play to gain trust and evaluate the child. The psychologist and foster mother agree on a treatment plan and then discuss the plan with the child in terms she can understand. Following the service, the psychologist provides a report to the patient's social worker.

Codes **90791** (psychiatric diagnostic evaluation) and **90785** (interactive complexity) are reported.

Chapter 10

Mental and Behavioral Health Services

Psychiatric Diagnostic Evaluation

★◀**90791** Psychiatric diagnostic evaluation
★◀**90792** Psychiatric diagnostic evaluation with medical services

Psychiatric diagnostic evaluation (**90791**) and psychiatric diagnostic evaluation with medical services (**90792**) include an integrated biopsychosocial assessment, including history, mental status, and recommendations. When medical services (ie, medical assessments and physical examination other than mental status, when indicated) are included, **90792** is reported by the physician or other QHP whose scope of practice includes medical services.

- Only psychiatrists and other physicians or QHPs who may independently provide and report E/M services may report **90792**.
- The same individual may not separately report E/M services on the same date as psychiatric diagnostic evaluation.
- Psychologists and other licensed mental health professionals working within their scope of practice may report **90791**.
- Psychiatric diagnostic evaluation or reevaluation (**90791**, **90792**) is reported once per day. Do not report psychotherapy codes (**90832–90839**) on the same DOS as **90791** or **90792**. Verify payer policy for the frequency of coverage for diagnostic reevaluations.
- Report **90785** for interactive complexity in addition to **90791** or **90792**, when applicable.

Health plans may not cover mental health consultation, testing, or evaluation that is performed to assess custody, visitation, or parental rights.

- **Verify health plan contractual obligations before providing services that may lack medical necessity and determine if a waiver of liability must be signed by the patient(s) before beginning the service.**
- **A waiver of liability (eg, Medicare's advance beneficiary notice) is the patient's agreement to pay out of pocket for services not covered by their health plan.**
- **Modifier GA (waiver of liability statement issued as required by payer policy, individual case) may be appended to the code reported to indicate that the waiver is on file.**

When services are requested for purposes that a health plan may not consider medically necessary, failure to obtain the responsible party's signature on a waiver of liability *before the service* may release the patient from the obligation to pay based on contractual agreement between the provider and health plan.

Examples

➤ **A 14-year-old girl is referred by her primary care pediatrician for evaluation and treatment of depression with suicidal ideation.** The psychologist obtains information on the presenting problem and situation. A statement of need and expectations is documented. Current symptoms and behaviors are documented. The patient has no history of previous psychiatric treatment. The patient does not describe previous or current substance use. Her current medication regimen of fluoxetine at 10 mg once a day is documented. She has no current medical problems and is not allergic to any medications. The patient's family and social status (current and historical), school status/functioning, and resources are obtained and documented. A diagnosis of moderate major depressive disorder, single episode with suicidal ideation, and parent-child relationship problem is documented.

Code **90791** is reported in conjunction with *ICD-10-CM* codes **F32.1** (major depressive disorder, single episode, moderate), **R45.851** (suicidal ideations), and **Z62.820** (parent-biological child conflict).

Chapter 10

Mental and Behavioral Health Services

➤ **A 15-year-old girl was admitted through the ED for new-onset psychosis.** The girl is evaluated by a psychiatrist. The psychiatrist performs a psychiatric diagnostic evaluation of this patient, who previously attempted suicide at age 13 years and has a history of recurrent major depressive disorder. The patient also expresses fear that she may be pregnant and has been exposed to a sexually transmitted infection. Medical history includes nausea with vomiting for the past week and most recent menstrual period of 6 weeks ago. Laboratory tests are ordered to rule out pregnancy and/or infection, and consultation with a gynecologist is ordered. Diagnoses are major depressive disorder, recurrent, severe with psychotic symptoms (**F33.3**); history of suicide attempt (**Z91.51**); nausea with vomiting (**R11**); and pregnancy test, unconfirmed (**Z72.40**).

Code **90792** is reported for combined psychiatric and medical evaluations.

➤ **A 17-year-old girl wishes to be evaluated to determine her ability to accept responsibility for herself.** The girl is seeking emancipation from her mother, who is currently living with an abusive boyfriend and will not allow her to move in with her aunt while finishing high school. An attorney has advised obtaining a psychological evaluation to support the girl's claims that she is psychologically prepared to take this action. The girl's health plan considers this service not medically necessary but allows for patient payment when a waiver of liability is obtained before the service. The patient agrees to sign the waiver and pay for the service. An evaluation is completed by a psychologist, and a report of the evaluation is provided to the girl and her attorney.

The service is reported to the health plan with modifier **GA** (waiver of liability statement issued as required by payer policy, individual case) appended to **90791**.

Psychotherapy

CPT defines *psychotherapy* as the treatment of mental illness and behavioral disturbances in which the physician or QHP (including clinical psychologists and clinical social workers), through definitive therapeutic communications, attempts to alleviate the emotional disturbances, reverse or change maladaptive patterns of behavior, and encourage personality growth and development.

Progress notes for psychotherapy services should include

- **Duration of psychotherapy (Some payers may require start and stop times of psychotherapy.)**
- **Service type**
- **Diagnosis**
- **Interval history (eg, increase/decrease in symptoms, current risk factors)**
- **Names and scores of standardized rating scales used in monitoring progress**
- **Therapeutic interventions (eg, type of therapy, medications)**
- **Summary of goals and progress**
- **An updated treatment plan**
- **Date and signature of performing provider**

These elements should be documented in the progress note in the patient record rather than the protected psychotherapy notes. Protected psychotherapy notes *are not disclosed* for the purpose of receiving or supporting accurate payment.

- Services include ongoing assessment and adjustment of psychotherapeutic interventions and may include involvement of informants in the treatment process. A payer's policy may require that the patient's treatment plan be updated after a specific period (eg, 3 or 6 months) or after a change in status (eg, after a change in medication).
- Codes differentiate psychotherapy services to individuals (with and without E/M services), an individual family or groups of families, and groups of patients. Codes for each are provided in the following discussions.
- Separate codes (**90839**, **90840**) are reported for psychotherapy for crisis (refer to the Psychotherapy for Crisis section later in this chapter).

Follow these instructions when selecting codes for any psychotherapy service.

- Select psychotherapy codes on the basis of face-to-face time with a patient and/or family member.
- Report family psychotherapy (**90846**, **90847**) for services that involve family psychotherapy techniques to benefit the patient (eg, attempting to improve family communication or alter family interactions that negatively affect the patient, encouraging interactions to improve family functioning).
  - Family psychotherapy includes sessions with the entire family and sessions possibly without the patient.
  - The patient must be present for all or some of the service except when reporting family psychotherapy *without the patient present* (**90846**). This allows for the participation of others in the psychotherapy session for the patient as long as the patient remains the focus of the intervention. Documentation must support that the patient was present for a significant portion of the session.
- In reporting, choose the code closest to the actual time (**Table 10-3**). Do not report psychotherapy of less than 16 minutes.
- ✖ Do not report psychotherapy codes in conjunction with codes for adaptive behavior assessment or treatment services (**97153–97158**, **0362T**, **0373T**).
- Psychotherapy of more than 45 minutes is often considered unusual and may require health plan precertification.

Table 10-3. Reporting Psychotherapy Services

Duration of Psychotherapy (min)	*Current Procedural Terminology* Codes
<16	Do not report.
16–37	**90832**, **90833**
38–52	**90834**, **90836**
53–89	**90837**, **90838**
≥26	**90846**, **90847** (family psychotherapy)

When time spent in psychotherapy exceeds time assigned to the highest level of psychotherapy service (individual or family), refer to codes for psychotherapy for crisis (90839, 90840).

Chapter 10

Mental and Behavioral Health Services

Psychotherapy With Evaluation and Management

★◀+90833 Psychotherapy, 30 minutes with patient when performed with an E/M service
★◀+90836 45 minutes with patient when performed with an E/M service
★◀+90838 60 minutes with patient when performed with an E/M service

Psychiatrists and other physicians who provide a combination of psychotherapy and E/M services (eg, 99213) on the same date may report an E/M code and an AOC for psychotherapy (90833, 90836, 90838).

- To report both E/M and psychotherapy, the 2 services must be significant and separately identifiable.
- Time may not be used as the basis of E/M code selection. E/M code selection must be based on the level of *MDM alone* when reported in conjunction with psychotherapy.
- ✖ Prolonged services *may not* be reported when psychotherapy with E/M (90833, 90836, 90838) is reported.
- For outpatient psychotherapy performed with an E/M service provided via synchronous audio-video or audio-only telemedicine, report outpatient telemedicine E/M codes (98000–98015) in addition to 90833, 90836, or 90838.

Examples

➤ **An 8-year-old boy presents for psychotherapy.** The psychiatrist provides not only 20 minutes of psychotherapy services (face-to-face time) but also an established patient E/M service to reevaluate the effectiveness and patient reaction to current medications. The office E/M service includes low-level MDM based on the low number and complexity of problems (1 stable chronic illness) with moderate risk of morbidity of prescription drug management. Codes reported are 99213 and 90833.

The 20 minutes of psychotherapy services does not include the time of the E/M service. Because the midpoint (at least 16 minutes) was passed, 90833 (30 minutes) is reported. No modifier is required (eg, modifier 25) because the AOCs were assigned values that account for the overlapping practice expense of the 2 services (eg, same clinical staff and examination room).

Physicians and other QHPs who can independently report E/M services may be limited to reporting E/M codes for behavioral health counseling, but this may not be a disadvantage. In 2025, the total non-facility relative value units (RVUs) assigned to 99213 (2.75) and 90833 (2.25) were 5.0. In contrast, when reporting only an E/M code based on the physician's total time on the date of the encounter, 99215 (40–54 minutes) is valued at 5.43 RVUs. If the physician's total time were to exceed 54 minutes, 99417 would be reported, adding another 0.92 RVUs for each 15-minute period beyond the 54 minutes included in 99215.

➤ **The same service as in the previous example is provided via audio-video–only telemedicine.** The service is reported with either 98005 (established patient synchronous audio-video visit with low MDM) and 90833 or, when a payer requires that a physician or QHP report only an E/M service, 99215.

Psychotherapy Without Evaluation and Management

★◀90832 Psychotherapy, 30 minutes with patient and/or family member
★◀90834 45 minutes with patient and/or family member
★◀90837 60 minutes with patient and/or family member
★◀90863 Pharmacologic management, including prescription and review of medication, when performed with psychotherapy services

When psychotherapy is provided without an E/M service on the same date, codes 90832, 90834, and 90837 are reported according to the face-to-face time of service.

- To accommodate reporting of pharmacologic management by psychologists who have prescribing privileges but who cannot provide E/M services, AOC 90863 is reported in addition to the appropriate code for psychotherapy without E/M. For providers who may report E/M services, pharmacologic management is typically reported with an E/M code, not 90863.

  Only a psychologist with prescribing authority may provide pharmacologic management. Other QHPs may provide psychotherapy but must collaborate with a physician or advanced practice professional who provides pharmacologic management.
- Physicians and QHPs providing pharmacologic management report the service with an E/M code.
- Code 90863 is an AOC and may be reported only in addition to one of the stand-alone psychotherapy codes (ie, 90832, 90834, 90837). Time spent providing medication management is not included in the time spent in psychotherapy.

• indicates a new code; ▲, revised; #, re-sequenced; +, add-on; ★, audiovisual technology; and ◀, synchronous interactive audio.

Example

➤ **An 8-year-old boy presents for psychotherapy.** The LCP, whose state scope of practice includes prescribing authority, provides not only psychotherapy services with face-to-face time of 40 minutes but also a pharmacologic management service to reevaluate the effectiveness and patient reaction to current medications. Codes reported are 90834 and 90863.

A physician or other QHP who may provide and report E/M services would report 90836 (psychotherapy with E/M, 40 minutes) for this service.

Psychotherapy With Biofeedback

90875 Individual psychophysiological therapy incorporating biofeedback training by any modality (face-to-face with the patient), with psychotherapy (eg, insight oriented, behavior modifying or supportive psychotherapy); 30 minutes

90876 45 minutes

When psychotherapy incorporates biofeedback training, 90875 or 90876 is reported according to the face-to-face time of the combined services. Do not separately report codes for psychotherapy (90832–90838) or biofeedback training (90901).

Example

➤ **A child with frequent tension headaches is provided psychotherapy and biofeedback training to help her cope with and control her pain.** The face-to-face time of service is 45 minutes.

Code 90876 is reported for the combined services. If biofeedback training was provided on a date when no psychotherapy was provided, 90901 would be reported. Time of service is not a factor in reporting 90901.

Psychotherapy for Crisis

★◀90839 Psychotherapy for crisis; first 60 minutes

★◀✚90840 each additional 30 minutes (List separately in addition to code 90839)

Psychotherapy for crisis is provided on an urgent basis to a patient requiring mobilization of resources to defuse a crisis and restore safety. It also incorporates implementation of psychotherapeutic interventions to minimize the potential for psychological trauma.

- This includes assessment and history of a crisis state, a mental status examination, and a disposition.
- The presenting problem is typically life threatening or complex and requires immediate attention to a patient in high distress.
- Codes 90839 and 90840 are reported according to the total face-to-face time the physician or QHP spends with the patient and/or family providing psychotherapy for crisis on a single DOS. Time is cumulative for all psychotherapy for crisis on the same date even if time is not continuous.
  - Code 90839 is reported for the first 30 to 74 minutes of psychotherapy for crisis on a single DOS. For psychotherapy for crisis with face-to-face time of less than 30 minutes, report individual psychotherapy codes (90832 or 90833).
  - Add 90840 for each additional block of up to 30 minutes (ie, 1 unit for 75–90 minutes and additional units for each period up to 30 minutes beyond 90 minutes).

✖ Do not report psychotherapy for crisis (90839, 90840) for service of less than 30 minutes or on the same date as other psychiatry services (90785–90899).

Example

➤ **A psychologist or psychiatrist is consulted in the ED for a patient who was brought to the hospital by his parents after threatening to harm others and exhibiting paranoia.** The psychologist obtains history from the patient's parents. The psychologist examines the patient, obtains agreement for inpatient treatment, and arranges for admission. The total face-to-face time of the encounter is 45 minutes.

Code 90839 is reported. Although the code descriptor states "first 60 minutes," the instructions for reporting psychotherapy for crisis instruct that 90839 be reported for the first 30 to 74 minutes of face-to-face service.

Family Psychotherapy

★◀90846 Family psychotherapy (without the patient present), 50 minutes
★◀90847 Family psychotherapy (conjoint psychotherapy) (with patient present), 50 minutes
90849 Multiple-family group psychotherapy

Although family members may act as informants during individual psychotherapy, psychotherapy using family psychotherapy techniques is reported with 90846 or 90847 depending on whether the patient is present for the service.

- The focus of family psychotherapy is on family dynamics and/or subsystems within the family (eg, parents, siblings) and on improving the patient's functioning by working with the patient in the context of the family.
- ✖ Do not report family psychotherapy for services of less than 26 minutes.
- Codes for individual psychotherapy (90832–90838) or group psychotherapy (90853) may be reported on the same day as family psychotherapy codes 90846 and 90847 when the services are separate and distinct. Append modifier 59 (distinct procedural service) to the psychotherapy code when both services are reported on the same date.
- When multiple families participate in family psychotherapy at the same session, 90849 is reported once for each family.

Group Psychotherapy

★◀90853 Group psychotherapy (other than of a multiple-family group)

Report 90853 with 1 unit of service for each group member. Documentation should support the individual patient's involvement in the group session, the duration of the session, and issues that were presented.

No time is assigned to 90853. This service is reported with 1 unit of service regardless of the time of service.

Chapter 10

Mental and Behavioral Health Services

Other Psychiatric Services

The following services are often bundled under payer contracts (ie, considered components of other services) or non-covered. However, check plan benefits, especially for Medicaid patients, as there may be circumstances in which these services are separate benefits. Plan-specific modifiers are often required when coverage of the following services is a health plan benefit:

90882 Environmental intervention for medical management purposes on a psychiatric patient's behalf with agencies, employers, or institutions

90885 Psychiatric evaluation of hospital records, other psychiatric reports, psychometric and/or projective tests, and other accumulated data for medical diagnostic purposes

Code 90885 may be reported in addition to psychotherapy services (90832–90838) when both services are provided by the same individual on the same DOS.

90887 Interpretation or explanation of results of psychiatric, other medical examinations and procedures, or other accumulated data to family or other responsible persons, or advising them how to assist patient

✖ Do not report 90887 in conjunction with adaptive behavior services (97151–97158, 0362T, 0373T).

90889 Preparation of report of patient's psychiatric status, history, treatment, or progress (other than for legal or consultative purposes) for other individuals, agencies, or insurance carriers

Code 90889 should not be reported in conjunction with psychological or developmental testing, as the codes for these services include time for report writing.

✚0770T Virtual reality technology to assist therapy

Code 0770T represents the practice expense of using virtual reality technology in conjunction with specified patient therapy. Report 0770T in addition to codes for psychotherapy (90832–90853); treatment of speech, language, voice, communication, and/or auditory processing disorder (92507, 92508); health and behavior assessment/intervention (96158–96171); physical therapeutic procedures (97110–97112, 97150, 97530–97537); therapeutic interventions that focus on cognitive function (97129); and adaptive behavior services (97153–97155, 97158).

To test your knowledge of the information presented in this chapter, complete the quiz found at the end of it, after the resources. Answers to each quiz are found in **Appendix II**.

Chapter Takeaways

A variety of services related to diagnosis and management of behavioral and mental health were discussed in this chapter. Following are some takeaways from this chapter:

- Services for behavioral and mental health conditions may include a variety of health care professionals working within their scope of practice.
- Billing and coding of behavioral and mental health services must align with not only coding guidelines but also state scope of practice and individual payer policies regarding credentialing, network participation, and contracting.
- When payers deny claims appropriately reported with codes **F01–F99**, limiting submission of these codes to providers in a mental or behavioral health network, pediatricians may report the issue through the AAP Coding and Payment Hotline (www.aap.org/en/practice-management/child-health-finance-payment-strategy/coding-payment-hotline) or seek the assistance of an AAP pediatric council (www.aap.org/en/practice-management/child-health-finance-payment-strategy/payment-and-finance-advocacy/aap-pediatric-councils).
- Codes **99408** and **99409** are reported for screening and an initial brief assessment and intervention for alcohol or substance use of at least 15 minutes (SBIRT).
- Separately report psychological/neuropsychological test administration and scoring services (**96136–96139**) provided on the same or different days (ie, each service is separately reported on the same claim) as testing evaluation services (**96130–96133**).
- At least 2 distinct psychological or neuropsychological tests must be administered and scored to report **96136–96139**. Do not separately count subtests in a multifaceted test (eg, Wechsler Preschool and Primary Scale of Intelligence is 1 test with 14 subtests).
- Code **96127** (brief emotional/behavioral assessment, with scoring and documentation, per standardized instrument) may be reported for administration and scoring of a single standardized psychological or neuropsychological test.
- Select psychotherapy codes based on face-to-face time with a patient and/or family member.
- AOC **90785** is reported when interactive complexity complicates delivery of psychiatric services. Interactive complexity applies only to the psychiatric portion of a service including both psychiatric and E/M components.

Resources

AAP Coding Assistance and Education

AAP Coding and Payment Hotline (www.aap.org/en/practice-management/child-health-finance-payment-strategy/coding-payment-hotline)

AAP pediatric councils (www.aap.org/en/practice-management/child-health-finance-payment-strategy/payment-and-finance-advocacy/aap-pediatric-councils)

AAP policy statement, "Addressing Early Childhood Emotional and Behavioral Problems" (https://doi.org/10.1542/peds.2016-3023)

Pediatric Mental Health: Coding Quick Reference Card 2026 (www.aap.org/Pediatric-Mental-Health-Coding-Quick-Reference-Card-2026)

AAP Pediatric Coding Newsletter™

"Connecting Coding and Policy: Managing Behavioral Health Problems With General Behavioral Health Integration," August 2023 (https://doi.org/10.1542/pcco_book232_document001)

Test Your Knowledge!

1. **Which terminology may be used to describe health care professionals who may independently provide and report non-E/M services?**
   a. Clinical staff
   b. NQHCPs
   c. Allied health professionals
   d. Physician or other qualified health care professional
2. **Which of the following services requires a team that includes a treating physician or QHP, a BHCM, and a psychiatric consultant?**
   a. All integrated behavioral health care management services
   b. Psychotherapy with E/M services
   c. General behavioral health integration care management (99484)
   d. Psychiatric collaborative care management (99492–99494)
3. **Which is true of the time used in code selection for psychological and neuropsychological testing evaluation services?**
   a. Time is not a factor in selecting codes for testing evaluation services.
   b. The time in the code descriptor must be met or exceeded.
   c. The standard *CPT* time rule applies (ie, midpoint rule)
   d. Time spent by technicians is included in the time of testing evaluation services.
4. **Which of the following is reported only by NQHCPs (ie, not physicians or QHPs who may report E/M services)?**
   a. Psychiatric collaborative care management
   b. Health and behavior assessment and intervention procedures (96156, 96158, 96159, and 96164–96171)
   c. Psychotherapy codes (90832–90839)
   d. Interactive complexity (90785)
5. **Which of the following is true of family psychotherapy services (90846, 90847 90849)?**
   a. Family psychotherapy is always reported when family members act as informants during psychotherapy.
   b. Codes for individual psychotherapy may not be reported on the same date as family psychotherapy.
   c. Family psychotherapy provided to multiple families is reported with group psychotherapy code 90853.
   d. Family psychotherapy techniques reported with 90846 or 90847 depend on whether the patient is present for the service.

CHAPTER 11

Common Testing and Therapeutic Services

Contents

Chapter Highlights

- Reporting service components: only professional, only technical, or both
- Reporting provision of supplies and medications
- In-office pathology, laboratory, and radiology service codes and modifiers
- Codes for respiratory testing and treatment services
- Allergy testing and allergen immunotherapy codes and reporting guidelines
- Reporting emotional/behavioral assessment instruments
- Codes reported for developmental testing

Professional and Technical Components

This chapter discusses codes for some of the most common tests and therapeutic services performed in physician offices and outpatient clinics. Certain procedures (eg, electrocardiography [ECG], radiography, diagnostic procedures) include a professional component and a technical component.

- The *professional component* includes the physician work (eg, interpretation of the test, writing of a report).
- The *technical component* includes the costs associated with providing the service (eg, equipment, salaries of technical personnel, supplies, expense of facility).

When reporting that the global service (professional and technical components) was provided by a physician or other qualified health care professional (QHP), no modifier is required.

When practicing in an outpatient setting in which a facility bears the practice expense of equipment, supplies, and clinical staff, physicians and QHPs report only the services that have a professional component (eg, interpretation and report). The facility will report charges for services such as laboratory tests that represent a practice expense. The physician's or QHP's analysis of test results that do not require interpretation and report is part of an evaluation and management (E/M) service.

Codes to which the professional and technical component guidelines apply are often designated in payer policy, including the Medicare Physician Fee Schedule (MPFS) on which many payers base policies. An MPFS lookup tool (www.cms.gov/medicare/physician-fee-schedule/search) can be used to determine if the professional and technical component applies to a specific code. The *How to Use the MPFS Look-Up Tool* booklet (www.cms.gov/sites/default/files/2021-04/How_to_MPFS_Booklet_ICN901344_0.pdf) explains the professional and technical component indicators used in the MPFS.

Interpretation and Report

Many tests include recording of results and a written report with interpretation. *Current Procedural Terminology* (*CPT®*) instructs that

- *Results* are the technical component of a service. Testing leads to results; results lead to interpretation.
- *Reports* are the written work product of the interpretation of test results.
- Certain procedures or services described in *CPT* involve a technical component (eg, tests) that produces results (eg, data, images, slides). For clinical use, some of these results require interpretation. Some *CPT* descriptors specifically require interpretation and reporting to report that code.

Do not separately report review of another physician's interpretation and report or personal review of the tracing that has been interpreted by another physician. These activities contribute, however, to the medical decision-making (MDM) for any related E/M service.

Pediatricians performing services that include an interpretation of results should become familiar with the types of reports typical for each test (eg, typical report produced for the interpretation of ECG tracings). A report generated by an automated system is not typically sufficient to support reporting a service described as "with interpretation and report."

Some tests do not require interpretation and report (eg, point-of-care laboratory tests) but, rather, provide results that require analysis of how the result does or does not influence patient management or treatment. Use of the results in MDM may be credited to the amount and/or complexity of data to be reviewed and analyzed for an E/M encounter. Refer to **Chapter 6** for more information on how ordered tests and results reviewed influence the level of MDM of an E/M service.

Professional and Technical Component Modifiers

26 Professional component: When the physician or other QHP is reporting only the professional component of a service, append modifier **26** to the procedure code.

TC Technical component: When reporting only the technical component of a service, append modifier **TC** to the procedure code.

Modifiers are used to indicate that either the professional component or the technical component (not both) was performed. Modifiers **26** and **TC** are not reported when both components of a service were provided by the physician or QHP in a non-facility setting.

When the physician owns the equipment and is performing the technical and professional services, the 26 or TC modifier should not be appended to the code.

- If a physician is performing a service or procedure with equipment owned by a facility or another entity and the codes are written as a global service, services are reported with modifier **26** (professional component).
- *CPT* does not include a modifier for reporting the technical component. But most payers recognize Healthcare Common Procedure Coding System (HCPCS) modifier **TC**. Appending modifier **TC** to the procedure code indicates that only the technical component was provided by the entity (eg, facility-owned clinic).
- Some codes distinguish between the technical and professional components (eg, routine ECG codes **93000–93010**) without use of a modifier; however, many do not and therefore require use of modifier **26** or **TC** to indicate which component is billed.

No modifier is appended when the code descriptor for the service identifies whether the professional, technical, or global service is being reported.

Examples

➤ **A physician orders 2-view chest radiography of a child.** The radiographs are provided in the physician's office, and the physician interprets and documents a formal interpretation of the images. (No other physician will provide or report an interpretation and report.)

71046 (radiologic examination, chest; 2 views)

The physician does not include a modifier because the physician's practice provided the global service (ie, both technical and professional components). In-office radiography may be more common in large or multispecialty practices. If the practice included a radiologist who provided interpretation and report of all imaging services, the ordering physician would not report a radiology service.

➤ **A physician orders 2-view chest radiography of a child.** The child is sent to a neighboring physician's office (or outpatient department) for the radiograph (without interpretation). The radiographs are then brought back to the office and the pediatrician interprets them and creates a report of the findings.

Physician: **71046 26** (radiologic examination, chest; 2 views).

Neighboring physician's office: **71046 TC**.

➤ **A physician orders 12-lead ECG of an adolescent patient.** The patient is sent to another office that has an ECG machine to perform the ECG. The tracings are taken back to the pediatrician for review and written interpretation and report.

Physician: **93010** (routine ECG with at least 12 leads; interpretation and report only).

Other office: **93005** (routine ECG with at least 12 leads; tracing only, without interpretation and report).

Modifiers **26** and **TC** are not appended because the codes designate the professional and technical components.

➤ **A primary care physician (PCP) orders 2-view chest radiography of a child at an outpatient clinic that is part of a hospital's outpatient campus (place of service [POS] code 22).** The child receives the imaging service in the outpatient clinic where the PCP provides E/M services. A hospital-based radiologist will interpret and report the findings of the imaging, but the report is unavailable at the time of the visit. The PCP personally views and documents an informal interpretation of the images at the patient's visit.

- Primary care physician: E/M code for service provided with the independent interpretation of the images contributing to MDM (if the E/M code is selected on the basis of MDM rather than total time)
- Outpatient clinic (facility charges): E/M visit code and **71046 TC** (radiologic examination, chest; 2 views)
- Radiologist: **71046 26** (radiologic examination, chest; 2 views)

The physician will report POS code **22** on the claim for the E/M service to indicate that the service took place in a facility site. (Off-campus outpatient hospital, POS code **19**, is also a facility site of service.) The facility POS will result in payment based on total facility relative value units (RVUs) to reflect that the physician did not incur the practice expense of the visit. The facility will also report the E/M service (for practice expense) in addition to the technical component of the radiology service on a facility claim form (UB-04).

When interpreting a test at a location remote from the site of the technical service, follow payer guidelines for reporting. The POS for remote interpretation and report is typically the site at which the technical component of the test was performed (eg, outpatient hospital). Payer guidelines may vary.

Supplies and Medications

Supplies and Materials

99070 Supplies and materials provided by the physician over and above those usually included with the office visit or other services rendered

99071 Educational supplies, such as books, tapes, and pamphlets, for the patient's education at cost to physician or other QHP

The practice expense RVUs assigned to most services include the value of supplies (eg, nebulizer masks and tubing, gauze, needles) that are typically required for each service.

If reporting 99070, identify the supplies or materials on the claim form and be prepared to submit an invoice.

- Supplies should be separately reported when a payer does not use a payment methodology based on the RVUs assigned to each code under the MPFS. But most payers today use a payment method based on RVUs and do not provide separate payment for supplies that are typically used to perform a service.
- Only the supplies purchased by an office-based practice may be reported. Supplies not typically included in the value assigned to a service include items such as splints, casts, or medications.
- Use HCPCS codes when they are more specific than **99070**. HCPCS codes are available for a number of supplies (eg, codes **Q4001–Q4051** for cast and splint supplies).
- Code **99071** may be reported when the physician incurs costs for educational supplies and provides these supplies to the patient at cost. This code may be denied because of payment policies that consider supplies reported with **99071** to be a practice expense of a related service.

Medications

Medications used in testing or treatment (eg, albuterol) are not included in the value of service and are separately reported with HCPCS codes (eg, **J7613**, albuterol, inhalation solution, US Food and Drug Administration [FDA]–approved final product, noncompounded, administered through durable medical equipment, unit dose, 1 mg).

Visit www.aap.org/cfp2026 for a table of the most used pediatric medications, associated HCPCS **J** codes, and related administration codes.

- Report medications when the practice incurred a cost for the medication.
- HCPCS codes for drugs are listed with a base dosage (eg, per 1 mg, up to 5 mg). When the dosage exceeds the amount listed, report additional units for the total dosage administered.
- Follow payer-specific instructions, which may require that units reflect the exact strength of the medication. For example, when the unit in the code descriptor is per 1 mg, a payer may require the exact strength (eg, 2.5 units for 2.5 mg) or may instruct to round up to the next full unit (eg, round 2.5 to 3 units).
- Report the National Drug Code (NDC) in addition to **J** codes to provide more precise information on the medication and dose administered. The NDC should always be reported in addition to **99070** or **J3490** (unclassified drug), when applicable. You can find a list of NDCs at www.fda.gov/drugs/drug-approvals-and-databases/national-drug-code-directory.

- Pay attention to NDC units, which are often different from HCPCS units (eg, units per milliliter rather than per milligram).

For more information on NDCs, refer to Chapter 1.

When administering a drug or biologic from a *single-dose* vial or package, be aware of a payer's requirements for modifiers JW (drug amount discarded/not administered to any patient) and JZ (zero drug amount discarded/not administered to any patient). Follow payer instructions for reporting these modifiers. Learn more about these modifiers in **Chapter 2**.

Laboratory Testing Services

Blood Sampling for Laboratory Testing

Report collection of blood samples for testing (eg, venipuncture) in a physician practice regardless of whether the laboratory test is performed in the office or at an outside facility. The *International Classification of Diseases, 10th Revision, Clinical Modification* (*ICD-10-CM*) code reported for blood sampling is the same code that represents the reason for the testing ordered that requires the blood sample.

Venipuncture

36400	Venipuncture, younger than age 3 years, necessitating the skill of a physician or other QHP, not to be used for routine venipuncture; femoral or jugular vein
36405	scalp vein
36406	other vein
36410	Venipuncture, age 3 years or older, necessitating the skill of a physician or QHP professional (separate procedure), for diagnostic or therapeutic purposes (not to be used for routine venipuncture)
36415	Collection of venous blood by venipuncture
36416	Collection of capillary blood specimen (eg, finger, heel, ear stick)
36591	Collection of blood specimen from a completely implantable venous access device

- When a physician's skill is required to perform venipuncture on a child younger than 3 years (eg, access is too difficult for other staff to attain), codes 36400–36406 are reported in relation to the anatomical site of the venipuncture.
- Report 36410 when a physician's skill is required to perform venipuncture on a child 3 years or older.

If the physician performs the venipuncture as a convenience or because staff is not trained in the procedure, 36415 is reported because the physician's skill was not required.

Some payers require that modifier 25 be appended to the E/M code if an E/M service is reported on the same day of service. This is not a common practice.

✖ Do not report an E/M code when *only* laboratory testing and/or venipuncture or capillary finger stick is provided.
  - It is inappropriate to report a nurse visit (99211) in these cases.
  - If a medically necessary nursing E/M service is performed in compliance with payer guidelines (eg, incident to a physician's service) on the same date as venipuncture, append modifier 25 to 99211.
- Report 36591 (collection of blood specimen from a completely implantable venous access device) only when performed in conjunction with a laboratory service.

Refer to Chapter 18 for discussion of arterial catheterization.

Arterial Puncture

36600	Arterial puncture, withdrawal of blood for diagnosis

Arterial puncture (eg, radial artery) with withdrawal of blood for diagnosis is reported with 36600.

Chapter 11 Common Testing and Therapeutic Services

Pathology and Laboratory Procedures

CPT laboratory codes may either be generic for a particular analyte that is independent of testing method or have a specific *CPT* code, depending on the method used for the particular analysis.

Specimen collection other than blood sampling (eg, nasal or oral swab, urine collection) is typically not separately reported. Follow payer guidelines when exceptions are made.

Clinical Laboratory Improvement Amendments–Waived Tests

The Clinical Laboratory Improvement Amendments (CLIA) establish quality standards for all laboratory testing to ensure the accuracy, reliability, and timeliness of patient test results regardless of where the test was performed. All laboratories, including those within a physician practice, must comply with CLIA and must typically report a valid (current) CLIA certificate number on claims.

- A *laboratory* is defined as any facility that performs laboratory testing on specimens derived from humans for the purpose of providing information for the diagnosis, prevention, and treatment of disease or impairment or assessment of health.
- The term *CLIA waived* refers to simple laboratory examinations and procedures that have an insignificant risk of an erroneous result when manufacturer instructions are followed. One typical test that is CLIA waived is urinalysis without microscopy (81002). Other tests require higher levels of CLIA certification (eg, provider-performed microscopy).
- The term *moderate complexity* refers to tests that are performed only by laboratories certified as meeting the CLIA quality system standards, such as those for proficiency testing, quality control and assessment, and personnel requirements. The difference between moderate- and high-complexity certification is the personnel required.

Not Sure How a Test Is Categorized?

Refer to the FDA CLIA database at www.accessdata.fda.gov/scripts/cdrh/cfdocs/cfCLIA/search.cfm for tests of all categories by test system, manufacturer, or analyte. If your practice provides only waived test systems and analytes, visit www.accessdata.fda.gov/scripts/cdrh/cfdocs/cfClia/analyteswaived.cfm.

  — Some codes represent both CLIA-waived and higher-complexity test systems.
- Laboratories and physician offices performing waived tests should append modifier QW to the *CPT* code for CLIA-waived procedures. The use of modifier QW originated in the Medicare program but is now required by some other payers.
- Only a small number of CLIA-waived tests are exempt from use of modifier QW (eg, 81002, non-automated urinalysis without microscopy; 81025, urine pregnancy test; 82272, occult blood by peroxidase for other than colorectal neoplasm screening).

General Guidance for Reporting Laboratory Services

- Report a test performed in the office's laboratory with the appropriate laboratory code and, if performed, the appropriate blood collection code (36400–36416).
- Link the appropriate diagnosis code to the laboratory procedure and/or venipuncture and handling fee. The diagnosis must support the medical necessity or reason for the test or service.
- ✖ Do not report any laboratory test that is *not performed* in the office (eg, thyroid function, laboratory panels, phenylketonuria). Instead, report the appropriate blood-drawing code (36415 or 36416), when applicable, and handling fee code (99000). *Exception:* Follow state regulations and payer policies for physician billing of laboratory services performed by an outside laboratory (ie, purchased laboratory services). Generally, if the laboratory bills the pediatrician for the test, bill the patient with the appropriate laboratory analysis code plus modifier 90 to indicate that the procedure was performed in an outside laboratory.

Example

➤ **The physician orders a laboratory test requiring a blood sample, and the nurse obtains the blood via venipuncture.** The specimen is sent to an outside laboratory for processing.

Only the venipuncture (36415) and handling fee (99000) would be reported in addition to the E/M service and other procedures performed on that day.

• indicates a new code; ▲, revised; #, re-sequenced; ✚, add-on; ★, audiovisual technology; and ◀, synchronous interactive audio.

Chapter 11

Common Testing and Therapeutic Services

- Report modifier 91 (repeat clinical diagnostic laboratory test) on the code for a test that is repeated multiple times on a single date of service (DOS) (eg, multiple blood glucose tests).

Practices must stay up to date on payer policies that may limit the opportunity to provide and receive payment for in-office laboratory testing. Policies for physician office testing may limit payment for tests included in a "short turnaround time" laboratory test code list. A short turnaround test is typically described as yielding a result needed to appropriately manage the patient's care at the time of the visit (eg, rapid streptococcal antigen test).

Laboratory Panel Coding

All laboratory test panels in *CPT* were specifically developed for coding purposes and should not be interpreted as clinical parameters. (Refer to 80047–80076 for a component listing of these panels.) For example, the lipid panel (80061) includes total cholesterol (82465), high-density lipoprotein cholesterol (83718), and triglycerides (84478). Any additional tests performed can be coded separately from the panel code. *Do not unbundle individual laboratory tests if a laboratory panel code is available except as required by a payer.*

Direct Optical Observation

Direct optical (ie, visual) observation is a testing platform that provides a result (ie, positive or negative) by producing a signal on the reaction chamber (eg, test strip with colored bands) that can be interpreted visually (eg, point-of-care influenza testing). (Refer to 87804, influenza; 87807, respiratory syncytial virus; 87880, group A *Streptococcus;* and 87811, COVID-19. New in 2026: report 87812 for a single test for COVID-19 and influenza A and B.)

Per *CPT,* when reporting tests performed through direct optical observation, the number of unique results (eg, 2 results: positive for influenza A and negative for influenza B) determines the units of service reported. For instructions for reporting other tests that may identify multiple infectious agents, refer to the Combination Testing for SARS-CoV-2 and Other Infectious Agent(s) section later in this chapter.

Cultures

- Use 87086 (culture, bacterial; quantitative colony count, urine) once per encounter for urine culture to determine the approximate number of bacteria present per milliliter of urine.
- Use of a commercial kit with defined media to identify isolates in a positive urine culture is reported with 87088 (culture, bacterial; quantitative colony count, urine with isolation and presumptive identification of each isolate).
- Code 81007 (urinalysis; bacteriuria screen, except by culture or dipstick) (CLIA waived) can be used for a bacteriuria screening by non-culture technique using a commercial kit. The type of commercial kit must be specified.
- Code 87070 (culture, bacterial; any other source except urine, blood, or stool) is reported for throat cultures.
- Use 87045 to report culture, bacteria of the stool, aerobic, with isolation and preliminary examination (eg, Kligler [triple sugar] iron agar, lysine iron agar) for *Salmonella* and *Shigella* species. Additional pathogens are reported with 87046 with 1 unit per plate.
- Culture, presumptive pathogenic organisms, screening only (87081), is reported for testing for a specific organism (eg, *Streptococcus*).
- Report services with the symptoms (eg, dysuria) or the confirmed diagnosis (eg, urinary tract infection).

Proprietary Laboratory Analyses and Multianalyte Assays With Algorithmic Analyses

To report testing performed through proprietary laboratory analyses or multianalyte assays with algorithmic analyses, refer to Appendix O of the American Medical Association *CPT* manual, and for quarterly code updates, visit www.ama-assn.org/practice-management/cpt/cpt-pla-codes. Code selection for these codes is based on the analysis performed and the proprietary name of the test. **Table 11-1** shows how these codes are listed in *CPT* Appendix O. Codes for genomic sequencing procedures are also listed in *CPT* Appendix O.

Table 11-1. Example of *CPT* Appendix O Proprietary Laboratory Analysis Code List

Test Name	Code	Code Descriptor[a]
HART KD, Complete Omics Inc, Prevencio	0310U	Pediatrics (vasculitis, Kawasaki disease [KD]), analysis of 3 biomarkers (NT proBNP, C-reactive protein, and T-uptake), plasma, algorithm reported as a risk score for KD

Abbreviations: *CPT, Current Procedural Terminology;* NT proBNP, N-terminal pro B-type natriuretic peptide; T-uptake, thyroid uptake.

[a] Revision effective January 1, 2025; publication: *CPT 2026.*

Laboratory Tests Frequently Performed in the Office

COVID-19 (SARS-CoV-2 Infection) Testing

Tests for coronavirus (SARS-CoV-2) include those to detect the virus and those to detect antibodies to the virus.

Some tests for SARS-CoV-2 were designated as CLIA waived under an emergency use authorization during the public health emergency caused by COVID-19. It is advisable to verify the current classification of a test before purchase.

Diagnosis coding for SARS-CoV-2 is based on the current *ICD-10-CM* codes and guidelines.

SARS-CoV-2 Infection Testing

When multiple specimens are collected from different anatomical sites (eg, nasopharyngeal and oropharyngeal swabs), verify payer instructions for reporting separate assays on each specimen (eg, report **87635** and **87635 59**).

87635 Infectious agent detection by nucleic acid (DNA or RNA); severe acute respiratory syndrome coronavirus 2 (SARS-CoV-2) (Coronavirus disease [COVID-19]), amplified probe technique

87426 Infectious agent antigen detection by immunoassay technique (eg, enzyme immunoassay [EIA], ELISA, fluorescence immunoassay [FIA], immunochemiluminometric assay [IMCA]), qualitative or semiquantitative; severe acute respiratory syndrome coronavirus (eg, SARS-CoV, SARS-CoV-2 [COVID-19]) (CLIA-waived)

#87811 Infectious agent antigen detection by immunoassay with direct optical (ie, visual) observation; severe acute respiratory syndrome coronavirus 2 (SARS-CoV-2) (Coronavirus disease [COVID-19]) (CLIA-waived)

Combination Testing for SARS-CoV-2 and Other Infectious Agent(s)

CPT includes combination codes for tests to distinctly report testing for SARS-CoV-2 infection (COVID-19) in combination with other seasonal respiratory infections (eg, influenza A and B viruses and/or respiratory syncytial virus [RSV]).

✖ Do not report **87631–87633** (multiple respiratory infectious agent detection by nucleic acid by number of targets) when one of the following codes describes the test performed:

#87428 Infectious agent antigen detection by immunoassay technique (eg, EIA, ELISA, FIA, IMCA), qualitative or semiquantitative; severe acute respiratory syndrome coronavirus (eg, SARS-CoV, SARS-CoV-2 [COVID-19]) and influenza virus types A and B

87636 Infectious agent detection by nucleic acid (DNA or RNA); severe acute respiratory syndrome coronavirus 2 (SARS-CoV-2) (Coronavirus disease [COVID-19]) and influenza virus types A and B, multiplex amplified probe technique

87637 Infectious agent detection by nucleic acid (DNA or RNA); severe acute respiratory syndrome coronavirus 2 (SARS-CoV-2) (Coronavirus disease [COVID-19]), influenza virus types A and B, and RSV, multiplex amplified probe technique

Report 1 unit of service when the code descriptor includes testing for multiple antigens (eg, **87637** × 1 for the single test for COVID-19, influenza A and B, and RSV). Report a combination COVID-19 and influenza A and B test performed with direct optical observation with **87812**.

✖ Do not report codes that describe a test for single infectious agent (eg, **87420**, infectious agent antigen detection by immunoassay technique; qualitative or semiquantitative; RSV) when reporting a single test that detects the presence or absence of multiple infectious agents.

Report **87631–87633** when testing for SARS-CoV-2 and additional viral pathogens beyond those described by the codes listed. Testing for bacterial pathogens is not included in codes **87631–87633**. Note that respiratory viral panels as described in **87631–87633** may have limited or no coverage in the outpatient/office setting. Verify payer policy before testing.

The most up-to-date proprietary laboratory analyses codes for detecting SARS-CoV-2 in addition to other pathogens are most easily found in *CPT* Appendix O and quarterly updates posted to www.ama-assn.org/practice-management/cpt/cpt-pla-codes. The specific test name is followed by the code and its descriptor, as illustrated in **Table 11-1** earlier in this chapter. Remember that the code descriptor and the proprietary name must match the test performed.

Glucose Tests

82947	Glucose, quantitative, blood (without a reagent strip) (CLIA waived)
82948	blood, reagent strip
82951	Glucose tolerance test (GTT), 3 specimens (CLIA waived)
+82952	each additional beyond 3 specimens (CLIA waived)
82962	Glucose, blood by glucose monitoring device(s) cleared by the FDA specifically for home use (CLIA waived)
83036	Hemoglobin; glycosylated (A1c) (CLIA waived)
83037	Hemoglobin; glycosylated (A1c) by device cleared by FDA for home use (CLIA waived)

Report 83037 for in-office hemoglobin A1c measurement using a device that is cleared by the FDA for home use. This test is not limited to use in a patient's home.

Code 82962 describes the method when whole blood is obtained (usually by finger-stick device) and assayed by glucose oxidase, hexokinase, or electrochemical methods and spectrophotometry using a small portable device designed for home blood glucose monitoring. The devices are also used in physician offices, during home visits, or in clinics.

Continuous glucose monitoring is reported with 95249–95251 (for discussion, refer to **Chapter 21**).

Hematology

85013	Spun microhematocrit (CLIA waived)
85018	Hemoglobin (CLIA waived)
85025–85027	Complete blood cell count, automated (85025 is CLIA waived.)
88738	Hemoglobin (Hgb), quantitative, transcutaneous

If using a complete blood cell count (CBC) machine to perform only a hemoglobin test, follow these guidelines.

- If the CBC is normal, only the hemoglobin level may be reported because that was the medically necessary test ordered.
- If the CBC reveals an abnormality that is addressed during the visit, the CBC may be reported. The abnormality would be linked to the procedure, and the medical record would need to include documentation for the ordering of the test and to support the medical necessity of the procedure.

Influenza Point-of-Care Testing

87502	Infectious agent detection by nucleic acid (DNA or RNA); influenza virus, for multiple types or sub-types, includes multiplex reverse transcription, when performed, and multiplex amplified probe technique, first 2 types or sub-types (CLIA waived)
87804	Infectious agent antigen detection by immunoassay with direct optical (ie, visual) observation; influenza (CLIA waived)

Code 87502 describes a test that already accounts for the first 2 types or subtypes; therefore, do not report multiple units of 87502 for the separate testing of influenza A and B.

- Code 87804 may be reported twice with modifier 59 appended to the second code when tests performed separately detect the influenza A and B antigen, providing 2 distinct results. This applies whether the test kit uses 1 or 2 analytic chambers to deliver 2 distinct results.
  - Check with payers; some do not recognize modifier 59 and may require reporting with 2 units of service and no modifier.
  - Some payers (eg, Medicaid plans) may limit units reported to the number of separate test kits used rather than following *CPT* instruction.

Refer also to the Combination Testing for SARS-CoV-2 and Other Infectious Agent(s) section earlier in this chapter for discussion of codes as related to combination testing of COVID-19 and other respiratory illnesses, including influenza.

Lead Testing

83655 Lead, quantitative analysis (CLIA waived)

- This test does not specify the specimen source or the method of testing. Alternative tests sometimes (although rarely) used for lead screening are 82135 (aminolevulinic acid, delta), 84202 (protoporphyrin, red blood cell count, quantitative), and 84203 (protoporphyrin, red blood cell count, screen).
- Some states provide lead testing at no cost to patients covered under the Medicaid Early and Periodic Screening, Diagnostic, and Treatment program. Check your Medicaid requirements for reporting this service.
- Report *ICD-10-CM* code Z13.88 (encounter for screening for disorder due to exposure to contaminants) when performing lead screening. A payer may require Z77.011 (contact with and [suspected] exposure to lead) in lieu of Z13.88.

***ICD-10-CM* allows separate reporting of special screening examinations (codes in categories Z11–Z13) in addition to the codes for routine child health examinations (eg, Z00.121, Z00.129) when these codes provide additional information. A screening code is not necessary if the screening is inherent to a routine examination.**

Mononucleosis Heterophile Antibodies Screening

86308 Heterophile antibodies; screening (CLIA waived)

This code may be appropriate for rapid mononucleosis screening.

Presumptive Drug Tests

#80305 Drug test(s), presumptive, any number of drug classes, any number of devices or procedures; capable of being read by direct optical observation only (eg, utilizing immunoassay [eg, dipsticks, cups, cards, or cartridges]); includes sample validation when performed, per DOS (CLIA waived)

#80306 read by instrument assisted direct optical observation (eg, utilizing immunoassay [eg, dipsticks, cups, cards, or cartridges]); includes sample validation when performed, per DOS

#80307 by instrument chemistry analyzers (eg, utilizing immunoassay [eg, EIA, ELISA, EMIT, FPIA, IA, KIMS, RIA]), chromatography (eg, GC, HPLC), and mass spectrometry either with or without chromatography (eg, DART, DESI, GC-MS, GC-MS/MS, LC-MS, LC-MS/MS, LDTD, MALDI, TOF); includes sample validation when performed, per DOS

- Presumptive drug class screening includes all drugs and drug classes performed by the respective methodology (eg, dipstick kit with direct optical observation) on a single DOS. Sample validation is included in presumptive drug screening service.
- Venipuncture to obtain samples for drug testing may be separately reportable with 36415 (collection of venous blood by venipuncture).
- When testing is performed with a method using direct optical observation to determine the result, 80305 is reported. Tests that have a waived status under CLIA may be reported with modifier QW (waived test).
- When a reader is used to determine the result of testing (eg, a dipstick is inserted into a machine that determines the final reading), 80306 is reported.
- Testing that uses a chemistry analyzer or more effort than tests represented by 80305 and 80306 is reported with 80307.

Chapter 11

Common Testing and Therapeutic Services

Respiratory Syncytial Virus Test

87634 Infectious agent detection by nucleic acid (DNA or RNA); RSV, amplified probe technique (CLIA waived)

87807 Infectious agent antigen detection by immunoassay with direct optical (ie, visual) observation; RSV (CLIA waived)

For assays that include RSV with additional respiratory viruses, refer to 87631–87633. Tests reported with 87631 and 87633 are CLIA waived. Append modifier QW if required. Refer also to the Combination Testing for SARS-CoV-2 and Other Infectious Agent(s) section earlier in this chapter for discussion of codes as related to tests for combinations of respiratory infectious agents, including SARS-CoV-2, influenza virus, and RSV.

Serum and Transcutaneous Bilirubin Testing

82247 Total bilirubin (CLIA waived)

88720 Transcutaneous total bilirubin

A direct bilirubin test (82248) is typically not provided in the office or outpatient setting and is typically performed in conjunction with total bilirubin testing. Indirect bilirubin levels are derived from the total (82247) and direct (82248) bilirubin measurements and is not a separately reported test.

Streptococcal Test

87880 Infectious agent antigen detection by immunoassay with direct optical (ie, visual) observation; streptococcus group A (CLIA waived)

87651 Infectious agent detection by nucleic acid (DNA or RNA); streptococcus, group A, amplified probe technique (CLIA waived)

87081 Culture, presumptive pathogenic organisms, screening only

87430 EIA, qualitative, streptococcus group A

- Report the code based on the test method rather than on the site of specimen collection.
- Culture plates using sheep blood agar with bacitracin disks should be coded with 87081.

Testing Stool for Occult Blood

82272 Blood, occult, by peroxidase activity (eg, guaiac), qualitative, feces, 1–3 simultaneous determinations, performed for other than colorectal neoplasm screening (CLIA waived)

- Code 82272 is reported when a single sample is obtained from a digital rectal examination or a multi-test card is returned from the patient and is tested for blood. Report 82272 with 1 unit when up to 3 cards are returned.

Tuberculin Test (Mantoux)

86580 Tuberculosis, intradermal

- This test is exempt from CLIA requirements.
- The tuberculosis (TB) skin test (Mantoux) using the intradermal administration of purified protein derivative is the recommended diagnostic skin test for TB.
  - This is not the BCG TB vaccine.
  - The American Academy of Pediatrics (AAP) supports the use of the Mantoux test (TB, intradermal) for TB screening when appropriate.
- ✖ Do not report an administration code in addition to 86580 when the purified protein derivative is placed.
- Code 99211 is appropriate to report the reading of a purified protein derivative test when that is the only reason for the encounter.

The appropriate *ICD-10-CM* code is Z11.1 (encounter for screening for respiratory TB). In the case of a positive test result when the physician sees the patient, the complexity may lead to a higher-level code.

- Because risk-based testing is recommended for pediatric patients, an E/M service to evaluate the need for testing may be indicated when testing is requested by a third party (eg, school, employer).
- If TB testing by cell-mediated immunity antigen response measurement, gamma interferon (86480), is ordered, and a specimen obtained, venipuncture (36415) may be separately reported.

Code 96160 (administration of a patient-focused health risk assessment instrument [eg, health hazard appraisal] with scoring and documentation, per standardized instrument) may be reported when a health risk assessment tool is used to screen for TB risk. Payer policies may vary on separate payment for 96160 when the assessment is provided on the same date as an E/M service.

Urine Pregnancy Test

81025 Urine pregnancy test, by visual color comparison methods (CLIA waived)

Report 81025 with *ICD-10-CM* codes Z32.00–Z32.02, depending on the finding of the test (unconfirmed, positive, or negative).

Urinalysis

81000 Urinalysis, by dipstick or tablet reagent for bilirubin, glucose, hemoglobin, ketones, leukocytes, nitrite, pH, protein, specific gravity, urobilinogen, any number of these constituents; nonautomated, with microscopy

81001 as per 81000 with microscopy, automated

81002 as per 81000 but without microscopy (CLIA waived)

81003 as per **81000** but without microscopy, automated (CLIA waived)

It is important to report the correct code for the urinalysis test performed.

- Code **81000** is reported when the results are shown as color changes for multiple analytes (eg, ketone levels, specific gravity) that are compared against those on a standardized chart (nonautomated) and when microscopy (in a second step, the urine is centrifuged and examined under microscope) is performed.
- Code **81002** is reported if the test results are obtained by the same method but microscopy is not performed.
- Codes **81001** and **81003** are reported for urinalysis performed by a processor that reads the results (automated).

For urinalysis, infectious agent detection, or semiquantitative analysis of volatile compounds, use **81099**.

✖ Do not report **99211** for the collection of a urine specimen and/or urinalysis in the absence of a separately identifiable E/M service. Code **51701** is reported when a non-indwelling bladder catheter (straight catheterization) is inserted for a urine culture collection, as discussed in **Chapter 13**.

To learn more about in-office laboratory services, refer to the March 2023 *AAP Pediatric Coding Newsletter*™ article "Selecting the Right Codes for In-office Laboratory Testing" (https://doi.org/10.1542/pcco_book227_document002).

Respiratory Function Tests and Treatments

Pulmonary Function Tests

National Correct Coding Initiative (NCCI) edits exist between office-based E/M services and all pulmonology services (**94010–94799**). Append modifier **25** to the E/M service code as appropriate when reporting a pulmonology service on the same claim.

There is no code for peak flow analysis or oxygen administration. These services are considered part of the E/M service and/or a component of pulmonary function testing.

- Codes include laboratory procedure(s) and interpretation of test results. If a separately identifiable E/M service is performed, the appropriate E/M service code may also be reported.
- Spirometry is reported with **94010**. When spirometry is performed before and after administration of a bronchodilator, however, report only **94060** (bronchodilation responsiveness, spirometry, pre- and post-bronchodilator administration).
  - Code **94640** (nebulizer treatment) is inherent to (ie, included as part of) **94060**. When an additional nebulizer treatment is performed as a distinct separate procedure on the same date as **94060**, NCCI edits allow use of a modifier (eg, **94640 59**), when applicable.
  - RVUs assigned to codes include typical supplies (eg, masks, tubing). Report codes for supplies only if the payer does not use an RVU payment methodology.
  - Medication is separately reported with the appropriate HCPCS code (eg, **J7613**, albuterol, inhalation solution, FDA-approved final product, noncompounded, administered through durable medical equipment, unit dose, 1 mg).

When a physician reports spirometry (94010, 94060) on the date of an E/M service, the test is not counted as ordered or reviewed for the purpose of determining the level of MDM because the test includes a professional component (ie, interpretation and report).

- Measurement of vital capacity (**94150**) is a component of spirometry and is reported only when performed alone.
- Measurement of spirometric forced expiratory flows in an infant or child through 2 years of age is reported with **94011**.
- Code **94012** is used to report measurement of bronchodilation spirometric forced expiratory flows (before and after bronchodilator) in an infant or a child.
- Code **94013** is used to report measurement of lung volumes (eg, functional residual capacity, expiratory reserve volume, forced vital capacity) in an infant or child through 2 years of age.

***CPT* guidelines allow reporting of pulse oximetry (94760, 94761), but health plans using the MPFS will pay only if no other service is paid to the same physician on the same date (ie, some plans consider this an examination component like determining blood pressure). Pulse oximetry is not counted toward the amount and/or complexity of data to be reviewed and analyzed as part of an E/M service.**

- Pulmonary stress testing (94618) includes measurement of heart rate, oximetry, and oxygen titration, when performed. When spirometry is performed before and following a pulmonary stress test, separately report 2 units of spirometry (94010).

Inhalation Treatment

94640 Pressurized or nonpressurized inhalation treatment for acute airway obstruction for therapeutic purposes and/or for diagnostic purposes such as sputum induction with an aerosol generator, nebulizer, metered dose inhaler or intermittent positive pressure breathing device

94644 Continuous inhalation treatment with aerosol medication for acute airway obstruction; first hour (For services of less than 1 hour, use 94640)

+94645 each additional hour (List separately in addition to code for primary procedure)

Report 94640

- When treatment such as aerosol generator, nebulizer, metered dose inhaler, or intermittent positive pressure breathing device is administered.
- With modifier 76 (repeat procedure) with the number of units (eg, 94640 76 × 2 units) when more than one treatment is given on a DOS. Some payers require reporting only with the number of units and no modifier (eg, 94640 × 2). Follow payer guidelines for reporting these services.
- When any treatment lasting 30 minutes or less is performed.

CPT code 94060 includes spirometry and pre- and post-bronchodilation. Report only 94060 when 94010 and/or 94640 is a component of the 94060 service. When reporting additional inhalation treatments on the same date as spirometry with pre- and post-bronchodilation, append modifiers 59 and 76 to 94640 (eg, 94060, 94640 59 76 × 2).

Report 94644 and 94645 when

- A treatment lasts 31 minutes or longer.
- The total time spent in the provision of continuous inhalation treatments is documented in the medical record.

Codes 94644 and 94645 are not reported by physicians when services are provided in a facility setting because no physician work value is assigned to these codes.

Nebulizer Demonstration or Evaluation

94664 Demonstration and/or evaluation of patient utilization of an aerosol generator, nebulizer, metered dose inhaler or intermittent positive pressure breathing device

- Code 94664 is reported only once per DOS.
- Report 94664 when an initial or subsequent demonstration and/or evaluation is performed and documented. This work may be performed by clinical staff under physician supervision.
- Physicians providing nebulizer instruction in conjunction with an E/M service may include the time of nebulizer instruction in the total physician time on the date of an office E/M service (99202–99205, 99212–99215) in lieu of reporting 94664. No physician work is attributed to 94664.

When demonstration and/or evaluation of patient use of a device such as a metered dose inhaler is reported with 94664 on the same day as a nebulizer treatment (94640), modifier 59 (distinct procedural service) should be appended to 94664 to indicate to the payer that the services were separate and distinct and that both were clinically indicated.

- Per the Medicaid NCCI manual, the demonstration and/or evaluation described by 94664 is included in 94640 if the same device (eg, aerosol generator) is used for both services. The NCCI edits pair 94664 with 94640 but allow an override of the edit with modifier 59 when both services are indicated (eg, treatment via nebulizer and teaching for metered dose inhaler). Some payers, however, allow the use of modifier 59 in this instance but only if the 2 services occur at separate encounters on the same date. Check with your Medicaid payers.

Modifier 25 should be appended to an E/M service code reported on the same date to signify a separately identifiable service. All services must be documented in the medical record as significant, separately identifiable, and medically necessary.

Car Seat/Bed Testing

94780 Car seat/bed testing for airway integrity, for infants through 12 months of age, with continual clinical staff observation and continuous recording of pulse oximetry, heart rate and respiratory rate, with interpretation and report; 60 minutes

+94781 each additional full 30 minutes (List separately in addition to 94780.)

To report 94780 and 94781, the following conditions must be met:

- The patient must be an infant (aged ≤12 months). Reassessment after the patient is 29 days or older may be necessary.
- Continual clinical staff observation with continuous recording of pulse oximetry, heart rate, and respiratory rate is required.
- Vital signs and observations must be reviewed and interpreted and a written report generated by the physician.
- Codes are reported according to the total observation time spent and documented.
- If less than 60 minutes is spent in the procedure, 94780 may not be reported.
- Each additional full 30 minutes (ie, not <90 minutes total) is reported with 94781.
- A significant, separately identifiable office or other outpatient E/M service [eg, 99213 25]) may be reported on the same date as car seat/bed testing, when provided.

Example

➤ **A neonate born at 34 weeks' gestation was released from the hospital 2 weeks ago with instructions to the parents to use only a car bed when transporting him until the pediatrician retests and determines that the neonate can safely ride in a car seat.** The newborn is seen in the outpatient clinic for a preventive medicine visit, and car seat testing is conducted for a period of 1 hour 45 minutes. The physician reviews and interprets the nurse's records of pulse oximetry, heart and respiratory rates, and observations during the testing period. The interpretation is documented in a formal report and plan of care clearing the neonate to begin use of a rear-facing car seat. The plan of care is discussed with the parents, who also receive further instruction on appropriate use of the car seat.

ICD-10-CM	*CPT*
Z00.111 (health examination for newborn 8–28 days old) P07.37 (preterm newborn, gestational age 34 completed weeks)	99391 25 (preventive medicine service, established patient <1 year)
Codes for conditions of the newborn and P07.37	94780 (car seat/bed testing; first 60 minutes) 94781 (each additional full 30 minutes)

Teaching Point: In this scenario, a total of 105 minutes of testing was conducted. This would be reported with 1 unit of 94780 for the initial 60 minutes of testing and 1 unit of 94781 for the last 45 minutes (only 1 full period of 30 minutes beyond the first 60 minutes was performed). The 15 minutes beyond the last full 30-minute period is not separately reported. Modifier 25 is appended to 99391 to report that the service was significant and separately identifiable in the documentation of services provided on that date.

Allergy and Clinical Immunology

Allergy Testing

95004 Percutaneous tests (scratch, puncture, prick) with allergenic extracts, immediate type reaction, including test interpretation and report, specify number of tests

95017 Allergy testing, any combination of percutaneous (scratch, puncture, prick) and intracutaneous (intradermal), sequential and incremental, with venoms, immediate type reaction, including test interpretation and report, specify number of tests

95018 Allergy testing, any combination of percutaneous (scratch, puncture, prick) and intracutaneous (intradermal), sequential and incremental, with drugs or biologicals, immediate type reaction, including test interpretation and report, specify number of tests

95024 Intracutaneous (intradermal) tests with allergenic extracts, immediate type reaction, including test interpretation and report, specify number of tests

Chapter 11 Common Testing and Therapeutic Services

• indicates a new code; ▲, revised; #, re-sequenced; ✚, add-on; ★, audiovisual technology; and ◀, synchronous interactive audio.

95027 Intracutaneous (intradermal) tests, sequential and incremental, with allergenic extracts for airborne allergens, immediate type reaction, including test interpretation and report, specify number of tests

95028 Intracutaneous (intradermal) tests with allergenic extracts, delayed type reaction, including reading, specify number of tests

- *CPT* codes for allergy testing are reported by type of test.
  - Percutaneous, immediate type reaction (**95004**)
  - Intracutaneous (intradermal) with immediate (**95024**, **95027**) or delayed type reaction (**95028**)
  - Any combination of percutaneous and intracutaneous, sequential and incremental tests with venoms (**95017**) or with drugs or biologicals (**95018**)
- Specification of the number of tests applied is required for accurate reporting of the units of service provided. Medicaid NCCI edits do not allow inclusion of positive or negative controls in the number of tests reported.
- Codes **95004**, **95017**, **95018**, **95024**, and **95027** include test interpretation and report. Code **95028** includes reading.

When a significant, separately identifiable E/M service is performed and documented (eg, counseling on allergy avoidance, treatment, and use of epinephrine auto-injector) on the same date as testing, it may be reported with modifier **25** appended to the appropriate E/M code. Do not include the time spent in allergy test administration or interpretation in the total time of an E/M service provided on the same date.

✖ Do not report an E/M service for the obtainment of informed consent and interpretation and report of the results of allergy testing.

Example

➤ **A patient with seasonal allergies undergoes percutaneous testing with 22 allergenic extracts and 2 controls.** A clinician administers the extracts per the physician's order and monitors the patient for signs of reaction. For each extract administered, the reaction (eg, size of wheal) or lack of reaction is noted. The physician interprets the test and creates a report of the findings.

The physician reports **95004** with 24 units of service or, if the payer does not allow payment for controls, with 22 units. If a significant E/M service is provided on the same date and is separately identifiable in the documentation from the preservice and postservice work of the testing (eg, interpretation and report), append modifier **25** to the code for the E/M service provided.

- Patch and photo patch testing are reported with **95044–95056**.
- Specific challenge testing (**95060–95079**) is coded according to target organ (eg, ophthalmic mucous membrane, nasal, inhalation bronchial challenges without pulmonary function testing, ingestion).
- Nasal cytology, a test for allergy-type cells (eosinophils) or infection-type cells (neutrophils) on a nasal scraping, is reported with **89190**.
- Nitric oxide–expired gas determination is reported with **95012**. Nitric oxide determination by spectroscopy should be reported with **94799**.

Allergen Immunotherapy

Codes for allergen immunotherapy are reported based on the service provided: only preparation and provision of allergen extract, only administration, or combined provision and administration.

An appropriate office or outpatient code may be reported with allergen immunotherapy codes. Modifier **25** is appended to the E/M service when it is performed and documented.

Only Preparation and Provision of Extract

95144 Professional services for the supervision of the preparation and provision of antigens for allergen immunotherapy, single-dose vials(s) (specify number of vials)

95145 Professional services for the supervision of the preparation and provision of antigens for allergy immunotherapy (specify number of doses); single stinging insect venom

95146 2 stinging insect venoms

95147 3 stinging insect venoms

95148 4 stinging insect venoms

95149 5 stinging insect venoms

95165 Professional services for the supervision of preparation and provision of antigens for allergen immunotherapy; single or multiple antigens (specify number of doses)

95170 Professional services for the supervision of preparation and provision of antigens for allergen immunotherapy; whole body extract of biting insect or other arthropod (specify number of doses)

- Codes **95144–95170** are used to report preparation and provision of antigens for allergen immunotherapy without administration of the allergenic extract.
  - Codes **95144–95170** describe the preparation of the antigen, the antigen extract itself, the physician's assessment and determination of the concentration and volume to use based on the patient's history and results of previous skin testing, and the prospective planned schedule of administration of the extract.
  - The number of vials must be specified when reporting **95144**.
  - Report **95145–95170** according to the *number of doses* (eg, preparation of 2 vials that will provide 20 doses of extract containing 4 insect venoms is reported with **95148** and 20 units of service).
  - Services may be reported at the time the allergenic extract is prepared because injections occur on later dates (prospectively planned) or may not occur at all.
  - Administration of the allergenic extract is not included.
- Report **95146–95149** for preparation of extracts containing more than one stinging venom (eg, **95146** is reported for 2; **95147** is reported for 3).

National Correct Coding Initiative Immunotherapy Edits

The Medicaid NCCI manual instructs that for the purpose of reporting units of service for antigen preparation (ie, *CPT* codes 95145–95170), the physician report "number of doses." The NCCI program defines a dose for reporting purposes as 1 mL. Thus, if a physician prepares a 10-mL vial of antigen, the physician may report only a maximum of 10 units of service for that vial even if the number of actual administered doses is greater than 10. Verify payer policies on units of service before reporting.

Only Administration of Extract

95115 Professional services for allergen immunotherapy not including provision of allergenic extracts; single injection

95117 2 or more injections

Either **95115** or **95117** (not both) are used to report only administration of the allergenic extract. Report according to the number of injections when another health care professional (eg, the patient's allergist) has prepared and supplied the allergenic extract or when a physician (usually an allergist) administers the prospectively prepared extract (ie, prepared with the intent to administer on a planned schedule).

Example

➤ **The pediatrician administers 3 injections of allergen extract for a patient with allergic rhinitis resulting from pollen.** The extract was prepared and supplied by an allergist.

The pediatrician will report **95117** with *ICD-10-CM* code **J30.1**.

Combined Provision of Allergenic Extract With Administration

***CPT* recommends 95120–95134 be reported only when specifically required by the payer. These codes are not assigned RVUs in the MPFS that many payers use as a basis for physician payment. The Medicare program will accept only 95115, 95117, and 95144–95170 and will not allow payment for 95120–95134. Medicaid and commercial payers may follow the Medicare guidelines or may have their own established guidelines. Therefore, before reporting these services, research the reporting policies of your major payers.**

Refer to your *CPT* code manual or other code reference for full code descriptors for 95120–95134.

- Codes **95120–95134** are reported when the entire service of preparing, providing, and administering (injection) allergenic extract is performed at 1 patient encounter.
- Codes **95131–95134** are reported for extracts containing more than one stinging insect venom.
- ✖ Codes **95115** and **95117** *cannot* be reported with **95120–95134**.

- Codes 95120 and 95125 are reported according to the number of injections administered (ie, a single injection or ≥2 injections).
- Codes 95130–95134 are reported per injection. Therefore, if 2 separate injections of 2 stinging insect venoms (eg, wasp and bee) are provided, 95131 will be reported 2 times.
- For rapid desensitization per hour, refer to 95180.

Example

➤ **An allergist prepares a 10-dose vial of allergen extract and administers 1 dose at the time of the visit (allergenic extract was prepared with the intent to administer on a planned schedule).**

The allergist will report 95165 with 10 units of service and 95115 with 1 unit of service and the specific diagnosis code. Allergic rhinitis resulting from pollen would be reported with *ICD-10-CM* code J30.1 or, if caused by food, J30.5. Alternatively, 95120 would describe provision of allergenic extract and a single injection if required by a payer.

Epinephrine Auto-Injector Administration

Administration of epinephrine via an epinephrine auto-injector in the office or other outpatient setting is reported with 96372 (therapeutic, prophylactic, or diagnostic injection [specify substance or drug]; subcutaneous or intramuscular). Follow payer guidance for reporting an epinephrine injector kit furnished by the practice.

Healthcare Common Procedure Coding System updates in 2025 resulted in deletion of epinephrine/adrenalin codes J0171 and J0173. Replacing code J0171 for medications that are brand name (eg, Adrenalin or EpiPen) or therapeutically equivalent to brand name adrenalin products is J0165 (injection, epinephrine, not otherwise specified, 0.1 mg). Codes J0166–J0169 are reported for epinephrine products that are not therapeutically equivalent to brand name products, Adrenalin or Epipen.

Example

➤ **The patient has a reaction to the allergenic extract.** The physician supplies and injects a dose of epinephrine based on the patient's weight.

The injection using an auto-injection device would be reported as an intramuscular (IM) injection with 96372. The appropriate code, J0165–J0169, is reported based on the epinephrine/adrenalin product administered. The HCPCS units for epinephrine/adrenalin products are 1 unit per 0.1 mg (eg, 0.15 mg equals 1.5 units). It is advisable to include the product NDC and NDC units (eg, 0.1 ML, 0.15 ML, or 0.3 ML) to specify the exact product and dose provided.

Immunoglobulins

This information does not apply to immunization products or services (eg, 90380–90382, seasonal RSV immunoglobulin products). Refer to Chapter 8.

When reporting 90281–90378 and 90384–90399, remember that they are only for the cost of the immunoglobulin, so the appropriate separate administration code should also be reported (eg, 96372, 96374).

- A significant, separately identifiable E/M service performed during the same visit may also be billed if indicated.
- *ICD-10-CM* diagnosis codes to support immunoglobulin services include codes from categories D80–D84 for certain disorders involving the immune mechanism or codes for specific conditions, such as mucocutaneous lymph node syndrome (M30.3).
- ✖ When reporting immunoglobulin products, include the product's NDC to identify the exact immunoglobulin administered. Refer to **Chapter 1** for more information on reporting NDCs.

Hearing Screening and Other Audiological Function Testing Codes

(For central auditory function evaluation, refer to 92620, 92621.)

Audiometric tests require the use of calibrated electronic equipment, recording of results, and a written report with interpretation (eg, chart of hertz and decibels with pass/fail result for each ear tested and overall pass/fail result). Services include testing of both ears. If the test is applied to only 1 ear, modifier 52 (reduced services) must be appended to the code.

Medicaid plans may offer coverage information and forms/requirements for documentation of hearing screening/testing.

- Code 92551 (screening test, pure tone, air only) is used when earphones are placed on the patient and the patient is asked to respond to tones of different pitches and intensities. This is a limited study to identify the presence or absence of a potential hearing problem. Code 92551 is not used to report hearing screenings performed in newborns and infants.

Report hearing tests conducted following a failed hearing screening with *ICD-10-CM* code Z01.110 if results are normal. If findings are abnormal, report Z01.118 and a code to identify the abnormality.

- Code 92552 (full pure tone audiometric assessment) is used when earphones are placed on the patient and the patient is asked to respond to tones of different pitches and intensities. The threshold, which is the lowest intensity of the tone that the patient can hear 50% of the time, is recorded at a number of frequencies.
- Air and bone thresholds (92553) may be obtained and compared to differentiate among conductive, sensorineural, or mixed hearing losses. Air and bone thresholds are obtained in a similar manner.
- Code 92583 (select picture audiometry) is typically used for younger children. The patient is asked to identify different pictures with the instructions given at different intensity levels.

Automated audiometry testing is reported with Category III codes 0208T–0212T.

- Code 92558 is reported for evoked otoacoustic emissions, screening (qualitative measurement of distortion product or transient evoked otoacoustic emissions), with automated analysis. This is used when the results are obtained automatically (ie, no interpretation and report is required). Coverage for this is typically limited to newborn screening, including follow-up newborn screening from a failed screening in the hospital and screening on younger children. Check with your payers, however.
- Distortion product evoked otoacoustic emissions codes are reported according to the number of frequencies used. Code 92587 is used to report testing for confirmation of the presence or absence of a hearing disorder, 3 to 6 frequencies. Code 92588 is reported when a comprehensive (quantitative analysis of outer hair cell function by cochlear mapping) diagnostic evaluation with a minimum of 12 frequencies is performed. Interpretation and written report are required. *Do not report these codes for automated analysis.*
- Other commonly performed procedures include 92567 (tympanometry [impedance testing]) and 92568 (acoustic reflex testing, threshold portion). Code 92550 is reported when tympanometry and reflex threshold measurements are performed.
- Optical coherence tomography of the middle ear with interpretation and report is reported with Category III codes based on whether the service was unilateral (0485T) or bilateral (0486T). Be sure to verify payer policy before provision of services.
- Most audiological procedures are bundled with impacted cerumen removal services (69209, 69210) and, therefore, will not be separately payable. Report only the audiology test to payers that bundle impacted cerumen removal services.

Chapter 11

Common Testing and Therapeutic Services

Example

➤ **A 5-year-old whose hearing does not meet screening criteria at school is referred to her pediatrician for additional evaluation.** The child has a history of recurrent otitis media before the age of 3 years but no recent illness. Parents report no family history of hearing loss and no concerns at home. Tympanometry reveals no evidence of effusion. Examination findings are negative for other abnormalities. Screening audiometry is performed, and its results are atypical, as indicated by the school screening. The child is referred to an audiologist for further evaluation. Diagnosis is abnormal auditory function with possible hearing loss in her right ear.

ICD-10-CM	*CPT*
Z01.118 (encounter for examination of ears and hearing with other abnormal findings) R94.120 (abnormal auditory function study)	99213 (established patient office E/M, low MDM) 92567 (tympanometry [impedance testing]) 92551 (screening test, pure tone, air only)

Teaching Point: *ICD-10-CM* instructs the physician to report Z01.118 and an additional code for abnormal findings. Although the result of the screening was abnormal, the physician did not diagnose a hearing loss at this encounter. Code R94.120 describes the abnormal screening result.

If the screening result at this visit had been negative, the physician would have been required to code Z01.110 (encounter for hearing examination following failed hearing screening).

For information on vision screening, refer to Chapter 8. Assessment of visual acuity is considered an integral part of the eye examination when performed to address a problem such as difficulty seeing writing on a board at school.

Emotional/Behavioral Assessment

96127 Brief emotional/behavioral assessment (eg, depression inventory, attention-deficit/hyperactivity disorder [ADHD] scale), with scoring and documentation, per standardized instrument

Code 96127

- Represents the practice expense of administering, scoring, and documenting each standardized instrument. No physician work value is included. Physician interpretation is included in a related E/M service.
- May be used for screening (eg, screening for anxiety and/or depression) or to monitor treatment efficacy and support clinical decision-making.
- ✖ Not reported in conjunction with 96105, 96125, and 99483.
- Multiple separate completions (eg, by teachers and parent) of the same form may be separately reported (eg, 3 units of service). When reporting multiple units of service, it is advisable to learn whether the payer has specific guidance for reporting the total number of units as a single-line item or requires splitting to multiple claim lines. Medically Unlikely Edits may apply.
- Be aware of potential bundling edits when reporting a health risk assessment (96160) and brief emotional behavioral assessment on the same date. Modifier 59 (distinct service) may be required (ie, 96160 59).

Chapter 11

Common Testing and Therapeutic Services

Example

➤ **A 16-year-old patient receiving treatment of an initial episode of major depressive disorder returns for follow-up.** The patient's mother contributes to the patient's history since the last visit. Three standardized instruments (anxiety instruments by parent and by child and a depression instrument by child) are administered to assess the status of the patient's depression. The physician reviews the documented scores and considers the patient's responses in MDM. The physician recommends continued medication and counseling with a licensed clinical social worker. The physician's total time on the date of the encounter is 25 minutes. Diagnosis is a moderate single episode of major depressive disorder.

The established patient office E/M code 99214 is reported in addition to 96127. The diagnosis code F32.1 (major depressive disorder, single episode, moderate) is reported.

Refer to

- **Chapter 2 for more information on Medically Unlikely Edits**
- **Chapter 8 for discussion of developmental screening, brief emotional and/or behavioral assessment, and health risk assessment as preventive services**
- **Chapter 10 for discussion of neuropsychological or psychological testing**

Developmental Testing

Refer to **Chapter 10** for discussion of neurobehavioral status examination (96116, 96121).

★96112 Developmental test administration (including assessment of fine and/or gross motor, language, cognitive level, social, memory and/or executive functions by standardized developmental instruments when performed), by physician or other QHP, with interpretation and report; first hour

★✚96113 each additional 30 minutes (List separately in addition to code for primary procedure)

Developmental screening services are described by 96110. Developmental screening using an objective standardized instrument, including scoring and documentation, is typically done by clinical staff. Interpretation and counseling on the score are included in the related E/M service.

Codes 96112 and 96113

- Allow reporting of developmental testing in which the child is observed doing standardized tasks that are then scored, with interpretation and report.
- Include assessment of motor, language, social, and/or cognitive function by standardized developmental instruments (eg, scales of infant and toddler development) and include objective assessments as well.
- Billing time includes the sum of all face-to-face time spent in test administration and observation and time of interpretation, clinical decision-making, and report preparation.
  - Although not specifically stated in the code descriptor, interpretation and report is included as intraservice work in the assignment of work RVUs for these services.
  - Payer policies may vary on reporting of time spent in interpretation and report. Check the policies of individual health plans when reporting.
- Code selection is based on time personally spent per hour by the physician or QHP.
- The midpoint rule applies to developmental testing; time is met when the midpoint is passed (≥31 minutes to report 1 hour of service and ≥16 minutes to report a service assigned a time of 30 minutes).
- If a developmental instrument does not meet the criteria of being an objective instrument with the subjective element or the service does not take a minimum of 31 minutes to complete (including time of interpretation and report), refer to 96110 instead.
- ✖ Do not report 96110 if also reporting 96112 or 96113 on the same day for the same patient.
- A clinically indicated and significant E/M service may be reported on the same date, but no component of the testing is used to determine the level of E/M code selection. Modifier 25 (significant and separately identifiable E/M service) is appended to the E/M code (eg, 99214 25).

Example

➤ **A 7-year-old patient presents for extended developmental testing to assess long-standing social and learning difficulties at school.** Developmental tests are administered, with total testing time on this date of 75 minutes. The child returns and spends a total of 60 minutes to complete testing 1 week later. After testing is completed, the developmental pediatrician spends another 60 minutes on the same date interpreting the test results and 60 minutes formulating a report of the findings and recommendations.

First date: 96112 is reported for the 75 minutes of testing.

Second date: 96112 (first 60 minutes of testing) and 96113 with 4 units of service (2 hours interpreting the testing results and developing the report) are reported.

Teaching Point: Code 96113 is not reported on the first date because the midpoint between 60 and 90 minutes (76 minutes) was not passed. On the final DOS (ie, the day of the feedback session), submit 1 claim for all cumulative services detailed by separate dates of service.

Some payers may require that the entire service be reported on a single claim and single DOS. For these payers, report 96112 (for the 60 minutes of testing on the first day) and 6 units of 96113 (for the remaining 195 minutes) on the date of the second session. It is important that staff are trained to submit the records for all dates that testing services were provided, when necessary, in response to a payer's request for records.

Remember, the midpoint must be passed for the additional units to be billed. In this case, the remaining time was only 15 minutes.

Appropriate diagnosis codes should be assigned and may be required to support payer authorization for future treatment. *ICD-10-CM* provides codes for autism spectrum disorder (F84.0), Asperger syndrome (F84.5), and other pervasive developmental disorders (eg, F84.2, Rett syndrome). Codes for any associated medical condition and intellectual disabilities should also be reported.

Radiology Services

The following general guidelines are for reporting radiology services:

- Report only the service provided. Refer to the Professional and Technical Components section earlier in this chapter for appropriate reporting when the physician does not provide the global service.

- A signed written report of the physician's or QHP's interpretation of imaging is an integral part of the professional component of a radiological service.
- A reference to *image* in *CPT* may refer to an image on film or in digital format. Images must contain anatomical information unique to the patient for which the imaging service is provided.
- Certain health plans, including Medicaid plans, may require use of modifiers **FX** (x-ray taken using film) and **FY** (x-ray taken using computed radiography technology/cassette-based imaging) when reporting the technical component or global radiology service (ie, combined professional and technical components). Verify health plan requirements, as payment may be reduced for radiographs taken through technology other than digital imaging.

Some commonly reported codes for radiological examination follow. Refer to your coding reference for a full listing of codes and reporting instructions for radiology services.

Abdominal Radiographs

74018	Radiologic examination, abdomen; 1 view
74019	2 views
74021	3 or more views
74022	Radiologic examination, complete acute abdomen series, including 2 or more views of the abdomen (eg, supine, erect, decubitus), and a single view chest

Report **74022** when a series of radiographs is obtained to view the abdomen and chest as workup of acute abdominal illness or pain. An acute abdomen series includes 2 abdominal views and a single chest view.

Chest Radiographs

71045	Radiologic examination, chest; single view
71046	2 views
71047	3 views
71048	4 or more views

- The types of views (eg, frontal and lateral) obtained do not affect coding of chest radiographs.
- ✖ Do not separately report a single-view chest radiograph when obtained in conjunction with an acute abdomen series (**74022**).

Hip Radiographs

73501	Radiologic examination, hip, unilateral, with pelvis when performed; 1 view
73502	2–3 views
73503	minimum of 4 views
73521	Radiologic examination, hips, bilateral, with pelvis when performed; 2 views
73522	3–4 views
73523	minimum of 5 views
73525	Radiologic examination, hip, arthrography, radiological supervision and interpretation
73592	Radiologic examination lower extremity, infant, minimum of 2 views

Codes **73501–73523** include radiograph of the pelvis when performed. Do not separately report a single-view radiograph of the pelvis (**72170**) when performed in conjunction with a radiograph of the hip.

Total Spine Radiographs

72081	Radiologic examination, spine, entire thoracic and lumbar, including skull, cervical and sacral spine if performed (eg, scoliosis evaluation); one view
72082	2 or 3 views
72083	4 or 5 views
72084	minimum of 6 views

Codes **72081–72084** describe imaging of the entire thoracic and lumbar spine and, when performed, the skull, cervical, and sacral spine.

- ✖ Do not separately report codes for views of the individual spinal segments or skull when performed in conjunction with radiological examination of the spine. Rather, select the code that represents the total number of views obtained.

Administrative Services

Codes in this section cover some of the administrative aspects of medical practice.

99075 Medical testimony

99082 Unusual travel (eg, transportation and escort of patient)

S9981 Medical records copying fee, administrative

S9982 Medical records copying fee, per page

Codes **99071–99082** are for administrative services.

- Code **99075** may be reported when a physician presents medical testimony before a court or other administrative body.
- None of these services is assigned Medicare RVUs.
- HCPCS codes **S9981** and **S9982** may be reported when it is appropriate to charge for copying medical records. Commercial payers and some Medicaid programs may accept **S** codes.
  - State medical insurance departments or medical associations determine the amount a practice can charge for copying medical records. Be sure to know the state charge limitations, and do not overcharge.
  - The Health Insurance Portability and Accountability Act (HIPAA) of 1996 regulations, where more stringent, will override state regulations. For information on charges to patients for copying medical records, visit www.hhs.gov/hipaa/for-professionals/privacy/guidance/access/index.html#newlyreleasedfaqs.

Physician Group Education Services

99078 Physician or other QHP qualified by education, training, licensure/regulation (when applicable), educational services rendered to patients in a group setting (eg, prenatal, obesity, or diabetic instructions)

Code **99078** is used to report physician educational services provided to established patients in group settings (eg, obesity or diabetes classes).

- For preventive medicine and risk factor reduction counseling to patients in a group setting, refer to **99411** and **99412**.
- There are no time requirements.
- ✖ Modifier **25** (significant, separately identifiable E/M service) should *not* be appended to the code for an E/M service on the same date because **99078** is an adjunct service.
- Documentation in each medical record includes the education and training provided, follow-up for ongoing education, and total time of the education (distinct from any E/M service).
- Health plans and parents/caregivers of each participating child may be charged.
- Payers may require that these services be reported differently.

To test your knowledge of the information presented in this chapter, complete the quiz found at the end of it, after the resources. Answers to each quiz are found in **Appendix II**.

Chapter Takeaways

This chapter covered codes and coding guidance for many diagnostic and therapeutic services when provided in an office or outpatient setting. Following are some takeaways from this chapter:

- There are many services that may be reported for the complete or global service or for only the professional or technical component, when provided.
- The practice expense RVUs assigned to most services include the value of supplies (eg, masks, tubing, gauze, needles) that are typically required for each service.
- Laboratories and physician offices performing CLIA-waived tests should append modifier **QW** to the *CPT* code for CLIA-waived procedures except when reporting certain exempt codes (eg, **81002**, non-automated urinalysis without microscopy; **81025**, urine pregnancy test; **82272**, occult blood by peroxidase for other than colorectal neoplasm screening).
- Obtaining a blood specimen is separately reportable in conjunction with performing a point-of-care test and/or an E/M service.
- ✖ Do not report **99211** for services to obtain a specimen and/or perform a laboratory test in the absence of an E/M service by clinical staff.
- ✖ Do not include time spent in separately reported testing or therapeutic services in the time of an E/M service reported on the same date. Append modifier **25** to significant and separately identifiable E/M services provided on the same date as tests that include an interpretation and report or as otherwise specified in *CPT*.

Resources

AAP Coding Assistance and Education

2026 Coding Card Toolbox (www.aap.org/2026-Coding-Card-Toolbox)

Pediatric Office Superbill 2026 (www.aap.org/Pediatric-Office-Superbill-2026)

AAP Pediatric Coding Newsletter

"Did You Know? The CLIA-Waived Test Modifier," February 2024 (https://doi.org/10.1542/pcco_book238_document003)

CLIA Test Categorization

"CLIA—Clinical Laboratory Improvement Amendments—Currently Waived Analytes" (www.accessdata.fda.gov/scripts/cdrh/cfdocs/cfClia/analyteswaived.cfm)

FDA CLIA database (www.accessdata.fda.gov/scripts/cdrh/cfdocs/cfCLIA/search.cfm)

"Provider-Performed Microscopy Procedures" from the Centers for Medicare & Medicaid Services (www.cms.gov/regulations-and-guidance/legislation/clia/downloads/ppmplist.pdf)

HIPAA Release of Patient Records

"Questions and Answers About HIPAA's Access Right" (45 CFR §164.524) (www.hhs.gov/hipaa/for-professionals/privacy/guidance/access/index.html#newlyreleasedfaqs)

Medicare Physician Fee Schedule

How to Use the PFS Look-Up Tool booklet (www.cms.gov/sites/default/files/2021-04/How_to_MPFS_Booklet_ICN901344_0.pdf)

MPFS Look-Up Tool (www.cms.gov/apps/physician-fee-schedule/overview.aspx)

National Drug Codes

FDA National Drug Code Directory (www.fda.gov/drugs/drug-approvals-and-databases/national-drug-code-directory)

Online-Exclusive Content at www.aap.org/cfp2026

"Medications for Pediatrics: Most Common"

Proprietary Laboratory Analyses

"*CPT* PLA Codes" (www.ama-assn.org/practice-management/cpt/cpt-pla-codes)

Test Your Knowledge!

1. **What modifier is appended to code 93010 (routine ECG with at least 12 leads; interpretation and report only) when a physician provides only the interpretation and report of the ECG?**
   a. 26 (professional component).
   b. TC (technical component).
   c. None; no modifier is necessary according to the code descriptor.
   d. 52 (reduced service).
2. **Which type of specimen collection is separately reported?**
   a. Nasopharyngeal swab
   b. Urine sample (collected without catheterization)
   c. Throat swab
   d. Venipuncture
3. **Which service is reported with modifier QW?**
   a. A laboratory service reported by a physician or QHP but provided by another entity
   b. All laboratory services provided in an office or outpatient setting
   c. Collection of a specimen for laboratory testing
   d. Performance of a laboratory test that is CLIA-waived (with a few exceptions)
4. **For which testing platform is code selection based on the analysis performed and the proprietary name of the test?**
   a. Direct optical observation
   b. Provider-performed microscopy
   c. Proprietary laboratory analyses
   d. Point-of-care testing
5. **Which of the following is true when reporting an E/M service and testing services on the same date?**
   a. The physician's or QHP's analysis of test results that do not require interpretation and report is part of an evaluation and management (E/M) service.
   b. Modifier 25 may be required on the E/M service to indicate the service was significant and is separately identifiable in the documentation.
   c. Time spent providing a separately reported testing service does not contribute to the total time of an E/M service.
   d. All of the above.

CHAPTER 12

Nonphysician Qualified Health Care Professional Services

Contents

• indicates a new code; ▲, revised; #, re-sequenced; ✚, add-on; ★, audiovisual technology; and ◀, synchronous interactive audio.

Chapter Highlights

- Terminology used to differentiate nonphysician qualified health care professionals (NQHCPs) from qualified health care professionals (QHPs) and clinical staff (and why this differentiation matters)
- Identifying the scope of practice for an NQHCP
- Recognizing the various NQHCPs who may perform and report services to pediatric patients
- *Current Procedural Terminology* (*CPT*®) and Healthcare Common Procedure Coding System (HCPCS) codes and modifiers that may apply to reporting services performed by NQHCPs

Services Provided by Nonphysician Qualified Health Care Professionals

In their quest to provide comprehensive and high-quality care to patients, pediatric physicians are including more NQHCPs (eg, dieticians) in their practices and utilizing clinical staff to their full potential.

This chapter focuses on medical services that are provided by health care professionals other than physicians and other QHPs, such as nurse practitioners (NPs) and physician associates (PAs) (formerly titled physician assistants), who are distinguished by the ability to provide and independently report evaluation and management (E/M) services.

Refer to Chapter 10 for information on reporting mental and behavioral health services provided by NQHCPs. Refer to Chapter 21 for information on remote therapeutic monitoring by NQHCPs.

Terminology

Throughout the *CPT* code set, use of terms such as *physician, QHP,* or *individual* is not intended to indicate that other entities may not report the service. In select instances, specific instructions may define a service as limited to professionals or other entities (eg, hospital, home health agency).

To help differentiate, the following definitions apply to discussions and examples in this chapter:

- **Qualified health care professional:** Advanced practice providers, such as advanced practice nurses, clinical nurse specialists, and PAs, whose scope of practice includes E/M services beyond minimal services incident to a physician (ie, 99211 or 99281, E/M visit not requiring physician face-to-face service).

Refer to Chapter 7 for detailed discussion of incident-to services and E/M services reported with 99211.

- **Nonphysician qualified health care professional:** A broad category of health care professionals who typically would not independently prescribe and manage, whose professional services are typically performed under the order and supervision of a physician or QHP, and whose scope of practice does not include E/M services beyond 99211. When providing services that do not require direct physician supervision, some NQHCPs are able to bill under their own National Provider Identifier (NPI). This category includes providers such as clinical psychologists, licensed counselors, dietitians/nutritionists, certain health educators, licensed therapists, and, sometimes, lactation consultants, among others.
- **Clinical staff member,** as defined by *CPT:* A health care team member who works under the supervision of a physician or other QHP and who is allowed by law, regulation, and facility policy to perform or assist in the performance of a specific professional service but *does not individually report that professional service.* These include, but are not limited to, registered nurses (RNs), licensed practical nurses (LPNs), and medical assistants.

CPT references *clinical staff member* mostly in the context of staff who provide components of physician or QHP services, such as obtaining patient history, and services that are always billed by a supervising physician or QHP (eg, nurse visit, medication administration).

Nonphysician Qualified Health Care Professional Services

Chapter 12

Staff who can perform *only administrative functions,* such as reception, scheduling, billing, dictation, or scribing, are not clinical staff for coding purposes.

Refer to the May 2025 *AAP Pediatric Coding Newsletter*™ article "Procedure Codes for Nonphysician Qualified Health Care Professional Services" (https://doi.org/10.1542/pcco_book253_document002) for additional discussion of codes for reporting services provided by NQHCPs.

Including Nonphysician Qualified Health Care Professionals in Your Practice

Services by NQHCPs, provided under a physician's or QHP's order within a physician group practice, can be an integral part of providing a full scope of care in the medical home.

- Billing and coding must align not only with coding guidelines but also state scope of practice (refer to the Scope of Practice Laws section later in this chapter) and individual payer policies on credentialing, contracting, and billing for services of the specific NQHCP.
- *Before including NQHCPs within your group practice,* it is important to seek expert advice on related state regulations for scope of practice and supervision requirements, enrollment and payment policies of the group's most common payers, and best practices in employment and/or contractual agreements.
- The number of services that may be provided can be estimated from current patient diagnoses or history of referral for services. Reports from electronic health records or billing software may be used in this estimation (eg, report of the number of unique patient accounts containing a diagnosis code for conditions that a nutritionist may address).

When physicians choose to arrange for services provided within their group practice by NQHCPs who are not employed or contracted with the group practice, additional counsel should be obtained to prevent conflict with anti-kickback and/or self-referral regulations.

Payment for NQHCP services begins with negotiating and contracting with payers for coverage and payment of services as described by *CPT* and/or HCPCS codes. (For a list of HCPCS codes that may be used to report nonphysician education services, refer to the Disease Management Program Services section later in this chapter.)

- Payers may pay separately for these services when your practice can demonstrate the overall cost savings (eg, decreased physician or emergency department visits, decreased hospital care) that may be achieved through expanded care in the physician practice.

For more on quality and performance measurement, refer to Chapter 3.

- If payers do not agree to directly compensate for individual services, consider opportunities for shared savings and other revenue that may be realized when NQHCP services support quality improvement initiatives (eg, per-member-per-month compensation for meeting certain quality measures) and redirection of physician and QHP time to services that are restricted to or best delivered within their scope of practice.
- Physicians should be especially aware of each payer's policy addressing use of E/M codes for services provided by NQHCPs or clinical staff. Other than 99211, Medicare and payers that adopt Medicare policy do not allow reporting of E/M codes for services provided by NQHCPs or clinical staff. Services that specifically indicate work of clinical staff under physician supervision (eg, transitional care management [TCM] or chronic care management [CCM]) are exceptions.

For more information on CCM and TCM, refer to Chapter 9.

Example

➤ ***CPT* describes 99401–99404 as representing services provided face-to-face by a physician or other QHP for the purposes of promoting health and preventing illness or injury.** Yet some payers directly instruct that codes such as 99401 be reported for specific services by specific clinical staff or by NQHCPs such as medical nutritionists or certified lactation consultants.

Teaching Point: Always keep a printed or electronic copy of payer guidance that conflicts with *CPT* or standard billing practices.

Scope of Practice Laws

Scope of practice is a term used by state licensing boards for various professions to define the procedures, actions, and processes that are permitted for a licensed individual. Scope of practice may also address the delegation of health care activities to unlicensed individuals who the delegating physician or other QHP/NQHCP has ascertained have the education, training, and/or certification necessary to safely perform the activity. Additional limitations on scope of practice of NQHCPs and on delegation to clinical staff may come from Medicaid programs, health care systems, or health care professional membership organizations.

Physicians, RNs, clinical NPs, PAs, LPNs, physical therapists, and licensed nutritionists are among some of the professions for which scope of practice laws are defined. Some states limit the autonomous practice of advanced practice professionals and require these QHPs to have written collaboration agreements and/or general or direct supervision by a physician. Prescribing authority may also be limited. Verify your state's requirements for all clinicians and appropriate inclusions in any collaboration/supervision agreements.

Every state has laws and regulations that describe the requirements of education and training for health care professionals. Some states, however, do not have different scope of practice laws for every level of professional (eg, LPN, lactation consultant). Health systems, government payers, and health care professional membership organizations may also define or limit the scope of practice or delegation to NQHCPs and clinical staff.

Scope of practice should be considered when delegating directly or through standing orders (eg, physician writes order that recommended screening instruments be completed for all patients presenting for well-baby/child [health supervision] examinations).

Although scope of practice provides guidance on what services may be performed by NQHCPs and clinical staff, certain codes also limit who can report specific services. For instance, nurses are allowed to counsel for and administer immunizations, but administration codes **90460** and **90461** are reported only when a physician or QHP has provided immunization counseling. Likewise, E/M services are reported only by a physician or QHP, although NQHCPs and clinical staff may perform tasks included in the service (eg, obtaining vital signs and initial history).

- Payers that follow Medicare policy on reporting E/M services will not accept **98000–98016**, **99202–99205**, **99212–99215**, or **99217–99499** performed and reported by NQHCPs. Codes **99211** and **99281** describe E/M services that may not require a physician's presence but are reported by a supervising physician or QHP. For full discussion of **99211**, refer to **Chapter 7**. Code **99281** is discussed in **Chapter 14**.

National Provider Identifier

The NPI is a unique ID number for covered health care professionals. The NPI is required on administrative and financial transactions under the Health Insurance Portability and Accountability Act of 1996 administrative simplification provisions.

- Anyone who directly provides health care services (eg, physical therapist, nutritionist, audiologist) can apply for and receive an NPI.
- Usually only those who will bill for services and/or order services or prescription drugs will need an NPI.
- The NPI is included on medical claims to indicate who ordered, provided, or supervised the provision of services.

Nonphysician Assessment and Management Services

An NQHCP whose scope of practice does not include providing and independently reporting E/M services may report assessment and management services. Assessment and management services may be provided in person (as discussed for specific types of services throughout this chapter), via online digital communication or telephone, or as a participant of a team conference. Each type of assessment and management service has specific reporting guidelines.

Online Medical Assessment (98970–98972)

98970 NQHCP online digital assessment and management service, for an established patient, for up to seven days, cumulative time during the 7 days; 5–10 minutes

98971 11–20 minutes

98972 21 or more minutes

An online electronic medical assessment (**98970–98972**) is a non–face-to-face assessment and management service by an NQHCP to an established patient using internet resources in response to a patient's online inquiry.

Online digital E/M services by a physician or other QHP (who may report E/M services) are reported with 99421–99423. Refer to Chapter 20 for information on online digital E/M services.

Online assessment and management refers to use of asynchronous communication technology such as secure email and other asynchronous digital communication.

This contrasts with *telemedicine services* provided via synchronous interactive audio-only or audio and video telecommunications systems that permit real-time communication between the NQHCP and the patient.

- Before providing online medical services, understand local and state laws, ensure that communications will be compliant with the Health Insurance Portability and Accountability Act (eg, conducted through a secure patient portal), establish written guidelines and procedures, educate payers and negotiate for payment, and educate patients.
- Codes 98970–98972 are time-based codes used by an NQHCP to report an online assessment and management service (eg, managing feeding problems in a patient with chronic illness).
- One code and 1 unit of service are reported for the sum of communications pertaining to the online encounter during a 7-day period.
- The 7-day service period begins with the initial, personal NQHCP review of the patient-generated inquiry.
- All time spent addressing the manifesting problem and any additional problems (including new unrelated problems addressed by online electronic communications) during the service period is cumulative and reported as 1 service.
- Online assessment and management includes
  - Review of the initial inquiry
  - Review of patient records or data pertinent to assessing the patient's problem
  - Personal NQHCP interaction with clinical staff focused on the patient's problem
  - Development of management plans
  - Timely reply to the patient's/caregiver's request for online service
  - Permanent record of the service (hard copy or electronic)
  - All related communications during a 7-day episode of care (eg, conducting related phone calls)
  - Cumulative time of NQHCPs in the same group who provide distinct portions of the online digital E/M service

Online digital assessment services (98970–98972) are *not* reported

- ✖ For services of less than 5 minutes' cumulative time.
- ✖ For new patient inquiries, although new problems may be addressed for established patients.
- ✖ For electronic communication of test results, scheduling of appointments, or other communication that does not include assessment and management.
- ✖ If the patient generates an online digital inquiry within 7 days of a previous treatment or assessment and management service and both services relate to the same problem.
- ✖ If a separately reported assessment service occurs within 7 days of the initial online digital inquiry.
- ✖ When care plan oversight (99374, 99375; 99377–99380), CCM (99487, 99489–99491), TCM (99495, 99496), or collection of physiologic data (99091) are provided in the same period, do not count the time of communications related to these services toward the time of online digital medical services.

Example

➤ **Parents of a patient with type 1 diabetes securely email a medical nutrition therapist who is a certified diabetes educator, requesting advice on preparing their child for adhering to the diabetes care plan on a weeklong trip with a sports team.** The diabetes educator responds to the request, and emails are exchanged to further clarify concerns and provide advice. The child is instructed to contact the diabetes educator or the treating physician by phone if questions or concerns arise during travel. The cumulative time of the communication is 15 minutes.

The diabetes educator reports 98971. But if the patient had been seen within the past 7 days or scheduled for an appointment within the 7-day period, this service would not have been separately reported.

Telephone Calls (98966–98968)

98966 Telephone assessment and management services provided by an NQHCP to an established patient, parent, or guardian not originating from related assessment and management service provided within the previous 7 days nor leading to an assessment and management service or procedure within the next 24 hours or soonest available appointment; 5–10 minutes of medical discussion

98967 11–20 minutes of medical discussion
98968 21–30 minutes of medical discussion

Codes **98966–98968** are used to report telephone assessment and management services by NQHCPs. The QHPs, who may independently provide and report E/M services, report **98008–98015** for an audio-only telemedicine E/M service, as discussed in **Chapter 20**.

Report **98966–98968** when

- The patient or caregiver initiates a call that is not in follow-up to a service by the same NQHCP within the past 7 days.
- Five minutes or more is spent in assessment and management services (*time must be documented*).
- No decision to see the patient within 24 hours or at the next available appointment is made during the telephone service.

Services Not Reported as Telephone Assessment and Management

Most telephone services provided by clinical staff (eg, relaying physician instructions) are included in the practice expense value assigned to NQHCP services and not separately reported.

Do not report telephone assessment and management services that

- ✖ Relate to a service provided by the NQHCP within the past 7 days (including another service reported with **98966–98968**), regardless of whether the service was planned or prompted by patient or caregiver concern.
- ✖ Result in scheduling an appointment within the next 24 hours or the next available appointment. When telephone assessment and management result in scheduling the patient for an appointment within 24 hours or the next available appointment, the service is considered preservice work to the face-to-face encounter.

Example

➤ **An adolescent patient with history of class 1 obesity and prediabetes, now overweight, contacts a licensed clinical social worker (LCSW) who has previously provided education and training for patient self-management. The patient has questions regarding a new diet plan.** The social worker spends 32 minutes on the phone with the patient discussing the risks and benefits of implementing the diet plan versus resuming a previously adopted plan.

The LCSW reports **98968** according to the time spent addressing the parents' concerns. Although the time of medical discussion exceeded 30 minutes, there is no code for reporting the time beyond 30 minutes. This service would not have been reported had the call happened within 7 days of a previous service by the same provider or resulted in an appointment within 24 hours or the next available face-to-face appointment.

Payer Use of Healthcare Common Procedure Coding System Codes

Disease Management Program Services

HCPCS Level II codes may be reported when the narrative differs from the *CPT* code for the service. What follows is a small sample of HCPCS codes and modifiers that may be used for services by NQHCPs when a payer accepts these codes to describe services rendered as part of a specific disease management program (eg, services specific to management of sickle cell anemia).

Payment for services reported with HCPCS codes may vary, especially for codes not assigned relative value units in the Medicare Physician Fee Schedule, on which many payers base their fee schedules.

Where a nonspecific term for a health care professional (eg, *nurse* versus *RN*) is included in a code descriptor, or when the code descriptor does not include identification of a health care professional, review the specific payer's policy for coverage of the service provided. It is advisable to retain copies of a payer's written policies and guidance for reporting HCPCS codes such as

S0315 Disease management program; initial assessment and initiation of the program
S0316 Disease management program, follow-up/reassessment
S0317 Disease management program; per diem
S0320 Telephone calls by a registered nurse to a disease management program member for monitoring purposes; per month
S9460 Diabetic management program, nurse visit
S9470 Nutritional counseling, dietitian visit

For an example of how to report services as part of a disease management program for diabetes, refer to the Payer-Specific Coding for Nutrition Assessment and Intervention section later in this chapter.

Payer policies, particularly Medicaid plan policies, often drive the decision between reporting with *CPT* and reporting with HCPCS.

Healthcare Common Procedure Coding System Modifiers

Payers may also instruct certain NQHCPs to report services by appending a HCPCS modifier to the *CPT* or HCPCS code for services provided.

HA Child/adolescent program
HN Bachelor's degree level
HO Master's degree level (eg, licensed master social worker)
HP Doctoral level
HQ Group setting
SW Services provided by a certified diabetic educator
UN Two patients served
UP Three patients served
UQ Four patients served
UR Five patients served
US Six or more patients served

Nutritional Support Services

Breastfeeding Support/Lactation Services (S9443, 99211)

Under the Patient Protection and Affordable Care Act, most health insurance plans must cover breastfeeding support, counseling, and equipment to mothers for the duration of breastfeeding. These services are not subject to a deductible, co-payment, or coinsurance. Access to benefits for lactation counseling, however, is not always straightforward.

Be aware that some plans bundle provision of breastfeeding support and counseling to the global obstetric service or postpartum care of the mother and do not pay separately for breastfeeding support or lactation counseling. It is important to understand contractual obligations that may limit a physician's or NQHCP's ability to bill the patient for these covered services.

Medicaid plans often ask that covered breastfeeding mothers be referred to the Special Supplemental Nutrition Program for Women, Infants, and Children for lactation counseling and other support services.

In the absence of feeding problems of an infant or health problems of the mother, **Z39.1** (encounter for care and examination of lactating mother) is the diagnosis code reported for lactation counseling.

Lactation consultation services do not have a specific *CPT* code, and billing is a source of confusion for many providers. Many states do not license lactation consultants. Also, many health plans do not include lactation consultants in their networks.

Code **S9443** is the code most specific to lactation services. This code is included in some health plan policies for preventive medicine services or breastfeeding/lactation counseling services.

S9443 Lactation classes, nonphysician provider, per session

Clinical staff services may be reported with **99211** when provided incident to a physician's plan of care for an established patient (health plan policies may or may not align with Medicare's incident-to policy). Refer to the "Lactation-Related Services by a Physician or Other Qualified Health Care Professional" box later in this chapter for more about E/M codes for lactation services.

Other specific codes used to report these services when provided by NQHCPs may include

S9445 Patient education, not otherwise classified, nonphysician provider, individual, per session
S9446 Patient education, not otherwise classified, nonphysician provider, group, per session
★98960 Education and training for patient self-management by a nonphysician qualified health care professional using a standardized curriculum, face-to-face with the patient (could include caregiver/family), each 30 minutes; individual patient

Refer to the Education and Training for Patient Self-Management (98960–98962) section later in this chapter for more information.

Key considerations for reporting lactation services include

- Unless the newborn or infant has been diagnosed with a feeding problem, the mother is typically the patient, and claims are filed to the mother's health benefit plan.
- Payer policies may not allow separate payment for lactation counseling on the same date as an E/M service.
- Challenges might be encountered in states where licensure is not yet enacted for lactation support professionals. Hurdles include credentialing and coverage by payers that cover only services provided by licensed health care professionals, although services provided incident to a physician or QHP (eg, 99211 or S9443) may be allowed.
- When a medical condition (eg, feeding problem) was diagnosed by the physician on an earlier date, an NQHCP may see the mother and patient to identify the psychological, behavioral, emotional, cognitive, and social factors important to the prevention, treatment, or management of physical health problems. Behavioral health assessment and intervention codes 96156, 96158 and 96159, and 96164–96171 may be reportable for these services. Again, payer policy determines who may provide these services and what is paid.
- Lactation counseling provided by an NQHCP in conjunction with a physician's or QHP's E/M service, although not always separately reported, may reduce the physician's time spent on history taking, counseling, and education. This may also support quality initiatives.

Lactation-Related Services by a Physician or Other Qualified Health Care Professional

Physicians and QHPs may report preventive medicine counseling codes 99401–99404 for personally performed lactation counseling services. When payer policy instructs that these codes be reported for services by an RN or an NQHCP (eg, lactation consultant), a written copy of the payer policy should be kept on file.

When a pediatrician provides services related to newborn or infant feeding problems or maternal health issues, report E/M codes by site of service (eg, office visit). E/M services provided to address maternal issues are reported to the mother's health plan. An *International Classification of Diseases, 10th Revision, Clinical Modification* (*ICD-10-CM*) code is used to identify the type of problem (eg, O92.5, suppressed lactation).

Nonphysician Qualified Health Care Professional Services

Chapter 12

Medical Nutrition Assessment and Intervention (97802–97804)

★◄97802 Medical nutrition therapy; initial assessment and intervention, individual, face-to-face with the patient, each 15 minutes

★◄97803 Reassessment and intervention, individual, face-to-face with the patient, each 15 minutes

★◄97804 group (2 or more individuals), each 30 minutes

Medical nutrition therapy is one of the services for which *CPT* instruction excludes reporting by a physician or QHP who may report E/M services.

- Codes are reported when provided by an NQHCP who may report medical nutrition therapy services under their individual state's scope of practice.
- Many states restrict the provision of medical nutrition therapy to certain NQHCPs (eg, registered dietitians, licensed medical nutritionists). Practices providing medical nutrition therapy services should be aware of state licensing and scope of practice regulations as well as health plan credentialing policies.
- HCPCS modifiers may be required to report the type of provider for medical nutrition therapy services, such as AE (registered dietitian).
- Coverage may also be limited to patients with certain conditions (eg, diabetes, kidney disease) and to a number of units of service or visits per year.
- When medical nutrition therapy is provided as a preventive service (eg, counseling a patient who has overweight), modifier 33 may be appended to 97802–97804.

For more on modifier 33, refer to Chapters 2 and 8.

- Services are reported according to time. Per *CPT* instruction, a unit of time is met when the midpoint is passed.
  - Report 97802 or 97803 with 1 unit for 8 to 22 minutes of service. An additional unit may be reported for each subsequent 15 minutes and the last 8 to 22 minutes of service.
  - Certain payers may require that the time in the code descriptor (eg, 15 minutes) be met or exceeded for each unit of service reported.
- Time must be documented.

● indicates a new code; ▲, revised; #, re-sequenced; ✚, add-on; ★, audiovisual technology; and ◄, synchronous interactive audio.

Examples

➤ **A physician refers a 28-month-old child to a registered dietitian for weight loss associated with cystic fibrosis and exocrine pancreatic insufficiency.** Assessment and intervention are requested out of concern for failure to thrive and related decrease in lung function. The child's body mass index (BMI) has fallen to the fifth percentile. Parents report feeding numerous high-fat meals a day and nonfat snacks. The dietitian meets with the family and spends 30 minutes discussing appropriate high-calorie and high-protein meals and snacks, enzyme use, and monitoring intake and weight gain/growth.

ICD-10-CM	*CPT*
Z71.3 (dietary counseling and surveillance) R63.4 (abnormal weight loss) E84.8 (cystic fibrosis with other manifestations) K86.81 (exocrine pancreatic insufficiency) Z68.52 (BMI pediatric, 5th–<85th percentile for age)	If payer allows billing under the registered dietitian's NPI, 97802 × 2 (medical nutrition therapy, initial assessment and intervention, individual, face-to-face with the patient, each 15 minutes) If payer requires billing under the NPI of a supervising physician, 97802 AE × 2 (medical nutrition therapy as above by a registered dietitian)

Teaching Point: Some Medicaid plans and/or private payers may require that medical nutrition therapy, when provided in the physician practice, be provided under a physician's order and general supervision. Services are reported as if provided by the physician, but modifier AE indicates that the service was provided by a registered dietitian.

➤ **A group of adolescent patients with type 1 diabetes is referred to a licensed medical nutritionist for reassessment and intervention.** The patients receive both individual reassessment and group therapy services for a total time of 50 minutes.

ICD-10-CM	*CPT*
Z71.3 (dietary counseling and surveillance) E10.- (type 1 diabetes mellitus [additional characters required to indicate manifestations or lack thereof])	If payer allows billing under the registered dietitian's NPI 97804 × 2 (medical nutrition therapy, reassessment and intervention, each 30 minutes) If payer requires billing under the NPI of the supervising physician 97804 AE × 2 (medical nutrition therapy as above by a registered dietitian)

Teaching Point: The service provided to a group, even with individual reassessments in the group setting, is reported to each patient's health plan with 97804 with 1 unit per 30 minutes. Because the time of service was 50 minutes, 2 units of service are reported (ie, the midpoint between the first and last 30-minute periods was passed).

Payer-Specific Coding for Nutrition Assessment and Intervention

HCPCS codes may be required by certain payers to report reassessment and subsequent intervention after a change in diagnosis, medical condition, or treatment.

G0270 Medical nutrition therapy; reassessment and subsequent intervention(s) following second referral in same year for change in diagnosis, medical condition, or treatment regimen (including additional hours needed for renal disease); individual, face-to-face with the patient, each 15 minutes

G0271 group (2 or more individuals), each 30 minutes

Documentation of services should include the physician or QHP order for services, information on the medical need for services, medical nutrition therapy evaluation and plan for intervention, time, correspondence with the referring provider, date of service (DOS), and name, credentials, and signature of the provider of the medical nutrition therapy.

Payers may also offer specific benefits for nutrition assessments and counseling under specific disease management programs. HCPCS codes may be required in lieu of *CPT* codes.

G0108 Diabetes outpatient self-management training services, individual, per 30 minutes

G0109 Diabetes outpatient self-management training services, group session (2 or more), per 30 minutes

S9449 Weight management classes, NPP, per session

S9452 Nutrition class, NPP, per session

S9455 Diabetic management program, group session
S9460 nurse visit
S9465 dietitian visit
S9470 Nutritional counseling, dietitian visit

Example

➤ **A group of adolescent patients with type 1 diabetes is referred to a licensed medical nutritionist for reassessment and intervention as part of a diabetes outpatient self-management training program.** The patients receive both individual reassessment and group therapy services for a total time of 50 minutes.

ICD-10-CM	CPT
E10.- (type 1 diabetes mellitus [additional characters required to indicate manifestations or lack thereof]) Z71.3 (dietary counseling and surveillance)	If payer allows billing with *CPT* 97804 × 2 (medical nutrition therapy, reassessment and intervention, each 30 minutes) If payer requires billing with HCPCS G0109 × 2 (diabetes outpatient self-management training services, group session [2 or more], per 30 minutes)

Teaching Point: The service should be reported per the individual payer's policy for the program. Note also that a payer may require that the time of service be met or exceeded (ie, a second unit of service will be reported only if time meets or exceeds 60 minutes).

Adaptive Behavior Assessment and Treatment Services

Adaptive behavior services address

- Deficient adaptive behaviors, such as impaired social, communication, or self-care skills
- Maladaptive behaviors, such as repetitive and stereotyped behaviors
- Behaviors that risk physical harm to the patient, others, and/or property

Codes for adaptive behavior services are a combination of Category I and Category III (emerging technology) *CPT* codes. Adaptive behavior services may be delivered by a physician or QHP but more typically are provided by a behavioral analyst and/or licensed psychologist working with assistant behavior analysts or technicians. Services are typically reported for conditions that develop with maladaptive behaviors, such as autism spectrum disorder (ASD).

It is important to verify health plan policies for coverage and payment of adaptive behavior services, including any required provider qualifications (eg, certification, licensure) and prior authorization before provision of services.

Most states mandate coverage of adaptive behavior services for patients diagnosed with ASD. Some states require that behavior analysts providing ASD-related assessment and/or treatment be licensed and/or certified by the Behavior Analyst Certification Board as a Board Certified Behavior Analyst or Board Certified Behavior Analyst–Doctoral.

- In the discussion of adaptive behavior services, Board Certified Behavior Analysts and licensed psychologists are QHPs who typically can independently report personally preformed services and services provided by technicians under the QHP's general supervision.

Refer to your procedure coding reference (eg, *CPT* coding manual) for specific instructions for reporting these services, including definitions of functional behavioral assessment, functional analysis, standardized instruments and procedures, and non-standardized instruments and procedures.

The general rule is that time is met when the midpoint is passed (eg, at least 8 minutes of service is required to support a service specified as 15 minutes).

Adaptive Behavior Assessment (97151–97152, 0362T)

#97151 Behavior identification assessment, administered by a physician or other QHP, each 15 minutes of the physician's or other QHP's time face-to-face with patient and/or guardian(s)/caregiver(s) administering assessments and discussing findings and recommendations, and non-face-to-face analyzing past data, scoring/interpreting the assessment, and preparing the report/treatment plan

#97152 Behavior identification supporting assessment, administered by one technician under the direction of a physician or other QHP, face-to-face with the patient, each 15 minutes

0362T Behavior identification supporting assessment, each 15 minutes of technicians' time face-to-face with a patient, requiring the following components:
- administration by the physician or other QHP who is on site;
- with the assistance of two or more technicians;
- for a patient who exhibits destructive behavior;
- completion in an environment that is customized to the patient's behavior.

Behavior identification assessment (**97151**) is conducted by a physician or other QHP and may include

- Analysis of pertinent past data, including medical diagnosis
- A detailed behavioral history
- Patient observation
- Administration of standardized and/or non-standardized instruments and procedures
- Functional behavior assessment
- Functional analysis
- Guardian/caregiver interview to identify and describe deficient adaptive behaviors, maladaptive behaviors, and other impaired functioning secondary to deficient adaptive or maladaptive behaviors

Documentation should include a report of the assessment and a person-centered treatment plan.

If the physician or other QHP personally performs the technician activities, their time engaged in these activities should be included as part of the required technician time to meet the components of the code.

- Codes **97151**, **97152**, and **0362T** may be repeated on the same or different days until the behavior identification assessment (**97151**) and, if necessary, supporting assessment(s) (**97152**, **0362T**) are complete.
- Code **97152** is reported for assessment by a technician. The reporting physician or QHP is not required to be on-site during the assessment. Refer to **0362T** when multiple technicians and a customized assessment environment are required for a patient's destructive behavior(s).
- Code **0362T** represents testing of a patient who demonstrates destructive behavior (ie, maladaptive behaviors associated with a high risk of medical consequences or property damage) and requires multiple technicians and an environment customized to the patient and behavior. *The reporting physician or QHP is required to be on-site* (ie, immediately available and interruptible to provide assistance and direction throughout the performance of the procedure). The reporting physician or QHP is not required to be in the room during testing.
- Count the time of only 1 technician when 2 or more technicians are present. Code **0362T** is reported according to a single technician's face-to-face time with the patient and not the combined time of multiple technicians (eg, 1 hour with 3 technicians equals 1 hour of service) despite the expectation that more than one technician will be needed.

Examples

➤ **A 3-year-old child with characteristics of ASD presents for assessment.** The physician/QHP spends 1 hour face-to-face with the patient and/or guardian(s)/caregiver(s) administering assessments and discussing findings and recommendations and 38 minutes of non–face-to-face time analyzing past data, scoring/interpreting the assessment, and preparing the report/treatment plan. The total time of service is 98 minutes. Code **97151** is reported with 7 units (1 for each full 15 minutes of service and 1 for the last 8 minutes).

Teaching Point: If less than 8 minutes past the last full 15 minutes of service were provided, only the number of 15-minute periods of service would be reported (eg, 1 hour 37 minutes equals 6 units).

➤ **An additional assessment of the 3-year-old from the previous example is required to assess behavior that interferes with acquisition of adaptive skills.** A technician, under the physician's or QHP's direction, observes and records occurrences of the patient's deficient adaptive and maladaptive behaviors and the surrounding environmental events several times in a variety of situations. The physician/QHP reviews and analyzes data from the technician's observations. The face-to-face time of the technician is 1 hour.

Code **97152** is reported with 4 units of service.

➤ **An 11-year-old child with ASD requires evaluation to assess increased self-injury and aggression toward others.** A team of technicians conducts the assessment session in a room that is devoid of any objects that might cause injury. A physician/QHP is on-site and immediately available throughout the session. The technicians implement functional analysis (ie, they systematically present and withdraw events to the patient multiple times while observing and measuring occurrence of a target behavior) as directed by the physician/QHP and record data. Graphed data are reviewed and analyzed by the physician/QHP to identify the environmental events in whose presence the level of behavior was highest and lowest. The technicians spend a total of 90 minutes face-to-face with the patient during the assessment.

Code **0362T** is reported with 6 units of service.

Adaptive Behavior Treatment

Adaptive behavior treatment services address specific treatment targets and goals based on results of previous assessments and include ongoing assessment and adjustment of treatment protocols, targets, and goals. Codes describe services to an individual patient, groups of patients, families, and an individual patient who exhibits destructive behavior.

Codes for adaptive behavior treatment specify services provided by protocol (**97153**, **97154**) or with protocol modification (**97155**, **97158**, **0373T**). Behavior treatment with protocol modification requires adjustments be *made in real time* rather than for a subsequent service.

Adaptive Behavior Treatment by Protocol (97153–97154)

#97153 Adaptive behavior treatment by protocol, administered by technician under the direction of a physician or other QHP, face-to-face with one patient; each 15 minutes

#97154 Group adaptive behavior treatment by protocol, administered by technician under the direction of a physician or other QHP, face-to-face with two or more patients, each 15 minutes

- Adaptive behavior treatment by protocol to a single patient (**97153**) and group adaptive behavior treatment by protocol (**97154**) are administered by a technician under the direction of a physician/QHP, with a treatment protocol *designed in advance* by the physician or other QHP, who may or may not provide direction during the treatment.
  - The service described by **97153** is face-to-face with only 1 patient.
  - Code **97154** is reported for services delivered face-to-face with 2 or more patients but not more than 8 patients.
- Codes **97153** and **97154** do not include protocol modification.
- If the physician/QHP personally performs the technician activities, their time spent engaged in these activities should be reported as technician time. The physician is not required to be on-site during the provision of these services.

Examples

➤ **A 4-year-old child with ASD presents with differences in language and social skills and emotional outbursts in response to small changes in routines or when preferred items are unavailable.** A QHP directs a technician in the implementation of treatment protocols and data collection procedures. The technician conducts a treatment session in the family home with multiple planned opportunities for the patient to practice target skills. The QHP reviews the technician's recorded and graphed data to assess the child's progress and determine if any treatment protocol needs adjustment. The technician spends 1 hour at the patient's home with face-to-face time of the treatment session lasting 50 minutes. Code **97153** is reported with 3 units of service.

Teaching Point: Only the technician's face-to-face time with the patient is used to determine the units of service. This service may also be conducted in a community setting (eg, playground, store).

➤ **Peer social skills training in a small group is recommended for a 7-year-old child with differences in social skills resulting from ASD.** A technician conducts the group session with treatment protocols and data collection procedures as previously designed by a QHP. The QHP reviews the technician's recorded and graphed data to assess the child's progress and determine if treatment protocols need adjustment. The total face-to-face time of the session is 60 minutes.

Code **97154** is reported with 4 units.

Adaptive Behavior Treatment With Protocol Modification (97155, 97158, 0373T)

#97155 Adaptive behavior treatment with protocol modification administered by physician or other QHP, which may include simultaneous direction of technician, face-to-face with one patient, each 15 minutes

#97158 Group adaptive behavior treatment with protocol modification, administered by physician or other QHP, face-to-face with multiple patients, each 15 minutes

0373T Adaptive behavior treatment with protocol modification, each 15 minutes of technicians' time face-to-face with a patient, requiring the following components:
- administration by the physician or other QHP who is on site;
- with the assistance of two or more technicians;
- for a patient who exhibits destructive behavior;
- completion in an environment that is customized to the patient's behavior.

- Adaptive behavior treatment with protocol modification (**97155**) is administered by a physician/QHP *face-to-face with a single patient.*
  - The physician/QHP resolves one or more problems with the protocol and may simultaneously direct a technician in administering the modified protocol *while the patient is present.*
  - Physician/QHP direction to the technician without the patient present is not reported separately.
- Group adaptive behavior treatment with protocol modification (**97158**) is reported when a physician/QHP provides *face-to-face* protocol modification services with up to 8 patients in a group. The physician/QHP monitors the needs of individual patients and adjusts treatment techniques during the group sessions, as needed.
- Adaptive behavior treatment with protocol modification (**0373T**) is reported for services to a patient who presents with one or more destructive behavior(s).
  - The service time is based on a single technician's face-to-face time with the patient and not the combined time of multiple technicians.
  - The physician/QHP must be on-site and immediately available during the service described by **0373T**.

Examples

➤ **A 5-year-old child previously showed steady improvements in language and social skills at home as a result of 1:1 intensive applied behavior analysis intervention, but skill development seems to have recently reached a plateau.** A QHP modifies the previously used written protocols to incorporate procedures designed to build the child's language and social skills into daily home routines (eg, play, dressing, mealtimes). The QHP demonstrates the procedures to the technician and directs the technician to implement the protocols with the child. The QHP then observes and provides feedback as the technician implements the procedures with the child. The technician's face-to-face time with the patient is 45 minutes. Code **97155** is reported with 3 units of service.

Teaching Point: Time spent by the technician and QHP without the patient present is not included in the time of service.

➤ **A 13-year-old teen is reported to be isolated from peers because of poor social skills and odd behavior.** The teen attends a group treatment session that focuses on peer social skills. A QHP begins the group session by asking each patient to briefly describe 2 of their recent social encounters with peers, one that went well and one that did not. The information is used to develop a group activity through which each patient can practice the skills they used in the encounters that went well and can problem-solve the interactions that did not go well. The QHP helps each patient identify social cues that were interpreted correctly and incorrectly and what they could have done differently. The QHP also provides prompts and feedback individualized to each patient's skills. The QHP ends the session by summarizing the discussion. The total time of the session was 70 minutes, including a 10-minute break (ie, 60 minutes of group session). Code **97158** is reported with 4 units of service.

Teaching Point: Only the QHP's face-to-face time spent providing the service is reported.

➤ **A 16-year-old teen has had 2 surgical procedures to relieve esophageal blockages caused by pica involving repeat ingestion of small metal objects (eg, paper clips, pushpins).** The patient's pica behavior has not responded to previous treatment. The QHP supervising the patient's treatment plan has previously developed written protocols for reducing the patient's pica. A technician carefully inspects the room before the session to make sure no potential pica items are accessible to the patient. Two technicians are present, with one guiding the patient through a series of trials in which the patient is presented with a food item and a nonhazardous item that resembles a pica item. The second technician prompts the patient to choose the food item and blocks attempts to choose the pica item. The patient's response to each trial is recorded. The QHP is on-site and available to assist as needed. The total session lasts 40 minutes. Code **0373T** is reported with 3 units.

Teaching Point: Although 2 technicians were present, time is counted only once. The midpoint rule allows reporting a unit of service for the final 10 minutes of service.

Family Adaptive Behavior Treatment Guidance (97156–97157)

Family adaptive behavior treatment guidance (97156) and multiple-family group adaptive behavior treatment guidance (97157) are administered by a physician or QHP face-to-face with guardian(s)/caregiver(s) and involve identifying potential treatment targets and training guardian(s)/caregiver(s) to implement treatment protocols designed to address deficient adaptive or maladaptive behaviors.

#97156 Family adaptive behavior treatment guidance, administered by physician or other QHP (with or without the patient present), face-to-face with guardian(s)/caregiver(s), each 15 minutes

#97157 Multiple-family group adaptive behavior treatment guidance, administered by physician or other QHP (without the patient present), face-to-face with multiple sets of guardians/caregivers, each 15 minutes

- Family adaptive behavior treatment guidance (97156) provided to the caregiver(s) of 1 patient may be performed with or without the patient present. Adaptive behavior treatment in which the parent(s) or guardian(s) are present but not part of the therapy would not qualify as family adaptive behavior treatment.
- Family adaptive behavior treatment guidance provided to the caregiver(s) of multiple patients (97157) is performed without the patients present. The group must be no larger than the caregiver(s) of 8 patients. *CPT* does not include a code for reporting services to a group of 9 or more patients.

Examples

➤ **The parents of a 6-year-old child seek training in procedures for helping the child communicate through picture cards during typical family routines, a skill he previously developed in adaptive behavior treatment therapy sessions with technicians.** A physician/QHP trains the parents. The service includes reviewing the written treatment and data collection protocols with the parents, demonstrating how to implement the cards in role-playing and with the child, and having the parents implement the protocols with the child while the provider observes and provides feedback. The time of service is 1 hour.

Code 97156 is reported with 4 units of service.

➤ **The parents of a 3-year-old child who has pervasive hyperactivity and no functional play, social, or communication skills seek training in how to manage his hyperactive and disruptive behavior and help him develop appropriate play, social, and communication skills.** The parents attend a group session (without the patient) led by a physician who asks each set of parents to identify 1 skill to be increased or 1 problem behavior to be decreased in their own child. The physician describes how behavior analytic principles and procedures could be applied to the behavior identified by the parents of the 3-year-old patient. The physician demonstrates a procedure (eg, prompting the child to speak instead of whining when he wants something; not giving him preferred items when he whines). The parents then role-play, implementing that procedure. Other group participants and the physician provide feedback and make constructive suggestions. That process is repeated for skills/behaviors identified by other sets of parents. The group session ends with the physician summarizing the main points, answering questions, and giving each set of parents a homework assignment to practice the skills they worked on during the session. The session lasts 110 minutes. Code 97157 is reported with 7 units.

Teaching Point: The last 5 minutes is not reported because the midpoint of 8 minutes beyond the last full 15-minute period (105 minutes) was not passed.

Habilitative and Rehabilitative Modifiers (96, 97)

Adaptive behavior services may be either habilitative or rehabilitative. *Habilitative* services help an individual learn skills not yet developed and keep and/or improve those skills. *Rehabilitative* services help a patient keep, get back, or improve skills that have been lost or limited because of illness, injury, and/or disability. Because the Patient Protection and Affordable Care Act requires that certain health plans provide equal coverage for habilitative and rehabilitative services and count each type of service separately, it may be necessary to indicate that a service is habilitative or rehabilitative. Modifiers 96 (habilitative services) and 97 (rehabilitative services) are appended to procedure codes to designate the nature of a service. Modifiers 96 and 97 may not be adopted for use by all payers or may have limited utility. Verify payer policies for these modifiers when providing habilitative and rehabilitative services.

Other Nonphysician Qualified Health Care Professional Services

Medical Team Conferences (99366, 99368)

99366 Medical team conference with interdisciplinary team of health care professionals, face-to-face with patient and/or family, 30 minutes or more; participation by nonphysician qualified health care professional

99368 Medical team conference with interdisciplinary team of health care professionals, patient and/or family not present, 30 minutes or more; participation by nonphysician qualified health care professional

Although included in the E/M section of *CPT*, 99366 and 99368 are reported for services by NQHCPs. Physicians and QHPs report team conference participation *without the patient or caregiver present* with 99367. Refer to Chapter 9 for more information.

Medical team conference codes are used to report participation by a minimum of 3 health care professionals, including physicians, QHPs, and NQHCPs, of different specialties in conferences to coordinate or manage care and services for established patients with chronic or multiple health conditions (eg, a child with ventilator dependence and developmental delays, seizures, and a gastrostomy tube for nutrition).

- Codes differentiate between face-to-face (**99366**) and non–face-to-face (patient and/or family is not present [**99368**]) team conference services.
- Medicaid and commercial payers may follow these Medicare requirements or have their own specific rules.
- One unit of service is reported for each conference of 30 minutes or more.

Medical team conferences require

- In-person participation by a minimum of 3 health care professionals (any combination of NQHCPs, physicians, and/or QHPs) from different subspecialties or disciplines (eg, speech pathologists, dietitians, social workers), with or without the patient, family member(s), community agencies, surrogate decision-maker(s) (eg, legal guardian), and/or caregiver(s) as *CPT* does not include **99366** and **99368** in the codes reportable for telemedicine services

Verify payer policies for care team conferences. Although payment for 99366 and 99368 is bundled into payment for other services in the Medicare Physician Fee Schedule, some benefit plans allow separate payment when an NQHCP participates either in person or virtually.

- Active involvement in developing, revising, coordinating, and implementing health care services needed by the patient by each participant
- That the participant has provided face-to-face evaluation(s) and/or treatment to the patient, separate from any team conference, within the previous 60 days
- Only 1 individual from the same specialty to report **99366–99368** for the same encounter
- Medical record documentation that supports the reporting individual's participation, the time spent from the beginning of review of an individual patient until the conclusion of review, and the contributed information and subsequent treatment recommendations

Medical team conferences *may not be reported* when

✖ The facility or organization is contractually obligated to provide the service, or the conferences are informal meetings or simple conversations between physicians and NQHCPs (eg, therapists).

✖ Less than 30 minutes of conference time is spent in a team conference.

Examples

➤ **A care team meets to discuss the care plans for a 4-year-old child with history of congenital heart disease, cerebrovascular injury with residual paraplegia, and developmental delays.** As the child nears entry to kindergarten, the pediatrician has requested input to the child's individualized education program and ongoing health care plan from all health care professionals. The pediatrician, cardiologist, physiatrist, occupational and physical therapists, speech pathologist, home care coordinator, and social worker attend the conference to discuss the child's current medical status, prognosis for the short and long term, and necessary accommodations for her education. The conference lasts 60 minutes. The patient and family are not present for the conference.

Nonphysician qualified health care professionals report participation using **99368** when the patient or caregivers are not present. Assign appropriate *ICD-10-CM* codes for the specified developmental delays (codes in categories **F80–F88**) and other health concerns addressed.

• indicates a new code; ▲, revised; #, re-sequenced; ✚, add-on; ★, audiovisual technology; and ◀, synchronous interactive audio.

➤ **A patient with cerebral palsy requires coordination with multiple health care professionals (eg, physical and occupational therapists, neurologist, pediatrician).** Each participant in the conference has completed their evaluation of the patient within 60 days before the conference, and a team conference of 40 minutes is held to assess the current plan of care and therapy. The patient's family is at this conference.

Code **99366** would be reported by the physical and occupational therapists. Physicians at the conference would report an E/M code that best describes their services on this date (eg, office or other outpatient E/M service based on face-to-face time with the family spent in counseling and/or coordination of care).

Education and Training for Patient Self-Management (98960–98962)

★**98960** Education and training for patient self-management by a nonphysician qualified health care professional using a standardized curriculum, face-to-face with the patient (could include caregiver/family) each 30 minutes; individual patient

★**98961** 2–4 patients

★**98962** 5–8 patients

Report **98960–98962** when

- The purpose of these services is to teach the patient and caregivers how to self-manage the illness or disease or delay coexisting conditions in conjunction with the patient's professional health care team.

Improved patient self-management may benefit a practice through payments received for quality initiatives related to management of complex and/or chronic conditions (eg, a percentage of patients aged 5–64 years and identified as having persistent asthma had a ratio of controller medications to total asthma medications of ≥0.50 during the measurement year). To learn more about how quality measurement may influence coding and payment, refer to Chapter 3.

- A physician prescribes the services and a standardized curriculum is used. A standardized curriculum is one that is consistent with guidelines or standards established or recognized by a physician or NQHCP society, association, or other appropriate source (eg, curriculum established or endorsed by the American Academy of Pediatrics).
- Qualifications of the NQHCPs and the content of the program are consistent with guidelines or standards established or recognized by a physician or NQHCP society, association, or other appropriate source.
  - These codes apply to diabetes and asthma self-management training—important categories of patient self-management education and training. Such training can be provided by nurse educators or other clinicians who have received special education and/or certification from accreditation societies or state licensing panels.
  - These services could be reported by the supervising physician when the services are rendered by the appropriately certified professional and acknowledged by the payer via the payer contract or published guidance. Some payers, however, include codes **98960–98962** in policies that allow payment only when reported directly by NQHCPs.
- Education and training services are provided face-to-face (including via audiovisual telemedicine service) to patients with an established illness or disease.
- When a standardized curriculum is not used in the provision of education and training for patient self-management, consider whether the service meets the requirements of health behavior assessment and interventions services by an NQHCP (**96156**, **96158**, **96159**, and **96164–96171**) as discussed in **Chapter 10**.

Qualifications of the NQHCPs and the content of patient self-management education (98960–98962) must be consistent with guidelines or standards established or recognized by a physician or NQHCP society, association, or other appropriate source.

Code selection is based on the number of patients receiving the service and the general *CPT* instruction for reporting services based on time. Time is met when the midpoint is passed (ie, report **98960** for ≥16 minutes of face-to-face time and with units of service for each additional full 30 minutes and the last 16–30 minutes).

Example

➤ **A 14-year-old patient was recently diagnosed with type 1 diabetes and is referred to the diabetes educator for continued training under an approved curriculum.** The certified nurse educator assesses what the patient and caregivers have learned since diagnosis and uses a standardized curriculum to provide additional education. The total documented time of service is 30 minutes.

Nonphysician Qualified Health Care Professional Services

Chapter 12

Code 98960 is reported for the 30 minutes of service. If the time of service extended 16 to 30 minutes beyond the first 30 minutes, an additional unit would be reported.

The content, type, duration, and patient response to the training must be documented in the medical record.

The payer contract will determine whether services are reported under the name of the diabetes educator, supervising physician, or QHP. If the payer credentials educators, report under the name and NPI of the educator. If the payer does not credential educators, follow payer guidance for reporting.

When the service is provided for multiple patients, either 98961 (2–4 patients) or 98962 (5–8) patients is reported.

Genetic Counseling Services (96041)

★◄96041 Medical genetics and genetic counseling services, each 30 minutes of total time provided by the genetic counselor on the date of the encounter

- Trained genetic counselors provide services that may include obtaining a structured family genetic history, pedigree construction, analysis for genetic risk assessment, and counseling of the patient and family.
- Report 96041 with a unit of service based on the *CPT* midpoint rule for time.
  - Report 1 unit for the first 16–45 minutes on the DOS.
  - Report an additional unit for each additional full 30 minutes and for the last 16 to 30 minutes.
- Services may include review of medical data and family information, face-to-face interviews, and counseling services. Education provided to the individual patient regarding genetic risks is reported with 96041.
- For education regarding genetic risks by an NQHCP to a group, refer to 98961 and 98962.
- Physicians and other QHPs may report E/M services for genetic counseling including
  - Problem-oriented E/M services (eg, 99212–99215) for counseling regarding symptoms or established disease
  - Preventive medicine counseling and risk factor reduction services (eg, 99401–99404) for counseling when a patient presents without symptoms or established disease

✖ Do not report 96041 for less than 16 minutes of genetic counselor time.

Nonphysician Qualified Health Care Professional Services

Chapter 12

Medication Therapy Management Services by a Pharmacist (99605–99607)

99605 Medication therapy management service(s) provided by a pharmacist, individual, face-to-face with patient, with assessment and intervention if provided; initial 15 minutes, new patient

99606 initial 15 minutes, established patient

✚99607 each additional 15 minutes (List separately in addition to 99605 or 99606)

Medication therapy management services

- Are provided only by a pharmacist face-to-face with the patient or caregiver and usually in relation to complex medication regimens or medication adherence in conditions such as asthma and diabetes.
- Are provided on request of the patient or caregiver, prescribing physician, other QHPs, or prescription drug benefit plan (not reported for routine dispensing-related activities).
- Are reported with codes selected according to the patient's status, new or established, and the pharmacist's face-to-face time with the patient.
- Include review of pertinent patient history (not limited to drug history).
- Include documentation of review of the pertinent patient history, medication profile (prescription and nonprescription), and recommendations for improving health outcomes and treatment adherence.
- *New patients* are those who have received no face-to-face service from the pharmacist or another pharmacist of the same clinic or pharmacy within 3 years before the current DOS.
- Unless otherwise specified by the payer policy, time is met when the midpoint is passed.
  - Report 99605 and 99606 for the first 8 to 22 minutes of face-to-face time with the patient.
  - When time exceeds 22 minutes, 99607 may be reported for subsequent 15-minute periods and the last 8 to 22 minutes.
- Under the Medicare program, pharmacists may also provide services incident to a physician or QHP and report E/M services with 99211 when allowed under the scope of practice as defined by state licensure.

Physical and Occupational Therapy (97161–97546)

Although many physical and occupational therapy services are included in a facility's charges, some states allow therapists to practice independently. There are codes for reporting therapy evaluations, reevaluations, and therapeutic activities/modalities. Payment for physical and occupational therapy services is often defined by not only the therapist's scope of practice but also the payer's credentialing and payment policies that often restrict the number of therapy services provided within a specific time frame.

Following are some of the codes commonly used for reporting evaluative and therapeutic services to create, revise, or carry out a therapy plan of care. Therapists use specific methods of evaluating (eg, occupational therapy profile with review of medical and therapy history and assessment of performance deficits) and providing therapeutic services based on clinical guidelines.

Therapeutic modalities are any physical agent applied to produce therapeutic changes to biological tissue including, but not limited to, thermal, acoustic, light, mechanical, or electric energy.

97161–97163 Physical therapy evaluations
97164 Physical therapy re-evaluation
97165–97167 Occupational therapy evaluations
97168 Occupational therapy re-evaluation
97010–97028 Supervised therapy modalities
97032–97039 Therapy modalities requiring constant attendance (one-on-one patient contact)
97110–97546 Therapeutic procedures

Refer to **97169–97172** for athletic training evaluations and reevaluations.

Modifiers for Services Provided by Therapists and Speech Pathologists

Medicaid and other payers may require specific modifiers for certain outpatient therapeutic services. Check with individual payers for guidance on reporting therapy modifiers.

GN **Services delivered under an outpatient speech language pathology plan of care**
GO **Services delivered under an outpatient occupational therapy plan of care**
GP **Services delivered under an outpatient physical therapy plan of care**

The following modifiers may be required in addition to either GO or GP when a therapy assistant provides a therapy service under a therapist's supervision:

CO **Outpatient occupational therapy services furnished in whole or in part by an occupational therapy assistant**
CQ **Outpatient physical therapy services furnished in whole or in part by a physical therapist assistant**

Speech Pathology Services (92507, 92521–92523, 92630, 92633)

Speech and language evaluation and therapy may be provided for the treatment of disorders of speech, language, voice, communication, and/or auditory processing. These services are often necessary in the care of children with developmental delay, ASD, injury, or congenital anomaly (eg, cleft palate).

Common codes for services by speech pathology services include

◄92507 Treatment of speech, language, voice, communication, and/or auditory processing disorder; individual
◄92521 Evaluation of speech fluency (eg, stuttering, cluttering)
◄92522 Evaluation of speech sound production (eg, articulation, phonological process, apraxia, dysarthria)
◄92523 with evaluation of language comprehension and expression (eg, receptive and expressive language)
92630 Auditory rehabilitation; prelingual hearing loss
92633 postlingual hearing loss

Take the quiz found at the end of this chapter to review and confirm your understanding of some of its takeaways. Answers to each quiz are found in **Appendix II**.

• indicates a new code; ▲, revised; #, re-sequenced; ✚, add-on; ★, audiovisual technology; and ◄, synchronous interactive audio.

Chapter Takeaways

This chapter reviewed health care services that might be provided by NQHCPs and independently reported in pediatric practice. Following are some takeaways from this chapter:

- For the purpose of reporting health care services, differentiation of physicians and QHPs whose scope of practice includes E/M services from NQHCPs whose scope of practice does not include E/M services is a key consideration.
- Nonphysician qualified health care professionals are distinct from clinical staff when regulations and payer policies allow independent reporting of services.
- Assessment and management services are reported with codes other than E/M service codes.
- HCPCS codes and modifiers may be required for reporting services provided by NQHCPs.
- It is important to understand both scope of practice and payer policies for provision and coding of the NQHCP's services before provision of services.

Resources

AAP Coding Assistance and Education

AAP Coding and Payment Hotline (www.aap.org/en/practice-management/child-health-finance-payment-strategy/coding-payment-hotline)

Supporting Breastfeeding and Lactation: The Primary Care Pediatrician's Guide to Coding (https://downloads.aap.org/AAP/PDF/coding_breasfeeding_lacation.pdf)

AAP News™

"Is this billable? How to report lactation counseling services in pediatric practice," April 1, 2024 (https://publications.aap.org/aapnews/news/28461)

AAP Pediatric Coding Newsletter

"Procedure Codes for Nonphysician Qualified Health Care Professional Services," May 2025 (https://doi.org/10.1542/pcco_book253_document002)

Test Your Knowledge!

1. **Which is indicated by the term *scope of practice*?**
   a. Procedures, actions, and processes that are permitted for a licensed individual
   b. The advertised services of a practice
   c. Specialty or subspecialty certification
   d. Services for which a health plan allows independent reporting
2. **Which service may be independently provided and reported by an NQHCP when allowed by regulation and payer policy?**
   a. Any office evaluation and management visit (eg, **99212–99215**)
   b. Online medical assessment (**98970–98972**)
   c. **99211**
   d. Immunization administration codes **90460** and **90461**
3. **Which of the following is reported with online assessment and management (A/M) service codes 98970–98972?**
   a. An online A/M service lasting 3 minutes
   b. An online A/M service provided 3 days after a prior service reported with **98970–98972**
   c. An online A/M service to answer questions related to a service provided 5 days ago
   d. The cumulative time of 2 online A/M services provided 3 days apart
4. **True or false? There is no *CPT* code specifically for reporting breastfeeding support and lactation services?**
   a. True
   b. False
5. **Which is a requirement of the services reported with code 98960?**
   a. Use of a standardized curriculum.
   b. The services are always prescribed and reported by an NQHCP.
   c. The service includes at least 60 minutes of face-to-face service.
   d. Code selection is not based on time.

CHAPTER 13

Surgery, Infusion, and Sedation in the Outpatient Setting

Contents

Chapter Highlights

- Components included in the surgical package for services assigned a global period
- Separately reportable medication and supply codes
- Evaluation and management (E/M) services provided in conjunction with procedures
- Reporting reduced or terminated services
- Discussion of codes for some commonly performed procedural services
- Reporting contraceptive services (ie, injection, insertion, or implant)
- Selecting appropriate initial and subsequent codes for hydration and infusion services
- Reporting moderate sedation by the same or different physician performing the procedure for which sedation is required

Procedural Services in the Office or Other Outpatient Setting

This chapter reviews coding for procedural services including minor surgical procedures, fracture care, and injections and infusions.

The commonly used Medicare global periods and total non-facility relative value units (RVUs) are provided for reference for many procedures discussed in this chapter. The RVUs included are from the 2025 Medicare Physician Fee Schedule (MPFS) and are not geographically adjusted (2026 RVUs were unavailable at the time of this publication). Individual payers may not use Medicare global periods and/or current-year Medicare RVUs. Check contract terms and payer policies for payer-specific information.

ICD-10-CM Coding for Procedures

International Classification of Diseases, 10th Revision, Clinical Modification (*ICD-10-CM*) codes linked to a procedure code should be the codes that most accurately reflect the reason for the service provided (eg, **S81.011D**, laceration without foreign body, right knee, subsequent encounter), and these codes may differ from ones linked to other services provided on the same date (eg, E/M service). Refer to **Chapter 1** for information on linking diagnosis codes to service lines on a claim.

Know Your A, D, and S Seventh Characters!

***ICD-10-CM* seventh characters A, D, and S define an encounter type for injuries and certain other diagnoses. Here are tips for remembering which character to use.**

- **Active management of the initial injury or complications**
- **During healing of an injury that does not require active management (eg, routine follow-up, suture removal)**
- **Scars and other sequelae (effects of an injury) (Always report the *sequelae code* before the injury code when the service is directed to the sequelae. Injury codes with seventh character S are never the first-listed diagnosis.)**

Seventh characters are also appended to codes for external cause of injury (eg, tripping). Additional seventh characters are provided for reporting types of fractures and fracture care.

Surgical Package Rules

Current Procedural Terminology (*CPT*®) surgical codes (**10004–69990**) are *packaged* or *global* codes. To understand documentation and coding of procedural services, it is necessary to know what is included in each service from a coding and payment perspective. *CPT* directs that each procedure code represents a "surgical package" of service components.

These include

- E/M services subsequent to the decision for surgery on the day before and/or day of surgery, including the history and physical examination
- Local or topical anesthesia, including metacarpal, metatarsal, and/or digital block
- Immediate postoperative care
- Writing of orders
- Evaluation of the patient in the recovery area
- Typical postoperative follow-up care

According to the *CPT* definition of the surgical package, RVUs are assigned to each procedure on the basis of the typical preoperative, intraoperative, and postoperative physician work; practice expense (eg, procedure room, instruments, supplies, support staff); and professional liability. Payers that use RVUs to calculate payments will typically not pay separately for any components of the surgical package.

The RVUs assigned to procedures include the typically used supplies under the practice expense component. Know your payer policies on this. To learn more about the RVUs, refer to Chapter 4.

Medicare Surgical Package Definition

Most Medicaid programs follow the Medicare definition of the surgical package. The Medicare definition differs from the *CPT* one.

- *CPT* defines neither global periods nor minor and major surgery. Global periods are defined in the MPFS Relative Value Files (www.cms.gov/medicare/payment/fee-schedules/physician/pfs-relative-value-files). Most payers use the MPFS, but some Medicaid plans assign a 30-day global period, and other payers may also assign different global periods.
- Throughout this chapter, when an assigned global period is noted, this refers to the period assigned in the MPFS.

Medicare defines procedures as *minor* (procedures assigned a 0- or 10-day global period or endoscopies) or *major* (procedures assigned a 90-day global period) as shown in **Table 13-1**. *The day of surgery is day 0 (zero); the postoperative period begins the next day.*

Table 13-1. The Medicare Surgical Package

Global Periods	0-Day Global Surgical Procedures	10-Day Global Surgical Procedures	90-Day Global Surgical Procedures
Services before date of procedure	Not included		All related services 1 day before surgery if after decision for surgery
Services on date of procedure	E/M services typically included regardless of when decision for surgery is made		All related services except E/M services at which decision for surgery is made
Postoperative services	Typical postoperative care on same date	All related care on DOS and 10 days following	All related care on DOS and 90 days following, including care for complications that does not require a return to the OR

Abbreviations: DOS, date of service; E/M, evaluation and management; OR, operating/procedure room.

- *CPT* does not include care related to surgical complications in the surgical package. Medicare considers care related to complications following surgery to be included in the surgical package unless a return to the operating/procedure room is necessary.

Most office and outpatient clinic procedures will have 0- or 10-day global periods. Exceptions are certain services such as care of fractures, as discussed in the Fracture and/or Dislocation Care section later in this chapter. For the number of global days and RVU values from MPFS 2025 for many commonly reported office procedures, refer to "Common Office Procedures and Global Days" at www.aap.org/cfp2026.

The day of surgery is day 0 (zero) of the global period; the postoperative period begins the next day.

Supplies and Materials

99070 Supplies and materials provided by the physician over and above those usually included with the office visit or other services rendered

- Items such as elastic wraps, clavicle splints, or circumcision and suturing trays may be reported with this code. Remember that some supplies (eg, circumcision and suturing trays) are included in the value of the surgical procedure when the payment is based on RVUs.
- Only the supplies purchased in an office-based practice may be reported.

If reporting 99070, identify the supplies or materials on the claim form and be prepared to submit an invoice.

- Some payers require the use of Healthcare Common Procedure Coding System (HCPCS) codes. More specific HCPCS codes are available for certain supplies (eg, codes Q4001–Q4051 for cast and splint supplies). Use HCPCS codes when they are more specific.

For more information on HCPCS codes, refer to Chapter 1.

Significant Evaluation and Management Service and Procedure

The Medicare Resource-Based Relative Value Scale is used by most private payers and Medicaid plans to determine RVUs and global periods for services. Under this payment methodology, procedural services include some preservice and post-service E/M by the performing physician. Payer edits, such as the National Correct Coding Initiative (NCCI) edits used by Medicare and Medicaid, also bundle E/M services with certain procedures.

For minor procedures, separate payment for a significant, separately identifiable E/M service is allowed when modifier 25 is appended to the E/M code. But care should be taken to use modifier 25 only when documentation supports *a significant, separately identifiable* E/M service. The separately reported E/M service may be indicated by the same problem for which a procedure is required (eg, neurological evaluation for open wound of the head that requires sutures).

- Medicare states that an E/M code may be reported on the same day as a minor surgical procedure only when a significant, separately identifiable E/M service is performed and modifier 25 is appended to the E/M code. *CPT* does not specifically include the initial E/M service before a minor procedure when the decision for surgery occurs at the visit.

Modifier 25 does not indicate that a decision for surgery was made at the visit. Modifier 57 may be appended when the decision for a procedure is made during the E/M service on the day before or same date as the procedure. (Medicare limits use of modifier 57 to major procedures.) Documentation should clearly show E/M of the problem resulting in the initial decision to perform the related procedure. E/M services provided on the day before or day of a procedure that take place *after a decision for surgery on an earlier date* are included in the surgical package.

Coding Conundrum: Procedure, or Evaluation and Management and Procedure?

The differences in the Centers for Medicare & Medicaid Services and *CPT* surgical package guidelines may lead to confusion. Answer the following questions when determining whether you should report a procedure alone or a procedure with an E/M service:

- Did you address a problem or condition before deciding to perform the procedure (above and beyond the usual preoperative care associated with the procedure) or a significant and separately identifiable problem? If yes, report an E/M service and procedure.
- Does the medical record documentation clearly support the performance of a medically necessary E/M service (and meet code descriptor requirements), the procedure (procedure note), the clinical indications for both, and the decision to perform the surgery? If yes, report an E/M service and procedure.
- Was the purpose of the visit only for the procedure (eg, decision for surgery made at an earlier visit) or a procedure requiring minimal E/M (eg, incision for splinter removal)? If yes, do not report an E/M service.
- Does the payer follow the *CPT* or Centers for Medicare & Medicaid Services guidelines for reporting surgical procedures? If the focus of an E/M service is related to the procedure, the history and physical examination are part of preoperative service, and only the surgical procedure should be reported.

Examples

➤ **A neonate returns for repeat cauterization of an umbilical granuloma.** The physician reviews patient history since the last visit and documents that there is still some drainage from the umbilical stump. Other documentation includes notation of the weight and vital signs, patient/caregiver consent, procedure including precautions to protect surrounding tissues, patient tolerance, outcome and post-procedural examination findings, and instructions for home care and follow-up visits.

ICD-10-CM	*CPT*
P83.81 (umbilical granuloma)	17250 (chemical cauterization of granulation tissue [ie, proud flesh])

Teaching Point: Although the physician performs a preoperative examination, this is included in the procedure performed on the same date.

➤ **A patient presents for reevaluation of asthma.** The patient requests evaluation of itching and hearing loss in the left ear. After evaluating the patient's current asthma status and determining that current management should be continued, the patient's ears are examined. Impacted cerumen is identified in the left ear. The cerumen is removed by clinical staff, under the physician's supervision, using lavage. On reexamination, the impacted cerumen is cleared and the patient reports improved hearing. The diagnoses are stable mild persistent asthma and impacted cerumen, left ear. The medical decision-making (MDM) of the encounter is low, supporting 99213.

ICD-10-CM	*CPT*
J45.30 (mild persistent asthma, uncomplicated) H61.22 (impacted cerumen, left ear)	99213 25 (office or other outpatient E/M) 69209 LT (removal of impacted cerumen using irrigation/lavage, unilateral)

Teaching Point: A significant and separately identifiable E/M service was provided to address the patient's asthma and is indicated by appending modifier 25 to the E/M code. If the E/M code were selected according to time, the work associated with the cerumen removal, including documentation of the procedure, would not be included in the time of the E/M service.

Modifier LT indicates that the unilateral procedure was performed on the left ear. Payer policies sometimes require use of modifiers to indicate laterality even when the linked *ICD-10-CM* code indicates the site of the procedure.

Reporting Postoperative Care

Postoperative Evaluation and Management

- Report *CPT* code 99024 (postoperative follow-up visit) for follow-up care provided during the global surgery period. No RVUs are assigned to 99024, as the RVUs were included in the total value of the related procedure.
  - Payment for postoperative care is included as part of the procedure. Payers track the postoperative care provided and reported with 99024.
  - If a physician is not providing or reporting the postoperative care typically performed for a procedure, payers may reduce payment for the surgical service.
  - Reporting 99024 allows tracking of the number of visits performed during the postoperative period of specific procedures. A practice can use this data to calculate office overhead expenses (eg, supplies, staff, physician time) associated with the procedure and potentially use the data to negotiate higher payment rates.

Payment of a surgical procedure may be reduced if the physician does not report 99024. For an example of 99024, refer to the Fracture and/or Dislocation Care section later in this chapter.

- When the physician who performed a procedure provides an unrelated E/M service during the postoperative period, modifier 24 (unrelated E/M service by the same physician during a postoperative period) should be appended to the E/M service code.
- When a physician *other than the surgeon* provides unrelated services to a patient during the postoperative period, the services are reported without a modifier. Despite the use of different National Provider Identifiers and diagnosis codes, some payers with assigned follow-up surgical periods will deny the service. The claim should be appealed for payment with a letter advising the payer that the service was unrelated to surgical care.

Example

➤ **A patient returns 1 month after initial closed treatment of a non-displaced clavicle fracture with concern of runny nose and cough.** History is provided by the child's mother and father. The physician not only diagnoses an acute upper respiratory infection (URI) but also reevaluates the patient's healing fracture. The patient's parents are instructed on home management of the URI.

ICD-10-CM	CPT
J06.9 (acute URI, unspecified) S42.024D (nondisplaced fracture of shaft of right clavicle, subsequent encounter for fracture with routine healing) A code for the external cause of injury will also be reported (eg, W07.XXXD, fall from chair, subsequent encounter).	99213 24 99024

Teaching Point: Modifier 24 is reported to identify that the service to evaluate the patient's respiratory illness was unrelated to the prior procedure. The MDM of the E/M service was low given the low number and complexity of problems addressed (acute, uncomplicated illness), limited data (history from independent historians), and low risk of complications, morbidity, or mortality associated with recommended home care. The evaluation of the healing fracture during the postoperative period is not included in determining the level of service for the encounter, because it is included in postoperative care when provided during the 90-day global period.

Suture Removal

The Medicare global surgery period of 0 days indicates that payment includes the procedure or service plus any associated care provided *on the same day of service.* Therefore, practices may separately report follow-up visits and removal of sutures or staples placed *as part of a procedure assigned a 0-day global period.*

The Medicare global surgery periods of 10 and 90 days include the procedure or service plus any associated follow-up care for 10 or 90 days following the date of the procedure. Therefore, the charge for the procedure already includes suture or staple removal by the same physician or a physician of the same group and specialty as part of the global surgical package, and 99024 is reported for this follow-up care during the 10- or 90-day global period.

- ✖ Do not separately report codes for suture or staple removal *during the global period of a procedure with a 10- or 90-day global period* performed by a physician or qualified health care professional (QHP) in the same group practice except when general anesthesia or moderate sedation is required.
- ✖ Do not separately report codes for suture or staple removal associated with postoperative care following 10- and 90-day global period services when a transfer of care results in postoperative care by a physician or QHP who did not provide the procedure. The code for the procedure is appended with modifier 55 (postoperative management only) and reported for the postoperative care.

Surgery, Infusion, and Sedation in the Outpatient Setting

Chapter 13

Removal Requiring General Anesthesia or Moderate Sedation

15851 Removal of sutures or staples requiring anesthesia (ie, general anesthesia, moderate sedation)

Code 15851 is reported only when the patient requires general anesthesia or moderate sedation during suture or staple removal. This code is assigned 1.10 physician work RVUs and 1.71 total non-facility RVUs.

- ✖ Do not report 15851 for reopening a wound to perform an additional procedure.

Removal Not Requiring General Anesthesia or Moderate Sedation

#+15853 Removal of sutures or staples not requiring anesthesia
#+15854 Removal of sutures and staples not requiring anesthesia

Codes 15853 and 15854 are

- Reported only when sutures and/or staples are removed in follow-up to a procedure with a 0-day global period (and possibly for codes assigned XXX global period indicator [global period does not apply] if sutures or staples were placed)
- Add-on codes (AOCs) that are reported in addition to an E/M service at the same encounter
- Reported in conjunction with E/M codes 99202–99205, 99211–99215, 99281–99285, 99341–99345, or 99347–99350

AOCs are assigned a global period status of ZZZ, which indicates that the global period of the primary procedure is applied to the AOC (ie, a new global period does not begin with removal of sutures or staples).

The total non-facility RVUs for codes 15853 (0.34) and 15854 (0.43) do not include physician work but represent practice expense and professional liability costs.

- ✖ Do not report 15854 in conjunction with 15853. As shown in **Figure 13-1**, the codes represent removal of either sutures or staples (15853) or removal of both sutures and staples (15854).

- ✖ Do not report **15853** or **15854** when provided in a facility setting (eg, place of service code **19**, off-campus outpatient hospital).
- ✖ Do not include time related to suture removal when selecting an E/M code according to total time (eg, extended time due to patient's anxiety about the procedure).

Some payers may require reporting of HCPCS code S0630. Code S0630 is for removal of sutures by a physician other than the one who originally closed the wound. Report S0630 in lieu of 15853 and 15854 when required by payer policy.

Figure 13-1. Differentiate 15853 From 15854

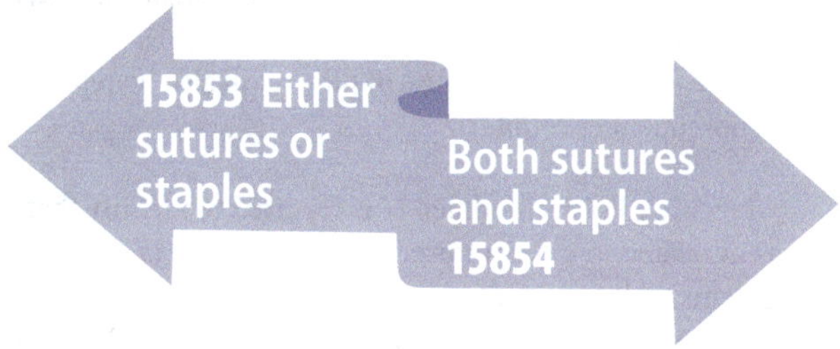

For aftercare of an injury, assign the acute injury code with the seventh character **D** (subsequent encounter). *ICD-10-CM* code **Z48.02** (encounter for removal of sutures) *is not reported* for removal of sutures previously placed to repair an injury but may be reported when removal of sutures is unrelated to care for an injury (eg, removal of sutures from a wound created during excision of a skin lesion).

Example

➤ **An 8-year-old sustained a 0.5-cm laceration on her forehead.** The wound on her face requires a simple repair. She is seen in follow-up 7 days later. The wound is clean, and the sutures are removed.

Visit	*ICD-10-CM*	*CPT*
Initial visit	**S01.81XA** (laceration without foreign body of other part of head, initial encounter)	**12011** (simple repair of the facial laceration 2.5 cm or less)
Follow-up visit	**S01.81XD** (laceration without foreign body of other part of head, subsequent encounter)	**99212–99215** (established patient E/M) according to MDM or the physician's total time not including time of suture removal **#+15853** (removal of sutures or staples not requiring anesthesia)

Teaching Point: Simple laceration repair has a 0-day global period, so any medically necessary follow-up care is separately reported. Code **15853** (removal of sutures) is reported in addition to the code for the E/M service to assess healing and provide any additional instructions for follow-up. No modifier is required on the E/M code because **15853** is an AOC.

Reporting Terminated Procedures

When a procedure is started but cannot be completed because of extenuating circumstances, physicians should consider the individual situation, including the reason for termination of the procedure and the amount of work that was performed, when determining how to report the service rendered.

When a procedure is performed but not entirely successful (eg, portion of foreign body removed), it may be appropriate to report the procedure code that represents the work performed without modification.

- Report reduced services (modifier **52**) or discontinued procedure (modifier **53**) only when the service is significantly reduced from the typical service.
- If the work performed before discontinuation is insignificant, it may be appropriate to not report the procedure. If you choose to not report the procedure, consider whether the level of a related E/M service was increased given the level of MDM associated with the attempted procedure, any complicating factors, and the revised management or treatment plan.

For an example of a discontinued service, refer to the Removal of Impacted Cerumen section later in this chapter.

Refer to Chapter 2 for more information on modifiers including 52, 53, 58 (staged procedure), and 76 (repeat procedure).

Common Pediatric Procedures

Minor Procedures That Do Not Have a Code

Some minor procedures are considered inherent to an E/M code or do not have separate *CPT* codes. But you may report any supplies used. The following procedures are included in an E/M service:

- Insertion or removal of an ear wick
- Removal of *nonimpacted* cerumen from the ear
- Nasal aspiration
- Nasogastric tube insertion without fluoroscopic guidance
- Removal of an umbilical clamp
- Removal of foreign bodies from skin not requiring an incision
- Puncture of abscess without aspiration
- Wound closure only with adhesive strips (eg, Steri-Strips, butterfly bandages)
- The use of fluorescein dye and a Wood lamp to examine for a corneal abrasion or foreign body of the eye

When significant time is spent performing a service that is not separately reported, documentation of the total time spent on the date of the encounter and code selection based on time may more adequately represent the level of E/M service than code selection based on MDM.

Identifying Separately Reportable Services

Some procedures, such as those requiring an incision and/or repair, are easily understood to be separately reported. For other procedural services, verify separate reporting through your procedure coding reference. There is value in capturing all procedural services that are distinct from E/M services.

Example

➤ **A physician removes a foreign body from a child's nose.** If the physician reports an office E/M visit with low-level MDM (**99213**, 2.75 total non-facility RVUs) in lieu of procedure code **30300** (foreign body removal from nose, 6.20 total non-facility RVUs), the service may be significantly undervalued.

Reporting the appropriate code for the foreign body removal will result in more appropriate payment for the service provided. Both services are reported only if a significant, separately identifiable E/M service, beyond the preservice work of the foreign body removal, is provided.

Examples of other procedural services that may be provided in a pediatric practice but are mistakenly included in or reported with an E/M code include the following services:

- Burn care for a first-degree burn (**16000**)
- Treatment of elbow dislocation (**24640**)
- Incision in lingual frenulum (**41010**)
- Urinary catheterization, straight (**51701**)

Remember that when reporting any procedures containing 0, 10, or 90 global days, modifier **25** or **57** is required on any separately identifiable E/M service provided on the same day (or, in some instances, the previous day before a planned major surgery).

Integumentary Procedures

Extraction

New in 2026! Code 10040 has been revised to reflect a change from "acne surgery" to a more specific description of the service, "extraction," which may be performed in the treatment of acne.

▲**10040** Extraction (eg, marsupialization, opening or removal of multiple milia, comedones, cysts, pustules)

The service reported with **10040** may include extraction of comedones and gentle lancing and draining of the pustular component of acne lesions.

Incision and Drainage

10060 Incision and drainage of abscess (eg, carbuncle, suppurative hidradenitis, cutaneous or subcutaneous abscess, cyst, furuncle, or paronychia); simple or single

10061 complicated or multiple

- The global period is 10 days for **10060** and **10061**.
- *CPT* does not differentiate between simple and complicated incision and drainage and leaves code selection to the physician's judgment.
- The difference in 2025 total non-facility RVUs for **10060** (3.84) and **10061** (6.44) indicates the significant additional work and practice expense associated with complicated or multiple incision and drainage procedures. Documentation should support the increased complexity when reporting **10061**.
- The simple incision and drainage procedure typically involves administering local anesthetic, making an incision, expressing purulent drainage, obtaining a culture, irrigating the wound, completely opening the cavity, and packing/dressing the wound.
- Complex incision and drainage often typically involves a deeper incision, breakdown of multiple loculations, placement of a drain, and/or debridement of the cavity.

Example

➤ **A 12-year-old presents with an abscess on his right lower leg.** The decision is made to perform incision and drainage. The physician documents administration of local anesthetic, incision of skin above the abscess, and expression of purulent material. The wound was irrigated and packed. The patient will return in 3 days for reevaluation.

Code **10060** is reported for the procedure. All related visits (eg, follow-up visit to recheck the wound) within the 10 days following the date of surgery may be reported with **99024** and no charge.

Removal of Skin Tags and Congenital Accessory Digits

11200 Removal of skin tags, multiple fibrocutaneous tags, any area; up to and including 15 lesions

A 10-day global period applies. The 2025 total non-facility RVUs were 2.79.

Code **11200** is used to report the removal of a sixth digit from a newborn. It is equivalent to a skin tag and is not assigned the code for an actual digit removal. The *ICD-10-CM* code for accessory digits would be **Q69.0** (accessory fingers), **Q69.1** (accessory thumb), **Q69.2** (accessory toes), or **Q69.9** (unspecified).

Destruction of Benign Lesions (eg, Warts)

17110 Destruction (eg, laser surgery, electrosurgery, cryosurgery, chemosurgery, surgical curettement) of benign lesions other than skin tags or cutaneous vascular proliferative lesions; up to 14 lesions

17111 15 or more lesions

A 10-day global period applies to **17110** and **17111**. The 2025 total non-facility RVUs were 3.40 for **17110** and 3.99 for **17111**.

Report destruction of flat or common warts (**B07.8**), plantar warts (**B07.0**), or molluscum contagiosum (**B08.1**) with **17110** or **17111** (with 1 unit of service), depending on the number of lesions removed. Do not report both **17110** and **17111** because they are mutually exclusive.

Chemical Cauterization of Granulation Tissue

17250 Chemical cauterization of granulation tissue (ie, proud flesh)

A 0-day global period applies. The 2025 total non-facility RVUs were 2.54.

Code **17250** is appropriately reported for cauterization of an umbilical granuloma.

- When reporting a significant and separately identifiable E/M service on the date, append modifier **25** to the E/M code reported (eg, **99391 25**, **99213 25**).
- ✖ Do not report **17250** with removal or excision codes for the same lesion, for achieving wound hemostasis, or in conjunction with active wound care management.

Example

➤ **A 2-week-old presents for her well-baby check.** On examination, a moderate-sized umbilical granuloma is noted. The physician takes a very brief history and decides to cauterize the umbilicus. The routine well-baby check is completed in addition to cauterization of the umbilical granuloma.

ICD-10-CM	*CPT*
Z00.121 (encounter for routine child health examination with abnormal findings) **P83.81** (umbilical granuloma)	**99391 25** **17250**

Teaching Point: Preservice work includes explanation of the procedure, obtaining informed consent, positioning and draping, preparing the site, and scrubbing in. Postservice work includes discussing follow-up care with parents and/or caregivers. Supplies and equipment, such as silver nitrate and an applicator, are included in the value assigned to the code when reporting to payers using RVUs. Follow-up visits and repeat procedures are separately reportable.

Laceration Repairs

12001–12018 Simple repair
12031–12057 Intermediate repair
13100–13160 Complex repair

- Most repairs performed in non-facility settings are simple or intermediate repairs, which are defined as follows:
  - *Simple:* Superficial wound and/or subcutaneous wound requiring a simple single-layer closure or tissue adhesives (eg, Dermabond). Wound closure requiring only adhesive strips is included in an E/M service. A 0-day global period applies. *When performed, local or topical anesthesia and hemostasis are not reported separately.*
  - *Intermediate:* Includes the repair of wounds that, in addition to the requirements for simple repair, require layered closure of one or more of the deeper layers of subcutaneous tissue and superficial (non-muscle) fascia, in addition to skin (epidermal and dermal) closure. Intermediate repair includes limited undermining (defined as a distance less than the maximum width of the defect, measured perpendicular to the closure line, along at least 1 entire edge of the defect). A 10-day global period applies.

Single-layer closure of heavily contaminated wounds that require extensive cleaning or removal of particulate matter also constitutes intermediate repair.

Refer to your *CPT* reference for the definition of complex repair and additional reporting instructions for wounds that require extensive debridement.

- Codes **12001–13160** are used to report wound closure using sutures, staples, or tissue adhesives (eg, Dermabond), singly or in combination with adhesive strips.
- Wound closure using chemical cauterization, electrocauterization, or adhesive strips (eg, Steri-Strips, butterfly bandages) only is considered inherent to the E/M service. Supplies may be separately reported, but payers may bundle supplies to the practice expense of the E/M service.
- Some payers may accept HCPCS code **G0168** (wound closure using tissue adhesive[s]) in lieu of simple repair codes (eg, **12001**, **12011**).
- Codes are reported according to difficulty of the repair, measured length of the wound, and location. To report wound repair, measure the length of the repaired wound(s) in centimeters.
  - If multiple wounds belong to the same category of difficulty and location, add the lengths and report with a single code.
  - If multiple wounds do not belong in the same category, report each repair separately with the more complicated repair reported as the primary procedure and the less complicated repair reported as the secondary procedure. Modifier **51** (multiple procedures) should be appended to the secondary code(s) when the payer does not recommend against reporting modifier **51**.
  - Simple ligation of vessels is considered part of the wound closure.
- Provision of topical or injected local anesthetic is included in the wound repair code.

Surgery, Infusion, and Sedation in the Outpatient Setting

Chapter 13

Examples

➤ **A 10-year-old sustained a 1.5-cm laceration on his left knee requiring a simple (single-layer) repair after a fall from playground equipment.**

ICD-10-CM	*CPT*
S81.012A (laceration without foreign body left knee, initial encounter) W09.8XXA (fall on or from other playground equipment, initial encounter) Y92.838 (other recreation area as the place of occurrence of the external cause)	12001 (simple repair of superficial wounds of scalp, neck, axillae, external genitalia, trunk and/or extremities [including hands and feet]; 2.5 cm or less)

Teaching Point: Simple repair includes only the care on the date of the repair (0-day global period). Follow-up E/M visits are separately reported and do not require a modifier. Codes W09.8XXA and Y92.838 are external cause codes that provide information about the cause and place of occurrence for the accident that may be used in injury research and evaluation of injury prevention strategies. Inclusion of codes for external cause of injury, although not required, may provide information that facilitates timely payment.

➤ **A 10-year-old fell from playground equipment and sustained a 1.5-cm laceration on his left knee and a 1.5-cm laceration on his left forearm. Each laceration required an intermediate repair.**

ICD-10-CM	*CPT*
S81.012A (laceration without foreign body left knee, initial encounter) S51.812A (laceration of left forearm without foreign body, initial encounter) W09.8XXA Y92.838	12032 (intermediate repair, extremities, 2.6–7.5 cm)

Teaching Point: A single code is reported when both wounds are in the same family of anatomical sites and both require the same level of repair (ie, simple, intermediate, or complex). If the patient returns for wound follow-up within 10 days following the date of repair, 99024 (postoperative follow-up visit) is reported for the encounter because intermediate repair has a 10-day global period. There is no separate charge for care within the global period.

Other Repairs

Code 11760 (repair of nail bed) is reported when part or all of the nail plate is lifted and a laceration of the nail bed is repaired. A 10-day global period applies. The 2025 non-facility total RVUs were 5.53.

Report 40650 (repair of lip, full-thickness, vermilion only) when a laceration of the full thickness of the lip and vermilion is repaired. A 90-day global period applies to this service. For less than full-thickness repair, refer to codes for repair of skin. For repair of a laceration that crosses the vermilion border, refer to 40652 (up to half vertical height) and 40654 (over half of vertical height).

Laceration repairs of the tongue (41250–41252) are reported according to size and location (eg, repair of laceration ≤2.5 cm, anterior two-thirds of the tongue, is reported with 41250). These codes are assigned a 10-day global period.

Refer to Chapter 18 for discussion of coding for negative pressure wound therapy (97605 and 97606 or 97607 and 97608).

Burn Care

CPT code 16000 (initial treatment, first-degree burn, where no more than local treatment is required) is reported for initial treatment for the symptomatic relief of a first-degree burn that is characterized by erythema and tenderness. The 2025 total non-facility RVUs were 2.42. Report a separate E/M service on the same date only when the service is both distinct and separately identifiable from the preservice work of the burn care.

16020 Dressings and/or debridement of partial-thickness burns, initial or subsequent; small or less than 5% total body (eg, finger)

A 0-day global period applies. The 2025 total non-facility RVUs were 2.58.

Code **16020**

- Is used to report treatment of burns with dressings and/or debridement of small partial-thickness burns (second degree), whether initial or subsequent.
- An E/M visit with modifier **25** appended may be reported if a significant, separately identifiable E/M service is clinically indicated, performed, and documented in addition to the burn care.

Refer to Chapter 18 for coding of larger partial- or full-thickness burns.

Examples

➤ **A 9-year-old with sunburn on her shoulders is seen by the physician.** There is redness and tenderness but no blistering. Topical treatment is applied, and an over-the-counter treatment of the first-degree burn is ordered.

ICD-10-CM	*CPT*
L55.0 (first-degree sunburn)	**16000** (first-degree burn requiring local treatment)

Teaching Point: Code **16000** was assigned 2.42 total non-facility RVUs in 2025 and is assigned a 0-day global period. For comparison, total non-facility RVUs for **99212** were 1.70.

➤ **A 4-year-old is seen in the office after sustaining a burn on the first finger of her right hand caused by touching a hot pan.** The area is red and blistered. Following examination by the physician, the finger is treated with a topical cream and bandaged.

ICD-10-CM	*CPT*
T23.221A (second-degree burn of single finger, initial encounter) **X15.3XXA** (contact with other heat and hot saucepan or skillet, initial encounter)	**16020**

Teaching Point: External cause-of-injury codes such as **X15.3XXA** are used to report the source, place, and/or intent of a burn injury. These codes are required only when state regulations mandate reporting of cause of injury (typically applies to emergency department [ED] services). But it is appropriate to report external cause-of-injury codes when the cause is known.

Removal of Foreign Bodies

Integumentary Foreign Bodies

10120 Incision and removal of foreign body, subcutaneous tissues; simple
10121 complex

A 10-day global period applies. The 2025 total non-facility RVUs were 4.55 (**10120**) and 7.95 (**10121**).

Incision and removal of a foreign body from within the subcutaneous tissues above the fascia is reported with a code from the integumentary system regardless of the site (eg, hand, foot).

Do not report **10120** or **10121** when a foreign body is removed with forceps alone, with no incision. Instead, report an E/M service. Incising of the skin can be accomplished by a scalpel or another instrument needed to "break open," or incise, the skin.

- Code **10120** includes the removal of splinters or ticks when the physician incises the skin to retrieve the foreign body.
- A complex removal may require extended exploration and removal of multiple foreign bodies (eg, pieces of glass), use of imaging to help locate the foreign body, or removal that is complicated by the anatomical site of the foreign body (eg, area that is not easily seen) and will have a greater intensity of physician work. The difference in physician work RVUs for the procedures may be used as an indicator of the difference—1.22 for **10120** versus 2.74 for **10121**.

The removal of an embedded earring or other jewelry requiring an incision would be reported with **10120** or **10121**, depending on the complexity of the procedure required to remove it. If the jewelry is removed by wiggling it out or another method that does not require incision, this work is included in the E/M service.

Musculoskeletal Foreign Bodies

Musculoskeletal codes are reported when a foreign body is removed from *within the fascia, subfascial area, or muscle.* Always check the *CPT* index to ensure you are reporting the most accurate code.

Codes in the musculoskeletal system are not reported for removal of foreign bodies within the skin and subcutaneous fat. Examples of codes for removal of foreign bodies within the musculoskeletal system are

- *Foot:* 28190 for foreign body removal from within the fascia, subfascial area, or muscle (10-day global period); from deep tissue of the foot, 28192 (90-day global period); or complex, 28193 (90-day global period)
- *Upper arm or elbow:* 24200 for removal of foreign bodies from subcutaneous tissues within the fascia (10-day global period); from deep tissue, below the fascia, or in the muscle, 24201 (90-day global period)

An object that is unintentionally placed (eg, trauma, ingestion) is considered a foreign body. An object intentionally placed by a physician or other QHP for any purpose (eg, diagnostic, therapeutic) is considered an implant. A broken or misplaced implant is a foreign body for coding purposes.

Foreign Bodies in Other Body Sites

CPT includes codes for reporting removal of foreign bodies from many different body sites. **Table 13-2** summarizes foreign body removal services from areas other than skin or muscle.

Table 13-2. Codes for Removal of Foreign Bodies From Sites Other Than Skin or Muscle

Site	Code(s)
Anal foreign body or fecal impaction	Use appropriate E/M code or 45999 (unlisted procedure, rectum) except when performed under anesthesia (45915, more than local anesthesia).
External auditory canal	69200 (removal foreign body from external auditory canal; without general anesthesia) (For removal of impacted cerumen, refer to the section by the same name later in this chapter.)
Eye	65205 (removal of foreign body, external eye; conjunctival superficial) 65220 (removal of foreign body, external eye; corneal, without slit lamp)
Nose	30300 (removal of intranasal foreign bodies when performed in the office) 30310 (removal of intranasal foreign bodies under general anesthesia)
Vagina	Use appropriate E/M code or 58999 (unlisted procedure, female genital system) except when performed under anesthesia (57415, more than local anesthesia).

Abbreviation: E/M, evaluation and management.

Fracture and/or Dislocation Care

Fracture and Dislocation Care Codes

Fracture and dislocation care codes are reported for care that is intended to begin the course of treatment of the injury. If a physician or QHP provides casting or strapping only for stabilization pending restorative treatment by another physician or QHP, refer to 29000–29799 (discussed in the Casts/Strapping/Splints section later in this chapter). A significant, separately identifiable E/M service to diagnose and manage the injury is separately reported.

Most fracture and dislocation care codes include a 90-day period of follow-up care under the Medicare global package. Modifiers are required when one physician or QHP provides initial care of a fracture or dislocation (eg, closed treatment of a fracture without manipulation in the ED) and another physician or QHP provides follow-up care.

- When a patient presents for follow-up care after initial fracture care is provided in another setting (eg, ED, urgent care), it is necessary to determine whether the provider of initial fracture care reported a code for fracture care with modifier 54 (surgical care only) or reported only casting/strapping for the initial care.
- If initial fracture care has been reported with modifier 54, the physician providing continued fracture care reports the fracture care code with modifier 55 (postoperative management only) appended.

Unrelated services that are provided during the global surgery period by the same physician (or physician of the same group and specialty) may be reported. Append modifier **24** to an unrelated E/M service.

Codes for fracture/dislocation care

- Are listed by anatomical location.
- Are provided (in most cases) for closed or open treatment, with or without manipulation, and with or without internal fixation.

Closed treatment of a nasal bone fracture without manipulation or stabilization is reported with an E/M code (eg, 99283, 99213) according to the site of service.

- Include the initial casting, splinting, or strapping.
- ✖ Do not include radiographs or E/M to determine the extent of injury and treatment options.

Fractures most seen in a primary care pediatric practice include closed fractures (ie, skin is intact on presentation), and treatment is typically closed (ie, fracture site is not surgically opened) without manipulation (an exception is treatment of nursemaid elbow).

- *Clavicular fracture:* Report closed treatment without manipulation with **23500**.
- *Nursemaid elbow:* Report closed treatment of radial head subluxation (nursemaid elbow) with manipulation with **24640**. (This code has a 10-day global period.)
- *Radial fracture:* Report **25500** for closed treatment of radial shaft fracture without manipulation and **25600** for closed treatment of distal radius fracture without manipulation.
- *Phalanx fracture:* Closed treatment of a proximal or middle phalanx, finger, or thumb (each) without manipulation is reported with **26720**. Closed treatment of a distal phalangeal fracture (each) without manipulation is reported with **26750**.
- *Great toe fracture:* Code **28490** is reported for the closed treatment of a fracture of the great toe, phalanx, or phalanges without manipulation.
- *Metatarsal fracture:* Report **28470** for closed treatment of a metatarsal fracture without manipulation.
- *Lesser toe fracture:* Closed treatment of fracture, phalanx, or phalanges, other than great toe without manipulation, is coded with **28510**.

Documentation matters: fractures not specified as displaced or non-displaced are reported with an *ICD-10-CM* code for a displaced fracture. Fractures not specified as open or closed are reported with a code for a closed fracture.

"Buddy taping" of a fractured digit may be reported as fracture care. When reporting fracture care, the code includes care during the global period. Buddy taping for an injury without fracture is included in the E/M service.

Examples

➤ **An urgent care physician performs and documents a comprehensive evaluation of a child (new patient) to assess for injuries following an unwitnessed fall from the stairs in her home. The child is diagnosed with a fracture of the shaft of the left clavicle and receives closed treatment without manipulation. The child will receive follow-up care from a physician of another practice.**

ICD-10-CM	*CPT*
S42.022A (displaced fracture shaft of clavicle, closed, initial encounter) **W10.9XXA** (fall [on] [from] unspecified stairs and steps, initial encounter)	**99202–99205 57**
S42.022A **W10.9XXA**	**23500 54** (closed treatment clavicle fracture without manipulation)

Teaching Point: Modifier **54** is appended to **23500** because the physician will not provide post-procedural care. A payer may require modifier **57** (decision for surgery) appended to the E/M code when performed in conjunction with a procedure that is assigned a 90-day global period. Individual payers may have different policies.

When follow-up care is provided by a physician or QHP of another group practice or specialty, **23500 55** is reported.

➤ **A physician evaluates a 22-month-old established patient whose parents report that she will not move her left arm after falling on steps while holding her father's hand.** After obtaining history and performing a physical examination to rule out other injuries, the physician diagnoses subluxation of the radial head that is reduced by manipulation. Reassessment after 10 minutes shows that the child uses both arms without difficulty. The parents are counseled about potential for recurrent injury and prevention. Follow-up will be at a previously scheduled 2-year-old visit unless otherwise indicated.

ICD-10-CM	*CPT*
S53.032A (nursemaid's elbow, left, initial encounter) **W10.9XXA** (fall [on] [from] unspecified stairs and steps, initial encounter)	**99213 25** (low MDM—acute, uncomplicated injury with assessment requiring an independent historian and low risk of morbidity) **24640** (closed treatment of radial head subluxation in child, nursemaid elbow, with manipulation)

Teaching Point: The physician provided a significant and separately identifiable E/M service to evaluate the extent of injury in addition to treatment of nursemaid elbow. Modifier **25** is required by most payers to indicate that the E/M service was significant and separately identifiable from the preservice work of the minor procedure (eg, 10-day global period) performed on the same DOS.

Casts/Strapping/Splints

- Codes for the application of casts, splints, or strapping (**29000–29590**) are reported only when they are replacements for the initial application *or performed as part of the initial E/M visit and fracture care is not reported.*
- ✖ Do not report codes **29000–29590** for the initial (first) application when a fracture or dislocation care code is reported because they are included as part of the global surgery package.
- *Strapping* refers to the application of overlapping strips of adhesive plaster or tape to a body part to exert pressure on it and hold a structure in place. Strapping may be used to treat strains, sprains, and dislocations, in addition to fractures.
- Refer to the Fracture Care Supplies section later in this chapter for information on reporting supplies such as slings.

The following codes are commonly used when treating a fracture or dislocation:

- Application of splints
  - Short arm splint (forearm to hand): static (**29125**); dynamic (**29126**)
  - Finger splint: static (**29130**); dynamic (**29131**)
  - Short leg splint (calf to foot): **29515**
- Strapping
  - Shoulder: **29240**
  - Elbow or wrist: **29260**

Verify payer policy for coverage of strapping procedures, as some policies prohibit payment for strapping of the shoulder, elbow, or wrist.

Example

➤ **An established adolescent patient returns to a physician for follow-up on an injury to the left wrist.** The patient was previously examined and a cast applied for a presumed scaphoid fracture (ie, diagnosed given the examination findings) that was not found on a radiograph. The service was reported with **25622** (closed treatment of carpal scaphoid [navicular] fracture; without manipulation). The diagnosis documented at the first visit was initial encounter for unspecified scaphoid fracture of the left wrist (**S62.001A**) caused by tripping while playing soccer with friends at a soccer field. The initial cast is removed and a 3-view radiograph of the wrist is ordered and obtained in the office. The physician interprets the radiograph, which now shows a fracture of the middle third (waist) of the left proximal scaphoid. The physician applies a replacement thumb spica cast. The patient will return in 4 weeks for reevaluation.

ICD-10-CM	*CPT*
S62.025D (nondisplaced fracture of middle third of navicular [scaphoid] bone of left wrist, subsequent encounter for fracture with routine healing) W01.0XXD (fall on same level from slipping, tripping and stumbling without subsequent striking against object, subsequent encounter)	99024 (postoperative follow-up visit) 29085 58 (application cast; hand and lower forearm [gauntlet]) Q4013 (cast supplies, gauntlet cast [includes lower forearm and hand], adult [11 years +], plaster) or Q4014 (same but fiberglass) 73110 (radiologic examination, wrist; complete, minimum of 3 views)

Teaching Point: Code 25622 is assigned a 90-day global period by most payers. The physician reports codes for follow-up during the global period (99024), radiograph, and application of the replacement cast. Diagnosis codes include the seventh character D to report subsequent care of this fracture; a more specific code for the confirmed diagnosis (S62.025D) is now used in lieu of S62.001D. Modifier 58 (staged or related procedure) is appended to 29085, as the service is related to the procedure performed by the same physician at the previous encounter.

Cast supplies are separately reported with either *CPT* code 99070 (supplies and materials [except spectacles], provided by the physician or other QHP over and above those usually included with the office visit or other services rendered) or, as shown here, more specific HCPCS codes.

If the initial care of the fracture had included only application of a splint to stabilize and protect the injury until a definitive diagnosis could be confirmed, codes for an E/M service and application of a splint would have been appropriate in lieu of fracture care. In that case, the return visit at which the fracture was diagnosed would have been initial fracture care, and 25622 would have been reported for this encounter in lieu of 99024 and 29085.

When reporting codes for radiographs, documentation should include a report of the indication for the test, number of views, findings, and, when applicable, comparison to previous radiographs.

- **✕ Do not report a charge for interpretation and report for review of images that have been or will be interpreted with creation of a formal report by a radiologist or other physician or QHP.**
- **The independent review of previously interpreted images is included in the amount and/or complexity of data to be reviewed and analyzed of an E/M service or in the follow-up during the global period of a service.**

Fracture Care Supplies

- Supplies associated with fracture care may be billed with every application, including the initial casting, splinting, or strapping performed in association with the global surgery procedure code when the service is performed in the private office setting.
- HCPCS codes A4580, A4590, and Q4001–Q4051 may be reported for cast supplies; E1800–E1841 may be reported for splints. Check with your major payers and/or review their payment policies for reporting these supplies.
- HCPCS codes are accepted by many Medicaid and commercial payers and are often specific to the age of the patient and type of supply and/or material.
- A description of supplies may be required when reporting special supplies code 99070.
- The following codes are commonly used:

99070	Supplies and materials (except spectacles)
A4565	Slings
A4570	Splint
L3650–L3678	Clavicle splints
Q4001–Q4051	Cast and splint supplies
S8450–S8452	Splint, prefabricated for finger, wrist, ankle, or elbow

Surgery, Infusion, and Sedation in the Outpatient Setting

Chapter 13

Ear, Nose, and Throat Procedures

Control of Nasal Hemorrhage

30901 Control nasal hemorrhage, anterior, simple (cautery or packing)
30903 Control nasal hemorrhage, anterior, complex (extensive cautery and/or packing) any method

A 0-day global period applies. The 2025 total non-facility RVUs were 4.67 (**30901**) and 7.22 (**30903**).

- If performing cautery or packing on both sides, report **30901** with modifier **50**.
- If bleeding is controlled with manual pressure or placement of a nasal clamp (clip), only the appropriate level of E/M service is reported.
- ✖ Do not report **30901** when packing is placed in the short term to administer medication (eg, insertion of medicated gauze into the nostrils) and not to serve a hemostatic and/or tamponade role following the encounter. Illumination and instrumentation (eg, suction, nasal speculum, forceps) are typically required for placement of packing to control nasal hemorrhage.

Removal of Impacted Cerumen

69209 Removal of impacted cerumen using irrigation/lavage, unilateral
69210 Removal of impacted cerumen requiring instrumentation, unilateral

A 0-day global period applies. The 2025 total non-facility RVUs were 0.47 (**69209**) and 1.44 (**69210**). Additionally, 0.61 work RVUs are assigned to **69210**.

Removal of cerumen that is not impacted is included in an E/M code regardless of how it is removed. Documentation of removal of impacted cerumen should include the indication for removal (eg, impairing examination, pain, itching, hearing loss).

Append modifier **25** to a significant, separately identifiable E/M service (eg, **99213**) provided on the same date as removal of impacted cerumen, as E/M codes are bundled to cerumen removal codes by NCCI edits.

Code **69209** is used to report removal of impacted cerumen by ear wash without direct visualization and instrumentation. This service may be provided by clinical staff under a physician's or QHP's supervision.

- This code is intended to capture the practice expense associated with the service and is not valued to include physician work.
- For a bilateral procedure, report **69209** with modifier **50**.
- ✖ Do not report **69209** for removal of cerumen that is not impacted.
- ✖ Do not report **69209** in conjunction with **69210** when performed on the same ear (modifiers **LT** and **RT** may be used to identify contralateral procedures).

Code **69210** is reported *only* when the physician or QHP, under direct visualization, removes impacted cerumen with, at a minimum, an otoscope and instruments such as wax curettes or with an operating microscope and suction plus specific ear instruments (eg, cup forceps, right angles).

- Medical record documentation must support that the cerumen was impacted and removed by the physician and include a description of what equipment and method were used to perform the procedure. Visualization of the impacted cerumen should also be documented.
- Report **69210** with modifier **50** when bilateral procedures are performed.
- NCCI edits bundle impacted cerumen removal (**69209**, **69210**) with some hearing assessments (eg, **92567**, tympanometry). There is no modifier to override this edit.

Note: Medicare does not recognize modifier **50** when reported with **69210** (impacted cerumen removal); therefore, payers that follow Medicare payment policy will not recognize it and may deny the claim outright. Check with your payers.

Examples

➤ **A physician orders removal of impacted cerumen from the right ear by lavage.** Clinical staff perform the lavage, removing the impacted cerumen. Because the child is uncooperative, the procedure takes 10 minutes.

ICD-10-CM	*CPT*
H61.21 (impacted cerumen, right ear)	**99202–99215 25** (Report if appropriate and use modifier **25** if required by payer.) **69209 RT** (**RT** indicates right ear.)

Coding Conundrum: Unsuccessful Removal of Impacted Cerumen

If a physician or other QHP attempts to remove impacted cerumen but finds the impaction too hard for safe removal, what code is reported for the attempt? The answer depends on the individual situation, including the amount of work that was performed and whether another procedure was successful.

- If the portion of the procedure completed required insignificant work and practice expense (eg, staff time), report only the services completed on that date (eg, E/M).
- If the patient was instructed to use softening drops and return later for removal, consider whether the effort and practice expense were sufficient to justify reporting the removal with reduced services modifier 52.
- If after significant effort and practice expense, the procedure was discontinued because of extenuating circumstances or concerns that the procedure might threaten the patient's well-being, report the procedure code with modifier 53 (discontinued procedure).
- If, after attempted removal by a physician is discontinued, softening drops were administered in the office and clinical staff performed removal of the impaction by lavage (69209), report only the completed procedure.

Teaching Point: This procedure was unilateral. If it were bilateral, modifier 50 would be appended to 69209. The anatomical modifier RT (right) is informational and may not affect payment. The extended time of service alone is not sufficient to support reporting increased procedural service (ie, modifier 22). Time spent by clinical staff does not contribute to the total time of the E/M service.

➤ **A physician documents "Impacted cerumen removed from both ears with an otoscope and curette" for a patient with concern of decreased hearing.** Following the procedure, the patient's hearing is assessed as normal.

ICD-10-CM	*CPT*
H61.23 (impacted cerumen, bilateral)	99202–99215 25 (Report if appropriate and use modifier 25 if required by payer.) 69210 50 (bilateral removal of impacted cerumen using instrumentation)

Teaching Point: Unless a payer instructs otherwise, modifier 50 is appended to 69210 to indicate a bilateral procedure. An E/M service is reported only if significant and separately identifiable. If selecting an E/M code based on time, do not include time spent performing the procedure. The diagnosis code for the condition(s) addressed by the E/M service is linked to the E/M code on the claim.

Digestive System Procedures

Incision in Lingual Frenulum

41010 Incision in the lingual frenum to free the tongue

A 10-day global period applies. The 2025 total non-facility RVUs were 6.36.

Note that 41115 (excision of lingual frenum) is inappropriate when an incisional release of tongue-tie is performed rather than excision (removal) of the frenum.

Example

➤ **A 14-day-old is seen for feeding difficulty caused by ankyloglossia.** The physician documents obtaining informed consent, positioning and restraining of the neonate, and gentle lifting of the tongue with a sterile, grooved retractor to expose the frenulum. The frenulum, adjacent to the ventral aspect of the tongue, is divided by 2 to 3 mm with sterile scissors. Afterward, the newborn is immediately returned to his mother for comfort and feeding. The latch appears improved. After feeding, the neonate is reevaluated with no evidence of complications. Code 41010 is reported for the procedure.

ICD-10-CM	*CPT*
Q38.1 (congenital ankyloglossia) P92.5 (neonatal difficulty in feeding at breast)	41010

● indicates a new code; ▲, revised; #, re-sequenced; ✚, add-on; ★, audiovisual technology; and ◀, synchronous interactive audio.

Teaching Point: If a significant and separately identifiable E/M service was provided in addition to the preservice work of the procedure, modifier **25** would be appended to the appropriate E/M code. Any related visit within the 10 days following the procedure may be reported (with no charge) with **99024**. An unrelated E/M service within 10 days following the procedure may be reported with modifier **24** (unrelated E/M service by the same physician or QHP during a postoperative period). When reporting modifier **24**, the diagnosis code(s) reported should be of an unrelated indication for the service.

Gastrostomy Tube Replacement

43762 Replacement of gastrostomy tube, percutaneous, includes removal, when performed, without imaging or endoscopic guidance; not requiring revision of gastrostomy tract

43763 requiring revision of gastrostomy tract

A 0-day global period is assigned. The 2025 total non-facility RVUs were 6.57 (**43762**) and 9.70 (**43763**).

- Report **43762** and **43763** only for percutaneous gastrostomy tube or gastrojejunal tube change without imaging or endoscopic guidance (eg, replacement gastrojejunal tube is placed into the stomach and anchored in place by inflating the gastric balloon with water or saline, and peristalsis carries the jejunal portion of the tube into the small intestine).
- Refer to other specific codes (eg, **49450–49452** and **43246**) for gastrostomy tube or gastrojejunal tube placement, conversion, or replacement *with imaging or endoscopic guidance.*
- A significant, separately identifiable E/M service on the same date may be reported with modifier **25** appended to the E/M code (eg, **99213 25**).
- ✖ Do not report an E/M service when the encounter is solely for replacement of the gastrostomy tube.
- Codes **43762** and **43763** include the gastrostomy tube kit.

Genitourinary System Procedures

Urinary Catheterization

51701 Urinary catheterization, straight

51702 Urinary catheterization, temporary

A 0-day global period applies. The 2025 total non-facility RVUs were 1.32 (**51701**) and 1.85 (**51702**).

- Code **51701** is reported when a non-indwelling bladder catheter (straight catheterization) is inserted (eg, for residual urine, for a urine culture collection).
- Code **51702** is reported when a temporary indwelling bladder catheter is inserted (ie, Foley).

Report 51701 when you insert a urinary catheter to collect a clean-catch urine specimen, after which the catheter is removed.

Lysis/Excision of Labial or Penile Adhesions

If lysis of labial or penile adhesions is performed by the application of manual pressure without the use of an instrument to cut the adhesions, it will be considered part of the E/M visit and not reported separately.

54450 Foreskin manipulation including lysis of preputial adhesions and stretching

A 0-day global period is assigned. The 2025 total non-facility RVUs were 2.10.
Code **54450** does not require general anesthesia.

- This procedure is performed on the uncircumcised foreskin and the head of the penis. Adhesions are broken by stretching the foreskin back over the head of the penis onto the shaft or by inserting a clamp between the foreskin and the head of the penis and spreading the jaws of the clamp.

54162 Lysis or excision of penile post-circumcision adhesions

This service includes a 10-day global surgery period. The 2025 total non-facility RVUs were 7.72. Code **54162** is reported only when lysis is performed under general anesthesia or regional block, with an instrument, and under sterile conditions.

- If post-circumcision adhesions are manually broken during the postoperative period by the physician who performed the procedure or a physician of the same group and specialty, it will be considered part of the global surgical package.

- Report the service with *ICD-10-CM* code **N47.0** (adherent prepuce in a newborn) or **N47.5** (adhesions of prepuce and glans penis [patients aged >28 days]).

56441 Lysis of labial adhesions

This procedure also includes a 10-day global surgery period. The 2025 total non-facility RVUs were 5.47. Code **56441** is performed with a blunt instrument or scissors under general or local anesthesia.

- *ICD-10-CM* code **Q52.5** (fusion of labia) would be reported with *CPT* code **56441**.
- When the service is provided without anesthesia, modifier **52** may be appended to indicate reduced services. Payer guidance may vary regarding use of modifier **52**. Refer to **Chapter 2** for more information on use of modifier **52**.

Newborn Circumcision

54150 Circumcision, using clamp or other device with regional dorsal penile or ring block

This service is assigned a 0-day global period. The 2025 total non-facility RVUs were 4.45.

When circumcisions are performed in the office,

- If the circumcision using a clamp or other device is performed without either dorsal penile or ring block, append modifier **52** (reduced services) to **54150**.
- If a payer does not base payment on a global surgical package, the surgical tray and anesthetic agents can be reported with **99070**. The description of the supplies (eg, circumcision tray and local anesthetic) would need to be included on the claim form.
- When an E/M service (eg, well-baby visit) is provided on the same date, append modifier **25** to the E/M code.
  - Link the appropriate *ICD-10-CM* code (eg, **Z00.110**, health check for newborn under 8 days old) to the E/M service and link *ICD-10-CM* code **Z41.2** (encounter for routine and ritual male circumcision) to the circumcision code.

Refer to **54160** and **54161** for circumcision performed with surgical excision other than a clamp, device, or dorsal split. These procedures are often provided in facility settings.

Refer to Chapter 15 for information on reporting circumcision in a facility setting.

Nervous System

Neurostimulators (Peripheral Nerve)

New in 2026! Code 64567 replaces temporary code 0270T for reporting noninvasive cranial nerve field stimulation.

●64567 Percutaneous electrical nerve field stimulation, cranial nerves, without implantation

Code **64567** is reported for percutaneous periauricular placement of a non-implanted electrical nerve field stimulator. The nerve field stimulation may be a covered service when provided for treatment of functional abdominal disorders in older children and adolescents.

- As with any new code, verification of coverage and fee schedule amounts prior to provision of services is recommended. Prior authorization and submission of records demonstrating failure of other treatment options (eg, diet modification, probiotics, medications) may be required.

Contraception

This section discusses codes for reporting contraceptive procedures such as injection, insertion, or implant of a contraceptive product. For discussion of codes for reporting contraceptive counseling, refer to the Preventive Medicine E/M for Contraceptive Counseling section in **Chapter 8**.

- Diagnosis codes in category **Z30** for contraceptive counseling or surveillance should be linked to the procedure code for contraceptive services. Refer to "Contraception: Diagnosis Codes for Counseling, Initiation, and Surveillance by Method" at www.aap.org/cfp2026.
- Refer to diagnosis codes in category **T83** for services to address complications associated with a contraceptive device and implant (eg, hemorrhage, pain, displacement, malposition). Codes for symptoms addressed (eg, **N64.4**, mastodynia) should be reported, when applicable.

- Medication and supplies are separately reported when purchased by the practice. Examples include
  - Etonogestrel (contraceptive) implant system, including implant and supplies (J7307)
  - Injection, medroxyprogesterone acetate, per 1 mg (J1050)
  - Intrauterine device (IUD) (J7296–J7298, J7300–J7301)
- When reporting supply of medications, including a contraceptive implant system, include the National Drug Code (NDC) and appropriate NDC units for the product supplied.
- Append modifier 25 to an E/M code when reporting an injection (96372) or other contraceptive procedure on the same date.
  - As with other procedures, codes for contraceptive services include typical preservice work. When patient was previously counseled and now presents for the procedure without an indication for counseling or other E/M service, report only the procedure and supply.
  - Separately report an E/M code only when a preventive medicine service or a significant problem-oriented E/M service is provided and documented. Link the appropriate diagnosis code for the preventive service or problem addressed to the E/M code.

Injectable Contraceptive

When a contraceptive is administered by injection, 96372 (subcutaneous or intramuscular injection) is reported in addition to the appropriate code for the medication (eg, J1050), an 11-digit NDC, and NDC units (eg, 1 unit per mL).

Long-Acting Reversible Contraception

Long-acting reversible contraception procedures include insertion, removal, or removal with reinsertion of an implantable subdermal contraceptive (11981–11983) or an IUD (58300–58301). Codes and 2025 total non-facility RVUs include

11981	Insertion, drug-delivery implant (ie, bioresorbable, biodegradable, nonbiodegradable) (3.03 RVUs)
11982	Removal, nonbiodegradable drug delivery implant (3.31 RVUs)
11983	Removal with reinsertion, nonbiodegradable drug delivery implant (4.25 RVUs)
58300	Insertion of IUD (3.25 RVUs)
58301	Removal of IUD (3.28 RVUs)

For a coding quick reference, refer to "Contraception: Codes for Services Related to Long-Acting Reversible Contraceptives" at www.aap.org/cfp2026.

- A single code, 11983, is reported for a procedure to remove and replace an implantable subdermal contraceptive when performed on the same date.
- Include a code for the implantable subdermal contraceptive (J7307) or IUD product (J7296–J7298, J7300–J7301) in addition to the code for an insertion or removal and reinsertion.
- Report both 58300 and 58301, removal and reinsertion of an IUD at the same encounter.
  - Be aware of payer policies when insertion and removal of an IUD take place on the same date. Some payers will allow payment for only 1 service despite the absence of NCCI code edits for IUD insertion (58300) and IUD removal (58301).
  - When a payer bundles same-date IUD insertion and removal, it may be advantageous to report first the higher-valued procedure. IUD removal (58301) was assigned 3.28 total non-facility RVUs in 2025, whereas IUD insertion (58300) was assigned 3.25 total non-facility RVUs.
- Clinically indicated ultrasonography services are separately reported. Although not commonly required, report limited pelvic ultrasonography (76857) or transvaginal ultrasonography (76830) to confirm placement following a difficult IUD insertion.

Hydration, Injections, and Infusions

Services included as inherent to an infusion or injection are the use of local anesthetic, starting the intravenous (IV) catheter, access to indwelling IV catheters or a subcutaneous catheter or port, flushing catheters at the conclusion of an infusion or between infusions, standard tubing, syringes and supplies, and preparation of chemotherapy agents.

These services are not assigned a global period.

- These codes are intended for reporting by the physician or other QHP in an office setting. They are not reported by a physician or other QHP when performed in a facility setting, because the physician work associated with these procedures involves only affirmation of the treatment plan and direct supervision of the staff performing the services.
- If a significant, separately identifiable E/M service is performed, the appropriate code may be reported with modifier 25 appended. The diagnosis may be the same for the E/M service and infusion or injection (96360–96379).

Documentation of medications administered in the outpatient pediatric practice should include

- **Order for medication**
- **Date and time of administration (Include start/stop times for timed procedures.)**
- **Medication, manufacturer, lot number, and expiration date**
- **NDC, if not captured elsewhere**
- **Dose**
- **Route (eg, intramuscular [IM]) and site of administration (eg, left deltoid)**
- **Observations (eg, held by mother, no sign of adverse reaction after 5 minutes)**
- **Signature and credentials of individual administering medication**

Subcutaneous or Intramuscular Injection (Therapeutic, Prophylactic, and Diagnostic)

96372 Therapeutic, prophylactic, or diagnostic injection (specify substance or drug); subcutaneous or IM

The 2025 total non-facility RVUs were 0.43.

Report **96372** for the administration of a diagnostic, prophylactic, or therapeutic (eg, antibiotic) subcutaneous or IM injection.

✖ Do not report for the administration of a purified protein derivative test.

For administration of immunizations, including administration of an immune globulin for passive immunization, refer to the Categories of Immunization Products and Associated Codes section in Chapter 8.

Hydration, Push Injections, and Infusions

The hydration and infusion codes reported are based on the time when medication administration begins to the time when administration ends. Time must be documented.

When reporting multiple infusions on the same date, physicians select an initial service on the basis of the service that is the primary reason for infusion services on that date. Refer to “Primary and Additional Infusion Codes” at www.aap.org/cfp2026 for a table of primary and additional IV infusion and IV push codes.

Hydration

Codes **96360** (IV infusion, hydration; initial, 31 minutes to 1 hour) and **96361** (each additional hour)

- Were assigned 0.93 (**96360**) and 0.36 (**96361**) 2025 total non-facility RVUs.
- Are intended to report IV hydration infusion using prepackaged fluid and/or electrolyte solutions (eg, physiological [normal] saline solution, D_5-0.45% physiological saline solution with potassium). HCPCS codes and NDCs for hydration solutions may be reported in addition to the procedure codes. Note that some plans may require submission of the invoice price paid for the hydration solution and will pay the lesser of a contractual rate or the amount of the invoice.
- Typically require direct physician supervision for the purpose of consent, safety oversight, or supervision of staff with little special handling for preparation or disposal of materials.
- Do not typically require advanced training of staff because there is usually little risk involved and little patient monitoring required.
- Are reported according to the actual time over which the infusion is administered and do not include the time spent starting the IV and monitoring the patient after infusion.

✖ Are not reported when IV infusions are 30 minutes or less.

Codes 96360 and 96361 are neither used to report infusion of drugs or other substances nor reported when hydration is incidental to non-chemotherapeutic/diagnostic or chemotherapeutic services.

Medical record documentation must support the time and service reported.

- **96360** may be reported for hydration infusion lasting longer than 31 minutes and up to 1 hour.
- **96361** is reported for each additional hour of hydration infusion and for a final interval of 31 to 59 minutes beyond the most recent hour reported.

Code **96361** is reported if an IV hydration infusion is provided secondary or subsequent to a therapeutic, prophylactic, or diagnostic infusion *and administered through the same IV access.*

✖ Do not report 96360 or 96361 when hydration is provided for the purpose of maintaining IV patency or when it is provided as a free-flowing IV infusion during a therapeutic or chemotherapy infusion.

Intra-Arterial and Intravenous Push Injections

96373 Therapeutic, prophylactic, or diagnostic injection (specify substance or drug); intra-arterial

Report 96373 for an initial intra-arterial injection. The 2025 total non-facility RVUs were 0.57.

96374 IV push, single or initial substance/drug

+96375 each additional sequential IV push of a new substance/drug

Codes 96374 and 96375 are reported for IV push or other short infusions of less than 15 minutes. The 2025 total non-facility RVUs were 1.05 (96374) and 0.44 (96375).

- Codes 96374 and 96375 are used only when the health care professional administering the substance or drug is in constant attendance during the administration *and* observing the patient. The IV push must be less than 15 minutes.

Short infusions of less than 15 minutes are reported as a push (eg, 96374).

- Sequential IV push of a new substance or drug is reported with AOC 96375.
- Each drug administered is reported separately with the appropriate infusion code.
- Code 96375 is reported in addition to codes for IV infusion (96365), initial IV push (96374), or chemotherapy administration (96409, 96413), when performed.
- Additional sequential IV push of the same substance or drug (96376) is not reported for services provided in the physician office (ie, is reported only by a facility).

Intravenous Infusions

96365 IV infusion, for therapy, prophylaxis, or diagnosis (specify substance or drug); initial, up to 1 hour

+96366 each additional hour

+96367 additional sequential infusion of a new drug/substance, up to 1 hour

+96368 concurrent infusion

Codes 96365–96368

- Are for infusions for the purpose of administering drugs or substances.
- Typically require direct physician supervision and special attention to prepare, calculate dose, and dispose of materials.
- If fluid infusions are used to administer the drug(s), they are considered incidental hydration and are not reported. Each drug administered is reported separately with the appropriate infusion code.

Subcutaneous Infusion

96369 Subcutaneous infusion for therapy or prophylaxis (specify substance or drug); initial, up to 1 hour, including pump setup and establishment of subcutaneous infusion site(s)

+96370 each additional hour

+96371 additional pump setup with establishment of new subcutaneous infusion site(s)

Subcutaneous infusion, 96369, is reported for services of 16 minutes to 1 hour and includes the pump setup and establishment of the infusion site. Report 96372 for a subcutaneous infusion of less than 16 minutes.

- Report AOC 96370 with 1 unit for each additional 31- to 60-minute period beyond the first hour reported with 96369.
- Do not report a unit of 96370 for a final period of 30 minutes or less.
- Report AOC 96371 when an additional pump setup and the establishment of a new subcutaneous infusion site are provided on the same date as the initial service reported with 96369.

Multiple Infusion Services

When services are performed in the physician's office, report as follows:

Initial Infusion

- Report the code that best describes the key or primary reason for the service regardless of the order in which the infusions or injections occur. Only 1 initial service code (eg, 96365) should be reported *unless the protocol or patient condition requires using 2 separate IV sites*. The difference in time and effort in providing this second IV site access is also reported with the initial service code with modifier 59 (distinct procedural service) appended (eg, 96365, 96365 59).

- If an injection or infusion is of a subsequent or concurrent nature, even if it is the first such service within that group of services, a subsequent or concurrent code from the appropriate section should be reported. For example, the first IV push given after an initial 1-hour infusion is reported with a subsequent IV push code.
- ✖ Do not report a second initial service on the same date caused by an IV catheter requiring a restart, an IV rate not being able to be achieved without 2 catheters, or a port of a multi-lumen catheter requiring access.

Sequential Infusion

This is an infusion or IV push of a new substance or drug following a primary or initial service. For example, if an IV push was performed through the same IV access after an IV infusion for therapy, the appropriate codes to report would be **96365** and **96375**. If an IV push was performed through a different IV access route, the services would be reported with **96365** and **96374**.

Sequential infusions are reported only 1 time for the same infusate. But if additional hours were required for the infusion, the appropriate "each additional hour" AOC would be reported. Different infusates can be reported with the same code as the original sequential code. All sequential services require that there be a new substance or drug; only a facility may report a sequential IV push of the same drug with **96376**.

Concurrent Infusion

AOC **96368** is used to report an infusion of a new substance or drug at the same time as another drug or substance, not including fluids for hydration. It is not time based and is reported only once per day. Concurrent administration of another new drug or substance (the third substance or drug) is not reported.

✖ Do not report hydration concurrently with any other infusion service.

Example

➤ **A 3-year-old established patient is seen with a concern of vomiting and fever for the past 24 hours.** She declined all food and liquids and last voided 12 hours before the visit. Her diagnosis is bilateral acute suppurative otitis media with fever and dehydration. Intravenous fluids are initiated with physiological (normal) saline solution, and IV ceftriaxone (750 mg) is infused over 30 minutes for her otitis media. After 1 hour 45 minutes of IV hydration, she urinates, begins tolerating liquids, and is released home. The problem addressed is 1 acute illness with systemic symptoms, and the risk of morbidity resulting from treatment is moderate, supporting moderate MDM.

ICD-10-CM	*CPT*
E86.0 (dehydration) **H66.003** (acute suppurative otitis media without spontaneous rupture of ear drum, bilateral) **R11.10** (vomiting) **R50.81** (fever in conditions classified elsewhere)	**99214 25** (established patient office E/M) **96365** (IV infusion, for therapy) **96361** × 1 (IV infusion, hydration, each additional hour) **J0696** × 3 units (ceftriaxone sodium, per 250 mg) **J7030** (infusion, normal saline solution, 1,000 cc)

Teaching Point: The initial 30 minutes of infusion is reported with **96365** for infusion of the IV ceftriaxone. The concurrent administration of saline solution is not separately reported. The nonoverlapping hydration infusion of 75 minutes is reported with 1 unit of AOC **96361**. One unit of **96361** is reported for each 31- to 60-minute period beyond the first hour of the infusion services. A period of 30 minutes or less (eg, the final 15 minutes of hydration beyond the last hour) is not reported with **96361**.

Link the appropriate diagnosis code to each procedure (eg, **H66.003** is linked to **J0696**). The medication should be reported with the appropriate NDC and NDC units in addition to the HCPCS codes. The fluid used to administer ceftriaxone is not reported because it is considered incidental hydration.

Other Injection and Infusion Services

96523 Irrigation of implanted venous access device for drug delivery systems

Code **96523** is used to report irrigation required for implanted venous access devices for drug delivery systems when services are provided on a separate day from the injection or infusion service.

✖ Do not report **96523** in conjunction with other services.

Chemotherapy and Other Highly Complex Drug/Biologic Agent Administration

Codes 96401–96549 are reported for chemotherapy administration. *CPT* defines *chemotherapy administration* as parenteral administration of non-radionuclide antineoplastic drugs, antineoplastic agents provided for treatment of non-cancer diagnoses and to substances such as certain monoclonal antibody agents and other biologic response modifiers.

Codes 96401–96549 represent services that require direct physician supervision of staff who have advanced practice training and competency as well as special considerations for preparation, dosage, or disposal. Commonly, these services entail significant patient risk and frequent monitoring. Although the codes may be appropriate for reporting administration of certain monoclonal antibody agents or other biologic response modifiers, the reporting physician or QHP should base code selection (eg, 96401, administration of non-hormonal anti-neoplastic versus 96372, subcutaneous or IM injection) on the complexity of the drug administration. Payer policies may also limit code selection.

New in 2026! To report mechanical scalp-cooling services that may be associated with chemotherapy, refer to *CPT* codes 97007–97009.

Moderate Sedation

Moderate sedation codes 99151–99153 and 99155–99157 are used for reporting moderate sedation when intraservice time is 10 minutes or more. **Table 13-3** contains sedation codes and descriptors.

Table 13-3. Moderate Sedation

	Intraservice Time	
Moderate Sedation by the Physician or QHP Performing the Diagnostic or Therapeutic Procedure	**First 15 min (10–22 min)**	**Each Additional 15 min and Last 8–22 min**
Moderate sedation services provided by the same physician or other QHP performing the diagnostic or therapeutic service that the sedation supports, requiring the presence of an independent trained observer to assist in the monitoring of the patient's level of consciousness and physiological status; initial 15 minutes of intraservice time, patient younger than 5 years of age	99151	+99153 (Report only in addition to 99151 or 99152.)
5 years or older	99152	+99153
Moderate Sedation by a Physician or QHP Other Than the Individual Performing the Diagnostic or Therapeutic Procedure		
Moderate sedation services (other than those services described by 00100–01999) provided by a physician other than the health care professional performing the diagnostic or therapeutic service that the sedation supports; patient younger than 5 years	99155	+99157 (Report only in addition to 99155 or 99156.)
5 years or older	99156	+99157

Abbreviation: QHP, qualified health care professional.

Moderate sedation is a drug-induced depression of consciousness. No interventions are required to maintain cardiovascular functions or a patent airway, and spontaneous ventilation is adequate.

Codes for moderate sedation are not assigned a global period. Code selection is based, in part, on the age of the patient (ie, <5 years or ≥5 years).

✖ Do not report moderate sedation codes for medication administration for pain control, for minimal sedation (anxiolysis), or for deep sedation or monitored anesthesia care (00100–01999).

Report 99151–99153 when

- The administration of moderate sedation is provided by the physician who is simultaneously performing a procedure (eg, fracture reduction, vessel cutdown, central catheter placement, wound repair).
- An independent trained observer is present (required element of service) to assist the physician in monitoring the patient during the procedure or diagnostic service.

An *independent trained observer* is an individual qualified to monitor the patient during the procedure but lacking other duties (eg, assisting at surgery) during the procedure.

Report **99155–99157** for moderate sedation

- By a second physician or QHP, other than the health care professional performing the diagnostic or therapeutic services, who administers the sedating agent(s) and monitors the patient (face-to-face) throughout the procedure and until the patient is stable for recovery status

Codes are selected according to intraservice time. Intraservice time

- Begins with the administration of the sedating agent(s)
- Ends when the procedure is completed, the patient is stable for recovery status, and the physician or other QHP providing the sedation ends personal continuous face-to-face time with the patient

Refer to your *CPT* reference for activities included in intraservice time.

For each additional 15 minutes of intraservice time, report either of the following codes:
99153 in addition to either **99151** or **99152**
99157 in addition to either **99155** or **99156**

The midpoint between the end of the previous 15-minute period must be passed to report an additional unit of intraservice time (ie, intraservice time must continue for at least 8 minutes beyond the last full 15 minutes of intraservice time).

✖ Do not report moderate sedation service of less than 10 minutes of intraservice time.

✖ Do not separately report the preservice work of moderate sedation services and do not include time spent in preservice work in the intraservice time. Refer to your *CPT* reference for activities included in preservice work.

✖ Do not separately report or include the time of postservice work in the intraservice time. Postservice work of moderate sedation includes

- Assessment of the patient's vital signs, level of consciousness, and neurological, cardiovascular, and pulmonary stability in the post-sedation recovery period
- Assessment of the patient's readiness for discharge following the procedure
- Preparation of documentation for sedation service
- Communication with the family or caregiver about sedation service

✖ Do not separately report pulse oximetry (**94760–94762**).

Documentation of moderate sedation services must include all the following items:

- **The description of the procedure**
- **Name and dosage(s) of the sedation agent(s)**
- **Route of administration of the sedation agent(s) and who administered the agent (physician or independent observer)**
- **The ongoing assessment of the child's level of consciousness and physiological status (eg, heart rate, oxygen saturation levels) during and after the procedure**
- **The presence, name, and title of the independent observer or performing physician or other QHP**
- **Total time from administration of the sedation agent(s) (start time) until the physician's face-to-face service is no longer required (end time)**

Examples

➤ **A 3-year-old requires incision and removal of a piece of glass from a puncture wound of the right foot.** Moderate sedation is required and is performed by the Pediatric Advanced Life Support–trained physician with an independent observer who has been trained in pediatric basic life support. The physician supervises the administration of the sedating agent; assesses the child until an effective, safe level of sedation is achieved; and continues to assess the child's level of consciousness and physiological status while performing the procedure. The procedure takes a total of 28 minutes from the time of administration of the agent until the physician completes the procedure and determines that the child's condition is stable and face-to-face physician time is no longer required.

ICD-10-CM	*CPT*
S91.341A (puncture wound with foreign body, right foot) Codes for external cause, activity, and place of injury are reported when documented.	**10121** (incision and removal of foreign body, subcutaneous tissues; complex) **99151** (moderate [conscious] sedation, patient younger than 5 years, first 15 minutes) **+99153** (moderate [conscious] sedation, each additional 15 minutes of intraservice time)

Teaching Point: If a medically necessary, significant, and separately identifiable E/M service had also been performed, an E/M visit with modifier **25** appended could have been reported. The agent itself should also be reported.

➤ **Same patient as previous example, except moderate sedation is performed by the Pediatric Advanced Life Support–trained physician while another physician performs the procedure.** The procedure, from the time of administration of the agent until the repair is complete and the child's condition is stable and no longer requires face-to-face physician time, takes a total of 28 minutes.

ICD-10-CM	*CPT*
S91.341A (puncture wound with foreign body, right foot) Codes for external cause, activity, and place of injury are reported when documented.	The physician repairing the wound reports **10121** (incision and removal of foreign body, subcutaneous tissues; complex) The physician performing moderate sedation reports **99155** (moderate [conscious] sedation, patient younger than 5 years, first 15 minutes) **+99157** (moderate [conscious] sedation, each additional 15 minutes of intraservice time)

Teaching Point: Each physician reports the service provided. The time of moderate sedation used in code selection is only the intraservice time.

For virtual reality procedural dissociation services to support and optimize patient comfort and tolerance during a procedure, refer to codes **0771T–0774T**. To learn more about these codes, read the December 2022 *AAP Pediatric Coding Newsletter*™ article "Category III Procedure Code Updates for January 2023" (https://doi.org/10.1542/pcco_book224_document002).

To test your knowledge of the information presented in this chapter, complete the quiz found at the end of it, after the resources. Answers to each quiz are found in **Appendix II**.

Chapter Takeaways

This chapter provided an overview of coding for procedures in the office and other outpatient settings. Following are some takeaways from this chapter:

- Many, but not all, payers use the RVUs and global periods assigned by the Medicare program. Learn how individual payers value and pay for procedural services.
- The practice expense component of RVUs assigned to procedural services includes supplies such as surgical trays and local anesthetics. Other supplies such as medications and splints may be separately reported when purchased by the practice.
- When a global service is provided, report follow-up visits during a global period with **99024**.
- Append modifier **24** to codes for unrelated E/M services during a postoperative period.
- Some minor procedures are included in E/M services and not separately reported (eg, removal of nonimpacted ear wax).
- All procedures include some preservice and postservice work. Only report an E/M service that is significant and separately identifiable in the documentation.

Resources

AAP Coding Assistance and Education

AAP coding webinar, "Burns, Foreign Bodies, and Beyond: Coding Acute Procedures in Pediatrics," May 2024 (https://publications.aap.org/codingnews/resources/27969/aap-coding-webinars)

AAP Pediatric Coding Newsletter

"Procedural Services: Modifiers to Report Site and Laterality," January 2025 (https://doi.org/10.1542/pcco_book249_document005)

"Reporting Care of Sunburn: Evaluation and Management or Procedure?" July 2024 (https://doi.org/10.1542/pcco_book243_document002)

Global Periods and Relative Value Units

MPFS Relative Value Files (www.cms.gov/medicare/payment/fee-schedules/physician/pfs-relative-value-files)

Online-Exclusive Content at www.aap.org/cfp2026

"Common Office Procedures and Global Days"

"Contraception: Codes for Services Related to Long-Acting Reversible Contraceptives"

"Contraception: Diagnosis Codes for Counseling, Initiation, and Surveillance by Method"

"Primary and Additional Infusion Codes"

Test Your Knowledge!

1. **What modifier is reported to indicate that an E/M visit on the day of surgery was significant and separately identifiable from the preservice and postservice work of a procedure?**
   a. Modifier 25
   b. Modifier 57
   c. Modifier 24
   d. None. An E/M service on the day before or day of surgery at which the decision for surgery is made is included in the surgical package.
2. **Which of the following is correct for reporting a visit for postoperative follow-up with removal of sutures (without anesthesia)?**
   a. 15853 and 15854 are reported whenever sutures and/or staples are removed.
   b. 15853 and 15854 are reported when a physician or QHP accepts a transfer of postoperative care and removes sutures and/or staples.
   c. An E/M code and both 15853 and 15854 are reported when provided for postoperative care of a procedure that has a 0-day global period.
   d. An E/M code and either 15853 or 15854 are reported when provided for postoperative care of a procedure that has a 0-day global period.
3. **Which procedure is included in an E/M service (ie, not separately reported)?**
   a. Burn care for a first-degree burn
   b. Incision in lingual frenulum
   c. Urinary catheterization for specimen collection
   d. Removal of an umbilical clamp
4. **Which of the following is true of laceration repair?**
   a. If multiple wounds belong to the same category of difficulty and location, add the lengths and report with a single code.
   b. Report separate codes for repair of each noncontiguous wound.
   c. Wound repair by dermal adhesive is included in an E/M service.
   d. Topical or injected local anesthetic is separately reported.
5. **Which is true of code 96360, initial hour of hydration infusion?**
   a. 96360 is reported if an IV hydration infusion is provided secondary or subsequent to a therapeutic, prophylactic, or diagnostic infusion.
   b. 96360 includes time spent starting the IV and monitoring the patient after infusion is completed.
   c. 96360 may be reported for hydration infusion lasting longer than 31 minutes and up to 1 hour.
   d. 96360 may be reported for hydration infusion of 15–30 minutes.

Part 3

Primarily for Hospital Settings

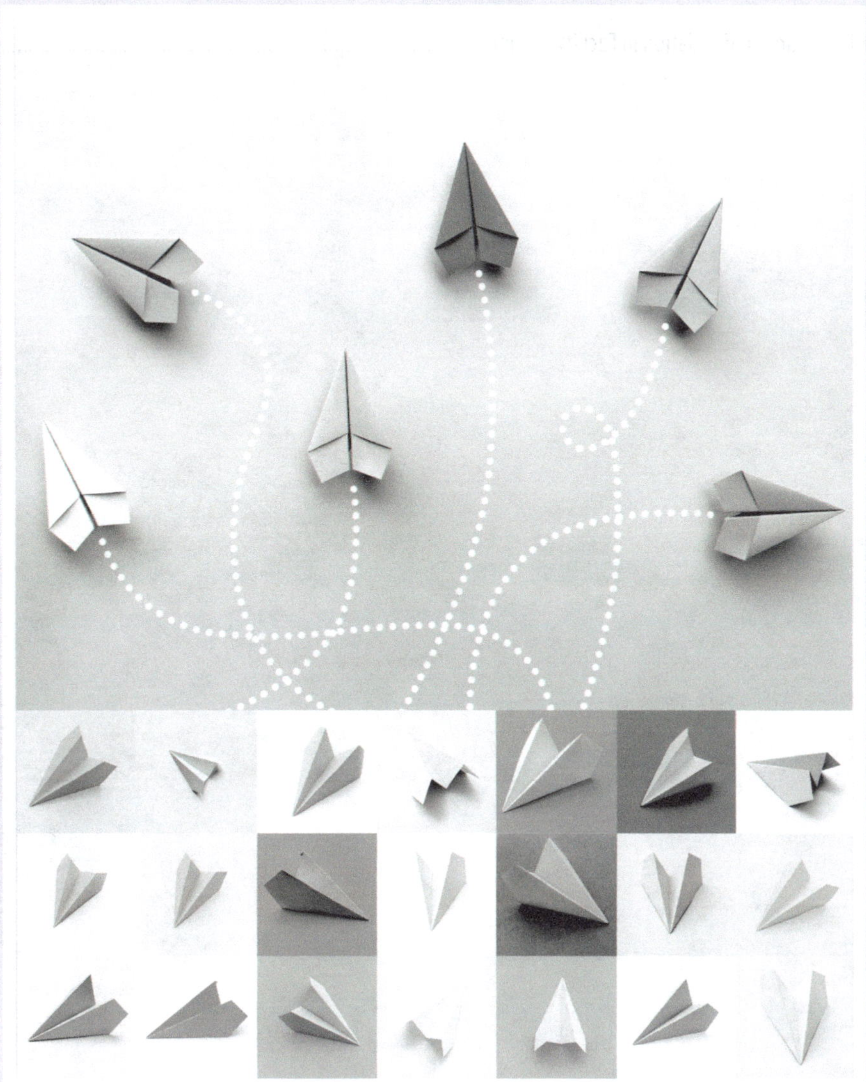

Part 3. Primarily for Hospital Settings

CHAPTER 14

Emergency Department Services

Contents

Chapter Highlights

- Documentation and coding of diagnoses for services in the emergency department (ED)
- Overview and examples of evaluation and management (E/M) code selection for ED services
- Use of procedure code modifiers
- Reporting procedures in the ED
- Directing emergency medical technicians
- Reporting provision of critical care services in the ED

Coding for Service Provided in the Emergency Department

This chapter reviews the importance of documentation and coding for services provided in the ED. This includes assigning codes based on the documented reason(s) for ED services and the problems addressed, selecting appropriate diagnosis and procedure codes, and determining when multiple services on the same date are separately reported.

Using Diagnosis Codes to Support the Level of ED Visits

ED physicians play critical roles in care and documentation. The reason for visit (ie, the chief complaint) may not be the principal discharge diagnosis. When multiple symptoms are listed as chief complaints during the ED triage process, the physician needs to designate only 1 sign, symptom, disease, or injury as the chief complaint (principal reason for the visit). Hospitals depend on the physician's designation of the chief complaint because only 1 diagnosis code may be reported for this category on the hospital claim form. This diagnosis is used to help support the urgency of the ED visit under prudent layperson guidelines as well as support resource utilization. This may be different from conditions that are "present on admission" that must be tracked by hospitals for inpatient admission.

The diagnoses on the physician's claim for professional services are equally important to support the level of ED service reported (99281–99285). Some health plans now compare diagnosis codes submitted on physician claims, especially those claims that include 99284 and 99285, to a predetermined list of diagnosis codes indicating conditions that the plan considers to typically require these levels of service. When a claim for 99284 or 99285 is submitted with diagnosis codes not included on the list, the claim may be down-coded (eg, changed to 99283) and/or paid at the rate of the lesser code. Billing staff should be alert for payment below the practice's contracted rates.

As shown in **Figure 14-1**, down-coding 99284 or 99285 to 99283 results in a significant corresponding decrease in relative value units (RVUs) and fee-for-service payment. RVUs listed are 2025 RVUs (not geographically adjusted), as 2026 RVUs were unavailable at the time of this publication. To learn more about payment based on RVUs, refer to **Chapter 4**.

Figure 14-1. Impact of Down-Coded Services by Relative Value Units

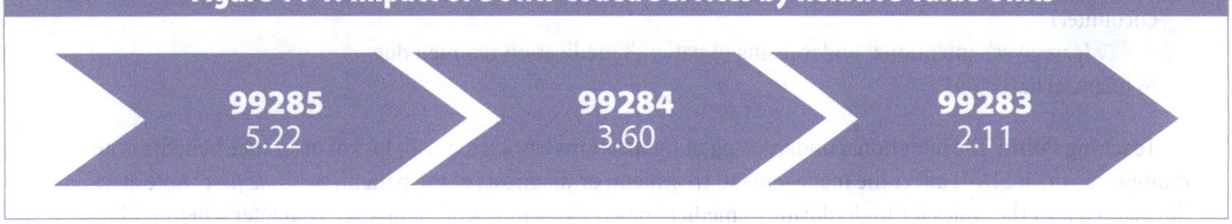

Medicaid plans also significantly limit the amount paid for any condition not included on a diagnosis list, regardless of the level of service reported. To receive the payment most appropriate under the health plan contract,

- List first the diagnosis that is most responsible for the level of service provided, and report the code for that diagnosis first on your claim.
- Document and report codes for all current conditions that require or affect patient care treatment or management.

Some plans consider only the first 1 or 2 diagnoses listed on the claim.

Some plans account for all diagnoses on the claim, including

- Complicating factors (eg, **F84.0**, autism spectrum disorder)
- Social determinants of health (SDoH; eg, **Z59.82**, transportation insecurity)
- External cause of injury (eg, **W04.XXXA**, fall while being carried or supported by other persons, initial encounter)

Physicians should clearly document all diagnoses, including factors that increased the level of medical decision-making (MDM) of an encounter (eg, in an assessment statement). This documentation can help a professional coder, if used, extract the appropriate diagnosis codes. It is important to note that a coder cannot extract diagnoses from an ED note or assessment when listed with "indeterminant" wording such as "consistent with," "possible," or "probable." However, the diagnosis can be extracted by the coder if it is listed as a definitive impression or diagnosis. To appeal a down-coded claim, medical records supporting the higher level of service must typically be submitted to the health plan.

For example, if the physician notes that the condition is "consistent with dehydration" in the MDM or assessment statement but lists "dehydration" under the discharge diagnosis, then the coder can use it as a definitive diagnosis.

The specificity of the secondary diagnosis can also have an impact on third-party payer determinations. For example, using the diagnosis of "fever" (**R50.9**, fever, unspecified) instead of "fever affecting a medical condition" (**R50.81**, fever presenting with conditions classified elsewhere) could potentially cause down-coding of the encounter. The more specific fever code is intended to be reported in conjunction with codes for conditions (eg, leukemia, sickle cell disease, or cystic fibrosis) for which fever indicates the need for prompt medical attention because of the patient's underlying medical problem.

Coding for Social Determinants of Health

When SDoH (eg, homelessness, food insecurity) influence a patient's health and/or limit the management and treatment options for a patient, the SDOH should be documented to support assignment of codes for the SDoH. Clinical staff and/or a patient or caregiver may document the SDoH in the medical record. Codes for SDoH are mainly found in categories **Z55–Z60** and **Z62–Z65**.

Emergency Department Services

Chapter 14

Example

➤ **A 10-year-old with severe persistent asthma presents with an acute exacerbation.** Twice-daily fluticasone and salmeterol inhaler were prescribed; however, the mother says she has been giving it once every other day because the child lost insurance benefits. The child improves after ED treatment. To promote compliance with the child's asthma treatment plan, the patient's mother is referred to an ED social worker for assistance in getting the child's medications filled. The child is discharged to home. Discharge diagnoses are severe persistent asthma with exacerbation and underdosing of fluticasone and salmeterol inhaler due to financial hardship.

ICD-10-CM	*CPT*
J45.51 (severe persistent asthma with (acute) exacerbation) **T48.6X6A** (underdosing of antiasthmatics, initial encounter) **T38.0X6A** (underdosing of glucocorticoids and synthetic analogues, initial encounter) **Z91.A20** (caregiver's intentional underdosing of patient's medication regimen due to financial hardship)	**99284** Moderate MDM

Teaching Point: The intentional underdosing of medications associated with loss of insurance benefits is an example in which SDoH affect the management, treatment, or diagnosis of the patient. A "*Code first*" note at **Z91.A20** directs to report the codes for underdosing of medications (**T36–T50**) with fifth or sixth character **6** before **Z91.A20**.

The level of MDM for this example is supported by the moderate complexity of an exacerbated chronic condition and moderate risk of morbidity or mortality of prescription drug management. Moderate risk is also supported when SDoH significantly limit diagnosis or treatment. The limitation of diagnosis or treatment associated with the SDoH must be documented to support moderate risk.

Reporting External Cause of Injury

States may require EDs to report codes describing the circumstances of an injury or another morbidity. These codes are referred to as *external cause* codes in *International Classification of Diseases, 10th Revision, Clinical Modification* (*ICD-10-CM*). These codes capture the cause, intent, place of occurrence, activity of the patient at the time of the event, and patient status (eg, employee, military, volunteer, student). External cause codes (categories **V00–Y99**) are indexed in the

ICD-10-CM External Cause of Injuries Index and found in Chapter 20 of the tabular list of *ICD-10-CM*. For example, under the term struck, sub-terms allow reporting of external causes such as struck by baseball (**W21.03-**) or baseball bat (**W21.11-**). An additional code can be used to show if the striking was intentional (**Y08.0-**). Combination codes allow for reporting multiple details, such as striking against an object with subsequent fall (**W18.0-**). *These codes are never listed as a principal diagnosis.*

Although the physician may not be required to add the specific external cause code with the discharge diagnosis, there should be sufficient documentation in the record to allow a coder to extract the proper diagnosis code.

External cause codes provide information that is valuable for research on the cause and occurrence of injuries as well as evaluation of injury prevention strategies (eg, reporting of head injuries reduced because of campaigns to encourage bicycle helmet use). This is particularly important in pediatrics, as injuries remain the leading cause of death and disability.

Examples of assignment of external cause codes are provided in the ED Evaluation and Management Codes section later in this chapter.

Key points for reporting external cause codes include

- External cause codes are never the principal or first-listed diagnosis code.
- External cause codes may be reported in conjunction with any health condition that is related to an external cause (eg, adverse effect of medical treatment).
- Report *ICD-10-CM* codes for the cause and intent of an injury or illness for the duration of treatment. The seventh character of the code indicates the nature of the encounter.
  - Initial or *active* care (**A**).
  - Subsequent care *during the healing phase or follow-up care* (**D**).
  - Care for a *sequela* (**S**) of the injury or illness.
  - Seventh characters in some code categories provide additional details (eg, type of open fracture).

For additional information and examples of seventh characters in use, refer to Chapter 1.

- External cause codes indicating place of occurrence, activity, and patient status are reported only at the initial encounter for treatment.
- If the intent (eg, accident, self-harm, assault) of the cause of an injury or another condition is unknown or unspecified, code the intent as *accidental*.
- No external cause code should be assigned when the cause and intent of an illness or injury are included in another reported code (eg, **T58.11XA**, initial encounter for toxic effect of carbon monoxide from utility gas, accidental).
- No external cause code should be assigned when an injury is ruled out after examination and observation (eg, **Z04.1**, encounter for examination and observation following transport accident).

In *ICD-10-CM*, the X character is used as a placeholder to allow for future expansion and must be included for the code to be valid. Refer to the American Academy of Pediatrics (AAP) *Pediatric ICD-10-CM 2026: A Manual for Provider-Based Coding* (www.aap.org/Pediatric-ICD-10-CM-2026-11th-Edition-Paperback) and *ICD-10-CM* resources (www.aap.org/en/practice-management/child-health-finance-payment-strategy/coding-and-valuation/icd-10-cm-resources) for more information on codes and code selection.

Reporting Suspected or Confirmed Abuse or Other Maltreatment

ICD-10-CM includes codes for reporting suspected or confirmed neglect or abandonment; physical, sexual, or psychological abuse; forced sexual exploitation; and forced labor exploitation. These codes are selected depending on the type of maltreatment, whether the patient is a child or an adult, and whether the maltreatment is suspected, confirmed, or ruled out at the encounter.

Suspected (**T76.-**) or confirmed maltreatment (**T74.-**) is reported as the first-listed diagnosis when this is the reason for the encounter. Codes for associated mental health or physical injury are reported secondary to the code for suspected or confirmed abuse.

- Codes are selected with documentation as the basis. The record should clearly state whether abuse is suspected, ruled out, or confirmed.
- Codes include seventh characters **A**, **D**, and **S**.

Examples

In each example, codes for diagnosed injuries, assault, and perpetrator are reported in addition to the T74 code.

➤ **Physical abuse is confirmed and initial active treatment is provided at an encounter.**
T74.12XA Child physical abuse confirmed, initial encounter

➤ **Follow-up care during healing of injuries caused by confirmed physical abuse is provided at an encounter.**
T74.12XD Child physical abuse confirmed, subsequent encounter

➤ **A child is evaluated for scar contracture that is a late effect of injuries caused by confirmed physical abuse.**
T74.12XS Child physical abuse confirmed, sequela

- When reporting confirmed abuse (T74.-), also report codes for assault (X92–Y04; Y08, Y09) and, when known, perpetrator (Y07.-).

Report T76 (suspected maltreatment or abuse) when maltreatment cannot be confirmed or ruled out. For example, a child says she is being bullied at school. You would code T76.32- (child psychological abuse, suspected).

Reporting Suspected Maltreatment When Ruled Out

Report one of the following codes from category Z04 for an encounter at which neglect, abuse, or exploitation is *suspected but ruled out* and not a code from category T74 or T76:

Z04.72 Encounter for examination and observation following alleged child physical abuse
Z04.42 following alleged child rape
Z04.81 of victim following forced sexual exploitation
Z04.82 of victim following forced labor exploitation

When maltreatment is ruled out but problems are addressed, however, report codes for the problems addressed in lieu of a category Z04 code.

Z04 codes may be reported when a patient is brought in for evaluation by a legal authority as well as when the patient presents with a parent or caregiver.

ED Evaluation and Management Codes

Refer to the full discussion of the E/M guidelines provided in **Chapter 6** to learn the guidelines and definitions that guide E/M code selection.

99281 ED visit for the E/M of a patient that may not require the presence of a physician or other qualified health care professional
99282 ED visit for the E/M of a patient, which requires a medically appropriate history and/or examination and straightforward MDM
99283 ED visit for the E/M of a patient, which requires a medically appropriate history and/or examination and low level of MDM
99284 ED visit for the E/M of a patient, which requires a medically appropriate history and/or examination and moderate level of MDM
99285 ED visit for the E/M of a patient, which requires a medically appropriate history and/or examination and high level of MDM

For coding purposes, an ED is defined as *an organized hospital-based facility for the provision of unscheduled episodic services to patients who present for immediate medical attention.* The facility must be available 24 hours a day, 7 days a week.

- ED E/M codes 99281–99285 are reported only when care is provided to a patient who has been admitted to an ED.
  - Some states allow for freestanding EDs that are not hospital affiliated. Payers may or may not allow the use of ED codes in these circumstances.
  - Physician services provided in a freestanding hospital-affiliated ED may be subject to specific billing rules. Check payer contracts for payment and billing policies.
- Report the appropriate *Current Procedural Terminology* (*CPT*®) office or other outpatient visit codes (99202–99215) and appropriate place of service code (eg, 20 for urgent care facility) for services performed in an urgent care center, a non-hospital facility, or a facility that is not open 24 hours a day. These facilities are not considered freestanding EDs.
- There is no differentiation between new and established patients for ED encounters.

- The level of ED codes 99282–99285 is based on the MDM. Time is not used in selection of 99282–99285.
- The highest 2 of 3 elements of MDM are used to select the level of an ED E/M code.
  1. **Problem(s):** the number and complexity of presenting problems
  2. **Data:** the amount and/or complexity of data to be reviewed and analyzed
  3. **Risk:** the risk of complications and/or morbidity or mortality of patient management
- The concept of the level of MDM does not apply to 99281 because this level of service does not require a physician's or other qualified health care professional's (QHP's) MDM.

Because 99281 represents a service that does not require the presence of a physician or other QHP and is likely performed by clinical staff employed by the facility, payment policies for the physician's or QHP's supervision may vary.

Medical necessity is an overarching criterion for selecting the level of E/M service. Physicians should always consider whether the nature of the presenting problem supports the medical necessity of services rendered when selecting the level of E/M service. All levels of ED service include a medically appropriate history and examination as determined by the treating physician or QHP.

Split or Shared ED Visits

When a physician and QHP of the same specialty and same group practice each participate in the E/M service provided to a patient, the service is reported by the individual who provided the substantial portion of the encounter (eg, made or approved the management plan for the number and complexity of problems addressed at the encounter and takes responsibility for that plan with its inherent risk of complications and/or morbidity or mortality of patient management). This can be documented either by placing a statement such as "I personally made/approved the management plan for this patient and take responsibility for the patient management" or by documenting the MDM elements performed (eg, plan of care, discharge instructions). Some payers may require that modifier FS (split or shared E/M visit) be appended to the E/M code when reporting a split/shared visit. Refer to Chapter 6 for additional discussion of reporting split/shared visits. Refer also to the Time-Based Critical Care in the ED section later in this chapter for discussion of split/shared critical care services.

Use **Table 14-1** to help you select the appropriate level of ED E/M service in the examples for each level of service that follow.

Emergency Department Services

Chapter 14

Examples

➤ **A 6-year-old presents with a splinter in their right forefoot.** The patient was playing on a wooden deck with bare feet about an hour ago and felt the splinter enter the foot. The mother wants assistance removing the splinter because the child has refused to be still for removal at home. Immunizations are up to date. The child appears well and is in no discomfort. Examination reveals a visible wood splinter that is readily grasped with tweezers and removed. Antibiotic ointment and a bandage are applied.

ICD-10-CM	*CPT*
S90.851A (superficial foreign body, right foot, initial encounter)	99282 Straightforward MDM

Problem(s) addressed ➡ ***Minimal*** (minor)
Data reviewed and analyzed ➡ ***Limited*** (independent historian)
Risk of patient management ➡ ***Minimal***

Teaching Point: The MDM elements support 99282. Although the data are limited, potentially supporting low MDM, the other 2 elements support straightforward MDM. Clinically indicated history and examination are documented but are not the basis of code selection. Because no incision was required to remove the splinter, removal of the foreign body is not separately reported.

If the splinter removal had required an incision, a code for incision and removal of a foreign body from subcutaneous tissue would have been reported with 10120 if simple or 10121 if complex. A separately reportable E/M service would not likely be supported (ie, would not likely be significantly beyond the typical preservice work of the procedure).

Table 14-1. Code Selection Requirements for Emergency Department Evaluation and Management Service (Excluding 99281)

Level/Codes	Medical Decision-Making (2 of 3 Required: Problems, Data,[a] Risk)		
	Problem(s) Addressed	**Data Reviewed and Analyzed[b]**	**Risk**
Low 99283	Low—*Any 1 of* ≥2 self-limited or minor problems 1 stable chronic illness 1 acute, uncomplicated illness or injury 1 stable acute illness 1 acute, uncomplicated illness or injury requiring hospital inpatient or observation level of care *Examples* • Acute gastroenteritis • Uncomplicated hand-foot-and-mouth disease • Recheck of wound repaired at previous encounter • Resolution of URI with continued cough	Limited (*Meet 1 of 2 categories*) Category 1: Tests and documents (*Any 2*)[a] • Review of prior external note(s)—each unique source • Review of the result(s) of each unique test • Ordering of each unique test Category 2: Assessment requiring an independent historian(s)	Low *Examples* • Over-the-counter medication(s) • Removal of sutures • Physical, language, or occupational therapy
Moderate 99284	Moderate—*Any 1 of* ≥1 chronic illness with exacerbation, progression, or side effects of treatment ≥2 stable chronic illnesses 1 undiagnosed new problem with uncertain prognosis 1 acute illness with systemic symptoms 1 acute, complicated injury *Examples* • Asthma with exacerbation but not hypoxia • Unexplained bruising • Acute gastroenteritis with dehydration • Intermittent headaches and confusion following concussion	Moderate (*Meet 1 of 3 categories*)[a] Category 1: Tests and documents (*Any 3*) • Review of prior external note(s)—each unique source • Review of the result(s) of each unique test • Ordering of each unique test • Assessment requiring an independent historian(s) Category 2: Independent interpretation of a test performed by another physician/other QHP[b] Category 3: Discussion of management or test interpretation with external physician/other QHP/appropriate source[b]	Moderate *Examples* • Prescription drug management or off-label use of over-the-counter medication • Decision about minor surgery with identified patient or procedure risk factors • Decision about elective major surgery without identified patient or procedure risk factors • Diagnosis or treatment significantly limited by SDoH

Table 14-1 (*continued*)			
	Medical Decision-Making (2 of 3 Required: Problems, Data,[a] Risk)		
Level/Codes	**Problem(s) Addressed**	**Data Reviewed and Analyzed[b]**	**Risk**
High 99285	High—*Any 1 of* ≥1 chronic illness with severe exacerbation, progression, or side effects of treatment 1 acute or chronic illness or injury that poses a threat to life or bodily function *Examples* • Asthma with hypoxia (status asthmaticus) • Infant fever, tachycardia, lethargy, and dehydration • Injury or illness with shock	Extensive (*Meet 2 of 3 categories*) Category 1: Tests and documents (*Any 3*)[a] • Review of prior external note(s) from each unique source • Review of the result(s) of each unique test • Ordering of each unique test • Assessment requiring an independent historian(s) Category 2: Independent interpretation of a test performed by another physician/other QHP[b] Category 3: Discussion of management or test interpretation with external physician/other QHP/appropriate source[b]	High *Examples* • Drug therapy requiring intensive monitoring for toxicity • Decision about elective major surgery with identified patient or procedure risk factors • Decision about emergency major surgery • Decision about hospitalization or escalation of hospital level of care • Decision not to resuscitate or to de-escalate care because prognosis is poor • Decision regarding parenteral controlled substances

Abbreviations: QHP, qualified health care professional; SDOH, social determinants of health; URI, upper respiratory infection.

[a] Each unique test, order, or document contributes to the combination of 2 or combination of 3 in Category 1.

[b] Do not count data review or communications reported with other codes (eg, electrocardiogram interpretation and report reported with 93010, interprofessional consultation referral service reported with 99452).

➤ **A 13-year-old patient presents with an injury to the left ankle.** The patient reports hurting the ankle by tripping during a basketball game approximately an hour earlier and is experiencing continued mild pain but without swelling. The patient can bear their full weight. Parents report no prior injuries. There is discussion with the patient and family that a requested radiograph is not indicated. A compression wrap is applied, and the patient and parents are instructed on home care including over-the-counter nonsteroidal pain medication. They are to follow up with the patient's primary care physician. Diagnosis is sprain of the anterior tibiofibular ligament of the left ankle.

ICD-10-CM	*CPT*
S93.432A (sprain of tibiofibular ligament of left ankle, initial encounter) W01.0XXA (fall on same level from slipping, tripping and stumbling without subsequent striking against object, initial encounter) Y93.67 (activity, basketball)	99283 Low MDM

Problem(s) addressed ➡ ***Low*** (acute, uncomplicated injury)
Data reviewed and analyzed ➡ ***Limited*** (Category 2—independent historian)
Risk of patient management ➡ ***Low***

Teaching Point: Low MDM supports 99283. All 3 elements of MDM support this level of service. If a physician or QHP personally performs ankle strapping, 29540 is reported in addition to 99283 25. Modifier 25 is appended to indicate the E/M service was significant and separately identifiable from the preservice and postservice work of the strapping procedure.

There is shared decision-making with the family regarding a lack of indication for and/or decision against testing that counts toward the amount of data as if the test had been ordered. The combination of 1 test considered and not ordered does not meet the Category 1 data (2 tests or documents). The need for an independent historian at this encounter supports a limited amount and/or complexity of data (Category 2 data).

Codes Y92.310 (basketball court as the place of occurrence of the external cause) and Y99.8 (other external cause status [leisure activity]) may also be reported to add to injury information that may be necessary for determining whether another party is responsible for the patient's medical expenses (eg, school injury policy).

When a test is considered but not ordered (after discussion with the patient and/or caregivers), document that it was considered but not ordered and the reason for not ordering it (eg, not indicated, unavailable). This documentation supports inclusion of the test that was not ordered in determination of the amount and/or complexity of data to be reviewed and analyzed.

➤ **An 11-year-old patient presents with an injury to the left ankle.** The patient reports hurting the ankle by tripping during a basketball game approximately an hour earlier and is not able to bear full weight on the ankle. The lateral aspect of the ankle is also swollen and tender to the touch. The parents also offer a history of a prior ankle fracture. A radiograph is ordered and images are reviewed. The ED physician chooses to speak with a radiologist about the interpretation of the radiograph. An acute fracture is not seen, but a Salter-Harris type I cannot be ruled out. The patient is placed in a prefabricated walking boot and instructed on home care and follow-up with the primary care physician for possible reimaging. Since a "rule out" cannot be used as a diagnosis, the highest level of clinical certainty at this point is sprain of the anterior talofibular and calcaneofibular ligaments of the left ankle.

ICD-10-CM	*CPT*
S93.412A (sprain of calcaneofibular ligament of left ankle, initial encounter) S93.492A (sprain of other ligament of left ankle, initial encounter) W01.0XXA (fall on same level from slipping, tripping and stumbling without subsequent striking against object, initial encounter) Y93.67 (activity, basketball) Y92.310 (basketball court as the place of occurrence of the external cause) Y99.8 (other external cause status [leisure activity])	99284 Moderate MDM

Problem(s) addressed ➡ ***Moderate*** (signs or symptoms of a fracture)

Data reviewed and analyzed ➡ ***Extensive*** (Category 2—independent visualization of images, Category 3—discussion with performing physician)

Risk of patient management ➡ ***Low*** (walking boot and follow-up with primary care physician)

Teaching Point: Moderate MDM is supported by the moderate complexity of the problem addressed and the extensive data analysis necessary to determine diagnosis and management. The order for and the independent review and interpretation of images each contribute to the amount and complexity of the data. Only 2 of 3 elements are required to support the level of MDM.

The final diagnosis for a condition does not, in and of itself, determine the complexity or risk, as extensive evaluation may be required to reach the conclusion that the signs or symptoms do not represent a highly morbid condition.

SDoH that affect management may indicate a higher risk of morbidity resulting from additional treatment than is otherwise associated with the plan of care (eg, documented consultation with case management to assist family with transportation to follow-up appointments with a community physician).

➤ **An adolescent is brought to the ED by ambulance after a noncollision rollover automobile accident.** Emergency medical technicians relay that the patient was driving and wearing a seat belt, but the older-model vehicle did not have airbags. Witnesses to the accident reported that the patient lost consciousness for several minutes before arrival of the ambulance. The ED physician comprehensively examines the patient, whose Glasgow Coma Scale score is 14 given the patient's confusion. Parenteral controlled substances are administered. Radiographs of the chest and left shoulder and a computed tomographic scan of the head are ordered. The patient is found to have a closed frontal skull fracture without underlying bleeding as well as a displaced fractured right clavicle. Neurosurgery and orthopedic consultations are obtained, and after discussion with the neurosurgeon and orthopedic surgeon, the patient is admitted for observation by the neurosurgeon.

ICD-10-CM	*CPT*
S02.0XXA (fracture of vault of skull, initial encounter for closed fracture) **S06.0X1A** (concussion with loss of consciousness of 30 minutes or less) **S42.021A** (displaced fracture of shaft of right clavicle, initial encounter for closed fracture) **R40.2142A** (coma scale, eyes open, spontaneous, at arrival to ED) **R40.2242A** (coma scale, best verbal response, confused conversation, at arrival to ED) **R40.2362A** (coma scale, best motor response, obeys commands, at arrival to ED) **V48.5XXA** (car driver injured in noncollision transport accident in traffic accident, initial encounter) **Y92.413** (state road as the place of occurrence of the external cause)	**99285** (ED visit code) High MDM

Problem(s) addressed ➡ ***High*** (trauma with altered mental status)

Data reviewed and analyzed ➡ ***Extensive*** (Categories 1–3—unique tests ordered, independent historians; Category 3—discussion of management with external physicians)

Risk of patient management ➡ ***High*** (decision regarding parenteral controlled substances)

Teaching Point: All 3 elements of MDM support a high level of MDM in this case.

E/M services provided by the orthopedist would be reported with office or other outpatient consultation codes (likely **99244** or **99245**). The neurosurgeon will report an outpatient consultation with modifier **25** (significant, separately identifiable E/M service) in addition to subsequent hospital inpatient or observation care (**99231–99233**) or may combine the total time or MDM of the services and report only initial hospital care, **99221–99223**. Each physician will report the diagnoses for the conditions confirmed at the conclusion of the encounter (eg, the ED physician reports what was known at the time the patient is transferred to the neurosurgeon's care).

ED codes may be reported by any physician or QHP providing unscheduled care to a patient who presents to an ED for immediate medical attention. But if a patient is seen in the ED for the convenience of a physician or QHP, use office or other outpatient services codes (99202–99215) or other appropriate codes (eg, initial hospital inpatient or observation services) to report the E/M service.

Observation in the ED Setting

Physicians in the ED setting may need to observe a patient for an extended period to determine whether admission to inpatient status or discharge is appropriate or while providing treatment in an effort to avoid inpatient admission (eg, repeat treatments for asthma exacerbation). The physician's dated and timed order for observation status is the starting point of the observation service. The order for admission to observation status should not be added at the time of discharge from a lengthy ED visit.

- In addition to the order for an observation stay, documentation includes a plan of care for nursing and other therapeutic services, documentation of physician reassessments, and planning for discharge or a decision for transition to inpatient status (or transfer to another facility).
- Observation services may be applicable when patients are observed pending transfer to a psychiatric facility.
- Append modifier **25** (significant, separately identifiable E/M service) to the ED service code (**99282–99285**) when the treating ED physician or QHP provides initial hospital inpatient or observation services (**99221–99223**) or same-date initial hospital inpatient or observation admission and discharge (**99234–99236**) on the same date of service as the ED encounter.
  - Report codes for subsequent (**99231–99233**) or discharge (**99238** and **99239**) services for continued care on subsequent dates of service.
  - Report **99234–99236** only when a patient is admitted to observation status and, after a stay of 8 hours or more and at least 2 visits by the admitting physician, is discharged on the same date. An observation stay of less than 8 hours duration or with a single visit by the admitting physician or QHP is reported with **99221–99223**.

Refer to **Chapter 16** for full discussion of codes reported for hospital inpatient and observation services.

Not all payer policies align with *CPT* instruction for reporting an ED E/M service and initial hospital care. When an ED visit provided on the same date as an inpatient or observation service by the same physician or QHP *is not separately reported* (eg, to comply with payer policy), the combined services may be reported according to the total time on the date of the encounter or the aggregate MDM. Although time is not used for selection of 99282–99285, the total time spent by the same individual(s) of the same specialty and same group practice providing ED care and inpatient or observation care on the same date may be used in code selection for the inpatient or observation service.

Modifiers Used With ED Codes

Physicians need to understand when it is appropriate to report modifiers in addition to E/M or procedural service codes. Modifiers **25** (significant, separately identifiable E/M service) and **57** (decision for surgery) may be appended to ED E/M codes to indicate E/M beyond the preservice work of a procedure. Procedures performed in the ED may require reporting of modifiers such as **26** (professional component), **54** (surgical care only), or **59** (distinct procedural service) or, when accepted by the payer in lieu of modifier **59**, modifier **XE** (separate encounter), **XP** (separate practitioner), **XS** (separate structure), or **XU** (unusual nonoverlapping service). Refer to **Chapter 2** for more detail on the use of modifiers.

Modifiers specifying the laterality (**RT**, right, or **LT**, left) of paired body sites or a specific anatomical site (eg, **F5**, right thumb) of a procedure may also be required by a payer (even when laterality or site is included in a reported *ICD-10-CM* code descriptor). For an example, refer to the Fracture Care section later in this chapter.

Example

➤ **The ED physician is caring for a 9-year-old who has a 4-cm–long, deep laceration of the right calf and a separate 1-cm–long laceration of the right ankle from broken glass in their backyard.** The physician obtains history from the child and parents. A radiograph of the extremity is obtained and reviewed with notation of no retained radiopaque foreign bodies. The child's immunizations are current, with the most recent tetanus booster having been administered less than 5 years ago. The physician irrigates, carefully explores both wounds, and performs a 2-layer repair on the calf. The ankle laceration requires only single-layer closure. The child is discharged with appropriate follow-up plans.

ICD-10-CM	*CPT*
S81.811A (laceration without foreign body, right lower leg, initial encounter) **S91.011A** (laceration without foreign body, right ankle, initial encounter) **W25.XXXA** (contact with sharp glass, initial encounter) **Y92.007** (garden or yard of noninstitutional residence)	**99283 25** **12032** (intermediate repair of the extremities, 2.6–7.5 cm) **12001 59** or **XS** (simple repair of the extremity, ≤2.5 cm)

Problem(s) addressed ➡ ***Low***
Data reviewed and analyzed ➡ ***Moderate*** (Category 2—independent interpretation of tests)
Risk of patient management ➡ ***Low***

Teaching Point: Modifiers are used to indicate that the laceration repairs were distinct procedures (**59**) or of a separate structure (**XS**). Append modifier **25** only when providing an E/M and other service with an E/M component (preservice and postservice work) on the same date to indicate that the E/M was significantly beyond the preservice work of the other service and distinctly documented. For further discussion of preservice and postservice work, refer to the Reporting Procedures in the ED section that follows.

For discussion of billing for follow-up care when the patient returns to the ED for services such as suture removal, refer to the "Coding Conundrum: The Surgical Package of Laceration Repair" box later in this chapter.

Refer to **Chapter 2** for more information on these modifiers and appropriate modifier placement.

Reporting Procedures in the ED

Many procedures performed in the ED have an associated global period assigned by Medicare and other payers and/or are subject to the *CPT* surgical package. The global period affects reporting of pre- and post-procedural care. The *CPT* surgical package defines the work included in each surgical procedure. (Refer to **Chapter 18** for the definition of the *CPT* surgical package and Medicare global period.)

Refer to "Common Emergency Department Procedures" at www.aap.org/cfp2026 for a list of procedures, with assigned Medicare global periods, commonly performed in the ED.

Any separately identifiable procedure that is personally performed by the physician may be reported, except for

- Procedures that are bundled in time-based critical care codes (Refer to **Table 17-1** for a list of services and procedures that are included in hourly critical care codes.)
- General supervision of services performed by hospital personnel because they are billed by the hospital facility (If a nurse or other clinical staff assist in part of a procedure, the ED physician may bill for the professional services if the ED physician provides the primary or key component of the procedure.)

Coding Conundrum: The Surgical Package of Laceration Repair

Per *CPT* instruction, if the patient returned to the ED for a recheck of the wounds or removal of sutures within 10 days following the day of laceration repair, these services would be part of the typical postoperative care included in the surgical package. Likewise, Medicare and payers that adopt Medicare policy assign a 10-day global period to intermediate or complex repair services, during which all postoperative care that does not require a return to the operating room are included in the fee paid for the repair.

For simple laceration repair, however, Medicare and payers that adopt Medicare policy assign a 0-day global period to the simple repairs, thus allowing separate billing of follow-up care. Physician groups may adopt a policy applying *CPT* instructions for inclusion of uncomplicated postoperative care following simple laceration repair in the fee for the laceration repair.

Modifier **54** (surgical care only) is appropriately appended to procedure codes with 10- or 90-day global periods when the patient will not return to the ED for follow-up care during the postoperative period. For example, full-thickness repair of a lacerated lip not involving the vermilion border is reported with **40650 54**. Modifier **54** is appended because this procedure is assigned a 90-day global period and the follow-up care will be provided by another physician. Some payers require modifier **54** only on codes assigned a 90-day global period.

To report an E/M service in addition to a procedure, there must be documentation of performance of a significant and separately identifiable E/M service beyond the pre- and post-procedural work typical for the procedure (eg, evaluation for a concussion and repair of wounds at 1 encounter). Post-procedural prescriptions for pain control or prophylactic antibiotics may be included in the procedure performed.

- ✖ Hydration, infusion, and/or injection procedures (**96360–96379**) because the physician work associated with the procedures involves only confirmation of the treatment plan and not direct supervision of staff
- ✖ Procedures involving use of hospital-owned equipment (eg, pulse oximetry), unless the procedure includes both technical and professional components (If performed and documented, the professional component, such as interpretation and report of radiographic findings, may be reported by appending modifier **26** [professional component] to the procedure code.)

Fracture Care

Fracture care in the ED is typically limited to initial care. Most codes for fracture care include a 10- or 90-day period of care related to the fracture. Correct coding requires appending modifier **54** (surgical care only) to codes for fracture care when follow-up care will be provided by another physician. The physician who assumes management during the follow-up period reports the same fracture care code with modifier **55** (postoperative management only) and the same date of service. Some payers require that both physicians document the transfer of care.

Casting, splinting, or strapping may be used solely to temporarily stabilize the fracture for the comfort of a patient who will receive fracture care by an orthopedist in the next few days. When this happens, it is not considered closed fracture treatment and is reported with a code for application of casts and strapping service (29000–29584) in addition to any significant E/M service reported with modifier 25, when applicable.

Example

➤ **A 16-year-old patient is seen in the ED for right shoulder pain that occurred following a fall while playing soccer at a community sports field.** The patient is examined for additional injuries. Diagnosis is anterior glenohumeral dislocation of the right shoulder. The patient agrees to an attempt at reduction without analgesia, which is successful. A sling is applied. The physician refers the patient to another physician for follow-up care and documents the transfer of care.

ICD-10-CM	*CPT*
S43.014A (anterior dislocation of right humerus, initial encounter) **W18.39XA** (other fall on same level, initial encounter) **Y93.66** (activity, soccer) **Y92.322** (soccer field as place of occurrence)	**99282–99285** with modifier **57** (decision for surgery), as appropriate **23650 54 RT** (closed treatment of shoulder dislocation, with manipulation; without anesthesia)

Teaching Point: The use of modifier **54** (surgical care only) alerts payers that another physician will report follow-up care for this procedure, which typically includes multiple services over a 90-day period of post-procedural care. Modifier **RT** indicates the right shoulder as the site of the procedure. Modifier **57** indicates the decision for surgery during an E/M service.

Nasal Fractures

Closed treatment of nasal bone fracture without manipulation is reported with an E/M code based on MDM performed and documented (ie, 99283 or 99284). Closed treatment with manipulation is reported with 21315 and 21320.

21315 Closed treatment of nasal bone fracture with manipulation; without stabilization
21320 with stabilization

Point-of-Care Ultrasound

Point-of-care ultrasound services performed by the ED physician are separately reportable in addition to the ED E/M service when *all 3 of the following conditions apply:*

1. Thorough evaluation of organ(s) or anatomical region is performed.
2. There is permanent image documentation (with measurements, when clinically indicated).
3. A written report equivalent to that typically produced by a radiologist is documented.

Use of handheld or portable ultrasound machine that does not include all 3 of the listed elements is not separately reported.

Without all these elements, the examination is not separately reported and would be considered part of any E/M service provided. (*Exception:* Permanent image documentation is not required for ophthalmic ultrasonography for biometric measurement.)

Point-of-care ultrasound services in the ED are reported by the physician only with the professional component modifier (26). The technical component (eg, equipment cost, facility overhead costs) is typically reported by the facility. (Payers may limit physicians to reporting the professional component only for all facility-based services even if the physician performs the ultrasonography and/or owns the equipment used for the service. The technical component includes all associated overhead costs. Check individual payer policies for reporting.)

One use of point-of-care ultrasound services in the ED is the focused assessment with sonography for trauma examination. This may consist of 3 distinct components: limited transthoracic echocardiography, limited chest ultrasound, and limited abdominal ultrasonography. When 3 distinct procedures are performed, 3 codes are reported.

76705 Ultrasound, abdominal, real-time with image documentation; limited
93308 Echocardiography, transthoracic, real-time with image documentation (2D), includes M-mode recording, when performed, follow-up or limited study
76604 Ultrasound, chest (includes mediastinum), real time with image documentation

Emergency Department Services

Chapter 14

Example

➤ **A child is seen in the ED for injuries sustained in an automobile accident.** The physician performs a trauma assessment, including a focused assessment with sonography for trauma examination. This examination includes limited transthoracic echocardiography, limited chest ultrasound, and limited abdominal ultrasonography.

Teaching Point: In addition to the appropriate E/M service code, the physician reports 76705 26, 76604 26, and 93308 26 (refer to code descriptors earlier in this section). Modifier 26 signifies that the physician is reporting the professional component of each service. The facility will report the same codes with modifier TC to indicate reporting of the technical component of each service. When applicable and when all requirements for reporting are met, ultrasonography performed with physician-owned equipment is reported without a modifier (ie, modifiers 26 and TC are not applicable).

Limited studies are defined in *CPT* as those that include examination of less than the required elements for a "complete" examination (eg, limited number of organs, limited portion of region evaluated). Refer to your *CPT* reference for required components of complete examinations.

Refer to the Central Venous Access section in **Chapter 18** for appropriate reporting of ultrasound guidance for vascular access (76937). This code is reported separately in addition to a code for primary vascular access procedure (eg, 36555) when imaging documentation is not included in the procedure.

When ultrasound guidance is used for needle placement for procedures such as aspiration of an abscess, 76942 is reported. Do not report 76942 in conjunction with a service for which the code descriptor includes ultrasound guidance (eg, joint aspiration). Code 76937 (ultrasound guidance for vascular access) is not reported in conjunction with 76942. Certain services, such as insertion of a peripherally inserted central venous catheter, include all imaging guidance and are reported with reduced service modifier 52 when imaging is not performed or imaging is performed by radiology (eg, chest radiograph) in lieu of the individual performing the procedure.

Sedation

Moderate Sedation

Moderate sedation (99151–99157) is a drug-induced depression of consciousness during which patients may respond purposefully to verbal commands, either alone or accompanied by light tactile stimulation. Moderate sedation may be necessary for the performance of certain procedures in the ED.

99151 Moderate sedation services provided by the same physician or other QHP performing the diagnostic or therapeutic service that the sedation supports, requiring the presence of an independent trained observer to assist in the monitoring of the patient's level of consciousness and physiological status; initial 15 minutes of intraservice time, patient younger than 5 years of age

99152 initial 15 minutes of intraservice time, patient age 5 years or older

+99153 each additional 15 minutes intraservice time (report with 99151 or 99152)

99155 Moderate sedation services provided by a physician or other QHP other than the physician or other QHP performing the diagnostic or therapeutic service that the sedation supports; initial 15 minutes of intraservice time, patient younger than 5 years of age

99156 initial 15 minutes of intraservice time, patient age 5 years or older

+99157 each additional 15 minutes intraservice time (report with 99155 or 99156)

Refer to Chapter 13 for a full discussion of coding for moderate sedation.

- Codes are selected according to intraservice time. Intraservice time
  - Begins with the administration of the sedating agent(s)
  - Ends when the procedure is completed, the patient is stable for recovery status, and the physician or other QHP providing the sedation ends personal continuous face-to-face time with the patient
  - Includes ordering and/or administering the initial and subsequent doses of sedating agents
  - Requires continuous face-to-face attendance of the physician or other QHP
  - Requires monitoring patient response to the sedating agents, including
    - Periodic assessment of the patient
    - Further administration of agent(s) as needed to maintain sedation
    - Monitoring of oxygen saturation, heart rate, end-tidal carbon dioxide levels, and blood pressure
- Moderate sedation services of less than 10 minutes' intraservice time are not separately reported.

Example

➤ **A 5-year-old requires a procedure in the ED.** A physician other than the ED physician performs the procedure. The ED physician provides the moderate sedation and documents 25 minutes of service, beginning with administration of the sedating agent and ending when the patient is sufficiently recovered so the physician's continuous face-to-face monitoring is no longer necessary.

CPT
99282–99285 25 99156 (moderate sedation by other than physician performing procedure, first 15 minutes) 99157 (moderate sedation, each additional 15 minutes)

Teaching Point: The ED physician reports an E/M code as appropriate for care before the pre-sedation evaluation (eg, initial evaluation of illness or injury) and appends modifier 25 to indicate that the service was significant and is separately identifiable in the documentation. Code 99157 is reported for the final 10 minutes because the midpoint between the first and second 15-minute period was passed.

• indicates a new code; ▲, revised; #, re-sequenced; ✚, add-on; ★, audiovisual technology; and ◀, synchronous interactive audio.

Deep Sedation

Deep sedation or analgesia is a drug-induced depression of consciousness during which patients cannot be easily aroused but respond purposefully after repeat verbal or painful stimulation (eg, purposefully pushing away a noxious stimuli). The ability to independently maintain ventilatory function may be impaired. Patients may require assistance in maintaining a patent airway, and spontaneous ventilation may be inadequate. Cardiovascular function is usually maintained. A state of deep sedation may be accompanied by partial or complete loss of protective airway reflexes.

Although ED physicians may provide deep sedation, payment for these services is limited. National Correct Coding Initiative (NCCI) edits do not allow payment of an ED visit (99281–99285) and deep sedation when provided by the same ED physician. No modifier will override the NCCI edits. Payers that have adopted Medicare or Medicaid NCCI edits may deny the ED visit when reported on the same date as deep sedation.

Deep sedation provided by a physician also performing the services for which the sedation is being provided is reported by appending modifier 47 (anesthesia by surgeon) to the procedure code for the service for which sedation is required. Many health plans do not pay separately for anesthesia by the physician or surgeon performing the procedure.

However, if the deep sedation is provided by another physician from the same specialty and same group, modifier XP (separate practitioner) should be added to the appropriate anesthesia code.

Refer to **Chapter 18** for more information on deep sedation.

Directing Emergency Medical Personnel

99288 Physician or other QHP direction of emergency medical systems (EMS) emergency care, advanced life support

- Code 99288 is designated as a bundled procedure (included in the work value of other services) by Medicare. There are no relative values assigned under the Medicare Resource-Based Relative Value Scale. Check with your major payers and negotiate for coverage of this service.
- Report 99288 (physician direction of EMS) when
  - The physician directing the services is in the hospital and in 2-way communication with EMS personnel who are in the prehospital setting providing advanced life support that requires direct or online medical control.
  - The documentation includes the times of all contacts, any orders provided, and/or directions provided to the EMS team.
- Code 99288 may be reported on the same day as ED E/M or hourly critical care services. Append modifier 25 to 99288 to alert payers that this was a significant and separately identifiable service from ED E/M (99282–99285) or the critical care (99291, 99292) service provided.
- The supervising physician cannot report the actual procedures and interventions performed by the EMS team because they are not physically present during the transport.
- When a QHP (eg, nurse practitioner) provides critical care services during transport and those services will be reported under the QHP's National Provider Identifier or by the employing hospital, the ED physician does not report 99288.
- Refer to 99485 and 99486 in **Chapter 17** for information on supervision of inter-facility transport of a critically ill or injured patient, 24 months or younger, via direct 2-way communication with a transport team.

Time-Based Critical Care in the ED

99291 Critical care, E/M of the critically ill or critically injured patient; first 30–74 minutes

+99292 each additional 30 minutes (Use in conjunction with 99291.)

To report 99291 and 99292, the patient's condition must meet the specific *CPT* definition of a critically ill or injured patient. Documentation must support that the patient's condition was critical and that the services provided involved high-complexity decision-making to assess, manipulate, and support vital system function(s) to treat single or multiple vital organ system failure and/or to prevent further life-threatening deterioration of the patient's condition.

A *critical illness* or *injury* is defined in *CPT* as acutely impairing one or more vital organs such that there is a high probability of imminent or life-threatening deterioration of the patient's condition.

Guidelines for reporting critical care codes 99291 (critical care, E/M of the critically ill or injured patient; first 30–74 minutes) and 99292 (each additional 30 minutes) are described in detail in **Chapter 17**. *CPT* instructs that add-on code 99292 be reported in conjunction with 99291 when critical care time extends *up to 30 minutes* beyond the first 74 minutes and for each additional period of up to 30 minutes. Report 1 unit of 99292 for critical care time of 75 to 104 minutes and then an additional unit for each additional period of up to 30 minutes.

Medicare policy requires a minimum of 104 minutes of service to report 99292 in addition to 99291. Coders should be aware of potential adoption of this policy by Medicaid programs and other payers.

- Time-based critical care codes (**99291** and **99292**) should be used to report the provision of critical care when performed in the ED. The daily codes for pediatric or neonatal critical care should not be reported by a physician providing critical care in the ED unless that physician (eg, an intensivist) will continue to provide critical care services in the inpatient setting.

Per *CPT*, time-based services that are continuously provided with time continuing past midnight do not restart at midnight. For example, an episode of critical care lasting from 11:20 pm to 12:15 am is reported with 1 unit of 99291. If the same patient receives another episode of critical care beginning at 2:00 am, the first 30 to 74 minutes of service for that episode is reported with 99291.

- Time spent providing critical care does not need to be continuous and includes time at the bedside as well as time in the ED reviewing data specific to the patient, discussing the patient with other physicians, and discussing the patient's management or condition with the patient's family.

Time of any learner (eg, student, resident) involved in the patient's care may not be reported by the attending physician. Only the time specifically spent by the attending physician may be reported.

- Time reported for critical care must be devoted to the critically ill or injured patient. Therefore, the "critical care clock" stops when attention is turned to the care of another patient or the physician is not readily available in the ED.

Medicare Policy for Time-Based Critical Care by Multiple Physicians

Medicare provides specific guidance for reporting critical care services provided by physicians and QHPs in the same group practice. Other payers may adopt Medicare policy.

Medicare considers physicians and QHPs to be in different specialties. A physician and QHP in the same group providing critical care to the same patient on the same calendar date report the services based on the combined total time of critical care furnished to a patient. The individual who furnishes the substantive portion of the cumulative critical care time reports the critical care service(s). Modifier FS (split or shared visit) may be required by some payers.

When multiple physicians or multiple QHPs in the same specialty and the same group practice furnish critical care services to the same patient on the same date, the physician or QHP who provides the initial episode of critical care time of 30 minutes or more reports 99291 Other physicians or QHPs in the same specialty and same group practice who continue the critical care services will report their time with appropriate units of 99292. However, when the physician or QHP who initially provides critical care spends less than 30 minutes in critical care services before care is assumed by another individual, the combined critical care time may support 99291 and is reported by the individual who spent the greater portion of time providing the critical care service.

- Refer to **Table 17-1** for a list of services and procedures that are included in hourly critical care codes.
- Those procedures *not bundled* with codes **99291** and **99292** and personally performed by the reporting provider may be reported separately (eg, starting an intravenous line on a child aged <3 years, placing an intraosseous or central venous catheter, endotracheal intubation, cardiopulmonary resuscitation [CPR], cardioversion). Time spent performing these separately reported services must be subtracted from the critical care time calculated and reported.

Example

➤ **A 13-month-old with apparent sepsis and hypotension is brought to the ED.** The child requires placement of an intraosseous needle to achieve vascular access and subsequently receives parenteral fluids, antibiotics, and vasopressors. The child experiences cardiopulmonary arrest, prompting the ED physician to intubate the child and provide CPR. Time spent in separately reported procedures is 20 minutes. The child is in the ED for a total of 45 minutes before transfer to the critical care unit.

Emergency Department Services

Chapter 14

ICD-10-CM	CPT
I46.9 (cardiac arrest) If the physician included sepsis in the diagnosis, A41.9 (sepsis, unspecified organism), R65.21 (severe sepsis with septic shock), and I46.8 (cardiac arrest due to other underlying condition) would be appropriate.	99285 25 92950 (CPR) 36680 (placement of intraosseous needle) 31500 (endotracheal intubation, emergency)

Teaching Point: Critical care time does not accrue during the performance of non-bundled, separately billable procedures. Twenty minutes of the 45-minute ED time was spent providing a separately billable, non-bundled service (CPR). Because the ED physician did not spend a minimum of 30 minutes providing critical care, an ED E/M service is reported rather than critical care. Coding is based on documented elements of MDM (high-complexity problem and high risk).

ICD-10-CM codes for severe sepsis (R65.20) and septic shock (R65.21) are reported secondary to the underlying infection (eg, A41.9, sepsis, unspecified organism) and followed by codes for related organ failure (eg, J96.01, acute respiratory failure with hypoxia).

Critical Care and ED E/M Services on the Same Date

Critical care and ED E/M services may both be reported on the same date when, after completion of the ED service, the condition of the patient changes and critical care services are provided. Modifier 25 should be appended to the ED E/M code when this occurs.

Examples

➤ **The ED physician performs a comprehensive history and physical examination on a 13-month-old patient with severe stridor and respiratory distress believed to be secondary to croup.** MDM is highly complex. The patient's condition does not improve with nebulized epinephrine and then worsens, as evidenced by progressive lethargy. The patient's capillary blood gas result shows hypercapnia. Critical care is provided for 40 minutes, not including 10 minutes spent performing endotracheal intubation.

ICD-10-CM	CPT
J96.02 (acute respiratory failure with hypercapnia) J05.0 (croup)	99285 25 (ED visit code) 99291 25 (critical care, first 30–74 minutes) 31500 (endotracheal intubation, emergency)

Teaching Point: Endotracheal intubation is not bundled with critical care; therefore, time spent in the provision of the service (10 minutes for this patient) is not considered in the total critical care time. Modifier 25 is appended to 99285 and 99291 to indicate that they were significant and separately identifiable services from each other and the endotracheal intubation.

➤ **The ED physician saw a 10-year-old for exacerbation of moderate asthma in the morning.** The child responded well to an aerosolized bronchodilator treatment and was discharged home. The child returns to the ED a few hours later with a more severe exacerbation and is seen by the same physician. The child now has respiratory failure with hypoxia. The child receives oxygen, a continuous bronchodilator nebulizer treatment, and, subsequently, a parenteral bronchodilation drug. The child's condition improves enough for them to be admitted to a monitored medical ward bed with diagnosis of respiratory failure caused by status asthmaticus. The ED physician spends a total of 60 minutes in patient-directed critical care.

ICD-10-CM	CPT
J96.01 (acute respiratory failure with hypoxia) J45.42 (moderate persistent asthma with status asthmaticus)	99284 25 99291

Teaching Point: The patient received oxygen, continuous inhalation treatment, and parenteral bronchodilator in the ED. But these services include no professional component. The facility will report the services because the costs of supplies and clinical staff time are an expense to the facility.

Special Service Codes

99053 Service(s) provided between 10:00 pm and 8:00 am at 24-hour facility, in addition to basic service

99056 Service(s) typically provided in office, provided out of office at request of patient, in addition to basic service

99060 Service(s) provided on an emergency basis, out of office, which disrupts other scheduled office services, in addition to basic service

Special service codes may be used to report services that are an adjunct to the basic service provided. *CPT* guidelines do not restrict the reporting of adjunct special service codes in the ED. But third-party payers have specific policies for coverage and payment. Communicate with individual payers to understand their definition or interpretation of the service and coverage and payment policies.

These codes are intended to describe services that are provided outside the normal time frame and location.

Code 99053 will be reported when services are provided between the designated time limits in an ED.

Although *CPT* does not restrict reporting of any procedure or service to any specific specialty, codes 99056 or 99060 are intended for services outside of the ED.

If appropriate, a non-ED physician could report *CPT* code 99056 or 99060 when they provide services in the ED in addition to an outpatient office or clinic visit, ED visit, or consultation E/M code.

Continuum Model for Fever

The continuum model is a teaching tool that gives examples of how common conditions in the ED might be reported according to the severity and/or complexity of the presenting problem(s). The following "Continuum Model for Fever in the Emergency Department" presents fever as the presenting concern across the continuum of codes 99282–99285 plus critical care.

Continuum Model for Fever in the Emergency Department
A clinically appropriate history and examination are required for each level of service

CPT Code Vignette	No. and Complexity of Problem(s) Addressed	Data to be Reviewed and Analyzed	Risk of Complications and/or Morbidity or Mortality of Patient Management
99282 4-year-old with temperature of 37.7 °C (99.8 °F), fussy before ED admission	**Minimal:** 1 self-limited problem	**Limited:** Required history obtained from independent historian	**Minimal:** Advice for home care
99283 5-year-old with temperature of 38.3 °C (101.0 °F) last night and URI symptoms	**Low:** Acute, uncomplicated illness	**Limited:** Required history obtained from independent historian	**Low:** Over-the-counter ibuprofen/acetaminophen as needed
99283 8-year-old with temperature of 38.3 °C (101.0 °F), cough, and sore throat	**Low:** Acute, uncomplicated illness considered and ruled out after evaluation	**Limited:** 1 unique test ordered (87636, influenza and SARS-CoV-2 test); required history obtained from independent historian	**Low:** Advice for home care and isolation
99284 5-year-old girl with temperature of 39.0 °C (102.2 °F) and abdominal pain disturbing sleep	**Moderate:** Acute illness with systemic symptoms	**Moderate:** CBC, urinalysis and urine culture; required history obtained from independent historian	**Moderate:** Antibiotic prescribed

Continued on next page

Continuum Model for Fever in the Emergency Department (*continued*)			
***CPT* Code Vignette**	**No. and Complexity of Problem(s) Addressed**	**Data to be Reviewed and Analyzed**	**Risk of Complications and/or Morbidity or Mortality of Patient Management**
99285 Neonate presenting with fever, not feeding well, and having ill appearance	**High:** Differential diagnosis that includes neonatal sepsis	**Moderate:** CBC, comprehensive metabolic panel, blood culture, urine culture, lumbar puncture; required history obtained from independent historian	**High:** Decision regarding admission to inpatient care
99291, 99292 Neonate with fever and gray appearance	1. Patient in critically ill, unstable condition; requires >30 minutes of directed patient care. 2. Physician assesses, manipulates, and supports vital system function(s) to treat single or multiple vital organ system failure and/or to prevent further life-threatening deterioration of the patient's condition.		

Abbreviations: CBC, complete blood cell count; *CPT*, *Current Procedural Terminology;* ED, emergency department; URI, upper respiratory infection.

Although the actual assignment of a code for an individual patient may vary from the examples, members of the AAP Committee on Coding and Nomenclature generally agree that these examples provide an accurate representation of how 1 condition typically flows across the family of codes. Examples are not provided for 99281 (typically reported for an encounter with clinical staff such as simple suture removal) because no MDM is required for services reported with this code.

Additional continuums for 3 common conditions—asthma, head injury, and laceration—are included at www.aap.org/cfp2026.

It is important to remember that 2 of 3 elements of MDM (ie, number and complexity of problems addressed, amount and/or complexity of data to be reviewed and analyzed, and risk of complications and/or morbidity or mortality of patient management) must be met to support the code selected.

To test your knowledge of the information presented in this chapter, complete the quiz found at the end of it, after the resources. Answers to each quiz are found in **Appendix II**.

Chapter Takeaways

- The physician's designation of the chief complaint is important because only 1 diagnosis code may be reported for this category on the hospital claim form and this diagnosis is used to help support the urgency of the ED visit under prudent layperson guidelines.
- SDoH that influence a patient's health and/or limit the management and treatment options should be documented to support assignment of codes for the SDoH. When applicable, the limitations to diagnosis or treatment should be documented to support an increased risk of patient management.
- The level of ED codes **99282–99285** is based on the highest 2 of 3 elements of MDM. Time is not used in selection of **99282–99285**.
- When a physician and QHP in the same specialty and same group practice each participate in the E/M service provided to a patient, the split/shared service is reported by the individual who provided the substantial portion of the MDM for the encounter.
- Append modifier **25** (significant, separately identifiable E/M service) to the ED service code (**99282–99285**) when the treating ED physician or QHP provides initial hospital inpatient or observation services on the same date as an ED service.
- When initial hospital inpatient or observation service is reported for combined ED and hospital care services by the same individual on the same date, in lieu of separately reporting each service (eg, to comply with payer policy), code selection is based on either the total time on the date of the encounter or the aggregate MDM.
- Modifier **54** (surgical care only) is appropriately appended to procedure codes with 10- or 90-day global periods when the patient will not return to the ED for follow-up care (eg, visits for follow-up care of a fracture).
- Documentation of critical service services must support that the patient's condition was critical and the services provided involved high-complexity decision-making to assess, manipulate, and support vital system function(s) to treat single or multiple vital organ system failure and/or to prevent further life-threatening deterioration of the patient's condition.

Resources

AAP Coding Assistance and Education

AAP *ICD-10-CM* resources (www.aap.org/en/practice-management/child-health-finance-payment-strategy/coding-and-valuation/icd-10-cm-resources)

AAP Payer Advocacy: Prepayment Downcoding Checklist (https://downloads.aap.org/AAP/PDF/Downcoding%20Checklist.pdf)

Pediatric ICD-10-CM 2026: A Manual for Provider-Based Coding (www.aap.org/Pediatric-*ICD-10-CM*-2026-11th-Edition-Paperback)

AAP Pediatric Coding Newsletter™

"Coding for Conditions Due to Heat Overexposure," July 2024 (https://doi.org/10.1542/pcco_book243_document001)

"Coding Hotline," April 2025 ("*CPT*: Prescription Drug Management) (https://doi.org/10.1542/pcco_book252_document005)

"Coding Hotline," October 2024 ("*CPT*: Emergency Department Observation") (https://doi.org/10.1542/pcco_book246_document006)

"Connecting Coding and Clinical Reports: Oral and Dental Aspects of Child Abuse and Neglect," February 2025 (https://doi.org/10.1542/pcco_book250_document001)

"Critical Care: What's Included? What's Not?" June 2025 (https://doi.org/10.1542/pcco_book254_document004)

"Learning Through Examples: Coding for Concerns Related to Child Abuse or Neglect," February 2025 (https://doi.org/10.1542/pcco_book250_document005)

"Procedural Services: Modifiers to Report Site and Laterality," January 2025 (https://doi.org/10.1542/pcco_book249_document005)

"You Code It! Cannabis Poisoning in a 4-Year-Old," April 2024 (https://doi.org/10.1542/pcco_book240_document005)

"You Code It! Answers: Cannabis Poisoning in a 4-Year-Old," April 2024 (https://doi.org/10.1542/pcco_book240_document006)

Online-Exclusive Content at www.aap.org/cfp2026

"Asthma, Head Injury, and Laceration: Coding Continuums"

"Common Emergency Department Procedures"

Test Your Knowledge!

1. **Which of the following must be designated in the documentation of an ED visit to help support the urgency of the ED visit under prudent layperson guidelines?**
   a. 1 sign, symptom, disease, or injury as the chief complaint
   b. All signs and symptoms noted during triage
   c. 1 definitive diagnosis (ie, not a sign or symptom)
   d. A diagnosis that typically requires at least moderate MDM
2. **Which service is appropriately reported with Z04.72, encounter for examination and observation following alleged child physical abuse?**
   a. A visit at which child physical abuse is suspected but not confirmed.
   b. A visit at which child physical abuse is confirmed.
   c. A visit at which a child's signs or symptoms of illness or injury are addressed and determined to not be due to abuse.
   d. A visit at which the child, who presents without signs or symptoms, is observed for alleged child abuse that is ruled out at the visit.
3. **Which of the following is the starting point for initial hospital inpatient or observation services (99221–99223) initiated by an ED physician or QHP?**
   a. The time at which the patient presented to the ED facility for care
   b. The time at which the ED physician or QHP first provided face-to-face care to the patient
   c. The time at which the ED physician or QHP wrote an order for the patient's admission to observation status
   d. Time beyond the first hour spent in the ED
4. **Which procedure would not be reported by a physician or QHP providing care in the ED?**
   a. General supervision of services performed by hospital personnel
   b. Hydration, infusion, and/or injection procedures
   c. Procedures involving use of hospital-owned equipment and have no associated professional component that would be reported with modifier 26
   d. All of the above
5. **Per CPT instruction, what is the minimum time of critical care service required to report 99292 in addition to 99291?**
   a. 104 minutes
   b. 61 minutes
   c. 75 minutes
   d. 89 minutes

CHAPTER 15

Hospital Care of the Newborn

Contents

Chapter Highlights

- Defining the perinatal and neonatal periods
- Diagnosis codes reported for conditions of the newborn
- Reporting attendance at delivery versus standby services
- Codes for normal newborn and hospital inpatient care
- Codes for services throughout the course of the birth admission
- Coding for circumcisions and car safety seat testing

Perinatal Care

This chapter focuses on coding for care of the normal newborn and newborns with conditions not requiring intensive monitoring or critical care.

The American Academy of Pediatrics (AAP) Section on Neonatal-Perinatal Medicine, in conjunction with state chapters and councils of the AAP, has developed successful strategies that address concerns about payment for neonatal care. Contact your state chapter, its pediatric council, your section district AAP Executive Committee representative, a neonatal trainer, or the AAP Committee on Coding and Nomenclature for assistance in addressing any payment inequities for neonatal services in your state.

You can also complete the AAP Coding and Payment Hassle Hotline Form (www.aap.org/en/practice-management/child-health-finance-payment-strategy/coding-payment-hotline).

Coding Definitions of the Perinatal and Neonatal Periods

For coding purposes, the *perinatal period* commences before birth and continues through the 28th completed day following birth. According to this definition, the *neonatal period* begins at birth and continues through *the completed 28th day after birth*, ending on the 29th calendar day after birth. The day of birth is considered day 0 (zero). Therefore, the day after birth is considered day 1. This definition is important for selection of the correct diagnosis codes for conditions that originate in the perinatal period. (It is also important for selection of codes for neonatal critical care and initial intensive care.)

Expectant Parent Visits

When expectant parents request a visit to choose a pediatrician and learn about the practice, these "meet and greet" visits are not typically considered a medically necessary service. But many pediatric practices establish policies for managing this type of visit, often at times when the practice is least busy, as a non-billable service used for marketing the practice.

Refer to the Consultations section later in this chapter for an example of a clinically indicated consultation provided to expectant parents at the request of another physician or other appropriate source (eg, to address risk reduction and plan newborn care in the presence of identified or suspected abnormalities). A service requested by an expectant parent is not a consultation.

Normal Newborn Care

Daily Care of the Normal Newborn

99460 Initial hospital or birthing center care, per day, for evaluation and management of normal newborn infant

99461 Initial care, per day, for evaluation and management of normal newborn infant seen in other than hospital or birthing center

99462 Subsequent hospital care, per day, for evaluation and management of normal newborn

99463 Initial hospital or birthing center care, per day, for evaluation and management of normal newborn infant admitted and discharged on the same date

99238 Hospital inpatient or observation discharge day management; 30 minutes or less on the date of the encounter

99239 more than 30 minutes on the date of the encounter

● indicates a new code; ▲, revised; #, re-sequenced; ✚, add-on; ★, audiovisual technology; and ◀, synchronous interactive audio.

Current Procedural Terminology (*CPT*®) codes for care of a normal newborn typically follow a pathway of daily care from initial care to subsequent care and/or discharge day management depending on the length of the newborn's hospital stay. Notable exceptions are newborns admitted and discharged on the same date (**99463**) and newborns receiving initial care in settings other than a hospital or birthing center (**99461**). Codes **99460–99463** are reported once per date of service (DOS) regardless of the number of visits or time spent, even when different physicians in the same specialty and same group practice see the newborn on the same date.

A *normal newborn* may be defined as a newborn who

- Completes a normal transition period after birth
- May require delivery room intervention, as discussed in the Attendance at Delivery section later in this chapter, but is normal after transition
- May require some testing or monitoring (eg, bilirubin, ABO and antiglobulin [Coombs] testing, complete blood cell count [CBC], culture[s])
- Does not require significant intervention(s)
- May be observed for illness related to maternal pregnancy or labor complication(s) but is not sick
- May be born with a nonthreatening anomaly (eg, polydactyly, undescended testes)
- May be late preterm (34 weeks–36 weeks 6 days) but requires no special care
- May be in house with their sick mother/twin

Normal newborn codes can be reported for care provided to neonates who are acting normally but recovering from intrapartum stress or a low Apgar score or who are being observed for a potential problem but are asymptomatic (eg, mother treated for group B streptococcal infection during labor).

Codes **99460**, **99462**, **99463**, **99238**, and **99239** are used to report evaluation and management (E/M) services provided to the healthy newborn in a health care facility such as a hospital, including birthing room deliveries, or birthing center. They are reported when the neonate is cared for in the mother's room (rooming-in), a labor and delivery room, a postpartum floor, or a traditional newborn nursery, as well as when a normal neonate is cared for after the mother is discharged (eg, awaiting foster care).

Code **99461** may be appropriate for E/M of a neonate born at home and evaluated in the physician practice soon after birth (ie, same day or next day).

Codes 99460–99463 are not reported for telemedicine services unless specified in payer policy. These codes are not included in the *CPT* listing of codes reported with modifier 95 (synchronous telemedicine service) or 93 (telemedicine service via real-time interactive audio-only telecommunications system).

Guidelines for reporting include

- Care or interventions provided in labor and delivery (eg, attendance at delivery or neonatal resuscitation) are reported separately from daily neonatal hospital, intensive, or critical care.
- Code **99463** (history and examination of the normal newborn, including discharge) should be reported when an initial history and physical examination and the discharge management are performed *on the same calendar date* for a normal newborn.
- ✖ Do not report **99463** when discharge occurs on the next calendar date even if less than 24 hours has passed since the initial newborn care.
- Code **99460** (history and examination of the normal newborn, initial service) is reported only once on the first day that the physician provides one or more face-to-face services in the facility. This date may not necessarily correlate with the date the patient is born or the hospital admission date.
- Code **99462** (subsequent hospital care, normal newborn) is reported once per calendar date, regardless of the number of visits, on the date(s) subsequent to the initial normal newborn care service but *not* on the date of a discharge management service.
- Discharge management services performed on a day subsequent to initial newborn care are reported with **99238** (hospital discharge day management; 30 minutes or less) or **99239** (hospital discharge day management; more than 30 minutes). Only time spent on the date of the discharge day management service is used in code selection. Time must be documented when reporting **99239**.
  - Include time spent in final examination of the patient, discussion of the hospital stay, instructions to parents/caregivers for continuing care, and preparation of discharge records, prescriptions, and referral forms.

Discharge day management codes 99238 and 99239 are valued higher than the subsequent newborn hospital care code (99462) to include the physician's time and work, such as reviewing and documenting the hospital stay and counseling parents about continuing care of their neonate.

- Any additional procedures (eg, 54150, circumcision using clamp or other device with dorsal penile or ring block) should be reported in addition to normal newborn care codes. Modifier 25 (significant, separately identifiable E/M service) should be appended to the E/M code when a procedure is performed on the same day of service.
- When reporting an E/M service based on time (eg, discharge day management), do not include the time spent providing a separately reported service (eg, circumcision) in the time of the E/M service (eg, obtaining consent, providing post-procedural care instruction).

ICD-10-CM Codes for Newborn Services

International Classification of Diseases, 10th Revision, Clinical Modification (*ICD-10-CM*) codes from category Z38 are used to report liveborn neonates and are the first-listed codes for care by the attending or admitting physician during the entire birth admission. Other physicians providing care during the birth admission do not report Z38 codes but, instead, report codes for the condition(s) they managed at each encounter. Category Z38 codes for single and twin liveborn neonates are shown in **Box 15-1**.

Box 15-1. *International Classification of Diseases, 10th Revision, Clinical Modification* Codes for Single and Twin Liveborn Neonates	
Z38.00 (single liveborn infant, delivered vaginally)	Z38.30 (twin liveborn infant, delivered vaginally)
Z38.01 (single liveborn infant, delivered by cesarean)	Z38.31 (twin liveborn infant, delivered by cesarean)
Z38.1 (single liveborn infant, born outside hospital)	Z38.4 (twin liveborn infant, born outside hospital)
Z38.2 (single liveborn infant, unspecified as to place of birth)	Z38.5 (twin liveborn infant, unspecified as to place of birth)

Refer to the *ICD-10-CM* manual for Z38 codes for other multiple-birth neonates.

Report *ICD-10-CM* code Z76.2 (encounter for health supervision and care of other healthy infant and child) when a healthy newborn continues to receive daily visits pending discharge of the mother or foster care placement or for other reasons. Code Z76.2 is useful for indicating the reason for an extended stay of a healthy newborn. Report Z76.2 as secondary to the appropriate Z38 code for services by the attending physician during the birth admission.

Code Z71.85 (encounter for immunization safety counseling) may be reported secondary to codes for liveborn infant and/or medical conditions addressed at a visit. When a monoclonal antibody to protect against respiratory syncytial virus (RSV) is ordered and administered during the newborn admission, Z29.11 (encounter for prophylactic immunotherapy for RSV) may be reported in addition to other diagnosis codes supporting newborn care. Code Z23 (encounter for immunization) is limited to administration of vaccine or toxoid products. *Physicians and qualified health care professionals (QHPs) do not report the administration of immune globulins or vaccine/toxoid products during the newborn admission.*

Examples

➤ **The physician receives a 10:00 pm call about the vaginal delivery of a healthy full-term boy.** A nurse relates that the newborn was admitted and seems fine. The physician's standing admission orders are followed, and the physician examines the newborn the following morning. The physician reviews the record, examines the neonate, and speaks with the mother. The physician performs circumcision of the newborn (54150) later that day as requested by the parents. The newborn and mother remain in the hospital until the next day, when both are then discharged home. Discharge management takes 25 minutes.

ICD-10-CM	*CPT*
Diagnosis code for all days Z38.00 (single liveborn, delivered vaginally)	**Birth date:** No charge (no face-to-face services provided) **Day 1:** 99460 25 (initial normal newborn care) 54150 (circumcision, using clamp or other device with regional dorsal penile or ring block) **Day 2:** 99238 (hospital discharge management; 30 minutes or less)

Teaching Point: Report newborn hospital care only when a face-to-face service is provided, regardless of any advice provided by phone. The date of the attending physician's first evaluation of the newborn is the date of initial newborn care (in this example, 1 day after the birth date). When a procedure (eg, circumcision) is provided on the same date as a newborn care service, modifier **25** is appended to the code for newborn care to signify that the E/M service was significant and separately identifiable from the preservice and postservice work of the procedure in the documentation. Code **Z41.2** (encounter for circumcision) is not required when reporting a **Z38.-** code.

➤ **A baby is born vaginally in the hospital on March 3 at 4:00 pm.** The physician first sees the baby on March 4 at 7:00 am and, later the same date, discharges the newborn as requested by the parents. A history and examination of the newborn, discussion of the hospital stay with the parents and the mother's doula (who will provide postpartum support to the family), instructions for continuing care, family counseling, and preparation of the final discharge records are performed.

ICD-10-CM	*CPT*
Z38.00 (single liveborn, delivered vaginally)	**99463** (initial normal newborn care and discharge on the same date)

Teaching Point: The physician's combined services are reported with **99463**.

➤ **A subsequent hospital visit is performed in the newborn nursery on a vaginally delivered 2-day-old who is being observed for jaundice caused by bruising received during delivery; however, no interventions are noted, and the baby is doing well. Diagnosis is neonatal bruising with risk for jaundice.**

ICD-10-CM	*CPT*
Z38.00 (single liveborn, delivered vaginally) **P54.5** (neonatal cutaneous hemorrhage [bruising])	**99462** (subsequent normal newborn care)

Teaching Point: The service is normal newborn care even though the newborn is being observed for risk of jaundice. The first-listed diagnosis code is **Z38.00**.

➤ **During a subsequent newborn care visit, the physician notes that the newborn failed the routine hearing screening.** The attending physician spends 15 minutes discussing the results with the parents, refers to an audiologist for testing to confirm or rule out hearing abnormality, and orders a screening test for cytomegalovirus.

ICD-10-CM	*CPT*
Z38.00 (single liveborn, delivered vaginally) **P09.6** (abnormal findings on neonatal screening for neonatal hearing loss) **Z11.59** (encounter for screening for other viral diseases)	**99462** (subsequent normal newborn care)

Teaching Point: The time spent providing the subsequent newborn care does not affect code selection, as normal newborn care services are reported per day, not per hour. Only **Z38.00** is reported when the result of an auditory screening is normal.

An audiologist performing confirmatory testing would report **Z01.110** (encounter for hearing examination following failed hearing screening) and codes for any identified conditions.

Hospital Care of the Ill Newborn

Choosing Normal Newborn Care or Hospital Care

The choice between coding for normal newborn care and coding for hospital care is based on the physician's judgment and the type and severity of symptoms demonstrated. Services to newborns that require an increased level of physician care, nursing observation, or physiologic monitoring (but not intensive care as described by 99477–99480) are typically reported with hospital inpatient or observation care codes (initial, 99221–99223; subsequent, 99231–99233).

- A sick-newborn visit includes a manifesting problem that supports the need for diagnostic investigation, enhanced observation and monitoring, or directed therapy. *Therapeutic intervention is typically necessary for the sick newborn (eg, antibiotics, intravenous [IV] fluids, oxygen, phototherapy).*
- The nature of the manifesting problem, testing, and extent of work required to diagnose and manage the problem should be considered when determining the appropriate procedure code.

Attendance at Delivery

99464 Attendance at delivery (when requested by the delivering physician or other QHP) and initial stabilization of newborn

Attendance at delivery (99464) is not reported when hospital-mandated attendance is the only basis for providing the service. When physician on-call services are mandated by the hospital (eg, attending all repeat cesarean deliveries) and not physician requested, report 99026 (hospital-mandated on-call service; in hospital, each hour) or 99027 (hospital-mandated on-call service; out of hospital, each hour).

Attendance at delivery (99464)

- Service is reported only when requested by the delivering physician and indicated for a newborn who *may* require immediate intervention (ie, stabilization, resuscitation, or evaluation for potential problems) even when no subsequent interventions were necessary.
- Medical record documentation must include the request for attendance at the delivery and substantiate the medical necessity of any services needed and performed. If there is no documentation by the delivering physician for attendance at delivery, the verbal request and the reason for the request should be documented in the attendance note.

Documentation of attendance at delivery should include the name of the requesting physician or QHP and the risks that prompted the request.

- Includes initial drying, stimulation, suctioning, blow-by oxygen, or transient continuous positive airway pressure (CPAP) or high-flow air/oxygen without positive pressure ventilation; a cursory visual inspection of the neonate; assignment of Apgar scores; and discussion of care for the newborn with the delivering physician and parents. A quick look into the delivery room or examination after stabilization has occurred is not sufficient to report 99464. Refer to the "Coding Conundrum: What Service Can Be Reported When a Physician Arrives After Delivery?" box later in this chapter for more information on reporting less than full attendance at delivery services.
- May be reported in addition to initial normal newborn (99460), initial sick newborn (99221–99223), initial intensive care of the neonate (99477), or critical care (99468; 99291, 99292) codes.
- Is not reported in conjunction with standby service codes 99026 and 99027.

When qualifying resuscitative efforts, including positive pressure ventilation, are provided to a neonate with respiratory or cardiac instability, report 99465 (delivery/birthing room resuscitation, provision of positive pressure ventilation and/or chest compressions in the presence of acute inadequate ventilation and/or cardiac output) instead of 99464. Do not report both 99464 and 99465 (ie, report only 99465, when provided).

Refer to Chapter 16 for guidelines for standby service codes 99026 and 99027. Standby services *may be* reported with the newborn resuscitation services (99465) per *CPT* guidelines. Refer to Chapter 17 for more information on reporting delivery/birthing room neonatal resuscitation and separately reported services (eg, E/M services after admission) and guidelines for coding intensive or critical care services.

Hospital Care of the Newborn

Chapter 15

Examples

➤ **A physician is called at the request of an obstetrician to attend a cesarean delivery because of meconium-stained fluid.** The physician stands by until the neonate is delivered and provides stabilization of the neonate, who initially requires blow-by oxygen but steadily becomes more vigorous (99464). The same physician then provides initial normal newborn care (99460) on that same day.

Teaching Point: The physician separately reports the 2 services. No modifier is reported on codes 99460 and 99464 because the codes are not bundled under National Correct Coding Initiative edits.

➤ **A delivering physician asks a neonatologist to be present at delivery of a neonate whose mother has an active infection.** In addition to reviewing the maternal and fetal history and having a discussion with the parents and delivering physician, the neonatologist documents stabilization including use of CPAP without positive pressure ventilation and a comprehensive examination of the neonate.

The newborn is admitted to the newborn nursery under the orders of another physician. The attending physician provides a comprehensive history and examination, orders screening tests and prophylactic interventions, and counsels the family that the neonate will be monitored closely for signs of illness. The physician also counsels about topics such as feeding, sleep, and safety. The attending physician would report 99460 or initial hospital inpatient or observation care (99221–99223) if the newborn experienced an abnormal transition and required significant intervention(s) on that date.

Teaching Point: Although a history and examination were performed, they do not equate to initial hospital care of the newborn. The neonatologist reports 99464 for attendance at delivery.

Coding Conundrum: What Service Can Be Reported When a Physician Arrives After Delivery?

There are no specific time requirements for reporting attendance at delivery. This service requires a request for attendance at delivery by the delivering physician and includes physician work, as described in the Attendance at Delivery section earlier in this chapter. When a physician arrives in the delivery room after the delivery and some or all of this work has been performed, should attendance at delivery be reported? Physicians might want to consider

- When the newborn continues to require significant or prolonged intervention or stabilization in the delivery room, reporting 99464 (attendance at delivery) if the physician work (eg, repetitive stimulation, brief reapplication of CPAP, or intermittent oxygen) is related to the initial transition or 99465 if the neonate requires more intensive resuscitative interventions (eg, bag and mask ventilation)
- When the work provided in the delivery room is related more to the initial hospital care (eg, neonate is examined and attending physician sends the neonate to the well-baby nursery), reporting only the initial normal newborn care code (99460)

For example, attendance at delivery was requested by the delivering physician and the physician arrives after the delivery.

- The 1-minute Apgar score was already assigned; the neonate was dried, stimulated, and suctioned by the nurses; and the neonate is ready to be sent to the newborn nursery by the time the pediatrician appears in the delivery room. The delivering physician acknowledges that assistance is no longer needed. The attending pediatrician reports initial normal newborn care (99460) after completing the initial examination of the newborn. But if the pediatrician is not the attending pediatrician, no service can be reported.
- In the previous example, the child requires continued attendance and assistance. The pediatrician assigns the 5-minute Apgar score, performs continued observation and a focused examination, reviews the birth history, and discusses care of the newborn with the delivering physician and parents. Code 99464 is reported because most of the basic elements of the attendance at delivery were performed and documented in the medical record.

When reporting services to the mother after a stillborn delivery or to a neonate when resuscitation services are unsuccessful, refer to the "Stillborn Deliveries and Unsuccessful Resuscitation" box in **Chapter 17**.

Diagnosis Codes for Perinatal Conditions

There are some important guidelines for reporting conditions that originate in the perinatal period. In *ICD-10-CM*, these conditions are classified to Chapter 16 and codes P00–P96. Codes in this chapter are used only in the neonate's record and not in that of the mother.

Following is the order for reporting codes for neonates at the birth hospital:

1. **Birth outcome (Z38-, reported only by the attending/admitting physician)**
2. **Codes from the perinatal chapter (P00–P96)**
3. **Codes from the congenital anomalies chapter (Q00–Q99)**
4. **Codes from all other chapters**

Other important guidelines include

- Perinatal condition codes are assigned for any condition that is clinically significant. In addition to clinical indications for reporting codes from other chapters, perinatal conditions are considered clinically significant if the condition has implications for future health care needs. Other clinical indications that apply to all conditions are those requiring
  - Clinical evaluation (eg, subspecialty consultation)
  - Therapeutic treatment
  - Diagnostic procedures
  - Extended hospital stay
  - Increased nursing care and/or monitoring
- Should a condition originate in the perinatal period and continue past the 28th day after birth, the perinatal code should continue to be used regardless of the patient's age.

Typical scenarios that may require exclusive use of perinatal or neonatal codes beyond the perinatal period are those related to care of a critically ill or recovering neonate, such as necrotizing enterocolitis in newborn (P77.-), chronic respiratory disease arising in the perinatal period (P27.-), and preterm birth (P07.-).

Perinatal codes are not reported for conditions with *onset after the patient is 28 days old.* For example, necrotizing enterocolitis with onset after the neonatal period is reported with K55.30–K55.33.

- If a newborn has a condition that may be caused by the birth process or community acquired, and documentation does not indicate which the cause is, the condition is reported as resulting from the birth process. Community-acquired conditions are reported with codes other than those in *ICD-10-CM* Chapter 16.
- Codes in categories P00–P04 (newborn affected by maternal factors and by complications of pregnancy, labor, and delivery) may be reported when the conditions are suspected but have not yet been ruled out.

If a neonate is suspected of having an abnormal condition that, after examination and observation, is ruled out, assign codes for signs and symptoms or, in the absence of signs or symptoms, a code from category Z05 (encounter for observation and evaluation of newborn for suspected diseases and conditions ruled out).

Example

➤ **A neonate was born at 37-weeks'-gestation to a mother whose group B β-hemolytic streptococcal culture result was still pending at the time of delivery.** The newborn was alert with excellent Apgar scores in the delivery room and was admitted to the newborn nursery. The newborn was treated per current group B streptococcal disease guidelines, with no indication of illness. The next day, the mother's group B streptococcal culture result was negative and the newborn continued to receive normal newborn care.

ICD-10-CM	*CPT*
Day 0: Z38.00 (single liveborn, delivered vaginally), P00.89 (newborn affected by other maternal conditions) **Day 1:** Z38.00 (single liveborn, delivered vaginally), Z05.1 (observation and evaluation of newborn for suspected infectious condition ruled out)	**Day 0:** 99460 **Day 1:** 99462

Teaching Point: On the date of birth (day 0), the patient was suspected of being affected by a localized maternal infection (P00.89). Normal initial newborn care is reported rather than hospital care because the neonate, although at risk of infection in this case, was asymptomatic and not treated but was observed and did not develop infection. By day 1, the condition was ruled out (Z05.1) and normal newborn services were continued (99462).

Hospital Care of the Newborn

Chapter 15

Daily Hospital Care of the Ill Newborn

Refer to Chapter 16 for full details on selecting and reporting hospital inpatient services 99221–99223, 99231–99233, 99234–99236, and 99238–99239.

Levels of hospital E/M services are based on all hospital care services provided on the same date by the same physician or QHP or by multiple physicians and QHPs of the same group practice (billing under the same tax ID number) and same exact specialty. Refer to discussion of split or shared visits in **Chapter 6** for information on determining which individual reports a hospital E/M visit that includes work by a physician and a QHP.

When multiple physicians of the same specialty and same group practice provide separate initial or subsequent hospital care to a newborn on the same date, report with a single code representing the combined medical decision-making (MDM) (eg, 99223, initial hospital inpatient or observation care with a high level of MDM) or combined total time on the date of the encounter.

Report an initial hospital or observation service when the patient has not received any professional services from the reporting physician or QHP, or another physician or QHP of the exact same specialty and subspecialty who belongs to the same group practice, during the current admission and stay. A prebirth consultation provided to the mother or attendance at delivery by the individual does not exclude separately reporting initial hospital care for services provided after admission to the newborn nursery.

Report a subsequent hospital or observation service when the patient has previously received professional service(s) from the physician or QHP or another physician or QHP of the exact same specialty and subspecialty who belongs to the same group practice, *during the current admission and stay.* Services provided by covering physicians are reported as if provided by the physician who is unavailable.

Once an initial-day care code for a higher service level (eg, intensive or critical care) has been reported, an *initial* code for a lower-level service within the same hospital stay will not be reported. Refer to the Coding for Transitions to Different Levels of Neonatal Care section later in this chapter for details.

When a neonate is not treated but only observed for the potential development of illness, normal newborn codes are reported.

Initial Inpatient Hospital or Observation Care

Codes 99221–99223 are used to report the initial hospital encounter with a sick neonate who does not require intensive observation and monitoring or critical care services.

Refer to Chapter 16 and Table 16-2 for the specific coding and documentation requirements for reporting initial hospital care.

Examples

➤ **A pediatrician is called to provide care to a 37-weeks'-gestation newborn, who developed respiratory distress during a nurse's initial assessment.** The pediatrician reviews the maternal and birth history and notes low concern about early-onset sepsis based on negative maternal screening results and a spontaneous vaginal delivery without meconium staining. Newborn examination findings are limited to respiratory distress with no indications of congenital heart disease or persistent pulmonary hypertension of the newborn. Oxygen saturation is 80% to 85% in room air despite good respiratory effort and muscle tone. Free-flow supplemental oxygen is administered at 25% to 30%. During 30 minutes of close monitoring, the newborn's oxygen saturation steadily increases to 90% and work of breathing improves. A portable chest radiograph is ordered and yields findings of retained fetal lung fluid. The newborn transitions to room air after 1 hour of supplemental oxygen. The pediatrician decides that close monitoring of the neonate in the mother's room is indicated in lieu of transfer to the intensive care nursery. The physician's total time on the date of the encounter is 95 minutes. Diagnoses of liveborn neonate and transient tachypnea of the newborn are documented.

ICD-10-CM	*CPT*
Z38.00 (single liveborn, delivered vaginally) P22.1 (transient tachypnea of the newborn)	99223 (initial hospital inpatient or observation care with moderate level MDM or ≥70 minutes of total time) 99418 (prolonged inpatient/observation E/M service[s] time with or without direct patient contact beyond the required time of the primary service when the primary service level has been selected using total time, each 15 minutes of total time)

Problem(s) addressed ➡ ***High*** (acute illness posing a threat to life or bodily function)
Data reviewed and/or analyzed ➡ ***Moderate*** (1 unique test ordered and history required from independent historian)
Risk of patient management ➡ ***High*** (decision regarding escalation of hospital level of care)

Teaching Point: Both MDM and total time support 99223. When selecting the code based on total time, 95 minutes supports additionally reporting 99418 for prolonged service.

For additional discussion, refer to the Prolonged E/M Service on the Date of a Hospital Encounter section later in this chapter.

➤ **The pediatrician admits a full-term neonate, born vaginally, with Rh incompatibility (mom O– and baby O+/Coombs test result positive).** The otherwise normal neonate is monitored with serial laboratory tests for bilirubin levels but requires no intervention on that date.

ICD-10-CM	*CPT*
Z38.00 (single liveborn, delivered vaginally) P55.0 (Rh isoimmunization of newborn)	99460 (initial newborn care)

Teaching Point: The neonate is being observed and monitored but not treated, supporting 99460.

Subsequent Hospital Care

Subsequent hospital care codes (99231–99233) are reported for each day of service subsequent to initial encounter for the newborn who continues to be sick (ie, not a typical neonate but not in critical condition and not requiring intensive observation and interventions).

Refer to Chapter 16 and Table 16-2 for detailed coding and documentation requirements for 99231–99233.

- Report the appropriate code for the highest acuity on each DOS, combining the times, if applicable, from more than one physician and multiple visits on the same date. On subsequent dates when a previously sick neonate's condition improves and they require no more than normal newborn care, the subsequent normal newborn care code (99462) should be reported.

Example

➤ **On day 2 of the birth admission, the attending pediatrician provides subsequent hospital care to a full-term neonate, born vaginally, with ABO incompatibility (mom O+/antibody test negative and baby B+/Coombs test result negative).** The total serum bilirubin level is elevated. The pediatrician orders phototherapy and follow-up total serum bilirubin and CBC tests. Clinically indicated history, obtained from the parents, and examination are documented.

ICD-10-CM	*CPT*
Z38.00 (single liveborn, delivered vaginally) P55.1 (ABO incompatibility)	99232 (subsequent hospital inpatient or observation care with moderate level MDM or ≥35 minutes of total time)

Problem(s) addressed ➡ ***Moderate*** (1 acute illness with systemic symptoms)

Data reviewed and/or analyzed ➡ ***Moderate*** (1 test reviewed, 2 tests ordered [total serum bilirubin and CBC], and history required from independent historian)

Risk of patient management ➡ ***Moderate*** (phototherapy)

Teaching Point: On day 2, the neonate continues to require therapeutic management, supporting subsequent hospital care.

Discharge Management

Dependent on total time involved in the discharge, either 99238 or 99239 (hospital discharge management) is reported when discharge occurs on a day separate from the initial hospital care. Codes 99238 and 99239 are reported only by the attending physician or QHP or a physician or QHP in the same specialty and same group practice.

- Time must be documented to support 99239 (ie, time of >30 minutes).

Codes for discharge services are not reported when

- ✖ A newborn dies on the date of birth. The attending physician should report a code for the level of hospital care provided (ie, initial hospital sick care, intensive care, or critical care) as appropriate.
- ✖ A neonate is transferred to another facility. The physician providing care before transfer reports the appropriate code for the type of care provided on that date (eg, hourly critical care 99291 and, when appropriate, 99292) before the transfer, but not discharge management.

Refer to Chapter 16 for more information on discharge management codes 99238 and 99239. Refer to the "Stillborn Deliveries and Unsuccessful Resuscitation" box in Chapter 17 for discussion of billing for services provided to a mother and/or neonate on the date of birth when the outcome is stillborn delivery or unsuccessful resuscitation of an ill neonate.

Examples

➤ **The physician performs a follow-up visit for a normal neonate (vaginally delivered) who will be discharged today.** The parents are counseled on home care and follow-up. The parents have general questions and some concerns about immunization, although consent was given for immunization against RSV and hepatitis B during the admission. All questions are answered, and the newborn is discharged. Documentation supports 40 minutes' total physician time on this date.

ICD-10-CM	*CPT*
Z38.00 (single liveborn, delivered vaginally) Z71.85 (encounter for immunization safety counseling)	99239 (discharge management, more than 30 minutes)

Teaching Point: Time (40 minutes unit/floor time dedicated to the patient) is the key controlling factor. If time spent in discharge day management is 30 minutes or less or is not documented, 99238 must be reported. Code Z71.85 indicates that time was spent in immunization safety counseling. Refer to the Coding for Counseling Without Same-Date Immunization section in **Chapter 8** for discussion of codes for reporting 3 minutes or more of immunization counseling without same-date administration.

➤ **The physician examines a 23-day-old full-term neonate who will be discharged with a home apnea monitor.** The parents are counseled on their neonate's condition and given instructions for home care and follow-up. Sixty minutes was spent reviewing the hospital course and expected follow-up, counseling the parents, completing orders, and documenting the service. Diagnoses are newborn delivered vaginally and newborn apnea.

ICD-10-CM	*CPT*
Z38.00 (single liveborn, delivered vaginally) P28.40 (unspecified apnea of newborn)	99239 (discharge management, more than 30 minutes)

Teaching Point: Discharge day management is reported for all care provided by the attending physician or QHP on the date of discharge. Although the time is significantly more than the 31 minutes or more required for 99239, there is no upper limit of time reported with 99239, and prolonged service codes are not applicable.

Consultations

A consultation is reported when a physician, other QHP, or other appropriate source (eg, attorney, nonclinical social worker) requests an opinion and/or advice from another physician or QHP. This request must be in writing or given verbally by the requester and documented in the consultation record. The consulting physician evaluates the patient, renders advice, records it, and returns a report to the requesting physician or appropriate source (either in a shared electronic health record or by separate written communication).

Codes 99252–99255 are reported for newborn care when the following circumstances are true:

- The encounter meets the definition of a consultation.
- The encounter is the first face-to-face professional service provided to the patient by the consulting physician or QHP (or another physician or QHP of the same exact specialty and same group practice) during the admission/stay.

A consulting physician's follow-up visits with a newborn (newly requested consultation or continuing care) during a single admission are reported as subsequent hospital care (99231–99233) unless the service meets the requirements for reporting hourly critical care (refer to **Chapter 17** for requirements of critical care).

Refer to Chapter 16 for details of the specific reporting, documentation, and coding requirements for inpatient consultations. Refer to Chapter 7 for discussion of consultations provided in office or other outpatient settings.

Examples

➤ **At the request of a primary care physician, a neonatologist evaluates a full-term–gestation neonate with moderate tachypnea after birth.** A detailed history is obtained from the mother, noting that she had a positive group B streptococcal screening result. Review of labor and delivery records reveals that she received 1 dose of IV ampicillin just prior to delivery. Because of fetal tachycardia and a non-reassuring fetal heart rate pattern, a cesarean delivery was performed. After birth, the newborn had Apgar scores of 7 and 9 and was noted to have tachypnea with mild substernal retractions. The neonatologist recommends obtaining a chest radiograph and blood cultures and beginning antibiotics pending the results of the cultures, as well as a follow-up CBC at 12 hours. The neonatologist counsels the baby's parents, writes a detailed medical record note, and discusses the recommendations with the attending physician by phone. The attending physician does not want the neonatologist to assume responsibility for all the patient's care but requests a follow-up visit to reevaluate risk for a developing infection.

At a follow-up visit later that day, the 12-hour CBC and C-reactive protein test results are reassuring, the blood culture result has remained negative, the tachypnea has resolved, and the chest radiograph is clear. The neonatologist recommends continuing the antibiotics until culture results are negative at 48 hours and otherwise signs off on the case, remaining available for further questions. The neonatologist's total time on the date of the encounter is 75 minutes.

ICD-10-CM	*CPT*
P22.1 (transient tachypnea of newborn) P00.82 (newborn affected by [positive] maternal group B streptococcus colonization)	99254 (hospital inpatient or observation consultation, with moderate level MDM or total time ≥60 minutes)

Problem(s) addressed ➡ ***Moderate*** (undiagnosed problem with uncertain prognosis)

Data reviewed and/or analyzed ➡ ***Moderate*** (3 tests reviewed and/or ordered and history required from independent historian)

Risk of patient management ➡ ***Moderate*** (IV antibiotics)

Teaching Point: Both the level of MDM and total time on the date of the encounter support 99254. If the payer policy does not allow payment for consultation codes, the 75 minutes of service supports initial hospital or observation care code 99223.

➤ **At the request of an obstetrician, a pediatric urologist provides a consultation to a family whose male fetus (single gestation) has an enlarged bladder and bilateral dilated ureters in the second trimester of pregnancy diagnosed through prenatal ultrasound.** The request for consultation is documented by the obstetrician and the urologist. The urologist spends 10 minutes reviewing records of this new patient provided by the obstetrician, including ultrasounds of the fetus before the consultation on the same date. The consultation with the family takes place via a secure, real-time audiovisual connection with the physician in an outpatient clinic and the patient at home. The service includes discussing how the mother's treatment will be affected (eg, follow-up testing and delivery will occur at a

Hospital Care of the Newborn

Chapter 15

facility with resources that may be required to care for the neonate). The time spent in consultation with the family is 34 minutes. The urologist documents the time spent and a summary of the discussion. Additionally, the urologist discusses ongoing patient management and delivery with the obstetrician via secure messaging. A written report is also produced and sent to the requesting obstetrician with a copy maintained in the patient's record. The urologist's total time on the date of the encounter is 65 minutes.

ICD-10-CM	*CPT*
035.8XX0 (maternal care for other [suspected] fetal abnormality and damage)	99245 95 (outpatient consultation with moderate MDM or total time ≥55 minutes, by telemedicine)

Teaching Point: The patient in this example is not a newborn but, rather, the expectant mother. The physician's total time supports 99245. Modifier 95 (synchronous telemedicine service rendered via a real-time interactive audio and video telecommunications system) is appended to indicate that the service met the requirements of a telemedicine service. If the consultation took place in person while the mother was hospitalized, 99254 (inpatient or observation consultation with moderate level MDM or total time ≥60 minutes) would be reported. If a payer requires submission of outpatient audio-video telemedicine codes in lieu of consultation codes, 98003 (synchronous audio-video visit with ≥60 minutes total time) and 99417 95 (prolonged outpatient E/M service, first 15 minutes, provided via synchronous audio-video telecommunication) would be reported.

Prolonged E/M Service on the Date of a Hospital Encounter

#★✚99418 Prolonged inpatient or observation E/M service(s) time with or without direct patient contact beyond the required time of the primary service when the primary service level has been selected using total time, each 15 minutes of total time

Code 99418 is reported in addition to a code for a face-to-face E/M service in a facility setting under the following circumstances:

- Only when the code for the primary E/M service was selected according to the physician's or QHP's total time on the date of the encounter
- Only in conjunction with highest-level hospital inpatient or observation services (99223, 99233, 99236, 99255) or nursing facility services (99306, 99310)
- Only when the total time required for the highest level of service in a code category (eg, 99223 for initial hospital or observation care) has been exceeded by at least 15 minutes

Refer to **Table 16-7** for illustration of required total time to report 99418 in conjunction with inpatient and observation E/M services.

Do not report 99418

- ✖ When the total time on the date of the encounter exceeds the required time of the primary service or the time included in the most recent unit of prolonged service by less than 15 minutes
- ✖ For any time spent providing a separately reported service (eg, a procedure or interpretation and report of a diagnostic test)
- ✖ For prolonged services on a date other than the date of a face-to-face E/M service (Refer to 99358–99359, discussed in the Prolonged E/M Service on a Date Before or After a Direct Service section later in this chapter.)

Example

➤ **A physician reports initial hospital care, 99223, according to the required total time of 75 or more minutes.** The physician's total time on the date of the encounter is 105 minutes. The physician reports 99223 and 99418 × 2 units (1 unit for each full 15-minute period beyond the first 75 minutes).

Teaching Point: The physician's total time of 105 minutes exceeds the required time of 75 minutes or more for 99223 by 30 minutes. Two units of 99418 are reported because the initial unit of service for 99418 includes 15 to 29 minutes beyond the 75-minute total time of the related service and the second unit is reported when the time beyond the primary service is 30 minutes or more.

The Medicare program implemented the separate Healthcare Common Procedure Coding System code G0316 for prolonged hospital inpatient service. Verify individual payer policies for prolonged E/M services to identify payable codes and time requirements that may differ from the requirements in *CPT*.

Prolonged E/M Service on a Date Before or After a Direct Service

99358 Prolonged E/M service before and/or after direct patient care; first hour (minimum 30 minutes)
+99359 each additional 30 minutes (minimum 15 minutes)

Prolonged service without direct patient contact (99358, 99359) may be reported only in relation to an E/M service *when it occurs on a date other than the date of a face-to-face E/M service.* Report 99358 and 99359

- For non–face-to-face E/M services of 30 or more minutes' total duration on a single DOS
- For prolonged services in relation to any E/M service *regardless of whether time was used to select the level of the face-to-face service*
- When the prolonged E/M service is related to a service during or after which (face-to-face) patient care has occurred or will occur and relates to ongoing patient management

Do not report 99358 and 99359 when

✖ An E/M service that is selected according to total time (eg, in-person or telemedicine E/M service) is provided on the same date.
✖ Less than 30 minutes of time is directed to the individual patient on the DOS or for a period of less than 15 minutes beyond the first hour.
✖ The same time is attributed to another service (eg, medical team conference or interprofessional telephone/internet/electronic health record consultation).

Example

➤ **An infant will be transferred from a Level III neonatal intensive care unit, following a 30-day hospital stay, to a community Level II unit to complete recovery before home discharge.** The receiving physician spends 1 hour 20 minutes reviewing the digitally provided extensive transfer records on the evening before the patient arrives at the receiving facility.

99358 (prolonged non–face-to-face services; first hour).
99359 × 1 (each additional 30 minutes).

Teaching Point: This service included 80 minutes of prolonged service time on a date when no direct E/M service was provided. Code 99358 represents the first 60 minutes. Code 99359 is reported for the final 20 minutes of prolonged service. If less than 75 minutes of prolonged services were provided, 99359 would not be reported.

Hospital Care of the Newborn

Chapter 15

Coding for Transitions to Different Levels of Neonatal Care

The *Newborn Coding Decision Tool 2026* (www.aap.org/Newborn-Coding-Decision-Tool-2026) provides a quick reference to help determine appropriate codes for transitions in care.

During a hospital stay, a newly born or readmitted neonate may require multiple levels of care as the severity of the illness waxes and wanes over a protracted hospital course. A normal newborn may suddenly become sick, progress to requiring an intensive level of care, or require critical care during the same hospital stay. As the neonate recovers, a progressively lower intensity of care is required (eg, level of monitoring, observation, interventions) before home discharge.

It is important to remember that

- When a patient initially qualifies after birth for normal newborn care and, at a subsequent encounter on the same day, becomes ill and requires neonatal intensive or critical care services, normal newborn care (99460 or 99462) may be reported in addition to the following codes on the same day:
  - Initial intensive care (99477)
  - Initial critical care (99468)
  - Time-based critical care (99291, 99292)
- *CPT* instructs to report the appropriate E/M code with modifier 25 for these services in addition to the normal newborn code.

CPT does not directly address reporting hospital care of a newborn who becomes ill following provision of hospital care of the normal newborn earlier on the same date by the same physician or QHP (or individuals of the same group practice) but who does not require intensive or critical care. Bundling edits may result in denial of either 99460 or the problem-oriented hospital E/M code (eg, initial 99221–99223 or subsequent 99231–99233) when both are reported on the same date by the same individual or individuals of the same specialty and same group practice, even when modifier 25 is appended.

- When reporting only hospital care of the ill newborn following provision of normal newborn care earlier on the same date, the total time of hospital care provided on the same date may be used in selecting the level of initial or subsequent hospital care based on total time on the date of the encounter. This applies only when normal newborn care is not separately reported.

Example

➤ **A physician admits a full-term neonate, born vaginally, with Rh incompatibility (mom AB– and baby B+/ Coombs test result positive).** The mother did not receive RhoGAM injection during her pregnancy. Findings from a complete examination of the neonate are normal, without anemia, hydrops, or hepatosplenomegaly. The initial hemoglobin level is at the lower end of normal levels and the reticulocyte count is elevated. The parents are counseled, and the initial plan is to monitor the bilirubin and hemoglobin levels every 4 hours. The physician documents 30 minutes spent providing newborn care at this visit. The physician is notified of a rise in the bilirubin level to 10 mg/dL at 8 hours after birth and returns to reevaluate the neonate. The neonate's initial course and feeding history is reviewed with the nurses and parents and the repeat examination is documented, noting the dermal progression of the jaundice but no other clinical findings. The parents are counseled that the neonate will require continued hospital care and phototherapy, which is initiated at the visit. All the parents' questions are answered. The physician's total time on the date of the encounter is 75 minutes.

ICD-10-CM	*CPT*
Z38.00 (single liveborn, delivered vaginally) P55.0 (Rh isoimmunization of newborn)	99223 (initial hospital care requiring high MDM or total time meeting or exceeding 75 minutes)

Teaching Point: The physician may select the initial hospital care code based on MDM or total time directed to care of the individual patient on the DOS. The documented total time of 75 minutes supports 99223. If the physician's total time meets or exceeds 90 minutes, prolonged service code 99418 may be reported with 1 unit per each additional 15 minutes. The initial visit might have been reported as initial hospital care of the normal newborn (99460) if the patient's condition had not progressed to require intervention on the same DOS.

When a payer instructs that normal newborn care is to be separately reported in addition to a problem-oriented E/M later on the same date, no time spent in the separately reported service would be included in the total time of the problem-oriented visit.

- Once an initial-day care code for a higher service level has been reported, an *initial* code for a lower service level within the same hospital stay will not be reported.
  - If an ill neonate has required intensive care (initial or weight based, 99477–99480) but no longer qualifies for intensive care and is transferred to the care of a physician of a different specialty or different group practice, the receiving physician will report subsequent hospital care (99231–99233) based on the level of service provided.
  - The receiving physician *will not report* initial hospital care (99221–99223) for the first encounter after the transfer. If the neonate is no longer ill but requires continued hospital observation, the receiving physician will report subsequent normal newborn care (99460, 99462). If the neonate is still ill but no longer requires intensive observation, the subsequent hospital care codes (99231–99233) will be reported.
  - The transferring physician may report initial neonatal intensive care (99477) if provided earlier on the date of transfer. But when the ill neonate improves and is transferred on a date after the initial day of intensive care, a transferring physician will report subsequent hospital care (99231–99233) and not subsequent neonatal intensive care (99478–99480). The level of care determines the code, not the location where newborn care takes place. Care provided in the neonatal intensive care unit does not automatically support intensive or critical care service codes.

Example

➤ **A neonate (2,600 g) is transferred internally (same hospital) from neonatal intensive care by Dr A to Dr B, who is of a different specialty (eg, pediatrician, hospitalist), to complete recovery before home discharge.** On the day of transfer, Dr A determines that the ill but recovering neonate no longer requires intensive care and documents hospital care with moderate MDM prior to the transfer. Dr B provides a face-to-face E/M service to the neonate, documenting 75 minutes of total time directed to the patient, including review of the patient's hospital stay prior to transfer.

Dr A reports	Dr B reports
99232 (subsequent hospital care, moderate MDM or total time 35 minutes)	99233 (subsequent hospital care, total time 50 minutes) 99418 × 1 (direct prolonged services, first 15 minutes)

Teaching Point: Dr B may not report initial hospital care for services to the patient who has received prior initial hospital services (eg, initial neonatal intensive care) in the same facility and same stay. The typical time of 99233 was exceeded by 25 minutes, supporting 99418.

Other Newborn Hospital Care

Circumcision

54150 Circumcision, using clamp or other device with regional dorsal penile or ring block

If the circumcision with a clamp or other device is performed without dorsal penile or ring block, append modifier 52 (reduced services) to 54150.

- Medicare has assigned a global period of 0 (zero) to 54150.
- When performing a circumcision and a separately identifiable E/M service on the same day (eg, 99462, subsequent normal newborn care; 99238, discharge services ≤30 minutes), append modifier 25 to the E/M code. Link the appropriate *ICD-10-CM* code (eg, Z38.00) to the E/M service and to the circumcision procedure code.
- The American Hospital Association *Coding Clinic* instructs that Z41.2 (encounter for routine and ritual male circumcision) *not be assigned* in addition to codes in category Z38.-, as it believes circumcision is a routine part of the newborn's hospital care.

54160 Circumcision, surgical excision other than clamp, device, or dorsal slit; neonate (28 days of age or less)
54161 older than 28 days

Unlike with 54150, Medicare has a global period of 10 days assigned to 54160 and 54161. A physician who performs a procedure with a 10-day global period must append modifier 24 (unrelated E/M service by the same physician or other QHP during a postoperative period) to the E/M code for subsequent newborn or hospital care or discharge management (eg, 99238 24) provided in the 10-day period following the procedure for general care of the newborn that is unrelated to the procedure.

Refer to Chapter 13 for information on coding for circumcisions performed in the office.

Frenotomy

40806 Incision of labial frenum (frenotomy)
41010 Incision of lingual frenum (frenotomy)

Uncommonly, a newborn experiences issues with latching on or sucking effectively because of a tight frenulum. If these issues are severe enough to warrant intervention by incision or clipping of the frenulum, report 41010 for lingual frenotomy or 40806 for labial frenotomy. This may be completed in the hospital before discharge. Link *ICD-10-CM* codes P92.5 (neonatal difficulty in feeding at the breast) and Q38.1 (ankyloglossia) to the procedure code on the claim.

- If the physician performing the incision is also performing newborn care on the same date, be sure to append modifier 25 to the code reported for the newborn E/M service. Link this service to the appropriate Z38 code followed by P92.5 and Q38.1.
- ✖ Do not report *CPT* code 41115 (excision of lingual frenum [frenectomy]) when the frenulum is only incised or clipped.

Car Safety Seat Testing

Codes **94780** and **94781** (car seat testing) are reported when determining whether *an infant through 12 months of age* may be safely transported upright in a car seat or must be transported by lying down in a car bed.

- Car seat testing codes may be reported in addition to the subsequent hospital or discharge day management codes when performed and documented. *Note:* These codes cannot be reported in addition to critical or intensive care services.
- Time spent in car seat testing is not counted as time spent in discharge day management.
- Car seat testing may also be provided to an infant in an outpatient setting to determine if the infant can safely move from car bed to car seat transportation.

Refer to Chapter 17 for more information on car seat testing.

To test your knowledge of the information presented in this chapter, complete the quiz found at the end of it, after the resources. Answers to each quiz are found in **Appendix II**.

Chapter Takeaways

This chapter addressed coding for services provided during a newborn's birth admission. Following are some takeaways from this chapter:

- The neonatal period begins at birth and continues through the completed 28th day after birth, ending on the 29th calendar day after birth. The day of birth is considered day 0 (zero).
- *ICD-10-CM* codes from category **Z38** are used to report liveborn neonates according to type of birth and are the first listed code for care by the attending or admitting physician during the entire birth admission.
- The choice between coding for normal newborn care and coding for hospital care is based on the physician's judgment and the type and severity of symptoms demonstrated.
- *CPT* codes for care of a normal newborn typically follow a pathway of daily care from initial care to subsequent care and/or discharge day management.
- Physicians and QHPs of the same specialty and same group practice may report only 1 initial E/M service per admission/stay.
- Procedures such as circumcision are separately reported when performed.

Resources

AAP Coding Assistance and Education

AAP Coding and Payment Hotline (www.aap.org/en/practice-management/child-health-finance-payment-strategy/coding-payment-hotline)

Newborn Coding Decision Tool 2026 (www.aap.org/Newborn-Coding-Decision-Tool-2026)

AAP Pediatric Coding Newsletter™

"Coding Review: Care of the Newborn During the Birth Admission," January 2024 (https://doi.org/10.1542/pcco_book237_document003)

"Connecting Coding and Practice Guidelines: Hyperbilirubinemia," March 2023 (https://doi.org/10.1542/pcco_book227_document003)

"*CPT* 2024: Revisions to Guidelines for Split or Shared Visits," November 2023 (https://doi.org/10.1542/pcco_book235_document003)

Test Your Knowledge!

1. **True or false? Monday is day 1 of the neonatal period for a newborn delivered on Sunday (ie, 1 day ago).**
   a. True
   b. False
2. **When is a perinatal condition reportable with a code in *ICD-10-CM* Chapter 16 clinically significant?**
   a. Only when the condition requires therapeutic treatment.
   b. Only when the condition is the main reason for the newborn's continued hospital stay.
   c. Always, any condition, symptom, or finding is clinically significant when documented during the perinatal period.
   d. When the condition has implications for future health care needs and/or any of the clinical indications for reporting codes from other *ICD-10-CM* chapters.
3. **How does a physician or QHP report normal newborn care provided at two separate visits on the same date?**
   a. Report the visits based on the combined medical decision-making or total time on the date of the encounter.
   b. Report a single normal newborn care code for all care provided on that date (eg, 99460).
   c. Report a code from 99460–99463 with modifier 22 (increased service).
   d. Codes for normal newborn care are reported per visit (eg, 99460 × 2 units).
4. **Which code(s) are reported when a physician or QHP spends an hour in the delivery room to be present at a birth solely because of hospital policy followed by provision of initial normal newborn care on the same date?**
   a. Only initial newborn care (99460) can be reported.
   b. Attendance at delivery and initial stabilization 99464
   c. 99460 and 99464
   d. Standby service 99026 and 99460
5. **Which of the following is true when reporting a newborn circumcision with 54150?**
   a. Because circumcision is a minor procedure, an E/M service cannot be reported on the same date.
   b. Modifier 22 (increased procedural service) is appended when the service includes a regional dorsal penile or ring block.
   c. Modifier 52 (reduced service) is appended when the service does not include a regional dorsal penile or ring block.
   d. Modifier 24 (unrelated E/M during a postoperative period) is appended to codes for normal newborn care provided within 10 days of the circumcision.

CHAPTER 16

Noncritical Hospital Evaluation and Management Services

Contents

Chapter Highlights

- Guidelines and descriptors for codes used to report services provided in hospital inpatient and observation settings other than normal newborn, intensive, or critical care services
- How 2 of 3 elements of medical decision-making (MDM) are used to select a level of MDM
- Code selection based on time including continuous time crossing midnight and prolonged service
- Guidelines for reporting split or shared visits
- Selecting the appropriate category of hospital evaluation and management (E/M) services
- Codes for reporting face-to-face consultations and interprofessional consultations through internet, telephone, or electronic health record (EHR)

Coding for Noncritical Hospital Evaluation and Management Services

This chapter discusses codes and guidelines for all E/M services that are provided in a hospital inpatient or observation setting except normal newborn, intensive care, and critical care services. (Refer to **Chapter 15** for hospital care of the newborn and **Chapter 17** for discussion of critical care services.) Hospital inpatient or observation care codes are used to report partial hospitalization services in addition to inpatient and observation services.

Codes for reporting hospital inpatient and observation services (other than consultations reported with **99252–99255**) are shown in **Table 16-1**. For separate discussion of consultation codes, refer to the Inpatient and Observation Consultations section and **Table 16-7** later in this chapter.

Refer to the American Academy of Pediatrics (AAP) *Pediatric Evaluation and Management: Coding Quick Reference Card 2026* (www.aap.org/Pediatric-Evaluation-and-Management-Coding-Quick-Reference-Card-2026).

Refer to **Chapter 6** for E/M guidelines for selecting a level of MDM and determining total time and for specific documentation requirements. Refer to **Chapter 1** for guidelines for reporting hospital services provided in part by a resident.

Although E/M codes for hospital inpatient and observation care are combined, admission orders should distinctly designate the patient's admission status, as this may be important for payer coverage and payment rates. Because observation care is considered an outpatient encounter, when a patient transitions from observation to inpatient status, an order for inpatient admission should be clearly documented in the patient record.

Except for same-date admission and discharge services, *Current Procedural Terminology* (*CPT*®) does not limit reporting of hospital inpatient or observation care codes to the admitting physician. But some payer policies may require submission of outpatient E/M services for services provided to patients in observation status when provided by any physician or qualified health care professional (QHP) other than the admitting physician(s) or QHPs of the same specialty and same group practice.

Table 16-1. Hospital Inpatient and Observation Evaluation and Management Codes

Except for **99238** and **99239**, codes are selected according to either MDM or meeting or exceeding the listed total time on the date of the encounter. (Consultation codes not included here. Refer to **Table 16-7**.)

All levels of initial and subsequent hospital or observation care include a medically appropriate history and/or examination, but neither is a component of code selection.

Category of Service	Straightforward or Low MDM	Moderate MDM	High MDM
Admit/discharge on the same date	**99234** Total time: ≥45 min	**99235** Total time: ≥70 min	**99236** Total time: ≥85 min
Initial inpatient or observation care	**99221** Total time: ≥40 min	**99222** Total time: ≥55 min	**99223** Total time: ≥75 min
Subsequent inpatient or observation care	**99231** Total time: ≥25 min	**99232** Total time: ≥35 min	**99233** Total time: ≥50 min
Inpatient or observation discharge management	**99238** ≤30 min **99239** >30 min		

Abbreviation: MDM, medical decision-making.

Guidelines for Inpatient and Observation Services

Professional services are the face-to-face services, including telemedicine services, rendered by physicians and other QHPs who may report E/M services.

Following are basic guidelines for reporting hospital inpatient or observation E/M services with the codes in **Table 16-1**:

- There are no distinctions between new and established patients. But most codes differentiate initial from subsequent hospital or observation care.
  - Report an initial hospital or observation service when the patient has not received any professional services from the reporting physician or QHP or another physician or QHP of the exact same specialty and subspecialty who belongs to the same group practice (ie, has the same tax ID number or group National Provider Identifier [NPI]) during the current admission and stay.
  - Report a subsequent hospital or observation service when the patient has received professional service(s) from the physician or QHP or another physician or QHP of the exact same specialty and subspecialty who belongs to the same group practice, on a prior date during the current admission and stay.
  - When physicians and QHPs are working together, they are considered to be in the same specialty and subspecialty (eg, endocrinology, hospital medicine).
  - A physician or QHP who is covering for another physician or QHP reports a service as if provided by the physician or QHP who is unavailable.
  - A hospital stay that includes a transition between observation and inpatient is considered a single stay.

Hospital inpatient and observation services are reported for face-to-face services, including services via telemedicine. A physician's initial hospital E/M service may occur on a date after the hospital's admission date (eg, the day after either admission orders are provided via telephone or initial care is provided by a resident without teaching physician supervision).

Examples

➤ **A neonate was born by cesarean delivery on Monday and received normal newborn care from Dr Parker of Pediatric Hospitalists, Inc, on Monday.** On Tuesday, the neonate is evaluated by Dr Drake (also an employee of Pediatric Hospitalists, Inc, and of the same exact specialty and subspecialty as Dr Parker) and found to have developed hyperbilirubinemia requiring initiation of phototherapy. Dr Drake's service includes clinically indicated history and examination with moderate MDM. The diagnosis is jaundice caused by ABO incompatibility.

ICD-10-CM	*CPT*
Z38.01 (single liveborn infant, delivered by cesarean) P55.1 (ABO isoimmunization of newborn)	99232 (subsequent hospital inpatient or observation with moderate MDM)

Teaching Point: The neonate's service by Dr Drake is a subsequent encounter because Dr Parker, of the same group practice and same specialty, has provided E/M services on the day of birth. Although screening for jaundice falls within newborn care, treating jaundice does not.

➤ **An adolescent was admitted late on Monday and received initial hospital care from Dr Ahmad of Pediatric Hospitalists, Inc, on that date.** On Tuesday, Dr Ahmad requests that a neurologist evaluate the patient for a possible neurological condition. To this point, neither the neurologist nor any other physician or QHP of the same specialty and same group practice has provided a professional service to the patient during this stay.

Teaching Point: Dr Ahmad reports an initial hospital E/M service (99221–99223) for the services on Monday and subsequent hospital care (99231–99233) for the services on Tuesday.

The neurologist's service is an initial service. If all requirements for reporting a consultation are met, a hospital consultation (99252–99255) is reported. If, however, the service does not meet the requirements of a consultation or the payer does not pay for services reported with consultation codes, the neurologist reports initial hospital services (99221–99223). Refer to the Medicare Consultation Guidelines section later in this chapter for further discussion of reporting to payers that do not allow payment for consultation codes.

- Codes are reported according to the cumulative inpatient or observation services (*MDM or total time on the date of service [DOS]*) provided by one or more physicians or QHPs
  - Of the same exact specialty
  - With the same tax ID number (or group NPI)
  - *On a single calendar date*
- Services may be performed and reported by any physician of any specialty (eg, hospitalist, primary care physician, specialist) or QHPs.
- Any professional service (eg, procedure, interpretation and report) with a *CPT* code may be reported separately when performed by the reporting provider or group and documented.
- ✖ Do not include the time spent performing separately reported procedures in the time of the E/M service.
- E/M services may be provided by the same physician or QHP in an outpatient (eg, office, emergency department [ED]) or other facility (eg, nursing facility) setting before admission to observation or inpatient status on the same date. *CPT* guidelines instruct that these services *be separately reported* with modifier **25** appended to the E/M code for the initial encounter on that date. Individual payer policies for more than one E/M service provided on the same date may vary. Refer to the "Multiple Sites of Evaluation and Management Services" box later in this chapter for further discussion of this topic.

Example

➤ **A physician provides an office E/M service for a 4-year-old in an office setting and determines that hospital admission is indicated for treatment and further evaluation of dehydration associated with fever, vomiting, and diarrhea for 3 days and a rash that first appeared on the date of the visit.** Later that day, a QHP who is of the exact same specialty and same group practice visits the patient and provides initial hospital care.

Teaching Point: The physician may report the outpatient E/M service with modifier **25** appended to the appropriate E/M code (eg, **99215 25**) and the QHP reports an initial hospital inpatient or observation E/M service code (without a modifier or, when required, with modifier **AI**, principal physician of record).

If only 1 service is reported (eg, to comply with payer policy), the combined total time on the date of the encounter or aggregate MDM determines the level of service reported with a single code by 1 individual. Refer to the Reporting Services Split or Shared by a Physician and a QHP section later in this chapter for guidance on determining which individual reports the combined services.

Multiple Sites of Evaluation and Management Services

If after providing care to a patient in an encounter in another site of service (eg, ED, office, nursing facility), a physician or QHP (or individuals of the same specialty and same group practice) provides initial hospital or observation care on that same date, the code for the E/M service provided prior to admission is separately reported with modifier 25 (significant, separately identifiable E/M service) appended (eg, 99215 25, 99223).

Note that some payer policies may not align with *CPT* guidance for reporting more than one E/M service on a single DOS. When a physician or QHP has provided care in another setting, including the ED, before providing inpatient or observation care on the same date *and does not separately report each service* (eg, to comply with payer policy), the code reported may be selected according to the total time on the date of the encounter or the aggregate MDM of the visits.

For separate discussion of consultations provided before admission to inpatient or observation status, refer to the Consultation Guidelines section later in this chapter.

General E/M Code Selection Guidelines

As detailed in **Chapter 6**, any initial or subsequent hospital inpatient or observation care service code *may be selected according to either MDM or total time.* The reported code is determined through whichever method most benefits the reporting physician or QHP. The following sections provide some key points about using either MDM or total time on the DOS to select codes.

Refer also to the AAP publication *Pediatric Evaluation and Management Coding Revisions: Facility and Office Services* (www.aap.org/pediatric-evaluation-and-management-coding-revisions-facility-and-office-services-paperback) for code selection guidance.

Medical Decision-Making

Code selection based on MDM always requires that 2 of 3 elements be met at the level reported. As a reminder, the 3 elements of MDM are

1. Number and complexity of *problems addressed* (problems addressed)
2. Amount and/or complexity of *data to be reviewed and analyzed* (data)
3. Risk of complications and/or morbidity or mortality of *patient management* (risk)

Do not select a code based on 1 element of MDM (eg, high risk alone does not support high MDM).

Problems Addressed

For subsequent hospital inpatient and observation care services, the problem addressed is the problem status on the date of the encounter, which may significantly differ from that prompted by admission (eg, a physician addresses a new problem that manifested after admission, or a consultant is asked to evaluate a problem that was not the problem that prompted admission).

A problem is addressed or managed when evaluated or treated at the encounter by the reporting physician or QHP. Do not count problems that are not evaluated and/or do not affect MDM at the current encounter.

Determining the highest-complexity problem(s) addressed is key to selecting the number and complexity of problems addressed. Addressing multiple problems of the same complexity affects the level of problems addressed only when addressing 2 or more self-limited or minor problems or 2 or more stable chronic illnesses. Otherwise, multiple problems of the same complexity (eg, 2 acute, uncomplicated illnesses) do not affect the number and complexity of problems addressed.

Examples

➤ **A patient is admitted with a diagnosis of type 1 diabetic ketoacidosis without coma (E10.10).**

Problem(s) addressed ➡ ***High*** (one or more chronic illnesses with severe exacerbation, progression, or side effects of treatment)

On the next date, the patient's condition has improved, but they are receiving follow-up care for the uncontrolled (or new) diagnosis of type 1 diabetes with hyperglycemia (**E10.65**).

Problem(s) addressed ➡ ***Moderate*** (one or more chronic illnesses with exacerbation, progression, or side effects of treatment)

Teaching Point: The problem addressed is the problem status on the date of the encounter; at subsequent encounters, the problem addressed may significantly differ from that on admission. It is the problem being managed or comanaged by the reporting physician or QHP, and not necessarily the cause of the admission or continued stay, that is to be coded on the encounter date.

➤ **A patient with cerebral palsy was admitted as an inpatient for orthopedic surgery and, during the hospital stay, developed a urinary tract infection (UTI).** A hospitalist who has been managing the patient's conditions unrelated to the surgery provides a subsequent hospital inpatient or observation service to address the UTI.

Teaching Point: The problem addressed by the hospitalist (UTI) was not the reason for the admission. The hospitalist's code selection, when based on MDM, will include selecting the number and complexity of the problem addressed (ie, the UTI and any other problem addressed at the encounter).

The underlying chronic condition, cerebral palsy, may influence the level of MDM when addressed and results in an increased amount and/or complexity of data to be reviewed and analyzed or an increased risk of complications and/or morbidity or mortality of patient management. An *International Classification of Diseases, Tenth Revision, Clinical Modification* (*ICD-10-CM*) diagnosis code for cerebral palsy will be reported in addition to the code for the UTI when the cerebral palsy influences MDM.

Data

Following are important guidelines for determining the amount and/or complexity of data to be reviewed and analyzed:

- The data counted toward the level of MDM are data that are analyzed (ie, used as part of the MDM) at the current encounter.
- Review of tests ordered by the same physician or QHP (or individuals covering for or of the same specialty and group practice) at a prior encounter are not counted toward the data analyzed at the current encounter.

Each unique test is counted once toward the amount and/or complexity of data. Do not count both the order for and the review of the same unique test.

When a test with multiple components can be reported with a single code (eg, basic metabolic panel, complete blood cell count [CBC] with differential, or a test with a specific number of images), count the test once for the purpose of data to be reviewed and analyzed.

- Any test for which the reporting individual or another individual of the same specialty and same group practice will separately report a code for interpretation and report is not counted toward the data analyzed at the encounter.

A test may contribute to both Category 1 (includes tests ordered) and Category 2 (independent interpretation of tests) of the amount and/or complexity of data to be reviewed and analyzed when a physician or QHP orders and performs independent interpretation of the test. When the physician or QHP separately reports interpretation and report, the service does not contribute to the amount and/or complexity of data to be reviewed and analyzed.

Examples

➤ **A cardiologist who provides subsequent hospital care to a patient also reports the interpretation and report of an electrocardiogram.**

Teaching Point: The cardiologist does not include the order for or review of the electrocardiogram in the amount and/or complexity of data to be reviewed and analyzed because the interpretation and report of test results are separately reported.

➤ **A physician independently views and documents an informal interpretation of an image or tracing for which a formal interpretation and report will be provided by a subspecialist.**

Teaching Point: The physician's independent interpretation, used in MDM of an E/M visit but not separately reported, is included in the amount and/or complexity of data to be reviewed and analyzed when determining a level of MDM.

Noncritical Hospital Evaluation and Management Services

Chapter 16

Risk

Determine the level of risk of management decisions made at each individual encounter. Following are a few key points regarding selection of the level of risk:

- The element of risk of MDM is the *risk of management* and not the risk of the problem itself. For example, a presenting problem may have a high complexity on the basis of high-risk differential diagnoses, but a management decision to further evaluate the patient's problem with an elective procedure that occurs without identified patient or procedure risks factors represents a moderate risk.
- Risk may be increased by a decision against a management option (testing, treatment, or escalation in the level of care) that was *considered but not selected.*
- The risk associated with a decision for surgery is not determined by the global period assigned to the procedure but, rather, by how trained clinicians would commonly classify the risks of the procedure, also considering the patient-specific risk factors. For example, an orthopedic heel-cord release would be a low-risk procedure, but that risk would be significantly increased if the patient had cerebral palsy with respiratory and neurological disease.
- A decision regarding escalation of the level of service (eg, a decision to transfer to intensive or critical care) indicates a higher level of risk in the patient's management.

For examples of code selection for initial, subsequent, and same-date hospital or observation admission and discharge services based on elements of MDM, refer to the Level of Service Selection section later in this chapter.

Time-Based Code Selection

The time used for code selection is the physician's and/or QHP's total time directed to the individual patient's care on the date of the encounter. Refer to **Chapter 6** for full discussion of activities that may contribute to the total time.

Inpatient hospital or observation care code descriptors include a *minimum amount of time that must be met or exceeded* to report the code based on total time.

Following are some key points regarding total time of service:

- Total time is not limited to time spent on the unit/floor. Count all time in activities necessary for care of the individual patient, omitting time spent performing separately reported services.
- When time is used as the controlling factor in the selection of the code, *the total time spent on the date of the encounter must be documented in the medical record.*
- Continuous service time that crosses midnight is counted as a single service on a single date. When there is no continuous episode of care crossing midnight, separately report the services provided on each calendar date.

Do not count time spent on

- ✖ The performance of other services that are reported separately (eg, bedside procedure)
- ✖ Travel
- ✖ Teaching that is general for any patient admitted to the hospital and not specific to the management of the patient's problem(s) presently being addressed
- ✖ Time spent in activities normally performed by clinical staff (eg, assisting the patient to the bathroom or changing a diaper)

For examples of code selection for initial, subsequent, and same-date hospital or observation admission and discharge services based on total time, refer to the Level of Service Selection section later in this chapter, which further expands on time-based code selection.

Table 16-2 provides guidance for selecting a code according to the level of MDM supported by 2 of 3 elements of MDM or according to total time on the date of the encounter. This table is useful when reviewing examples of services provided in discussions of each category of hospital inpatient or observation E/M service.

For ease of reference, a printable version of Table 16-2 is included at www.aap.org/cfp2026.

Hospital or Observation Services by Multiple Physicians and QHPs

Concurrent Care

Concurrent care is defined by *CPT* as the provision of similar services to the same patient by more than one physician on the same day. Concurrent care may be provided by physicians from different practices or physicians from the same practice but different specialties. When concurrent care is provided, the diagnosis code(s) reported by each physician should reflect the medical necessity for the provision of services by more than one physician on the same DOS. Although it is easier to justify concurrent care when each treating physician reports different diagnoses, if the diagnosis codes reported by each physician are for the same condition, it does not prevent billing for the services.

Example

➤ **The attending physician requests that a consultant manage a patient's pulmonary care (eg, drainage of pleural effusion) while the attending physician provides ongoing treatment of complicated community-acquired pneumonia.**

Teaching Point: Both physicians report subsequent hospital care codes according to their individual total time or MDM and link the *CPT* codes to the appropriate diagnosis codes.

Refer to **Figure 1-1** for an example of linking diagnoses to procedure codes on a claim.

Reporting Services Split or Shared by a Physician and a QHP

In general, a split/shared E/M service is one in which a physician and a QHP from the same specialty and group practice, who could otherwise independently report an E/M service, each personally perform a medically necessary portion of one or more face-to-face E/M services on the same date. Split/shared billing may allow a physician to report the combined

Table 16-2. Hospital or Observation Evaluation and Management Services: Code Selection Requirements

Level/Codes/Total Time (min)[a]	Medical Decision-Making (2 of 3 Required: Data,[b,c] Problems, Risk)		
	Problem(s) Addressed	**Data Reviewed and Analyzed[b]**	**Risk**
Low *Same-date admission and discharge* **99234** (≥45) *Initial service* **99221** (≥40) *Subsequent service* **99231** (≥25) *Consultation* **99253** (≥45)	Low—*Any 1 of* • ≥2 self-limited or minor problems • 1 stable chronic illness • 1 acute, uncomplicated illness or injury • 1 stable acute illness • 1 acute, uncomplicated illness or injury requiring hospital inpatient or observation level of care	Limited (*Meet 1 of 2 categories*) Category 1: Tests and documents (*Any 2*) • Review of prior external note(s)—each unique source • Review of the result(s) of each unique test • Ordering of each unique test Category 2: Assessment requiring an independent historian(s)	Low *Examples* • Over-the-counter medication(s) • Removal of sutures • Physical, language, or occupational therapy
Moderate *Same-date admission and discharge* **99235** (≥70) *Initial service* **99222** (≥55) *Subsequent service* **99232** (≥35) *Consultation* **99254** (≥60)	Moderate—*Any 1 of* ≥1 chronic illness with exacerbation, progression, or side effects of treatment ≥2 stable chronic illnesses 1 undiagnosed new problem with uncertain prognosis 1 acute illness with systemic symptoms 1 acute, complicated injury	Moderate (*Meet 1 of 3 categories*) Category 1: Tests and documents (*Any 3*) • Review of prior external note(s)—each unique source • Review of the result(s) of each unique test • Ordering of each unique test • Assessment requiring an independent historian(s) Category 2: Independent interpretation of a test performed by another physician/other QHP[c] Category 3: Discussion of management or test interpretation with external physician/other QHP/appropriate source	Moderate *Examples* • Prescription drug management or off-label use of over-the-counter medication • Decision about minor surgery with identified patient or procedure risk factors • Decision about elective major surgery without identified patient or procedure risk factors • Diagnosis or treatment significantly limited by SDoH
High *Same-date admission and discharge* **99236** (≥85) *Initial service* **99223** (≥75) *Subsequent service* **99233** (≥50) *Consultation* **99255** (≥80)	High—*Any 1 of* ≥1 chronic illness with severe exacerbation, progression, or side effects of treatment 1 acute or chronic illness or injury that poses a threat to life or bodily function	Extensive (*Meet 2 of 3 categories listed in the previous row*)	High *Examples* • Drug therapy requiring intensive monitoring for toxicity • Decision about hospitalization or escalation of hospital level of care • Decision about elective major surgery with identified patient or procedure risk factors • Decision about emergency major surgery • Decision not to resuscitate or to de-escalate care because prognosis is poor • Decision regarding parenteral controlled substances

Abbreviations: QHP, qualified health care professional; SDoH, social determinants of health.

[a] Include only time personally spent by physicians and QHPs of the same specialty and same group practice directed to the individual patient's care on the date of the encounter.

[b] Each unique test, order, or document contributes to the combination of 2 or combination of 3 in Category 1.

[c] Do not count data review or communications reported with other codes (eg, test interpretation, interprofessional consultation).

work and receive payment at a higher fee schedule rate than would be paid if reported by the QHP. (Some health plans pay <100% of the plan's physician fee schedule [eg, 85%] for services reported by QHPs.)

Split/shared billing policy may not apply when a payer does not allow direct billing by a QHP. In this event, follow the payer's policy for reporting (eg, always bill for the combined work under the physician's NPI).

Current Procedural Terminology Guidelines for Split/Shared Services

CPT defines a "shared or split visit" as a visit in which a physician and QHP(s) jointly provide the face-to-face and non–face-to-face work related to a visit.

- Each individual should independently document their work (eg, history, examination, and MDM) and/or time spent on the date of the encounter.
- A physician cannot merely sign off on the documentation of the work by the QHP.
- Shared services are generally not permitted if the QHP is a hospital employee. (Exceptions may apply under value-based care payment arrangements.)

The *CPT* guidelines for split/shared services address use of time for code selection as follows:

- When time is used to select the appropriate level of hospital or observation service, the time personally spent by the physician and QHP(s) assessing and treating the patient and/or counseling, educating, or communicating results to the patient or family/caregiver on the date of the encounter is summed to define total time.
- When 2 or more individuals of the same specialty and same group practice jointly meet with or discuss the patient, only the time of 1 individual should be counted.
- The combined documentation must support the total time of the combined service when selecting a code on the basis of time.

When physicians and QHPs work together to provide care that is reported with a single E/M code, the service is reported by the professional who performed the substantive portion of the service. The substantive portion of the service is defined in either of the following ways:

- When code selection is based on time, the professional who spent the most time on that date in activities of an E/M service to the individual patient will report the service.
- When code selection for a split/shared visit is based on MDM, the professional who performed 2 of 3 elements of MDM has performed the substantive portion and reports the E/M service.
  - When the number and complexity of problems addressed at the encounter are one of the elements supporting the level of MDM, the professional who made or approved the management plan for the problem(s) addressed and who accepts the inherent risks of the management plan has performed the substantive portion of the service.
  - When the amount and/or complexity of data to be reviewed and analyzed is one of the elements on which the level of MDM is determined, the following guidance applies:
    - Consider an assessment of the documented history from an independent historian and documented tests ordered or results/documents reviewed to have been considered by the professional in formulating the management plan. The professional reporting the service does not have to personally perform these activities.
    - An independent interpretation of a test or discussion of management with an external physician is used in selecting the amount and/or complexity of data to be reviewed and analyzed only *when personally performed by the individual reporting the service.*

Medicare Guidelines for Split/Shared Services

Under Medicare policy, a split/shared service must be reported with modifier **FS** (split or shared E/M visit) appended to the code reported for the split/shared encounter.

Payers other than Medicare may require use of modifier FS to identify that a service was provided as a split/shared service. Practices should review payer policies to determine when this modifier is required.

- Per Medicare instructions, documentation must include
  - The identity of the physician and the QHP who perform the visit
  - Who performed the substantive portion of the visit
- The reporting physician or QHP must authenticate/sign the documentation of the service per Medicare policy.

Medicare policy states that at least 1 of the individuals providing a split/shared service must have face-to-face (in-person) contact with the patient, but this individual does not necessarily have to be the physician, or the individual who performs the substantive portion and bills for the visit. The substantive portion can be entirely with or without direct patient contact, and it is determined by the proportion of total time, not whether the time involves patient contact.

Examples

➤ **A physician orders admission of a patient at 8:00 am after reviewing the patient's medical record via remote access.** At 8:30 am, a nurse practitioner (NP) in the physician's group practice and exact same specialty provides an initial E/M service and documents 40 minutes of service. Later that day, the physician reassesses the patient and documents the visit, including references to the NP's note and that the combined total time of service on this date is 90 minutes (40 minutes by the NP and 50 minutes by the physician). The codes selected for the split/shared service are **99223 FS** (first 75 minutes) and **99418 FS** (1 unit of prolonged service for the final 15 minutes of service).

Teaching Point: Because both health care professionals are from the same group practice and have documented and signed off on their individually provided services, the split/shared guidelines apply. Because the physician spent the majority of the total time of service, the service is billed by the physician. Some payers may not require modifier **FS** to be appended to the reported codes. Refer to the Prolonged Hospital E/M Services section later in this chapter for more information on **99418**.

➤ **A physician associate (PA) provides a subsequent hospital visit to an uncircumcised 8-month-old patient admitted the prior afternoon for management of acute gastroenteritis with dehydration after a failed oral challenge.** The patient is reevaluated by the PA, who is concerned about possible UTI and sepsis on the basis of history from the patient's parents and examination findings. The PA orders urinalysis obtained by catheterization, basic metabolic panel, and blood and urine cultures. Later the same day, the attending physician reviews records of the patient's stay, including results of the urinalysis and basic metabolic panel. A working diagnosis of acute pyelonephritis with suspected acute kidney injury and a concern regarding congenital urinary tract abnormality are documented. Antibiotics are started, intravenous (IV) fluids are managed to avoid the risk of hyperkalemia, and renal bladder ultrasonography and a urology consultation are ordered. Still later on the same date, the urologist and the attending physician discuss renal bladder ultrasonography findings and plan urinary catheterization to relieve obstruction and, after the patient's fever resolves, a voiding cystourethrogram. The combined total time of service is not documented.

Teaching Point: Code selection based on total time is not an option because of lack of documentation. However, the elements of MDM that the physician may include are

Problem(s) addressed ➡ ***High*** (an acute illness that poses a threat to life or bodily function)

Data reviewed and/or analyzed ➡ ***Extensive*** (Category 1—review/order of multiple tests and independent historian, Category 3—discussion of management with physician of another specialty)

Risk of patient management ➡ ***Moderate*** (prescription drug management)

The MDM is high given the problem addressed and data reviewed and analyzed. The physician reports subsequent hospital inpatient or observation care with high-level MDM (**99233 FS**). Had the discussion of management with the urologist been performed by the PA, the higher level of MDM would have been attributed to the PA and the service would have been reported under the PA's name and NPI.

Reporting Hospital Inpatient or Observation Care

Selecting the Appropriate Code Categories

This section provides an overview of each category of hospital inpatient or observation E/M service. Code(s) reported by the physician or QHP, and same specialty/same group practice team who ordered the patient's admission, are based on the length of the patient's stay. Additional details for reporting codes in these categories are discussed later in this section. **Table 16-3** provides guidance for code selection based on duration of the patient's hospital stay.

Table 16-3. Hospital Inpatient and Observation Code Categories by Length of Stay	
This guidance does not apply to services provided to normal newborns admitted and discharged on the same date (99463).	
Stay of less than 8 hours	Report only an initial hospital care code (99221–99223) This applies whether the patient is discharged on the date of admission or the next day.
Stay of 8 hours or more with discharge on the same date	Report only a same-date admission and discharge service code (99234–99236) An additional requirement for 2 distinct visits by the attending physician or QHP applies.
Stay of 8 hours or more with discharge on a subsequent date	Report both initial hospital care (99221–99223) and discharge day management services (99238, 99239).

Level of Service Selection

Total time and MDM reporting criteria and examples of each level of service are included in discussion of each category of hospital services. Following are key points to remember in code selection:

- Examples given are not clinical recommendations, and levels of service supported may vary depending on documentation and patient age and presentation (eg, ill appearance beyond what is typical for concern).
- Select a code based on either total physician/QHP time on the DOS or MDM.
- Report an initial service when the patient has not received any professional services from the physician or QHP (or another physician or QHP of the exact same specialty and subspecialty who belongs to the same group practice) during the current hospital or observation stay.

Same-Date Admission and Discharge Services

99234 Hospital inpatient or observation care, for the E/M of a patient including admission and discharge on the same date, which requires a medically appropriate history and/or examination and straightforward or low level of medical decision making.

When using total time on the date of the encounter for code selection, 45 minutes must be met or exceeded.

99235 Hospital inpatient or observation care, for the E/M of a patient including admission and discharge on the same date, which requires a medically appropriate history and/or examination and moderate level of medical decision making.

When using total time on the date of the encounter for code selection, 70 minutes must be met or exceeded.

99236 Hospital inpatient or observation care, for the E/M of a patient including admission and discharge on the same date, which requires a medically appropriate history and/or examination and high level of medical decision making.

When using total time on the date of the encounter for code selection, 85 minutes must be met or exceeded.

(For services ≥100 minutes, refer to discussion of prolonged service add-on code (AOC) 99418 in the Prolonged Service on the Date of an E/M Service section later in this chapter.)

Prolonged service may be reported only in addition to the highest-level code in the category of E/M service (eg, 99418 is reported in addition to 99236 but not 99234 and 99235) and only when code selection is based on total time.

Codes 99234–99236 are reported when a physician or QHP provides a hospital inpatient or observation admission service during *a stay lasting 8 hours or more* and, *after reevaluation later on the same date,* provides discharge management services.

- Only the physician or QHP team (ie, members of the same specialty and same group practice) who ordered the admission and provided the discharge service on the same date report 99234–99236.
- Two or more encounters are required *on the same calendar date.* Report 99234–99236 only when one encounter consists of an initial admission service and another consists of a discharge management.
- For a patient admitted and discharged at a single face-to-face encounter, report only initial hospital inpatient or observation service codes 99221–99223.

- ✖ Do not report discharge management codes 99238 and 99239 in conjunction with 99234–99236 or in conjunction with 99221–99223 for admission and discharge services performed on the same calendar date.

Report 99463 for admission and discharge services provided to normal newborns on the same calendar date.

- When a patient receives hospital inpatient or observation care for less than 8 hours, report only an initial hospital inpatient or observation care code (99221–99223) on the date of admission. Do not report a separate code for hospital discharge (99238, 99239) for services during this admission.
- ✖ Do not report 99234–99236 when a patient was admitted to hospital inpatient or observation care and discharged on a different date. Instead, report either
  - Initial hospital care (99221–99223) for services during a stay of less than 8 hours
  - Initial hospital care (99221–99223) and hospital discharge day management (99238, 99239) for services during a stay of 8 hours or more

  Code selection is based on *either MDM or total time* on the date of the encounter.
- Include the combined MDM or total time provided by the same physician or physicians of the same specialty and same group practice provided on a single DOS.
- Except where payer guidance specifies otherwise, reporting of initial observation or inpatient care is based on the date of the face-to-face assessment and not the date of admission or designation of a status by a facility (eg, when changed on physician order).

  Use **Tables 16-2** and **16-4** to assign codes for the services based on MDM or total time on the date of the encounter.

For ease of reference, a printable version of Table 16-2 is included at www.aap.org/cfp2026.

Table 16-4. Codes for Admission and Discharge on the Same Date

Medical Decision-Making	Straightforward or Low	Moderate	High
Code/Total Time (min)	99234 ≥45	99235 ≥70	99236 ≥85

Examples

➤ **A 14-year-old patient with an acute exacerbation of asthma is admitted to an observation stay.** The attending physician performs the initial history and physical examination at 1:00 am and orders IV fluids, inhalation treatments every 4 hours, and continued close monitoring. Another physician from the attending physician's same specialty and group practice returns to the hospital at 12:00 pm and stops the IV fluids. At 5:00 pm that same day, after further evaluation of the child by the same physician, the patient is discharged home with new prescriptions for asthma control and emergency use medications.

ICD-10-CM	*CPT*
J45.41 (moderate persistent asthma with exacerbation)	99235 (initial inpatient E/M service with moderate MDM)

Problem(s) addressed ➡ *Moderate* (an exacerbated chronic condition)
Data reviewed and/or analyzed ➡ *Minimal or none*
Risk of patient management ➡ *Moderate* (prescription drug management)

Teaching Point: Because the physicians of the same specialty and same group practice provided inpatient admission and discharge services on the same date, 99235 is reported by one of the physicians. Determination of who reports the service may be based on the attending physician of record or practice policy. If the service were split/shared by a physician and QHP, the service would be reported by the individual who provided the substantial part of the MDM on which code selection was based.

Noncritical Hospital Evaluation and Management Services

Chapter 16

➤ **A 5-year-old patient is evaluated in the ED for admission to observation for treatment of diarrhea with moderate dehydration. At 5:00 am, a hospitalist provides the initial observation encounter in the ED and documents the admission order with the date and time.** The hospitalist orders include a time-based oral rehydration plan using an electrolyte solution. The patient is reevaluated by the hospitalist at 7:00 am and again at 10:00 am and determined to be sufficiently recovered for discharge home at the 10:00 am encounter. The hospitalist orders the discharge and documents all the services, including 50 minutes of total time spent directed to care of the patient. Diagnosis is viral gastroenteritis with moderate dehydration.

ICD-10-CM	*CPT*
A08.4 (viral intestinal infection, unspecified) E86.0 (dehydration)	99222 (moderate MDM) is reported for the 5-hour stay. The viral gastroenteritis with moderate dehydration and a decision for observation support moderate MDM.

Teaching Point: Although the service provided otherwise supports same-date admission and discharge (ie, the patient was evaluated at >1 encounter, and both an admission and a discharge management service were provided on the same date), the patient's stay did not meet the 8-hour minimum required for reporting 99234–99236.

The physician's total time on the DOS is 50 minutes, supporting 99221, but the physician selects the code on the basis of the most favorable method, total time, or MDM. Here, moderate MDM supports 99222.

When Payers Use Medicare Policy for Observation Services

Medicaid and private payers may adopt a Medicare policy requiring a medical observation record for the patient that contains dated and timed physician's orders for the inpatient or observation services the patient is to receive, nursing notes, and progress notes prepared by the admitting physician or QHP indicating physical presence and personal performance of services. This record must be in addition to (and not a copy-and-paste of) any record prepared as a result of an ED or outpatient clinic encounter before the admission.

Initial Inpatient Hospital Care

99221 Initial hospital inpatient or observation care, per day, for the E/M of a patient, which requires a medically appropriate history and/or examination and straightforward or low level medical decision making.

When using total time on the date of the encounter for code selection, 40 minutes must be met or exceeded.

99222 Initial hospital inpatient or observation care, per day, for the E/M of a patient, which requires a medically appropriate history and/or examination and moderate level of medical decision making.

When using total time on the date of the encounter for code selection, 55 minutes must be met or exceeded.

99223 Initial hospital inpatient or observation care, per day, for the E/M of a patient, which requires a medically appropriate history and/or examination and high level of medical decision making.

When using total time on the date of the encounter for code selection, 75 minutes must be met or exceeded.

(For services ≥90 minutes, refer to discussion of prolonged service AOC 99418 in the Prolonged Service on the Date of an E/M Service section later in this chapter.)

- Initial hospital inpatient or observation service codes are used to report initial face-to-face services provided to a patient admitted as a hospital inpatient or in observation status.
- Initial hospital encounters may be reported by more than one physician. For discussion of consultations in hospital inpatient or observation settings, refer to the Consultation Guidelines section later in this chapter.
- The code is reported on the first day that a face-to-face (physician-patient) service is provided and for the combined admission and discharge services provided during any inpatient or observation stay of less than 8 hours.
- The date of initial hospital inpatient or observation care that the physician reports does not need to correlate with the facility's date of admission.
- Only 1 initial hospital inpatient or observation care code is reported per physician or QHP team per stay. A transition from observation to inpatient does not constitute a new stay.

Use **Tables 16-2** and **16-5** to review the requirements used to select level of service in the examples that follow.

Table 16-5. Codes for Initial Hospital Inpatient or Observation Services			
Medical Decision-Making	**Straightforward or Low**	**Moderate**	**High**
Code/Total Time (min)	99221 ≥40	99222 ≥55	99223 ≥75

Examples

➤ **A 60-day-old girl is admitted from the ED to Dr Admit's service.** The patient's mother reported that the infant seemed warm to the touch and irritable, breastfed much less than normal, and had fewer wet diapers and 1 normal stool in the past 24 hours.

Laboratory evaluation: Complete blood cell count with white blood cells at 12,000/mcL, no left shift on differential count, and normal absolute neutrophil count. Urinalysis results normal or negative with a pH of 7.0 and a specific gravity of 1.020. Urine and blood culture results pending. C-reactive protein level normal (<3.1). Comprehensive metabolic panel findings normal except for a carbon dioxide level of 16 mEq/L. COVID-19 test result negative.

Assessment: 8-week-old with fever, mild dehydration, and acute metabolic acidosis. Because of the patient's age and continued symptoms, there is concern regarding sepsis or undetected bacterial infection. Pyelonephritis is doubtful given the normal urinalysis results, meningitis is less likely given the mild clinical findings, and bronchiolitis is doubtful given the lack of viral symptoms.

Plan: Admit the patient for IV antibiotics and IV fluids. Closely observe her for sepsis and pyelonephritis, but note that the examination findings, CBC, urinalysis results, and C-reactive protein level were normal. Follow blood and urine cultures. Breastfeeding can continue ad lib.

Dr Admit discusses the current diagnostic and treatment plans with the parents and explains that a QHP from the same group practice will visit later today to reevaluate the patient and plan for any needed overnight changes in management or for home discharge. Dr Admit's total time is 45 minutes.

ICD-10-CM	*CPT*
E86.0 (dehydration) E87.21 (acute metabolic acidosis) R50.9 (fever, unspecified)	99222 (moderate MDM)

Problem(s) addressed ➡ ***Moderate*** (undiagnosed new problem with uncertain prognosis)
Data reviewed and/or analyzed ➡ ***Moderate*** (Category 1—3 tests reviewed and independent historian)
Risk of patient management ➡ ***Moderate*** (prescription drug management) ***or High*** (if Dr Admit made the decision for hospitalization)

Teaching Point: Moderate MDM and 99222 are supported by all 3 elements of MDM.

➤ **Later that same calendar day, a QHP of the same specialty and same group practice reexamines the infant.** The QHP spends 35 minutes in care of the patient, including time reviewing records, examination of the infant (who shows signs of improvement), discussion with the parents and clinical staff, and documenting the service.

Plan: Reevaluate tomorrow; continue IV antibiotics pending result of cultures.

The total time of service for the 2 separate encounters is 70 minutes (45 + 35 = 80).

ICD-10-CM	*CPT*
E86.0 (dehydration) E87.21 (acute metabolic acidosis) R50.9 (fever, unspecified)	99223 (high MDM or ≥75 minutes). Modifier FS (split/shared service) is appended if required by the payer.

Teaching Point: The hospital E/M services provided on this date include the total time spent by the 2 individuals of the same specialty and same group practice. Dr Admit, who spent most of the total time of service and ordered the tests reviewed by the QHP, submits the bill for the calendar day's service. In this scenario, both the physician's total time and their level of MDM were higher than those of the QHP, as the problem was improving at the time of the QHP's visit, review of test results was included in the order by a physician of the same group and specialty, and the risk of management is unchanged.

● indicates a new code; ▲, revised; #, re-sequenced; ✚, add-on; ★, audiovisual technology; and ◀, synchronous interactive audio.

Modifier FS is reported, when required by a payer, to indicate that the visit was split/shared by the physician and/or QHP.

Tests are counted toward the level of data for the encounter at which the tests are ordered because review of results is included in the order. However, when a physician or QHP reviews results of tests ordered by a physician or QHP of another specialty or other group practice, the review is counted toward the amount and/or complexity of data for that visit.

➤ **A 14-year-old patient is admitted to inpatient status from the ED at 8:00 pm on Tuesday with an acute asthma exacerbation requiring IV methylprednisolone in addition to inhalation treatments.** The admitting physician's documentation includes notes of a discussion with an ED physician and decision for admission to the general pediatric unit rather than the intensive care unit. She reviews the results of 3 unique tests (eg, basic metabolic panel, CBC, spirometry, and/or blood gas analysis). The admitting diagnosis is acute asthma exacerbation, stable when the patient is receiving albuterol inhalation treatments and IV methylprednisolone. *Plan:* Continue albuterol inhalation therapy and IV methylprednisolone. Monitor peak expiratory flow rate, serum electrolyte levels, and glucose level overnight. Will reevaluate tomorrow morning or sooner, as indicated.

ICD-10-CM	*CPT*
J45.41 (moderate persistent asthma with acute exacerbation)	99223 (initial inpatient E/M service with high MDM)

Problem(s) addressed ➡ ***High*** (severe exacerbation of a chronic condition)

Data reviewed and/or analyzed ➡ ***Extensive*** (2 of 3 categories of data: Category 1—order or review of ≥3 tests, Category 3—discussion of management with an external physician [physician of another specialty])

Risk of patient management ➡ ***High*** (decision to admit to a unit/floor)

Teaching Point: The high-level MDM in this example is supported by all 3 elements of MDM. If the conversation between the admitting and ED physicians were limited to arranging transfer of the patient's care and not about determining the patient's admission status, the discussion would not be a discussion of management for purposes of determining the amount and/or complexity of data in MDM.

Subsequent Hospital Care

★99231 Subsequent hospital inpatient or observation care, per day, for the E/M of a patient, which requires a medically appropriate history and/or examination and straightforward or low level of medical decision making.

When using total time on the date of the encounter for code selection, 25 minutes must be met or exceeded.

★99232 Subsequent hospital inpatient or observation care, per day, for the E/M of a patient, which requires a medically appropriate history and/or examination and moderate level of medical decision making.

When using total time on the date of the encounter for code selection, 35 minutes must be met or exceeded.

★99233 Subsequent hospital inpatient or observation care, per day, for the E/M of a patient, which requires a medically appropriate history and/or examination and high level of medical decision making.

When using total time on the date of the encounter for code selection, 50 minutes must be met or exceeded.

(For services ≥65 minutes, refer to discussion of prolonged service AOC 99418 in the Prolonged Service on the Date of an E/M Service section later in this chapter.)

- Codes include all E/M services by a physician or QHP of the same specialty and same group practice provided on a subsequent day of inpatient or observation service. The level of service reported will depend on the total services provided and documented.
- Codes 99231–99233 are also reported by consulting physicians when reporting an inpatient or observation consultation code is inappropriate (eg, when an outpatient consultation was provided before admission on the same date). For additional discussion of consultations, refer to the Consultation Guidelines section later in this chapter.
- Selection of the code is based on either MDM or total time on the date of the encounter.

Use **Tables 16-2** and **16-6** to help select the appropriate codes in the examples that follow.

Table 16-6. Codes for Subsequent Hospital Inpatient or Observation Services

Medical Decision-Making	Straightforward or Low	Moderate	High
Code/Total Time (min)	99231 ≥25	99232 ≥35	99233 ≥50

Examples

➤ **A physician reevaluates an 8-week-old who has fever, dehydration, and lethargy and received initial hospital care from a physician of the same specialty and same group practice on the prior day.** *Progress note:* "No new reported problems overnight; breastfeeding has improved, but patient continues to have low-grade fever (38.2 °C [100.8 °F] maximum temperature) overnight; no reported apnea or cyanosis; no respiratory distress. Feeding better, more wet diapers, more alert, less irritable, and more active."

Laboratory: No growth in blood or urine cultures at less than 24 hours. Glucose level normal. Radiograph appearance normal.

Assessment/plan: Continued fever and continued concern for sepsis. A viral etiology is suspected given the negative workup so far for common serious bacterial infections such as pyelonephritis, pneumonia, and bacteremia. Continue IV antibiotics until culture results are negative for 48 hours. Breastfeeding can be continued ad lib.

The physician speaks with the mother and reviews overnight events, morning laboratory results, the current plan, and possible discharge home tomorrow.

Problem(s) addressed ➡ ***Moderate*** (undiagnosed with uncertain prognosis)

Data reviewed and/or analyzed ➡ ***Limited*** (if tests were ordered by the physician of the same specialty and same group practice) ***or Moderate*** (if the 3 unique test results reviewed were ordered by a physician of another group practice or other specialty)

Risk of patient management ➡ ***Moderate*** (managing IV antibiotics)

ICD-10-CM	*CPT*
R50.9 (fever, unspecified)	99232 (moderate MDM, ≥35 minutes)

Teaching Point: This visit is a subsequent visit without discharge management on this date.

In this example, the MDM is moderate (3 of 3 elements may support moderate, although only 2 of 3 are required). Time cannot be used as the controlling factor in code selection because the documentation does not indicate the total time spent on the date of the encounter. If another physician or QHP of the same care team provided care to the patient on this same date, the level of MDM of the combined services would be used in code selection unless the later visit included documentation of time to support a higher level of service.

➤ **A physician reevaluates a 14-year-old who was seen in consultation late on the prior evening following admission to observation for a first-time tonic-clonic seizure.** The physician obtains additional history from the patient and parents, completes a focused examination, reviews new laboratory test results, and explains a suspected diagnosis of juvenile myoclonic epilepsy based on the patient's description of muscle jerks occurring in the morning. Additional testing is planned for early the next morning. Anticonvulsant therapy is held as the workup is undertaken. The physician's total time devoted to the patient's care on this date is 45 minutes.

ICD-10-CM	*CPT*
R56.9 (unspecified convulsions)	99232 (≥35 minutes)

Teaching Point: The physician's total time supports 99232. Fifty minutes or more is required to report 99233 according to total time.

Hospital Inpatient or Observation Discharge Management

99238 Hospital inpatient or observation discharge day management; 30 minutes or less on the date of the encounter

99239 more than 30 minutes on the date of the encounter

As discussed in the Selecting the Appropriate Code Categories section earlier in this chapter, when a patient's stay lasts less than 8 hours, report only initial hospital or observation care (99221–99223) for the E/M services provided during the admission.

Codes 99238 (≤30 minutes) and 99239 (>30 minutes) are reported for discharge management services by the physician or QHP who is responsible for discharge services (the attending physician). Services by other physicians or QHPs who may have interacted with the patient/family and who provided additional instructions to the patient/family and coordinated post-discharge services may be reported with subsequent care codes 99231–99233.

Although discharge day management may be provided as a split/shared service (combining separate times spent on the date of discharge management), do not include any time spent by a QHP who is not in the same group practice (eg, hospital-employed NP working as part of a discharge management team).

Discharge management codes are reported for services on a date subsequent to the date of admission and only when the patient's inpatient or observation stay lasted a minimum of 8 hours.

- Same-date admission and discharge services for a patient stay of 8 hours or more, performed at 2 distinct encounters, are reported with 99234–99236.
- For admission and discharge services provided during a stay of less than 8 hours, report only 99221–99223.

Reporting is based on the total time (does not have to be continuous) spent performing all final discharge services, including, *as appropriate,* examination of the patient, discussion of the hospital stay, patient and/or family counseling, instructions for continuing care to all relevant caregivers, and preparation of referral forms, prescriptions, and medical records.

If the total time spent performing discharge management is not documented in the medical record, 99239 is not supported.

- Although time is the total time spent in discharge management on the date of the encounter (eg, time of documentation), a face-to-face physician-patient encounter in the hospital is required.
- Only the physician's total time spent on the date of the discharge management is reported with 99238 and 99239. Do not include time spent documenting discharge on a date after the service was rendered.
- Time spent on the day of discharge performing separately reported services (eg, newborn circumcision) is not included in the discharge management time.
- Report discharge management services 99238 or 99239 provided to patients who die during their hospital stay *when the service is provided on the date of death.* An exception is a neonate who dies on the date of birth; report only the appropriate level of hospital care (ie, initial hospital care, intensive care, or critical care) in this instance.
- The date of discharge management may or may not coincide with the date that the patient leaves the facility. It is the work of the discharge management service that defines the service. If the physician provides a face-to-face service on the day after discharge management is provided (eg, brief visit to verify the patient is still ready for discharge), it is reported with a code for subsequent hospital care (99231–99233).

Discharge codes are not reported

- ✖ For completion of a death certificate without a face-to-face visit or for completion of records *on a date after the date of death.*
- ✖ When a patient is transferred to another physician or another unit in the same facility or for transitions between observation and inpatient status.
- ✖ When a patient is transferred to another hospital and receives care from the same physician or a physician of the same group and specialty. Report subsequent hospital care in lieu of discharge management (and initial hospital care).
- ✖ When the duration of the patient's hospital stay is less than 8 hours.
- ✖ When reporting 99234–99236 for same-date admission/discharge.

Examples

➤ **An attending physician provides a final inpatient visit to a child who is ready for discharge home.** The physician documents 30 minutes' total time, including time spent with the patient and parents reviewing the hospital stay, providing instructions for follow-up care, and entering discharge orders.

Noncritical Hospital Evaluation and Management Services

Chapter 16

Teaching Point: The total time of the discharge management service supports 99238. Code 99239 is reported only for more than 30 minutes on the date of discharge day management services.

➤ **An attending physician visits a child who was admitted for an exacerbation of asthma.** The patient had gone 2 weeks without control medication owing to parental inability to pay the out-of-pocket costs for the medication. The patient's asthma control plan and instructions for follow-up in the asthma and allergy clinic are reviewed. Prior to discharging the patient, the physician verifies that the child's parents are now enrolled in a prescription discount program that will reduce out-of-pocket costs. The total time on the date of the encounter is 40 minutes.

Teaching Point: The total time of the discharge management service supports 99239.

Reporting *ICD-10-CM* codes for the social determinants of health that affected patient management (eg, Z59.868, other specified financial insecurity; Z59.71, insufficient health insurance coverage) can help demonstrate the complexity of the service (ie, reason for time spent) and alert a payer that a patient may require care coordination and other benefits as available under health plan policy. Also, the Medicare program recognizes homelessness (Z59.00–Z59.02) as a complication or comorbidity that may affect hospital payment.

➤ **An attending physician is notified by phone of the death of a patient who was an inpatient.** The physician comes into the facility the next morning and completes documentation.

Teaching Point: Discharge management services (99238, 99239) are not reported when no face-to-face encounter (eg, pronouncement of death or hospital discussion with family) is provided by the attending physician. Most health plans do not pay for services provided after the date of the patient's death (ie, the date that the patient's coverage ended).

Inpatient or Observation Consultations

Consultation Guidelines

CPT defines consultations as *initial encounters* provided by a physician or QHP at the request of another physician, QHP, or appropriate source (eg, nonclinical social worker, educator, lawyer, insurance company) to recommend care for a specific condition or problem. Codes 99252–99255 represent consultations provided to hospital inpatients, observation-level patients, nursing facility residents, or partial hospital setting patients.

Services requested by patients or by parents or other caregivers are not reported as consultations.

Consultation codes should not be reported by the physician who has agreed to accept transfer of care before an initial evaluation. Consultation codes are appropriate to report if the decision to accept transfer of care is not made until after the consultant's initial evaluation, regardless of site of service.

- When the role of attending physician is transferred to the consultant after the initial encounter, report subsequent hospital care codes (99231–99233) to indicate the level of service provided until the day of discharge management (99238, 99239).

Codes 99252–99255 are not reported when the patient has received any face-to-face professional services from the consultant or another physician or QHP of the exact same specialty and subspecialty who belongs to the same group practice during the stay.

In past guidance, a consultation code was reported when a physician with expertise in diagnosis and management of a specific problem was consulted by a physician of the same specialty and same group practice. Current *CPT* guidance, however, instructs to report subsequent hospital care in lieu of consultation codes as stated above.

Consultation Following a Related E/M Service

If a consultation is performed in anticipation of, or related to, an admission by another physician or QHP and then the same consultant performs an encounter after the patient is admitted, report the consultant's inpatient or observation encounter with the appropriate subsequent care code (99231–99233). Report subsequent hospital care even when the prior consultation was reported with an alternative to office or other outpatient consultation codes (eg, reported with office or other outpatient codes as required by a payer).

- Report subsequent care codes (99231–99233) for follow-up visits provided by the same physician or QHP (or individuals of the same group practice and same exact specialty). Examples of a follow-up visit might be to complete the initial consultation when test results become available or to respond to a change in the patient's status.

- When a consultant has provided an outpatient E/M service to a patient before performing an inpatient or observation consultation on the same date, the consultant reports the outpatient E/M service with modifier 25 appended (eg, 99245 25 for outpatient consultation) and a subsequent hospital inpatient or observation care code (99231–99233) for the second service on the same date.

Examples

➤ **A surgeon consulted with a pulmonologist, requesting clearance for surgery for a patient who has cystic fibrosis and may benefit from gastrostomy and enteral feeding.** The pulmonologist sees the patient in the office and recommends that the patient undergo the procedure as an inpatient with the pulmonologist's medical management. A few days later, the surgeon admits the patient and consults the pulmonologist for medical management.

Teaching Point: The pulmonologist reports the outpatient consultation (eg, 99244 or, if the payer does not allow payment for consultation codes, 99214) for the initial consultation and an applicable subsequent hospital inpatient or observation code (99231–99233) for the initial encounter in the hospital setting.

➤ **A pediatrician consulted a pulmonologist for advice on treating a patient who has cystic fibrosis and whose pulmonary function is worsening.** After evaluating the patient, the pulmonologist calls the pediatrician by phone and recommends hospital admission. The pediatrician, who does not provide hospital care, agrees with admission under the care of a hospitalist, who will consult the pulmonologist for pulmonary E/M. The pulmonologist provides an initial inpatient E/M service on the same date as the outpatient consultation.

Teaching Point: The pulmonologist reports the outpatient consultation (eg, 99244 25 or, if the payer does not accept a consultation code, 99214 25) and an applicable subsequent hospital inpatient or observation code (99231–99233) for the initial encounter in the hospital setting on the same DOS.

Medicare Consultation Guidelines

The Centers for Medicare & Medicaid Services policy for Medicare does not recognize consultation codes but pays for the services with codes for other E/M services. For detailed information on the *CPT* and Medicare guidelines for reporting consultations for office and outpatient consultations, refer to **Chapter 7**. Review those guidelines carefully as general guidelines that apply for all consultations.

Payers that adopt Medicare guidelines require that initial consultations provided to patients in observation or inpatient hospital status be reported with hospital inpatient or observation care codes (eg, 99221–99223). The admitting physician must report the initial hospital care services with modifier AI (principal physician of record) appended to the appropriate code to distinguish the services from the consulting physician's service. Subsequent face-to-face services, including new consultations within the same admission, are reported with subsequent inpatient or observation care codes 99231–99233 (refer to **Table 16-6**). Modifier AI is not required when reporting subsequent care codes.

Check with your commercial payers to learn if they follow Medicare consultation guidelines or have otherwise adopted consultation guidelines that differ from *CPT*.

Inpatient and Observation Consultations

99252 Inpatient or observation consultation for a new or established patient, which requires a medically appropriate history and/or examination and straightforward medical decision making.

When using total time on the date of the encounter for code selection, 35 minutes must be met or exceeded.

99253 Inpatient or observation consultation for a new or established patient, which requires a medically appropriate history and/or examination and low level of medical decision making.

When using total time on the date of the encounter for code selection, 45 minutes must be met or exceeded.

99254 Inpatient or observation consultation for a new or established patient, which requires a medically appropriate history and/or examination and moderate level of medical decision making.

When using total time on the date of the encounter for code selection, 60 minutes must be met or exceeded.

99255 Inpatient or observation consultation for a new or established patient, which requires a medically appropriate history and/or examination and high level of medical decision making.

When using total time on the date of the encounter for code selection, 80 minutes must be met or exceeded.

(For services ≥95 minutes, refer to discussion of prolonged services AOC 99418 in the Prolonged Service on the Date of an E/M Service section later in this chapter.)

Codes 99252–99255 are reported only for an initial encounter, as defined previously in this chapter, per hospital inpatient or observation admission. There are no specific guidelines for the length of stay.

- Procedures performed by the consultant will be separately reported, although the time spent performing the procedure is not added to the total time of the E/M service.

Use **Tables 16-2** and **16-7** to help select the appropriate codes in the example that follows.

Table 16-7. Codes for Hospital Inpatient or Observation Consultation Services

Medical Decision-Making	Straightforward	Low	Moderate	High
Code/Total Time (min)	99252 ≥35	99253 ≥45	99254 ≥60	99255 ≥80

Example

➤ **A 7-year-old was admitted to inpatient status from the ED by a hospitalist for left orbital cellulitis with a small subperiosteal abscess.** The hospitalist consults a pediatric ophthalmologist, regarding management (eg, IV antibiotics vs surgery). The pediatric ophthalmologist's consultation includes review of the patient's medical, family, and social history with the patient's parents, review of results of multiple laboratory tests ordered in the ED, independent review and interpretation of computed tomographic imaging of the sinuses and orbits, and a decision for continued IV antibiotics with close monitoring. The pediatric ophthalmologist's diagnosis is left orbital cellulitis with subperiosteal abscess without emergent visual compromise. The pediatric ophthalmologist will follow the patient with serial ophthalmic examinations.

ICD-10-CM	*CPT*
H05.012 (cellulitis of left orbit) H05.022 (osteomyelitis of left orbit)	99255 (inpatient or observation consultation with high-level MDM or ≥80 minutes)

Problem(s) addressed ➡ ***High*** (acute illness that poses a threat to bodily function)

Data reviewed and analyzed ➡ ***High*** (Category 1—review of ≥2 unique laboratory test results reviewed and independent historian; Category 2—independent interpretation of computed tomography)

Risk of patient management ➡ ***Moderate or high*** (decision regarding emergency surgery—minor or major)

Teaching Point: The pediatric ophthalmologist's service is a consultation based on the hospitalist's request to recommend care for the patient's specific problem. The total time is not included in this example. At least 2 elements of MDM support the high level. This supports 99255. If a decision for surgery had been made at this encounter, modifier 57 (decision for surgery) would be appended.

If the patient's health plan did not pay for services reported with consultation codes, the pediatric ophthalmologist would report initial hospital or observation care 99223 in accordance with the high MDM.

Interprofessional Telephone/Internet/Electronic Health Record Consultation

A consultation request by a patient's physician or QHP soliciting opinion and/or treatment advice by telephone, internet, or EHR from a physician with specialty expertise (consultant) is reported by the consultant with interprofessional consultation codes 99446–99451. No face-to-face contact between the patient and consultant is required. The patient may be in an inpatient or outpatient setting. Codes are selected according to the minutes of medical consultative discussion and review.

- When reporting 99446–99449 (consultation with verbal and written report), the consultant must spend at least 5 minutes, with more than 50% of the time reported as interprofessional consultation spent in medical consultative verbal or internet discussion rather than review of data (eg, medical records, test results).
- The service time for 99451 (consultation with written report only) is based on total review and interprofessional communication time.

Noncritical Hospital Evaluation and Management Services

Chapter 16

Code 99452 (interprofessional telephone/Internet/EHR referral service) may be reported *by a requesting physician or QHP* who spends 16 to 30 minutes preparing for and communicating with the consultant *on a date when no daily hospital E/M service is reported*. When the interprofessional consultation referral service takes place on the same date as an E/M service by the requesting physician or QHP, the referral service is included in either the MDM or total time of service on that date.

For full code descriptors and a detailed discussion of interprofessional consultation, refer to **Chapter 9**.

Prolonged Hospital E/M Services

Prolonged Service on the Date of an E/M Service

#★✚99418 Prolonged inpatient or observation E/M service(s) time with or without direct patient contact beyond the required time of the primary service when the primary service level has been selected using total time, each 15 minutes of total time

(List separately in addition to the code for the primary E/M service.)

Code 99418 is used to report prolonged total time provided by the physician or QHP on the date of an inpatient or observation service (or nursing facility service). Report 99418 only when

- The code for the primary E/M service was selected according to the physician's or QHP's total time on the date of the encounter.
- The total time exceeds the minimum total time of the highest level of service in the code category (ie, 99223, 99233, 99236, 99255, or nursing facility services 99306 and 99310) *by no less than 15 minutes.*
- Time spent performing other separately reported services (eg, procedures, interpretation and report of test results) is not included in the total time of the E/M service.

Table 16-8 provides time ranges for reporting 99418 in conjunction with each applicable code.

Table 16-8. Direct Prolonged Service Codes for Inpatient and Observation Care

Primary Service Code (min)	Time Range (min) = Codes × Unit(s)
99223 (≥75)	90–104 = 99223, 99418 × 1 105–119 = 99223, 99418 × 2
99233 (≥50)	65–79 = 99233, 99418 × 1 80–94 = 99233, 99418 × 2
99236 (≥85)	100–114 = 99236, 99418 × 1 115–129 = 99236, 99418 × 2
99255 (≥80)	95–109 = 99255, 99418 × 1 110–124 = 99255, 99418 × 2

Do not report 99418

- ✖ For any unit of less than 15 minutes beyond the required time of the primary E/M service or prior unit of prolonged service
- ✖ On the same DOS as psychotherapy services (eg, 90833, 90836, 90838)
- ✖ On the same date as prolonged service on a date when no E/M service is provided (99358, 99359)

Examples

➤ **A physician or QHP spends a total of 140 minutes reviewing extensive medical records and providing initial hospital care to a patient whose condition required multiple episodes of care throughout the day.**

Teaching Point: Codes 99223 (≥75) and 99418 × 4 units are reported. Each additional unit of 99418 is supported by at least 15 minutes beyond the prior unit.

➤ **A physician or QHP spends 40 minutes reviewing extensive medical records in addition to an initial inpatient E/M service reported on the same date.** The code for the initial inpatient E/M service (99223) was selected given the high MDM and is not supported by the physician's total time.

• indicates a new code; ▲, revised; #, re-sequenced; ✚, add-on; ★, audiovisual technology; and ◀, synchronous interactive audio.

Teaching Point: Code 99418 would not be reported. Prolonged service is not reported when the code for the related E/M service is not selected according to total time. Because a face-to-face E/M service was provided on this date, 99358 and 99359 are not reported.

Alternative Prolonged Service Code

The Centers for Medicare & Medicaid Services has implemented Healthcare Common Procedure Coding System code G0316 for reporting prolonged service in conjunction with inpatient and observation services reported with 99223, 99233, or 99236. Report G0316 when code selection is based on the total time of service and the total time meets or exceeds the time specified in payer policy. Use of G0316, in lieu of 99418, may be adopted by Medicaid plans or other payers. Refer to individual payer policy for reporting prolonged service to verify payable codes and time requirements.

Time requirements for G0316 as defined for the Medicare program are

99223 ≥90 minutes on date of visit
99233 ≥65 minutes on date of visit
99236 ≥110 minutes on date of visit and within 3 days after the visit

Refer to the April 2023 *AAP Pediatric Coding Newsletter*™ article "Prolonged Services: *CPT* Guidelines and Medicare/Medicaid Policy" (https://doi.org/10.1542/pcco_book228_document003) for more information on use of G0316 and other prolonged service Healthcare Common Procedure Coding System codes.

Prolonged Service on a Date Other Than the Face-to-Face E/M Service Without Direct Patient Contact

99358 Prolonged E/M service before and/or after direct patient care; first hour
+99359 each additional 30 minutes (Use 99359 in conjunction with 99358.)

Report 99358 and 99359 only when a prolonged service is *provided on a date other than the date of a face-to-face E/M encounter* with the patient and/or family/caregiver. Services are indirect but related to care of a single patient (eg, reviewing medical records, imaging, and/or developing and coordinating a patient management plan).

Codes 99358 and 99359

- Represent the total time spent by a physician or QHP (ie, not by clinical staff) on a single DOS.
- Must relate to a face-to-face professional service provided or planned to be provided by a physician or QHP and must be relevant to ongoing care.
- Are always provided and reported on a different date than the related E/M service. The related primary service may be any E/M service whether or not time was used to select the level of the face-to-face service.
- ✖ Are not reported for a physician's or QHP's time attributed to other services such as care plan oversight (99374–99380), chronic care management by a physician or QHP (99491, 99437), or principal care management by a physician or QHP (99424, 99425).

Prolonged service of less than 30 minutes' total duration on a given date is not separately reported. **Table 16-9** shows the required time for reporting 99358 (30–74 minutes) and 99359 (1 unit for each 30 minutes beyond the 1st hour and each additional 30 minutes). Code 99359 may be reported for the last 15 to 30 minutes of service beyond the prior reported unit of service.

✖ Do not add times of services *provided on different dates* to meet the time requirements for 99358 and 99359.

Table 16-9. Indirect Prolonged Service Codes and Time Units

Time of Service (min)	Code(s) × Unit(s)
<30	Not reported separately
30–74	99358 (always reported with 1 unit of service)
75–104	99358, 99359 × 1
≥105	99358, 99359 × ≥2 (have an additional unit added for each 15–30 min beyond the prior unit)

Noncritical Hospital Evaluation and Management Services

Chapter 16

• indicates a new code; ▲, revised; #, re-sequenced; +, add-on; ★, audiovisual technology; and ◀, synchronous interactive audio.

Examples

➤ **A consulting physician or QHP reviews extensive medical records received on the day after an initial inpatient consultation with the patient.** The physician or QHP uses the information to form opinion/recommendations that are provided to the requesting physician in a written report. Total time on this date is 45 minutes.

Teaching Point: Code 99358 would be reported on the date that 30 or more minutes were spent reviewing the medical records. Prolonged service of less than 30 minutes' total duration would not be separately reported. An inpatient consultation code (99252–99255) is reported on the date of the patient visit.

➤ **A consulting physician or QHP spends 40 minutes reviewing extensive medical records before an initial inpatient consultation provided later on the same date.**

Teaching Point: Code 99358 would not be reported. The time spent reviewing the medical records is included in the total time on the date of the encounter when selecting a code for the consultation service.

Hospital-Mandated On-Call Services

99026 Hospital mandated on-call service; in-hospital, each hour
99027 out of hospital, each hour

- Codes 99026 and 99027
- Describe services provided by a physician who is on call per hospital mandate (eg, hospital-required standby by a pediatrician during cesarean delivery) as a condition of medical staff privileges rather than a response to an individual patient's clinical indications.
- Are not covered by most payers because they consider this a contract issue between the hospital and physician. These codes may, however, be used for either tracking purposes or credit in larger groups by assigning the code a relative value unit when determining annual bonuses based on individual relative value unit production.
- Used to report on-call time spent by the physician when they are not providing other services.
- Time spent performing separately reportable services should not be included in time reported as mandated on-call services.

For attendance at delivery at the request of the delivering physician or QHP (and not per hospital mandate), refer to code 99464.

Continuing Care After Hospitalization

Preventing readmittance and/or ED visits following hospitalization is a key goal of many quality improvement programs. In recent years, *CPT* and payers have recognized a need for codes to capture services related to care coordination and management of chronic and episodic conditions that may lead to unnecessary emergency and inpatient care. For physicians continuing patient care after hospital discharge, services such as transitional care management, principal (ie, single serious disease) care management, or chronic (ie, multiple chronic illnesses) care management offer opportunities to provide and be compensated for care aimed at reducing the risk of decline, exacerbation, and/or functional decline.

Refer to **Chapter 9** for more information on care management services and other indirect services such as medical team conferences, care plan oversight, and advance care planning.

To test your knowledge of the information presented in this chapter, complete the quiz found at the end of it, after the resources. Answers to each quiz are found in **Appendix II**.

Chapter Takeaways

This chapter examined many aspects of code selection for services provided to patients in hospital inpatient or observation status.

- When time is used as the controlling factor in the selection of the code, the total time spent on the date of the encounter must be documented in the medical record. Continuous service time that crosses midnight is counted as a single service on a single date.
- *CPT* guidelines address who reports split/shared E/M services based on a substantive portion of either total time or MDM. Documentation should support the code(s) reported and provide details to support identification of the provider of the substantive portion of the service. Payers may require modifier **FS** (split or shared E/M service) to be appended to codes for split/shared services.
- **99234–99236** are reported only when 2 distinct encounters are provided for admission and discharge on the same DOS and only when the length of stay is no less than 8 hours. Report only initial hospital care for services provided during stays of less than 8 hours.
- **99252–99255** are reported only when the service qualifies as a consultation, is the initial encounter during the hospital stay, and does not relate to another E/M service by the same physician or QHP provided to the patient on the same or different date.
- A consultation request by a patient's physician or QHP soliciting opinion and/or treatment advice by telephone, internet, or EHR from a physician with specialty expertise (consultant) is reported by the consultant with interprofessional consultation codes **99446–99451**.
- Prolonged service in a facility setting is reported with **99418** when the required time of the associated E/M service, which was selected according to time, has been exceeded by at least 15 minutes.
- Prolonged service codes **99358** and **99359** are not reported on the same date as a face-to-face E/M service that may be reported according to the total time on the date of the encounter.
- *Pediatric Evaluation and Management: Coding Quick Reference Card 2026* (www.aap.org/Pediatric-Evaluation-and-Management-Coding-Quick-Reference-Card-2026) is an easy-to-use card that will help users navigate the steps to ensure proper code-level reporting for many E/M services (eg, it provides tables showing key component and time requirements for each type of code).

Resources

AAP Coding Assistance and Education

Pediatric Evaluation and Management: Coding Quick Reference Card 2026 (www.aap.org/Pediatric-Evaluation-and-Management-Coding-Quick-Reference-Card-2026)

Pediatric Evaluation and Management Coding Revisions: Facility and Office Services (www.aap.org/pediatric-evaluation-and-management-coding-revisions-facility-and-office-services-paperback)

AAP Pediatric Coding Newsletter

"Coding Challenge: Hospital Evaluation and Management Services," March 2024 (https://doi.org/10.1542/pcco_book239_document003)

"Coding Challenge Answers: Hospital Evaluation and Management Services," March 2024 (https://doi.org/10.1542/pcco_book239_document006)

"Coding Review: Social Determinants of Health," November 2023 (https://doi.org/10.1542/pcco_book235_document006)

"*CPT* 2024: New Guidelines for Brief Hospital Stays," November 2023 (https://doi.org/10.1542/pcco_book235_document004)

"*CPT* 2024: Revisions to Guidelines for Split or Shared Visits," November 2023 (https://doi.org/10.1542/pcco_book235_document003)

"Endocrinology: Updated *ICD-10-CM* Diabetes and Hypoglycemia Codes," October 2024 (https://doi.org/10.1542/pcco_book246_document001)

"You Code It! Adolescent Weight Loss Due to a Suspected Eating Disorder," October 2024 (https://doi.org/10.1542/pcco_book246_document005)

"You Code It! Answers: Adolescent Weight Loss Due to a Suspected Eating Disorder," October 2024 (https://doi.org/10.1542/pcco_book246_document007)

"You Code It! Stage 2 Hypertension, Hematuria, and Edema," May 2024 (https://doi.org/10.1542/pcco_book241_document002)

"You Code It! Answers: Stage 2 Hypertension, Hematuria, and Edema," May 2024 (https://doi.org/10.1542/pcco_book241_document004)

Test Your Knowledge!

1. **True or false? Because the codes for inpatient and observation E/M services are the same, it is not necessary for a physician or QHP to document a change in admission status.**
   a. True
   b. False
2. **Which type of hospital E/M service is reported by a physician or QHP providing inpatient care to a patient who has received services from a physician of the same exact specialty and subspecialty and same group practice on a prior date during the current stay?**
   a. Initial hospital inpatient or observation services
   b. An inpatient or observation consultation
   c. Subsequent inpatient or observation services
   d. Any of the above, but the code is appended with modifier FS
3. **What type of code is reported for hospital care when the physician who ordered the admission provides initial care and discharge management at the same time (ie, at a single visit)?**
   a. Same-date admission and discharge services
   b. Initial hospital care
   c. Initial hospital care and hospital discharge day management
   d. Hospital discharge day management
4. **Which of the following is a consultation?**
   a. A physician or QHP provides an initial E/M service to a child whose physician requested advice on management of an infection by an unidentified agent.
   b. A physician or QHP provides a follow-up visit to a child whose test results indicate need for additional advice or opinion on management.
   c. A QHP requests that a physician who has provided outpatient behavioral health care to a hospitalized patient assume inpatient management of the patient's behavioral health needs during an admission for an unrelated condition.
   d. A physician provides continuing care to a patient while covering for the patient's physician who is of the same specialty and same group practice.
5. **Which is true of prolonged service code 99418?**
   a. 99418 is reported for each additional hour beyond the total time required to report the related E/M service.
   b. 99418 is reported in addition to any hospital inpatient or observation code when the physician's total time exceeds that required for the primary E/M service.
   c. 99418 is reported only when the primary E/M service code is selected on the basis of total time and the total time is exceeded by at least 15 minutes.
   d. 99418 is reported for prolonged service within 24 hours of the primary E/M service.

CHAPTER 17

Critical and Intensive Care

Contents

Chapter Highlights

This chapter focuses on correctly coding critical and intensive care services, including

- Defining critical care and included services
- Hourly critical care
- Attendance at delivery and neonatal resuscitation
- Critical care of the neonate, infant, and child younger than 6 years
- Intensive care of the recovering or low-birth-weight neonate and infant
  - Services commonly reported before and after intensive or critical care services, such as care during emergency transport, are also included.

For discussion of evaluation and management (E/M) of the child requiring hospital care but no longer requiring intensive or critical care, refer to **Chapter 16**.

Defining Critical Care

- A *critical illness or injury* is defined by *Current Procedural Terminology* (*CPT*®) as acutely impairing one or more vital organs such that there is a high probability of imminent or life-threatening deterioration of the patient's condition.
- Services qualify as critical care *only if both* the injury or illness *and* the treatment being delivered meet the following criteria:
  - The illness or injury acutely impairs one or more vital organs as defined previously.
  - The treatment delivered involves high-complexity medical decision-making (MDM) to prevent life-threatening deterioration of the patient's condition.
- Critical care involves high-complexity MDM to assess, manipulate, and support vital organ system function(s); treat single- or multiple-organ system failure; and/or prevent further life-threatening deterioration of the patient's condition.
- Although immaturity alone does not define critical care, the complex decision-making applied to manage the therapeutic challenges manifesting in many preterm babies can support critical care.

An ill neonate who does not require critical care may require neonatal intensive care, as discussed in the Initial and Continuing Intensive Care section later in this chapter, or hospital care, as discussed in Chapter 16.

- Coding critical care is not determined by the location in which the care is delivered but by the nature of the care being delivered and the condition of the patient requiring care.
- Critical care is not limited to an inpatient setting or a critical care area, and a physician of any specialty can provide these services. Services must be provided directly by the physician or other qualified health care professional (QHP).
- Many typically performed procedures are included (bundled) in the work valuation of each critical care code and cannot be reported separately (**Table 17-1**). (Refer also to the next section of this chapter for commonly provided services not bundled with hourly and/or neonatal and pediatric critical care service.)

Critical and Intensive Care

Chapter 17

Procedures *Not* Bundled With Critical/Intensive Care Services

When reporting hourly critical or neonatal and pediatric critical and intensive care services, many services commonly performed in the provision of critical care are not bundled into the intensive or critical care services. However, claim edits may require appending a modifier to indicate that the services were distinct. Examples (not all inclusive) of procedures that are not bundled with critical care services include

- Thoracentesis (**32554**, **32555**) (via needle or pigtail catheter)
- Percutaneous pleural drainage with insertion of indwelling catheter (**32556**, **32557**)
- Complete (double volume) exchange transfusion (**36450**, newborn; **36455**, other)
- Partial exchange transfusion (**36456**)
- Abdominal paracentesis (**49082**, **49083**)
- Bone marrow aspiration (**38220**)
- Circumcision (**54150**)
- Cardioversion (**92960**)

- Cardiopulmonary resuscitation (CPR) (92950)
- Extracorporeal membrane oxygenation (ECMO) (33946–33949)
- Peripherally inserted central catheter (36568–36573)
- Insertion of non-tunneled centrally inserted central venous catheter, older than 5 years (36556)
- Replacement (rewire) of non-tunneled centrally inserted central venous catheter (36580)
- Therapeutic apheresis (36511–36514)
- Insertion of cannula for hemodialysis, other purpose (separate procedure); vein to vein (36800)
- Placement of needle for intraosseous infusion (36680)
- Initiation of selective head or total body hypothermia in the critically ill neonate (99184)

Example

➤ **In addition to directing subsequent neonatal critical care for a preterm neonate with a current weight of 2.8 kg, a physician places a peripherally inserted central catheter (PICC) without subcutaneous port or pump and without imaging guidance.** The PICC insertion is documented and distinctly identifiable in the patient record from the daily critical care service.

99469 25	Subsequent inpatient neonatal critical care, per day, for the evaluation and management of a critically ill neonate, 28 days of age or younger
36568 63	Insertion of peripherally inserted central venous catheter (PICC), without subcutaneous port or pump, without imaging guidance; younger than 5 years of age

Insertion of a PICC is not included in daily neonatal critical care services. Because the neonatal critical care service entails work significantly beyond the preservice and postservice work of PICC placement, modifier 25 is appropriately appended to code 99469.

Modifier 63 (procedure performed on infants less than 4 kg) is appended to code 36568 because the procedure is not specific to patients weighing less than 4 kg, as in this example.

Emergency cardiac defibrillation is included in CPR (92950). Per the Medicaid National Correct Coding Initiative (NCCI) manual, if emergency cardiac defibrillation without CPR is performed in the emergency department (ED) or critical/intensive care unit, the cardiac defibrillation service is not separately reportable. Report 92960 only for elective cardioversion.

Many practice management and billing systems include claim scrubbers to alert coders that claim edits apply and a modifier may be appropriate given the clinical circumstances. Payers may also offer online tools for determining when code pair edits apply.

Hourly Critical Care

99291	Critical care, E/M of the critically ill or critically injured patient; first 30–74 minutes
+99292	each additional 30 minutes (Use in conjunction with 99291.)

Guidelines for reporting 99291 and 99292 are as follows:

- Report only when critical care is provided for 30 minutes or more
  - In the outpatient setting (eg, ED, office, clinic) *regardless of age*
  - To an inpatient 6 years or older (For discussion of daily critical care of a child aged <6 years, refer to the Neonatal and Pediatric Daily Critical Care Codes section later in this chapter.)
  - Concurrently by a second physician from a different specialty to a critically ill or injured patient, regardless of age
  - To an inpatient 5 years or younger when the patient is being transferred to another facility in which a receiving physician of the same specialty but different medical group will be reporting the daily inpatient critical care service codes (99468 and 99469, 99471 and 99472, 99475 and 99476)
  - By the physician physically transporting a critically ill child older than 2 years or when payer policy does not recognize 99466 and 99467 (face-to-face transport care of the critically ill or injured patient aged ≤24 months as discussed in the Face-to-Face Pediatric Critical Care Patient Transport section later in this chapter)
- Refer to **Table 17-1** to determine which services are bundled (ie, included in the value assigned to critical care services) and to the Procedures *Not* Bundled With Critical/Intensive Care Services section, presented earlier in this chapter, to determine which ones are separately reported (eg, lumbar puncture, endotracheal intubation, thoracentesis).

Table 17-1. Critical Care Bundled Services

An x indicates that the services in that row are bundled to the corresponding critical care service. Services that are not bundled with a critical care service are separately reported only when personally performed by a physician or other QHP (ie, not clinical staff of the facility).

CPT Code and Procedure (An x in any column applies to all codes within the same row)	Hourly Critical Care 99291, 99292	Pediatric Transport 99466, 99467	Neonatal/Pediatric Critical and Intensive Care 99468–99476, 99477–99480
Interpretation and Monitoring			
71045 X-ray, chest; single view 71046 X-ray, chest; 2 views	X	X	X
+93598 Cardiac output measurement(s), thermodilution or other indicator dilution method, performed during cardiac catheterization for the evaluation of congenital heart defects	X	X	X
94760 Pulse oximetry; single determination[a] 94761 multiple determinations (eg, during exercise)[a] 94762 by continuous overnight monitoring[a]	X	X	X
Vascular Access Procedures			
36000 Introduction of needle or intracatheter, vein	X	X	X
36140 Catheterization extremity artery			X
36400 Venipuncture, <3 years, requiring physician or QHP skill; femoral or jugular vein 36405 scalp vein 36406 other vein		X	X
36410 Venipuncture, ≥3 years, requiring physician or QHP skill	X		X
36415 Collection of venous blood by venipuncture[a]	X	X	X
36420 Venipuncture, cutdown; younger than age 1 year			X
36430 Transfusion, blood or blood components[a] 36440 Push transfusion, blood, 2 years or younger			X
36510 Catheterization of umbilical vein, newborn			X
36555 Insertion of non-tunneled centrally inserted central venous catheter; <5 years of age			X
36591 Collection blood from venous access device[a]	X	X	X
36600 Arterial puncture, withdrawal of blood for diagnosis	X	X	X
36620 Arterial catheterization, percutaneous 36660 Catheterization, umbilical artery, newborn			X
Other Procedures			
31500 Endotracheal intubation, emergency			X
43752 Nasogastric or orogastric intubation, fluoroscopic guidance	X	X	X
43753 Gastric intubation including lavage if performed	X	X	X
51100 Aspiration of bladder; by needle			X
51701 Insertion of non-indwelling bladder catheter 51702 Temporary indwelling bladder catheter; simple			X

Continued on next page

Table 17-1 (*continued*)

Other Procedures (*continued*)			
62270 Spinal puncture, lumbar, diagnostic			X
92953 Temporary transcutaneous pacing	X	X	X
94002 Ventilation initiation; inpatient/observation, initial day **94003** each subsequent day	X	X	X
94004 Ventilation initiation; nursing facility, per day	X		X
94375 Respiratory flow volume loop			X
94610 Intrapulmonary surfactant administration			X
94660 CPAP, initiation and management	X	X	X
94780 Car seat/bed testing, infants through 12 months; 60 minutes **94781** each additional full 30 minutes			X

Abbreviations: CPAP, continuous positive airway pressure; *CPT, Current Procedural Terminology;* QHP, qualified health care professional.

[a] This procedure is not valued to include physician work. This code is reported to account for practice expense in a non-facility setting or reported by a facility for overhead expense.

The reported time of critical care cannot include any time spent performing procedures or services that are reported separately.

- Report **99291** and, when appropriate, **99292** when another physician or QHP of a *different specialty* (from either the same or a different group practice) provides neonatal or pediatric critical care services (**99468–99476**) on the same date.
- A teaching physician may report time-based critical care services only when personally present for the entire period for which the claim is submitted and that time is supported in documentation of the service.
- When inpatient and outpatient critical care services are provided to a neonate, infant, or child younger than 6 years on the same date by the same physician (or physician of the same group and specialty), only the daily *inpatient* critical care codes are reported (**99468–99476**). For exceptions, refer to the Neonatal and Pediatric Daily Critical Care Codes and the Emergency Medical Services Supervision and Patient Transport sections later in this chapter.
  - **Figure 17-1** illustrates the indications for reporting **99291–99292** as previously mentioned.

Figure 17-1. Indications for Reporting Time-Based Critical Care (99291–99292)

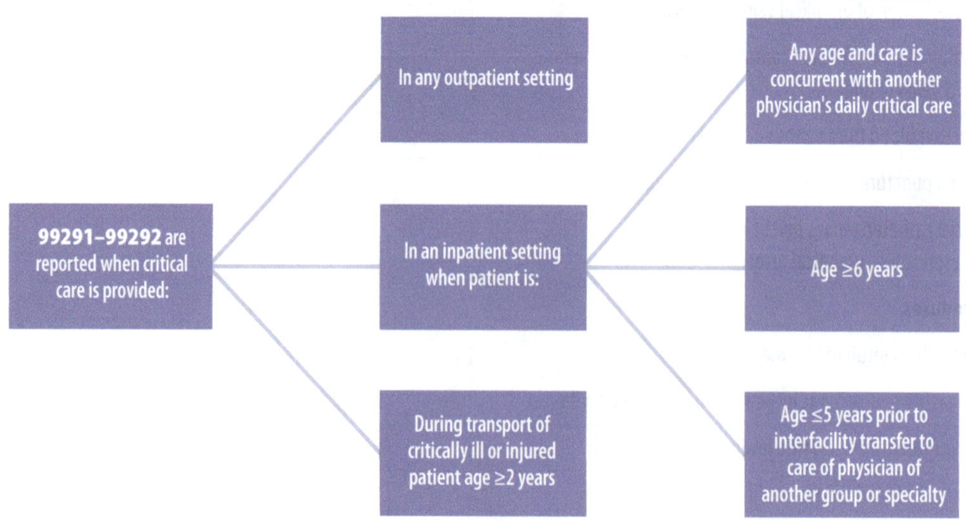

- Other significant, separately identifiable E/M services (eg, 99282–99285 for ED E/M services) can be reported in addition to time-based critical care services as appropriate. Do not count time spent in separately reported E/M services in critical care time.

Payer policies for same-date/same-physician critical care and other E/M services may vary. Medicare policy limits payment of ED services 99281–99285 and other E/M services on the same date as critical care services when all the following circumstances are true:

1. **The other E/M visit was provided before the critical care services at a time when the patient did not require critical care.**
2. **The services were medically necessary.**
3. **The services were separate and distinct, with no duplicative elements from the critical care services provided later in the day.**

Modifier 25 (significant, separately identifiable E/M service) is appended to the code for the noncritical care service.

Time Units of Hourly Critical Care

Reporting for 99291 and 99292 is based on time. **Table 17-2** lists times and billing units. The total floor or unit time devoted to the patient in the provision of critical care is used in code selection.

Table 17-2. Reporting Hourly Critical Care Services

Do not report services of <30 minutes as critical care; report the appropriate E/M service for the site at which service is provided.

Duration of Face-to-Face Critical Care (min)	30–74	75–104	105–134	135–164	165–194
***CPT* Codes and Units of Service**	99291	99291 × 1, 99292 × 1	99291 × 1, 99292 × 2	99291 × 1, 99292 × 3	99291 × 1, 99292 × 4

Abbreviations: *CPT, Current Procedural Terminology;* E/M, evaluation and management.

Medicare policy requires a minimum of 104 minutes spent in critical care activities to report 99292 (ie, completion of a full 30 minutes of critical care services beyond the first 74 minutes of service). Except where a payer's policy specifically aligns with Medicare policy, continue to report according to *CPT* instruction.

Critical care time is counted *when the physician or QHP is immediately available to the patient,* including face-to-face time spent between the physician and patient and other time spent directly related to the patient's care (eg, reviewing test results, discussing care with other medical staff or family, documenting services in the medical record).

- Time spent in the provision of critical care does not need to be continuous. The cumulative time of critical care provided on a single date of service (DOS) is used to calculate the units of service provided.

When a *continuous period* of critical care occurs before and after midnight, report the total time on the date that the period of care was initiated. Do not report a second unit of 99291 for the period that continues beyond midnight.

- Code 99291 is reported once on a given DOS when 30 to 74 minutes of critical care is performed. If less than 30 minutes of critical care is provided, an appropriate E/M service (eg, 99202–99215, 99282–99285 for ED services) is reported.
- Code 99292 is reported with 1 unit for each additional period up to 30 minutes beyond the previous period. Time spent providing critical care services must be documented in the medical record.

Unless otherwise indicated in payer policy, services of physicians and QHPs of the same group practice and exact same specialty are typically considered to be provided by a single physician or QHP.

- Code 99291 is reported once for 30 to 74 minutes of critical care performed by one or more physicians or QHPs of the same group practice and same exact specialty.
- When the combined times of physicians and QHPs in the same group practice and specialty support reporting 99292, follow payer guidelines regarding reporting by each individual physician or QHP (eg, the same physician reports 99291 and 99292, or the first physician reports 99291 and the other physician reports 99292, as indicated).

Critical and Intensive Care

Chapter 17

Medicare Guidelines for Critical Care Services

Medicare policy is often adopted by other payers (eg, Medicaid plans, group health plans). For example, Medicare policy requires a minimum of 104 minutes spent in critical care activities to report **99292** (ie, completion of a full 30 minutes of critical care services beyond the first 74 minutes of service). For this reason, it is good to be aware of Medicare policies that may affect how services are reported.

Medicare's Assignment of a Qualified Health Care Professional's Specialty

When QHPs work with physicians, *CPT* considers the QHPs to be working in the exact same specialty and exact same subspecialties as the physician. This guideline is not consistent with Medicare policy. Under Medicare policy, distinct specialty codes are assigned to QHPs such as nurse practitioners (NPs) (**50**), physician associates (**97**), and clinical nurse specialists (**89**). When adopted by other payers (eg, Medicaid plans), specialty differentiation affects how critical care is reported when provided in part by a physician and in part by a QHP. Reporting by the correct individual is important when there are differences between fee schedule payments to physicians and those to QHPs.

Hourly Critical Care by Physicians of the Same Specialty and Same Group Practice

As with *CPT,* when 2 physicians of the same specialty and same group practice or 2 QHPs of the same group practice provide hourly critical care services on the same date, Medicare policy allows reporting based on the combined times of each physician or each QHP.

Refer to the Split or Shared Critical Care Services section later in this chapter for Medicare payment policy that may apply to hourly critical care services provided *by a physician and QHP* in the same group practice on the same DOS.

Under the Medicare policy for reporting critical care services provided by 2 or more individuals of the same specialty and same group practice,

- The time of critical care services by 2 physicians or by 2 QHPs may be combined to support **99291**.
- A second physician cannot report **99291** when the initial 30 to 74 minutes of critical care services on the same date was provided by another physician of the same specialty and same group practice. The physician who provided the initial period of critical care services reports **99291**. If the requirements for reporting **99292** are met by the combined critical care service times of the 2 physicians, the second physician may report **99292**.

All the time attributed to critical care services must be medically necessary, and each visit must meet the definition of critical care to combine the times for the purpose of code selection.

Examples

➤ **Dr A spends 20 minutes providing initial critical care services to a 3-year-old child and orders a transfer to another facility.** Dr B, a physician of the same specialty and same group practice, assumes management and provides 45 minutes of critical care to the child during transport to the receiving facility.

Dr A or Dr B reports **99291** × 1 (critical care, first 30–74 minutes).

Teaching Point: Dr A's time does not support **99291**. But because Dr B is in the same group practice and same specialty, the time spent by each physician is combined (20 + 45 = 65) to support **99291**. Medicare does not designate which physician reports the service.

➤ **A 13-year-old adolescent is admitted to the intensive care unit in respiratory distress.** Nurse practitioner A, who specializes in pulmonology, spends 50 minutes providing initial critical care services. Later, on the same date, NP B, of the same group practice and who specializes in infectious disease, provides 40 minutes of critical care.

If a payer credentials NPs by specialty or subspecialty of practice and follows *CPT* instructions	When the payer follows Medicare policy considering NPs to be of a single specialty and requiring ≥104 minutes to report **99292**
NP A reports **99291** (critical care, first 30–74 minutes). NP B reports **99291**.	NP A reports **99291** (critical care, first 30–104 minutes).

Critical and Intensive Care
Chapter 17

Teaching Point: When the NPs are considered to be of the same specialty, only the first period of critical care services is reported with 99291. When payer policy aligns with Medicare, requiring a total of 104 minutes of critical care services to report 99292, only 99291 is reported by NP A, who spent the greater portion of the total time.

Split or Shared Critical Care Services

Because Medicare does not consider QHPs to be working in the same specialty as physicians, Medicare's split or shared services policy is applied when physicians and QHPs of the same group practice, not hospital employees, jointly provide E/M services in a facility setting. (In an office setting, incident-to policy, as discussed in **Chapter 7**, applies, rather than split/shared.)

Under the split/shared policy, hourly critical care services (ie, the service times of a physician and QHP of the same group practice) are combined and reported as a single service. But the policy requires that the service be reported by *the individual who spent the greater amount of time providing critical care services.*

- Modifier FS (split or shared E/M visit) must be appended to the critical care code(s) on the claim (ie, 99291 FS and, when applicable, 99292 FS).
- When 2 or more physicians and QHPs spend time jointly meeting with or discussing the patient as part of a critical care service, the time can be counted only once for the purpose of reporting the split/shared critical care visit.
- The physician and the QHP must document their personally performed services, but the reporting individual (the one who spent the greater portion of time) is responsible for authenticating and dating the record.

Example

➤ **A 4-year-old arrives to the ED in critical condition.** The ED physician provides 40 minutes of critical care before the child's condition is stabilized so they may be transferred to another facility. Pending transfer, a QHP of the same group practice assumes treatment of the patient, who is in stable condition at that time. The patient's condition deteriorates, and the QHP provides another 30 minutes of critical care before a team arrives to accept treatment of the patient during transport.

The ED physician reports 99291 FS.

Teaching Point: The ED physician who provided the substantive or greater amount (ie, 40 of 70 minutes) of the total time reports the critical care services with modifier FS appended to indicate that the services were split/shared. The physician and the QHP each document the individually provided services and time spent. Under Medicare policy, the individual reporting the service must authenticate/sign and date the record of the split/shared services reported. Any separately reportable procedure is reported by the physician or QHP who provided the service. Modifier 25 may be required in addition to FS.

Critical Care During the Neonatal Period

Defining the Neonatal Period

For coding purposes, the neonatal period begins at birth and continues through the completed 28th day after birth, ending on the 29th calendar day after birth. The day of birth is considered day 0 (zero). Therefore, the day after birth is considered day 1.

This definition is important in selecting the initial- and subsequent-day neonatal critical care codes 99468 and 99469 as well as 99477 for the initial hospital care of the neonate, 28 days or younger, who requires intensive observation, frequent interventions, and other intensive care services.

Refer to the American Academy of Pediatrics (AAP) *Newborn Coding Decision Tool 2026* (www.aap.org/Newborn-Coding-Decision-Tool-2026) for a quick code selection for services provided to newborns during the birth admission.

ICD-10-CM Guidelines and Neonatal Critical Care

It is important to correctly assign *International Classification of Diseases, 10th Revision, Clinical Modification* (*ICD-10-CM*) codes that reflect the diagnoses for which critical care services were required. Assign codes for neonatal conditions that require treatment or further investigation, prolong the length of stay, or require resource utilization, as well as codes for conditions that have implications for future health care needs.

When care is provided by the attending physician during the birth admission, report first a code from category Z38 (liveborn infants according to place of birth and type of delivery). Codes for abnormal conditions are reported secondary to the code for live birth. When a neonate is transferred to another facility after birth, the admission to the receiving facility is not a birth admission and Z38 codes are not reported.

- *ICD-10-CM* contains codes (P00–P96) for conditions originating in the perinatal period. These codes are reported for conditions described as having their origin in the fetal or perinatal period (before birth through the first 28 days after birth) even if morbidity occurs later. Again, this period includes the completed 28th day after birth with the day of birth being counted as day 0 (zero).
  - These codes are to be reported only when the condition originates in this time, but they can be reported beyond the perinatal period if the condition(s) causes morbidity or is the primary reason for or contributing to the reason the patient is receiving health care.
  - The perinatal code should continue to be used regardless of the patient's age if a condition originates in the perinatal period and continues throughout the patient's life.

Example

➤ **A 30-day-old who was a 26-weeks'-gestation preterm neonate continues to require critical or intensive care to address a condition originating in the perinatal period.**

Teaching Point: Although the patient is no longer a neonate, the *ICD-10-CM* code that is linked to the critical or intensive care service is the appropriate perinatal code (P00–P96) for the condition(s) currently managed or treated. When care is provided during the birth admission, the appropriate Z38 code is listed first.

- ✖ Do not report perinatal codes for any condition *originating* after the perinatal period (29th calendar day after birth and beyond). For example, report necrotizing enterocolitis with onset on the 30th calendar day after birth with codes in category K55.3-, not a code from category P77.- (necrotizing enterocolitis in newborn).
- A diagnosis of prematurity must be documented to support reporting a code for prematurity. Coders cannot assign codes for prematurity solely on the basis of documented gestational age.
- Codes in category P05 are reported for the newborn affected by fetal growth restriction or slow intrauterine growth. Note that head circumference is not a factor in these diagnoses.
  - Codes in subcategory P05.0 are used to report that the neonate is light for gestational age but not small (weight below but length above the 10th percentile). These neonates have often been said to exhibit *asymmetrical growth restriction.*
  - Codes in subcategory P05.1 are used to report that the neonate is small and light (both weight and length below the 10th percentile) for gestational age. These newborns have often been said to exhibit *symmetrical growth restriction* or *intrauterine growth restriction.*
- Code P05.2 is provided for reporting fetal (intrauterine) malnutrition affecting a newborn whose weight is not below the 10th percentile and has a significant disparity between weight and length percentiles.
- Codes from category P07 (disorders of newborn related to short gestation and low birth weight [not due to fetal malnutrition]) are reported according to the recorded birth weight (*not* <*10th percentile*) and estimated gestational age to indicate that these conditions are the cause of morbidity or reason for additional care of the newborn.
  - When both are documented, weight is sequenced before age.
  - These codes may be reported for a child as well as for an adult who was preterm or had a low birth weight as a newborn and whose current health status is affected.

Codes in subcategory P07.3- (preterm newborn) should be reported for neonates born at 36 weeks' gestation who stay in the newborn nursery or who are cared for in the neonatal intensive care unit (NICU).

- ✖ Do not report codes in subcategory P07.0- (extremely low birth weight newborn) and P07.1- (other low birth weight newborn) in conjunction with codes in category P05 (disorders of the newborn due to slow fetal growth and fetal malnutrition). Subcategory P07.2- (extreme immaturity of newborn) and P07.3- (preterm newborn), however, may be reported in addition to category P05.

Codes for congenital malformation or deformity (Q00–Q99) may also be used throughout the life of the patient. After a congenital malformation or deformity has been corrected, a personal history code should be used to identify the history of the malformation or deformity.

Attendance at Delivery and Neonatal Resuscitation

Attendance at Delivery

99464 Attendance at delivery (when requested by the delivering physician or other QHP) and initial stabilization of newborn

Attendance at delivery (**99464**) is reported only when the physical presence of the provider is requested by the delivering physician and indicated for a newborn who may require immediate intervention (ie, stabilization, resuscitation, or evaluation for potential problems).

- Includes initial drying, stimulation, suctioning, blow-by oxygen, or continuous positive airway pressure (CPAP) without positive pressure ventilation; a cursory visual inspection of the neonate; assignment of Apgar scores; and discussion of care of the newborn with the delivering physician and parents. A quick look in the delivery room or examination after stabilization is not sufficient to support reporting of **99464**.
  - When qualifying resuscitative efforts are provided, **99465** (delivery/birthing room resuscitation) is reported instead. Codes **99464** and **99465** cannot be reported on the same day of service.

Refer to **Chapter 15** for further discussion and coding examples for **99464**.

Neonatal Resuscitation

99465 Delivery/birthing room resuscitation, provision of positive pressure ventilation and/or chest compressions in the presence of acute inadequate ventilation and/or cardiac output

Attendance at delivery with neonatal resuscitation (**99465**)

- Is a service that mirrors CPR but is specific to a neonate. Positive pressure ventilation, delivered by any means (resuscitation bag or T-piece resuscitator), and/or cardiac compressions are required for **99465**.
- May be reported in addition to any initial care service, including initial daily inpatient critical care (**99468**), hourly critical care (**99291** and **99292**), initial neonatal intensive care (**99477**), or, if the resuscitation results in a stable full-term neonate, normal newborn care (**99460**).

Payers may require modifier 25 (significant, separately identifiable E/M service) appended to the code for E/M services reported in addition to 99464 or 99465. But NCCI edits do not bundle these services.

- Medically necessary procedures (eg, **31500**, intubation, endotracheal, emergency procedure; **31515**, laryngoscopy, direct, for aspiration; **36510**, catheterization of umbilical vein for diagnosis or therapy, newborn; **94610**, surfactant administration) essential to successful resuscitation that are performed in the delivery room before admission may also be reported in addition to codes **99465** and **99468** or **99477** (initial daily inpatient neonatal critical or intensive care).
- ✖ Do not report **99465** when a T-piece resuscitator is used only to provide CPAP. If the neonate responds to provision of CPAP with an adequate respiratory effort, **99464** should be reported.
- ✖ Do not separately report services performed as a convenience before admission to the NICU.
  - Medical record documentation must clearly support that the services are provided as a required measure for emergency resuscitation and not as part of an admission protocol.

Documentation of neonatal resuscitation should explicitly state that the neonate demonstrated respiratory and/or cardiac instability requiring intervention, including apnea or inadequate respiratory effort to support gas exchange; that the provider instituted positive pressure ventilation; and the neonate's response to the positive pressure ventilation.

Refer to the "Stillborn Deliveries and Unsuccessful Resuscitation" box later in this chapter for discussion of billing for services provided to a mother and/or neonate when the outcome is stillborn birth of a neonate or an ill neonate who was unresponsive to resuscitation.

Critical and Intensive Care

Chapter 17

Example

➤ **A neonatologist attends an emergency cesarean delivery of a 34-weeks'–gestation neonate whose mother has known, poorly controlled diabetes and a history of drug misuse. The neonate is born limp and cyanotic with no spontaneous respiratory activity.** The resuscitation includes positive pressure ventilation, intubation, and placement of an umbilical vein catheter with a normal saline bolus. The newborn, who is continuously bradycardic and pale, is admitted to the NICU, after which the neonatologist administers surfactant.

The intubation and umbilical vein catheterization are separately reported procedures provided as part of the resuscitation and not solely in anticipation of use after admission.

ICD-10-CM	*CPT*
Diagnoses are not stated in this example but may include the following: Z38.- (liveborn infant, additional characters required) P07.37 (preterm newborn, gestational age 34 completed weeks) P22.0 (respiratory distress of newborn) P70.1 (syndrome of infant of a diabetic mother)	99465 (delivery/birthing room resuscitation) 31500 (endotracheal intubation, emergency) 36510 (catheterization of umbilical vein for diagnosis or therapy, newborn) 99468 25 (initial daily neonatal critical care)

Teaching Point: Modifier 25 is appended to 99468 to signify a significant, separately identifiable E/M service provided in addition to 31500 and 36510 because these services are bundled by NCCI edits. Codes 99465 and 99468 are not bundled by NCCI edits, but individual payers may require modifier 25 to designate separately identifiable critical care services on the same date. The surfactant administration is not separately reported when performed in conjunction with neonatal critical care.

Stillborn Deliveries and Unsuccessful Resuscitation

Questions arise on documentation, coding, and billing for services provided to a baby who is stillborn or is thought to be viable (eg, showing fetal distress before delivery) but who, shortly after birth, despite resuscitative efforts, never shows active signs of a heartbeat.

If a baby is delivered but is known to have expired in utero, a separate medical record will not be created. Therefore, any services performed by a pediatrician or neonatologist will be documented in the maternal record. The physician could be called on to perform an examination and/or discuss any known or discovered fetal anomalies. In this circumstance, the physician could charge an initial hospital inpatient or observation encounter (99221–99223) or inpatient consultation (99252–99255) to the mother, which includes the physician's total time devoted to this service on the date of the encounter. In practice, physicians may not provide or may elect not to charge for this service.

As with a known intrauterine fetal demise, a neonate who was felt to be viable may be born without evidence of a heart rate or respiratory effort. Resuscitative efforts may be started and then stopped after a determined amount of time. Although neonatal resuscitation (99465) could be coded and billed for, a separate medical record might not be created for the neonate. The service may be billed with the mother as the patient; however, medical records would likely have to accompany the claim. Most payers will deny this claim, so an appeal would be required. It would be best to create a record for the baby so the services can be documented for both the physician and nursing staff. Again, in practice, many physicians do not charge for this service.

For a liveborn neonate who experiences distress and dies in the delivery room, an individual medical record should be created to document the care. This service will be reported as neonatal resuscitation services (99465) with the deceased neonate as the recipient of care. Remember to also document and report any other separately billable services (eg, surfactant administration), when performed.

Although all services and procedures performed must be clearly documented in the maternal or neonatal medical record (if one is created), billing for the services will be up to the individual physician.

Neonatal and Pediatric Daily Critical Care Codes

Codes are

- Reported for critical care of children younger than 6 years in the inpatient setting.
- Global. They encompass all E/M services by an attending physician or QHP, including individuals of the exact same specialty in the same group practice, *on 1 calendar date.* (For exceptions [eg, critical care transport], refer to the Guidelines for Reporting Neonatal or Pediatric Inpatient Critical Care section later in this chapter.)

Only the attending or principal physician or QHP reports daily critical or intensive care services. Other physicians and QHPs providing concurrent critical care, and not participating as part of the integrated health care team under direction and supervision of the attending or principal physician or QHP, report critical care codes 99291 and 99292 according to the total time spent in provision of critical care services.

- Bundled. They have commonly performed procedures included in the E/M codes. Refer to **Table 17-1** for services and procedures that are included with neonatal critical care codes.
- Reported according to postnatal age (refer to the Defining the Neonatal Period section earlier in this chapter) and initial or subsequent care (**Table 17-3**).
- ✖ Not time based. Prolonged services *may not* be reported in conjunction with neonatal or pediatric critical care services.
- ✖ Not based on typical E/M rules as applied to services for which codes are selected according to a level of MDM or total time on the date of an encounter.

Table 17-3. Neonatal and Pediatric Daily (Global) Critical Care

Daily (Global) Critical Care	28 Days or Younger	29 Days Through 24 Months of Age	2 Through 5 Years of Age
Initial daily critical care	99468	99471	99475
Subsequent daily critical care	99469	99472	99476

Guidelines for Reporting Neonatal or Pediatric Inpatient Critical Care

- The physician or neonatal NP (subject to state regulations, scope of practice, and hospital privilege credentials) primarily responsible for the patient on the DOS should report the neonatal or pediatric critical care codes. When both the physician and the neonatal NP provide critical care services to a patient, only one may report the code.
- If critical care is provided in both outpatient and inpatient settings by the same physician or a physician of the same specialty and group, only the inpatient code is reported.
- Daily critical care codes are reported only once per day, per patient.
- When the same physician or physicians of the same specialty and group practice provide pediatric critical care during transport of a child 24 months or younger (99466, 99467, 99485, 99486) and critical care after admission to the receiving facility, both services are reported and modifier 25 is appended to the transport code.
- Only 1 initial daily inpatient critical care code (99468, 99471, 99475) is reported per calendar day and *per hospital stay* for a given patient. For a second episode of critical care during the same hospital stay, report a subsequent critical care code (99469, 99472, 99476).
- Continued daily critical care to a patient who reaches the age of 29 days or of 2 years is also reported with a code for subsequent pediatric critical care (99472, 99476).
- Subsequent critical care may be reported on multiple days even if there is no change in the patient's condition if the patient continues to meet the critical care definition and documentation supports this level of service.
- Care may be provided on any unit of a hospital facility.

Subsequent-day intensive care codes (99478–99480, discussed in the Initial and Continuing Intensive Care section later in this chapter) are reported when critical care is no longer required and the neonate or infant who weighs 5,000 g or less on the day of service requires a higher level of care than what is typically provided under routine subsequent hospital care (99231–99233). Once a neonate weighing at least 5,001 g no longer requires critical care services, report an appropriate level of subsequent-day inpatient hospital care codes (99231–99233).

Neonatal Critical and Intensive Care Supervision Requirements

CPT states that codes 99468, 99469, and 99471–99476 are used to report services provided by a single individual "directing the inpatient care" of a critically ill neonate, infant, or child through 5 years of age. Constant in-house attendance by the supervising physician or QHP is not a requirement of neonatal critical and intensive care. But the codes' values were established under the assumption that the reporting individual is physically present and participating directly in the patient's care.

- Documentation in the patient's medical record should reflect this active participation, including documentation of hands-on care, such as a personal physical examination, and of the patient's condition that requires critical or intensive care.

- Medical record documentation must support the need for and meet the definition of critical care (eg, complex MDM, high probability of imminent or life-threatening deterioration, organ system failure).
- Care must be provided by the reporting individual, but it includes the services provided by the health care team functioning under the direct supervision of the physician *or a QHP (eg, neonatal NP) who is practicing independently and is not otherwise providing care under the direct supervision of the physician.* The concept of a split/shared service does not apply to daily critical or intensive care services.
- Typically, a neonate or an infant is evaluated during numerous intervals throughout a calendar day, depending on the clinical needs of the patient. The extent of the reporting individual's personal service (eg, overnight in-house care) and presence is determined by the complexity of the total population of neonates cared for in a nursery or the changes in a specific neonate's or infant's condition that cannot be adequately assessed or managed over the telephone.

For more information, refer to "Global Per Diem Critical Care Codes: Direct Supervision and Reporting Guidelines" at www.aap.org/cfp2026.

Coding Conundrum: Selecting the Appropriate Code

Many diagnoses or conditions, such as respiratory distress, infection, seizures, mild to moderate hypoxic-ischemic encephalopathy, and metabolic disorders, can be reported with **99468**, **99477**, or **99221–99223**. The patient's clinical status, required level of monitoring and observation, and present body weight determine which of these codes is chosen. Selection of the service must be justified by medical record documentation.

Neonatal Critical Care

99468 Initial inpatient neonatal critical care, per day, for the E/M of a critically ill neonate, 28 days of age or younger

99469 Subsequent inpatient neonatal critical care, per day, for the E/M of a critically ill neonate, 28 days of age or younger

Selection of the appropriate code will depend on the patient's condition and the intensity of the service provided and documented on a particular day of service.

- Report **99468** and, when appropriate, **99469** in addition to normal newborn care (**99460**, **99462**) when these services are provided on the same date that the patient later requires a separate encounter for critical care. Each service should be reported with the appropriate diagnosis code to support the service (eg, diagnosis codes for well newborn and the critical illness).

When reporting multiple E/M services provided by the same individual(s) of the same specialty and same group practice, refer to the payer's code edits (eg, NCCI edits) to determine if modifier 25 (significant, separately identifiable E/M service) is required to designate the separately reportable services.

- If the neonate or infant becomes critically ill on a day when initial or subsequent intensive care services (**99477–99480**) have been provided and the same physician(s) or QHP(s) from the same group practice provide critical care services, report only initial or subsequent critical care (**99468–99476**) according to the patient's age and whether this is the first or subsequent admission for critical care during the same hospital stay.

Coding Conundrum: Applying the Critical Care Definition

Although immaturity commonly leads to many levels of organ dysfunction that will increase the risk of a critical illness in a newborn, immaturity alone does not qualify for reporting critical care. The physician must use their experience and judgment in assigning the *CPT* definition of critical care. In summary, these are patients presently at clear risk of experiencing death or serious morbidity, requiring close observation and frequent interventions and assessments, and high-level MDM is apparent in the medical record documentation. Although immaturity alone does not define critical care, the complex decision-making applied to manage the therapeutic challenges manifesting in many preterm babies can support critical care. The most convincing way to demonstrate the appropriate application of a critical care code is to clearly document the neonate's condition in the medical record, noting the risks to the patient, frequency of needed assessments and interventions, degree and type of organ failure(s) the patient is presently experiencing, and level of the MDM.

- Only 1 individual reports daily critical care services for each patient per DOS. Other physicians and QHPs of different specialties and/or different group practices report critical care services with **99291** and, when appropriate, **99292**.

Examples

➤ **A 4-day-old (born at 39 weeks' gestation) is admitted following a pediatrician's outpatient evaluation of the neonate for decreased urine output and yellow skin tone.** A neonatologist accepts the pediatrician's referral for direct admission. The result of a bilirubin level ordered by the pediatrician is 32 mg/dL. On examination, the baby is sleepy, has difficulty feeding, and has a high-pitched cry. The mother's and baby's blood type is O Rh positive. The baby's Coombs (antiglobulin) test result is negative. After 4 hours of phototherapy, there is no change in bilirubin, and the neonatologist decides to do a total exchange transfusion given the risk of kernicterus. The neonatologist places umbilical catheters for the procedure.

Teaching Points: It is important to remember that respiratory and/or cardiovascular support (ie, mechanical ventilation) is not required to report critical care services. In this case, the risk of deterioration from bilirubin-induced neurological dysfunction qualifies as critical care. Code **99468** would be reported for the neonatologist's initial date of neonatal critical care services. The umbilical vessel catheterization is bundled with **99468**. The double-volume transfusion is reported with **36450**.

➤ **A 6-day-old born at 31 weeks' gestation with respiratory distress syndrome continues to require respiratory support via CPAP for apnea of prematurity.** The neonate continues to receive caffeine, partial parenteral nutrition by a peripheral vein, and intravenous (IV) antibiotics.

Code **99469** is reported because the medical record continues to document the neonate's continuous need for significant respiratory support and the continued need for critical care services.

Coding Conundrum: Apnea in Neonates

Apnea in neonates may be an expected component of preterm birth and may be effectively managed by manual stimulation, pharmacologic stimulation, high-flow nasal oxygen, or CPAP. At other times, this symptom is associated with a serious underlying problem(s) and reflects the instability of a critically ill neonate. When this is the case, one or more of the same interventions will be required. The physician must apply their best clinical judgment and clearly document the factors that make the patient's present condition critical (or require intensive care). The same requirements for organ failure, risk of imminent deterioration, and complex MDM apply. With apnea and many other conditions, the following information drives correct code selection: the total picture of the neonate with the diagnosis, clinical presentation, and immediate threat to life; the amount of hands-on and supervisory care provided by the physician; and the level of intervention needed to manage that neonate's conditions on a given day. When critical care codes are reported, the documentation must support the physician's judgment that the patient is critically ill and services provided are commensurate with the condition on the day of service on which critical care codes are reported.

Pediatric Critical Care

99471	Initial inpatient pediatric critical care, per day, for the E/M of a critically ill infant or young child, 29 days through 24 months of age
99472	Subsequent inpatient pediatric critical care, per day, for the E/M of a critically ill infant or young child, 29 days through 24 months of age
99475	Initial inpatient pediatric critical care, per day, for the E/M of a critically ill infant or young child, 2 through 5 years of age
99476	Subsequent inpatient pediatric critical care, per day, for the E/M of a critically ill infant or young child, 2 through 5 years of age

Services are provided to patients who are at least 29 days of age (postnatal age with day of birth being 0 [zero]) until the child reaches 6 years of age. Time-based critical care services (**99291**, **99292**) are reported for critical care services provided to children who are 6 years or older on the DOS.

Initial pediatric critical care codes (**99471**, **99475**) are reported by a single physician or QHP only once *per hospital stay* for a given patient. If the patient is stepped down from critical care to continued hospital care and then requires a subsequent episode of critical care during the same hospital stay, report a subsequent critical care code (**99472** or **99476**) for services on each date the child's condition remains critical.

Critical and Intensive Care

Chapter 17

Examples

➤ **A 22-month-old girl with status epilepticus is initially treated by the ED physician (1 hour of critical care).** Although seizures were initially controlled, pharmacologic management led to irregular respiratory activity, lethargy, and hypotension. The patient was admitted to the pediatric intensive care unit at 11:00 pm by the critical care attending physician, who intubated her, placed her on a ventilator, began fluid expansion, used dobutamine to control her blood pressure, and planned for a bedside electroencephalogram (EEG).

Teaching Point: The pediatrician or intensivist would report the initial inpatient pediatric critical care code (99471) for that calendar day, even though only 1 hour of care was provided. One hour later, after midnight, a new DOS would begin. The intubation is bundled with 99471 and cannot be separately billed.

The ED physician would report 1 hour of critical care (99291). Had the ED physician provided the intubation (31500) in addition to an hour of critical care, the ED physician would report both services.

➤ **A hospitalist admits a 5-year-old to observe for exacerbation of asthma that initially improved with treatment.** Later the same day, the patient is found to be in respiratory failure, and the hospitalist provides 35 minutes of critical care services before transferring the patient's care to a pediatric intensivist. The pediatric intensivist assumes management of the critically ill patient at 10:00 pm.

Teaching Point: The hospitalist reports initial hospital inpatient or observation care (99221–99223) according to the level of service provided and appends modifier 25 to indicate that this service is significant and separately identifiable from critical care services reported with 99291. The intensivist reports 99475 (initial inpatient pediatric critical care, per day, for the E/M of a critically ill infant or young child, 2 through 5 years of age). The intensivist will report 99476 for each subsequent calendar day on which critical care services are provided prior to the child's 6th birthday.

Daily critical care codes do not apply to children 6 years or older. If the child in this example were 6 years old, the intensivist would report 99291 and 99292 for time spent providing critical care services on each date that the child remained critically ill. If less than 30 minutes of critical care were provided on any date, hospital inpatient or observation care codes would be reported (initial, 99221–99223; subsequent, 99231–99233).

Patients Critically Ill After Surgery

Postoperative care of a surgical patient is included in the surgeon's global surgical package. For some neonatal surgical care, critical care days are included in the work values assigned to surgical procedures (eg, 39503, repair of diaphragmatic hernia; 43314, esophagoplasty, thoracic approach; with repair of tracheoesophageal fistula; 49605, repair of large omphalocele or gastroschisis; with or without prosthesis). Typically, the critical care represented within the surgical service is focused on care related to the patient's surgical condition and procedure and allows for additional, concurrent critical care by nonsurgical providers as needed to comprehensively address the patient's clinical requirements.

However, if a second physician (eg, intensivist, hospitalist) provides routine postoperative care for the patient, the surgeon must append modifier 54 (surgical care only) to the surgical code. (A formal transfer of care should be documented.)

When a payer has adopted Medicare policy, the intensivist accepting a transfer of care from a surgeon during a postoperative period reports modifier 55 (postoperative management only) and, if a critical care is unrelated to the surgical procedure, modifier FT (unrelated E/M visit during a postoperative period). The diagnosis code(s) reported should reflect the problem(s) addressed and may differ from the diagnosis for which the patient underwent surgery.

Example

➤ **A 1-month-old underwent bowel resection for volvulus and was recovering well 8 days after surgery.** On day 9, the patient's temperature is 38.4 °C (101.1 °F). The incision area is swollen and erythematous. Sepsis evaluation is initiated and antibiotics are started. Within hours, the patient becomes hypotensive, requiring vasopressors. The surgeon requests a transfer of care to an intensivist, who accepts the transfer and provides critical care to the critically ill patient.

Teaching Point: The services provided by the intensivist are beyond routine postoperative care. The intensivist reports 99471 (initial inpatient pediatric critical care, per day, for the E/M of a critically ill infant or young child, 29 days through 24 months of age). The intensivist will report 99472 for each subsequent calendar day on which critical care services are provided. The surgeon's postoperative care, other than a return to the operating/procedure room, is included in the global period of the surgery.

Initial and Continuing Intensive Care

99477 Initial hospital care, per day, for the E/M of the neonate, 28 days of age or younger, who requires intensive observation, frequent interventions, and other intensive care services

99478 Subsequent intensive care, per day, for the E/M of the recovering very low birth weight infant (present body weight less than 1500 grams)

99479 Subsequent intensive care, per day, for the E/M of the recovering low birth weight infant (present body weight of 1500–2500 grams)

99480 Subsequent intensive care, per day, for the E/M of the recovering infant (present body weight of 2501–5000 grams)

Continuing intensive care services provided to an infant weighing more than 5,000 g (approximately 11.02 lb) are reported with subsequent hospital care codes (99231–99233). Codes 99231–99233 are reported according to the documented level of MDM or the physician's or QHP's total time directed to the individual patient's care on the DOS.

Neonatal and pediatric intensive care codes (99477–99480) may be used to report daily care of neonates or infants who are not critically ill but have a need for intensive monitoring, observation, and frequent assessments by the health care team and supervision by the physician or QHP. This includes

- Neonates who require intensive but not critical care services from birth
- Neonates who are no longer critically ill but require intensive physician and health care team observation and interventions
- Recovering low-birth-weight infants who require a higher level of care than that defined by other hospital care services

These neonates or infants often have a continued need for oxygen, parenteral or gavage enteral nutrition, treatment of apnea of prematurity, and thermoregulation from an Isolette or radiant warmer and may be recovering from cardiac or surgical care. The intensive services described by these codes include one or more elements of intensive care such as intensive cardiac and respiratory monitoring, continuous and/or frequent vital sign monitoring, heat maintenance, enteral and/or parenteral nutritional adjustments, and laboratory and oxygen saturation monitoring when provided. Patients are under constant observation by the health care team, which is under direct supervision by a physician or QHP. Refer to the AAP *Newborn Coding Decision Tool 2026* (www.aap.org/Newborn-Coding-Decision-Tool-2026) for a continuum of care from normal newborn to neonatal critical care.

- **Table 17-4** illustrates codes for initial- (99477) and subsequent-day (99478–99480) neonatal and pediatric intensive care services by age and present body weight.

Table 17-4. Neonatal and Pediatric Intensive Care

Description	Present Weight <1,500 g	Present Weight 1,500–2,500 g	Present Weight 2,501–5,000 g	Present Weight ≥5,001 g
Initial intensive care of a neonate (28 days or less)	99477 (10.01 RVUs[a])			
Initial intensive care of an infant (29 days or older)	99221–99223 (2.46, 3.88, 5.17 RVUs)			
Subsequent intensive care	99478 (3.92 RVUs)	99479 (3.56 RVUs)	99480 (3.43 RVUs)	99231–99233 (1.43, 2.36, 3.52 RVUs)

Abbreviation: RVU, relative value units.

[a] Values shown are 2025 total facility RVUs, unadjusted for geographic area. Values for 2026 were unavailable at the time of this publication.

- Intensive care services (99477–99480) are bundled services and include the same procedures that are bundled with neonatal and pediatric critical care services (99468–99476). Refer to **Table 17-1** for a list of all the services and procedures that are included.

Code 99477 is used to report the more intensive services that an ill but not critically ill neonate (aged ≤28 days) requires on the day of admission to inpatient care. Code 99477 includes all E/M services on that date, excluding

- Attendance at delivery (99464) or newborn resuscitation (99465), which may be reported in addition to 99477, when performed.
- Normal newborn care (99460–99462), when performed.

Append modifier 25 to 99477 when reporting on the same date as 99460–99462, 99464, or 99465. Individual payer policies and code edits for multiple E/M services on the same date may vary.

- If the infant is older than 28 days at admission, codes 99221–99223 should be used for intensive care on the date of hospital admission (typically 99223, under the assumption that documentation supports high-level MDM or the documented total time is ≥75 minutes).
- Services are typically (but not required to be) provided in a NICU or special care unit and require a higher intensity of care than would be reported with 99221–99223 (initial hospital care of sick patient).
- ✖ Do not report 99477 twice in the same hospital admission. If a patient requires a new episode of intensive care during the same hospital stay, report subsequent intensive care services (99478–99480) for the first and each successive day that the patient requires intensive care services.
- Codes 99478–99480 depend on the *present* body weight of the infant, not the infant's age, on the DOS. Therefore, code selection may change from one day to the next depending on the infant's present body weight and condition.
- Codes 99478–99480 are typically used for subsequent days, as long as the neonate or infant continues to require intensive care, and include all the attending physician's or QHP's E/M services (and bundled procedures) provided to the patient on each DOS.
- Once the baby's weight exceeds 5,000 g, subsequent hospital care codes (99231–99233) are reported until the date of discharge (99238 –99239).

Examples

In these examples, the neonate is not critically ill but continues to require intensive monitoring and constant observation by the health care team under direct supervision by the reporting physician or QHP.

➤ **A neonate has mild respiratory distress on the initial date of hospital care at 2 days of age.** She is receiving 30% oxygen by low-flow nasal cannula, cardiorespiratory monitoring, and continuous pulse oximetry. Laboratory tests and radiographs are ordered, and IV fluids and antibiotics are started. Frequent monitoring and observation are required and ordered.

Code 99477 (initial hospital care for the ill neonate, 28 days of age or less, who requires intensive observation and monitoring) is reported by the attending physician or QHP. Procedures bundled with intensive care services (refer to **Table 17-1**) are not separately reported.

➤ **A 1,250-g infant, now 40 days old, is in stable condition while receiving 1 L of nasal cannula oxygen with fraction of inspired oxygen at 30%. The patient is receiving caffeine for apnea of prematurity, tolerates orogastric feedings, and requires use of an Isolette for temperature stability.**

Code 99478 is reported because the infant weighs less than 1,500 g.

➤ **A 15-day-old, 1,600-g neonate remains in an Isolette for thermoregulation and is receiving caffeine for intermittent apnea and bradycardia, for which the neonate requires continuous cardiorespiratory and pulse oximetry monitoring.** The physician adjusts the neonate's continuous gavage feedings according to tolerance and weight.

Code 99479 is reported for the infant whose present body weight is 1,500 to 2,500 g.

➤ **A baby requires intensive care and weighs 2,500 g on Monday.** The following day, she continues to require intensive care and her weight is 2,504 g.

Code 99479 is reported for the care provided on Monday. Code 99480 is reported for the continuing intensive care provided the following day.

Coding for Transitions to Different Levels of Neonatal Care

During a hospital stay, a newborn or readmitted neonate may require different levels of care. A normal newborn may end up becoming sick, intensively ill, or critical during the same hospital stay. Neonates who were initially sick may also improve to require lower levels of care (eg, normal neonatal care).

An initial-day critical or intensive care code (eg, 99468, 99477) is reported only once per hospital stay. If the patient recovers and is later stepped up again to that higher level of care, only the subsequent-level codes (99469, 99478–99480) are reported.

Refer to the AAP *Newborn Coding Decision Tool 2026* (www.aap.org/Newborn-Coding-Decision-Tool-2026) for numerous scenarios of coding for newborn care throughout admissions and transfers of care.

Emergency Medical Services Supervision and Patient Transport

Pediatric Critical Care Patient Transport

Face-to-Face Pediatric Critical Care Patient Transport

99466 Critical care face-to-face services, during an interfacility transport of critically ill or critically injured pediatric patient, 24 months of age or younger; first 30–74 minutes of hands-on care during transport

99467 each additional 30 minutes (List separately in addition to code 99466)

Codes 99466 and 99467 are used to report the physical attendance and direct face-to-face care provided by a physician or QHP during the inter-facility transport of a critically ill or injured patient 24 months or younger.

- The patient's condition must meet the *CPT* definition for critical care.
- Face-to-face time begins when the physician or other QHP assumes primary responsibility for the patient at the referring hospital or facility and ends when the receiving hospital or facility accepts responsibility for the patient's care. Only the time the physician spends in direct face-to-face contact with the patient during transport should be reported.
  - Time must be documented.
  - Code 99467 is used to report each additional 30 minutes of physician face-to-face time of critical care provided on the same day of service beyond the first 74 minutes reported with 99466.
- ✖ Less than 30 minutes of face-to-face time cannot be reported.
- Codes include the bundled services listed in **Table 17-1**. Codes 99466 and 99467 may be reported separately from any other procedures or services that are not bundled and performed on the date of transfer. The time involved in performing any procedures that are not bundled and are reported separately should not be included in the face-to-face transport time.
- Procedures or services that are performed by other members of the transport team with the physical presence, participation, and supervision of the accompanying physician may be reported by the physician. Documentation must support the physician's participation.
- Medical record documentation must include the total face-to-face time spent with the patient, the critical nature of the patient's condition, and any performed procedures that are not bundled.
- The pediatric critical care transport codes are preadmission codes and may be reported in addition to neonatal (99468) or pediatric (99471) initial-day critical care codes. For payers that have adopted NCCI edits, modifier 25 is required to indicate the significant and separately identifiable E/M services. Append modifier 25 to 99466 when reporting in conjunction with daily critical care codes.
- Face-to-face critical care services provided during an inter-facility transport of a child older than 24 months are reported with hourly critical care codes (99291 and 99292).
- If a neonatal NP employed by the neonatal group is on the transport team, the neonatal NP may report 99466 and 99467 if independent billing by a neonatal NP is allowed by the state and the activities are covered in the scope of practice. The neonatologist from that same group would not report 99485 and 99486 (physician direction of pediatric critical care transport) or 99288 (physician direction of emergency medical systems emergency care).
- If a neonatal NP employed by the hospital is on the transport team, the facility (hospital) could report 99466 and 99467. In this case, the neonatologist would report 99485 and 99486 for supervision of inter-facility transport because the neonatal NP is not of the same group practice.
- *CPT* does not include specific codes for face-to-face transport of a patient when criteria for critical care are not met. When face-to-face care during transport of a patient is medically necessary but critical care is not, report 99499 (unlisted E/M service).

Example

➤ **A 4-week-old with tetralogy of Fallot is brought to the local ED with concerns of feeding intolerance, blue lips, labored breathing, and crying.** Transport is dispatched from the regional neonatal center. On arrival, the transport neonatologist intubates the patient and administers morphine, which, over time, improves oxygen saturation. The neonatologist spends 50 minutes face-to-face evaluating and stabilizing the newborn at the transferring facility followed by 45 minutes during transport to the receiving nursery. Frequent assessments of vital signs and ventilator settings are performed during the transport. The neonatologist spent a total of 95 minutes of face-to-face critical care time with the neonate; 10 minutes is subtracted for time of the separately reported intubation. The time spent in critical care during the transport is 85 minutes. The neonatologist continues care of the newborn in the NICU.

99466 25 (first 74 minutes).

99467 25 × 1 unit (final 11 minutes).

31500 (endotracheal intubation, emergency).

99468 25 (initial daily inpatient neonatal critical care).

Modifier 25 is appended to each of the codes for E/M services to designate a significant and separately identifiable E/M service provided by the same physician on the same DOS. Endotracheal intubation is bundled with daily neonatal critical care but is separately reported when provided during transport of the critically ill or injured neonate.

Non–Face-to-Face Pediatric Critical Care Patient Transport

#99485 Supervision by a control physician of interfacility transport care of the critically ill or critically injured pediatric patient, 24 months of age or younger, includes two-way communication with transport team before transport, at the referring facility and during the transport, including data interpretation and report; first 30 minutes

#99486 each additional 30 minutes (List separately in addition to code 99485)

Code 99485 is used to report the first 16 to 45 minutes of a control physician's documented non–face-to-face supervision of inter-facility critical care transport of a patient 24 months or younger, which includes all 2-way communication between the control physician and the specialized transport team before transport, at the referring facility, and during transport to the receiving facility.

Each additional 30-minute period of communication is reported with add-on code 99486.

- The patient's condition must meet the *CPT* definition of critical care.
- Only report for patients 24 months or younger who are critically ill or injured.
- The control physician does not report any services provided by the specialized transport team.
- The control physician reports only cumulative time spent communicating with the specialty transport team members during an inter-facility transport. Communication between the control physician and the referring facility before or following patient transport *is not* counted.
- Reportable time begins with the initial discussions with the transport team, including discussions of the best mode of transport and strategies for therapy on arrival. Time ends when the patient's care is handed over to the receiving facility team.
- Time spent with the individual patient's transport team and reviewing data submissions should be recorded. Time spent discussing the patient with the referring physician or facility is not counted.
- Total communication time of 15 minutes or less is not reported with 99485. Code 99288, discussed in the Direction of Emergency Medical Services section later in this chapter, may be reported when requirements for 99485 are not met.
- Codes 99485 and 99486 represent preadmission services and may be reported by the same or different individual(s) of the same specialty and same group when neonatal or pediatric critical care services (99468–99476) are reported for the same patient on the same day.

✖ Do not report 99485 or 99486 for services of 15 minutes or less or for any time spent in supervision of a QHP from the same group who is reporting 99466 or 99467.

Example

➤ **A 3-week-old with respiratory distress and possible sepsis requires transfer.** The pediatric intensivist dispatches the transport team, consisting of a hospital-employed transport nurse and a respiratory therapist. On the trip to the referring hospital, the intensivist converses by telephone for 10 minutes with the team, explaining the neonate's condition and formulating an initial treatment plan. After arrival, the nurse evaluates the neonate and telephones the intensivist to discuss the findings. The decision is made to transport the patient. Because of the critical nature of the

Critical and Intensive Care

Chapter 17

neonate, the intensivist elects to remain on the telephone until transport is in motion and the patient's condition is critical but stable (15 minutes). On the return trip, another telephone contact lasting 10 minutes is made to receive additional guidance from the intensivist on the neonate's worsening respiratory status. The transport is completed and the neonate is admitted.

The intensivist spent a total of 35 minutes in direct 2-way telephone communication with the team in 3 discrete episodes. The intensivist carefully documents the time spent in communication with the transport team, the nature of the neonate's critical illness, and what decisions were made during each contact in the medical record. Code **99485** is used to report this service.

Direction of Emergency Medical Services

99288 Physician or other QHP direction of emergency medical systems (EMS) emergency care, advanced life support

Refer to the Non–Face-to-Face Pediatric Critical Care Patient Transport section earlier in this chapter for discussion of physician non–face-to-face supervision of inter-facility transport of a critically ill or injured pediatric patient 24 months or younger (**99485–99486**).

Code **99288**

- May be reported by any physician of any specialty or QHP when advanced life support services are provided via 2-way voice communications (eg, cardiac and/or pulmonary resuscitation; administration of IV fluids, antibiotics, or surfactant).
- This code reflects all the services provided by the directing physician and is not based on any time requirements. Code **99288** may be reported when less than 16 minutes is spent in physician non–face-to-face supervision of inter-facility transport of a critically ill or injured pediatric patient (ie, requirements for reporting **99485** are not met).
- The directing physician should maintain documentation of the times of all contacts, orders, and/or directions for treatment or management of the patient.
- Services or procedures performed by EMS personnel are not reported by the physician because the physician was not physically present.
- When an advanced practice professional provides and reports face-to-face services during transport, the physician does not report **99288**.
- The appropriate diagnoses are linked to the service.

If, after directing EMS personnel, the physician performs the initial critical care, the appropriate critical care code (eg, **99468**, initial daily inpatient neonatal critical care) will also be reported. Modifier **25** may be required to indicate that 2 separate and distinct E/M services were provided by the same physician on the same day of service.

There is no Medicare relative value unit (RVU) assigned to this service, so it is carrier priced and payments will vary by payer.

Medicare considers **99288** a bundled service and does not pay separately for the service. Check with your Medicaid program and other payers to determine their coverage policy.

Total Body Systemic and Selective Head Hypothermia

99184 Initiation of selective head or total body hypothermia in the critically ill neonate, includes appropriate patient selection by review of clinical, imaging and laboratory data, confirmation of esophageal temperature probe location, evaluation of amplitude EEG, supervision of controlled hypothermia, and assessment of patient tolerance of cooling

(Do not report **99184** more than once per hospital stay)

Code **99184** describes a service provided to a neonate and is not applicable to use of therapeutic hypothermia in older children.

Example

➤ **A full-term neonate born with evidence of hypoxic-ischemic encephalopathy is admitted to the NICU and receives critical care services.** Laboratory, EEG, blood gas, and imaging studies confirm that the neonate meets objective criteria for *total body cooling.* Continuous total body cooling is undertaken on the same date.

Code **99184** is reported for total body systemic hypothermia in addition to **99468** (initial day of neonatal critical care).

Code 99184 is also reported when selective head hypothermia is initiated (rather than total body systemic hypothermia).

When total body systemic or selective head hypothermia is used in treatment of a critically ill neonate, 99184 represents the work of initiating the service.

Documentation for use of total body systemic hypothermia and selective head hypothermia should include the neonatal criteria that support initiating this service.

- During either cooling approach, monitoring includes
  - Radiographic confirmation of core temperature probe (either esophageal or rectal probe)
  - Continuous core temperature assessment and adjustment
  - Repeat assessment of skin integrity
  - Recurrent objective evaluation of evolving neurological changes (eg, Sarnat stage), which may also include assessment of continuous amplitude EEG monitoring
- In addition, cooling-related laboratory evaluations are required to monitor for cooling-specific complications, including metabolic and coagulation alterations.

The physician providing interpretation and report of an EEG performed during hypothermia will report the appropriate code appended with modifier 26 (professional service). For discussion of modifier 26, refer to Chapter 2.

Extracorporeal Membrane Oxygenation or Extracorporeal Life Support Services

Prolonged extracorporeal membrane oxygenation (ECMO) and extracorporeal life support (ECLS) services commonly involve multiple physicians and supporting health care personnel to manage each patient. ECMO and ECLS codes differentiate components of initiation and daily management of ECMO and ECLS from daily management of a patient's overall medical condition.

These services include cannula insertion (33951–33956), ECMO or ECLS initiation (33946, 33947), daily ECMO or ECLS management (33948, 33949), repositioning of the ECMO or ECLS cannula(e) (33957–33964), and cannula removal (33965–33986).

ECMO/ECLS Cannula Insertion, Repositioning, and Removal

Codes for insertion, repositioning, and removal of ECMO and ECLS are reported according to the patient's age, with separate codes for procedures performed in newborns and children through 5 years of age and in patients 6 years and older. Codes for these services are shown in **Table 17-5**. Although these services are typically performed only by surgeons, other pediatric providers may perform them as well.

- ✖ Do not separately report repositioning of the ECMO or ECLS cannula(e) (33957–33964) at the same session as insertion (33951–33956).
- Report replacement of ECMO or ECLS cannula(e) in the same vessel with only the insertion code (33951–33956).
- If a cannula(e) is (are) removed from one vessel and a new cannula(e) is (are) placed in a different vessel, report the appropriate cannula(e) removal (33965–33986) and insertion (33951–33956) codes.
- ✖ Fluoroscopic guidance used for cannula(e) repositioning (33957–33964) is included in the procedure when performed and should not be separately reported.
- Extensive repair or replacement of an artery may be additionally reported (eg, 35226, 35286, 35371, 35665).
- Direct anastomosis of a prosthetic graft to the artery sidewall to facilitate arterial perfusion for ECMO or ECLS is separately reported with 33987 in addition to 33953–33956.

+33987 Arterial exposure with creation of graft conduit (eg, chimney graft) to facilitate arterial perfusion for ECMO/ECLS (List separately in addition to code for primary procedure)

- ✖ Do not report 33987 in conjunction with codes for open arterial exposure services (34714, 34716, or 34833).

ECMO/ECLS Initiation and Daily Management

33946 ECMO/ECLS provided by physician; initiation, venovenous
33947 initiation, venoarterial
33948 daily management, each day, venovenous
33949 daily management, each day, venoarterial

• indicates a new code; ▲, revised; #, re-sequenced; +, add-on; ★, audiovisual technology; and ◀, synchronous interactive audio.

Table 17-5. Extracorporeal Membrane Oxygenation or Extracorporeal Life Support Cannula(e) Procedures

Approach	Birth Through 5 Years of Age	6 Years and Older	Do Not Report With (not a comprehensive list)
Insertion			
Percutaneous peripheral (arterial/venous) cannula(e)[a]	33951	33952	33957–33964
Open peripheral (arterial/venous) cannula(e)	33953	33954	33957–33964, 34714–34716, 34812, 34820, 34833–34834
Central cannula(e) by sternotomy or thoracotomy	33955	33956	33957–33964, 32100, 39010
Reposition[b]			
Percutaneous, reposition peripheral (arterial and/or venous) cannula(e)[a]	33957	33958	33946, 33947, 34713
Open, reposition peripheral (arterial and/or venous) cannula(e)[a]	33959	33962	33946, 33947, 34714–34716, 34812, 34820, 34834
Central cannula(e) reposition by sternotomy or thoracotomy[a]	33963	33964	33946, 33947, 32100, 39010
Removal[c]			
Removal of peripheral (arterial and/or venous) cannula(e), percutaneous	33965	33966	Not applicable
Removal of peripheral (arterial and/or venous) cannula(e), open	33969	33984	34812, 34820, 34834, 35201, 35206, 35211, 35216, 35226
Removal of central cannula(e) by sternotomy or thoracotomy	33985	33986	35211

[a] Includes fluoroscopic guidance when performed.
[b] Repositioning of cannula(e) at the same session, as insertion is not separately reported.
[c] Report only the insertion when cannula(e) is replaced in the same vessel.

Initiation of the ECMO or ECLS circuit and setting parameters (33946, 33947) involves determining the necessary ECMO or ECLS device components, blood flow, gas exchange, and other necessary parameters to manage the circuit.

Daily care for a patient receiving ECMO or ECLS includes managing the ECMO or ECLS circuit and related patient issues. These services may be performed by one physician while another physician manages the patient's overall medical condition and underlying disorders, but a single physician may provide both services. Regardless of the patient's condition, the basic management of ECMO and ECLS is similar. Documentation for each service should be distinct in the medical record.

- ✖ Do not report modifier 63 (procedure performed on infants <4 kg) when reporting codes 33946–33949.
- The physician reporting daily ECMO or ECLS oversees the interaction of the circuit with the patient, management of blood flow, oxygenation, carbon dioxide clearance by the membrane lung, systemic response, anticoagulation and treatment of bleeding, cannula positioning, alarms and safety, and weaning the patient from the ECMO or ECLS circuit when heart and/or lung function has sufficiently recovered.
- Daily management of the patient may be separately reported with the relevant hospital observation services, hospital inpatient services, or critical care E/M codes (99221–99223, 99231–99233, 99234–99236, 99291, 99292, 99468–99480).
- Daily management (33948, 33949) or cannula repositioning (33957–33959, 33962–33964) may not be reported on the same date as initiation (33946, 33947) by the same or different physician.
- Conversion of venovenous to venoarterial ECMO on a date subsequent to the venovenous initiation may be reported by the managing physician with the initial venoarterial management code (33947) on the day of conversion (rather than a subsequent-day service).

Each physician providing part of the ECMO/ECLS services may report the services they provide except when prohibited by *CPT* instruction (eg, cannula repositioning is not reported by the same or another physician on the same date as initiation of ECMO/ECLS).

● indicates a new code; ▲, revised; #, re-sequenced; ✚, add-on; ★, audiovisual technology; and ◀, synchronous interactive audio.

Example

➤ **Venoarterial ECMO is initiated for a 10-year-old patient with cardiac and respiratory failure.** Physician A inserts the cannulae. Physician B manages the initial transition to ECMO, including the work with Physician A, ECMO specialists, and others to initiate an ongoing assessment of anticoagulation, venous return, cannula positioning, and optimal flow. Physician B also provides daily management of the patient's overall care. When ECMO is discontinued, Physician A returns and removes the cannulae.

Physician A will report codes for insertion and later removal of the ECMO cannulae (eg, 33952 and 33966) with the appropriate dates of each service. Physician B will report the code for initiation of venoarterial ECMO (33947), the appropriate hospital and/or critical care codes for overall treatment of the patient for each day provided (eg, 99468–99476; 99291, 99292; or 99231–99233), and the code for daily management of ECMO (33949) for each day provided.

Sedation

Refer to **Chapter 13** for specific guidelines for reporting moderate (conscious) sedation (99151–99157). Refer to **Chapter 18** for guidelines for reporting deep sedation.

Car Seat/Bed Testing

94780 Car seat/bed testing for airway integrity, for infants through 12 months of age, with continual clinical staff observation and continuous recording of pulse oximetry, heart rate and respiratory rate, with interpretation and report; 60 minutes

+94781 each additional full 30 minutes (List separately in addition to 94780.)

Neonates who required critical care during their initial hospital stay are most often the patients who require monitoring to determine whether they may be safely transported in a car seat or must be transported in a car bed. This testing is often performed in anticipation of discharge on a date when the neonate is receiving intensive care services. Codes 94780 and 94781 are bundled under neonatal and pediatric critical and intensive care codes (99468–99472, 99477–99480) and not separately reported.

However, the testing can be reported in conjunction with normal newborn or other hospital care services (eg, subsequent hospital care services 99231–99233; hospital discharge services 99238, 99239), when performed.

Report 94780 and 94781 when the following conditions are met:

- The patient must be an infant (ie, aged ≤12 months). Assessment is not limited to neonates and may be necessary in older infants.
- Continual clinical staff observation with continuous recording of pulse oximetry, heart rate, and respiratory rate is required.
- Inpatient or office-based services are reported.
- Vital signs and observations must be reviewed and interpreted and a written report generated by the physician.
- Codes are reported according to the total observation time spent and documented.
- If less than 60 minutes is spent in the procedure, 94780 may not be reported.
- Each additional full 30 minutes (ie, not <90 minutes total) is reported with 94781.
- ✖ Do not include the time of car seat/bed testing in time attributed to discharge day management services (99238, 99239).
- These codes may be reported in addition to hospital E/M services other than those reported with neonatal and pediatric critical and intensive care codes (99468–99472, 99477–99480).

Example

➤ **A neonate with Down syndrome who previously required neonatal intensive care has improved and requires a car seat test prior to anticipated discharge from the hospital.** A nurse places the neonate into the car seat and records the neonate's pulse oximetry, heart rate, and respiratory rate. The test is discontinued at 70 minutes in response to an episode of low oxygen saturation. The ordering physician reviews the data and creates a report and recommendations based on the findings. Not including time spent in the separately reported test interpretation and report, the physician's documented total time on this date is 40 minutes (eg, revising a plan of care, counseling parents, documenting the E/M service).

99232 25 Subsequent hospital inpatient or observation care with total time ≥35 minutes
94780 first 60 minutes

Code 94780 is reported for the first 60 minutes of testing. The last 10 minutes of testing is not reported with 94781 because only periods of no less than 30 minutes are reported.

Subsequent hospital care code 99232 is reported with modifier 25 appended to indicate that the E/M service was significant and separately identifiable from the physician's work associated with the test. If the newborn were receiving neonatal intensive or critical care on the date of car seat testing, the testing would not be separately reported.

Values and Payment

Although not exact or applicable for every patient, the preservice, intraservice, and postservice times assigned to codes for neonatal and pediatric critical and intensive care services provide a point of reference for differentiation of the services. RVUs for each code also allow for comparison of the work and time included in each service. "RUC Times and Values for Pediatric Critical Care/Intensive Care Services" is included at www.aap.org/cfp2026.

Payment Advocacy

The AAP encourages chapter development of pediatric councils as forums to discuss pediatric issues with payers. Pediatric councils have the potential to facilitate better working relationships between pediatricians and health insurance plans and to improve quality of care for children. To learn more about AAP pediatric councils, visit www.aap.org/en/practice-management/child-health-finance-payment-strategy/payment-and-finance-advocacy/aap-pediatric-councils.

The AAP Section on Neonatal-Perinatal Medicine, in conjunction with state chapters and councils of the AAP, has developed strategies that have been successful in addressing payment concerns for neonatal care. Contact your state chapter, its pediatric council, your section district AAP Executive Committee representative, a neonatal trainer, or the AAP Committee on Coding and Nomenclature for assistance in addressing any payment inequities for neonatal services in your state.

To test your knowledge of the information presented in this chapter, complete the quiz found at the end of it, after the resources. Answers to each quiz are found in **Appendix II**. Add to your knowledge through the information provided in other chapters that discuss codes for specific types of service.

Chapter Takeaways

This chapter reviewed the definitions of critical care and neonatal intensive care and code assignment for many services often provided to a critically ill or injured patient. Following are some takeaways from this chapter:

- A critical illness or injury is defined by *CPT* as one acutely impairing one or more vital organs such that there is a high probability of imminent or life-threatening deterioration of the patient's condition.
- Physicians should be aware of services that are included in the critical and intensive care services and those that can be reported separately in addition to codes for critical or intensive care services.
- When multiple physicians and QHPs provide critical or intensive care services on the same date, it is important to report the correct codes for the service provided (eg, daily critical or intensive care by the attending physician vs concurrent time-based critical care or hospital care by consulting physicians or QHPs).
- When reporting multiple E/M services provided by the same individual(s) of the same specialty and same group practice, refer to the payer's code edits (eg, NCCI edits) to determine if modifier 25 (significant, separately identifiable E/M service) is required to designate the separately reportable services.
- Payer guidelines, state regulations, and other factors, such as employment status, affect how services provided by QHPs are reported in conjunction with a physician's services on the same date. Neonatal NPs, who are not employed by a facility, may be able to independently report services.

Resources

AAP Coding Assistance and Education

AAP pediatric councils (www.aap.org/en/practice-management/child-health-finance-payment-strategy/payment-and-finance-advocacy/aap-pediatric-councils)

AAP Section on Neonatal-Perinatal Medicine Coding Corner (www.aap.org/en/community/aap-sections/sonpm/neonatologists/coding-corner)

AAP Section on Neonatal-Perinatal Medicine coding trainers are available to provide coding education through local educational seminars and continuing education events. Contact section manager Jim Couto (jcouto@aap.org) for additional information about these valuable services.

Newborn Coding Decision Tool 2026 (www.aap.org/Newborn-Coding-Decision-Tool-2026)

AAP Pediatric Coding Newsletter™

"Coding for Abnormalities in Fetal Growth," December 2020 (https://doi.org/10.1542/pcco_book200_document002)

"Coding Examples: Neonatal Critical Care and Intensive Care Services," February 2024 (https://doi.org/10.1542/pcco_book238_document004)

"Neonatal Coding Review: Daily Intensive or Critical Care Services," February 2024 (https://doi.org/10.1542/pcco_book238_document002)

"Understanding Age Ranges in *Current Procedural Terminology*," May 2023 (https://doi.org/10.1542/pcco_book229_document005)

Online-Exclusive Content at www.aap.org/cfp2026

"Global Per Diem Critical Care Codes: Direct Supervision and Reporting Guidelines"

"RUC Times and Values for Pediatric Critical Care/Intensive Care Services"

Test Your Knowledge!

1. **Which must be provided to support a neonatal resuscitation service reported using 99465?**
   a. Positive pressure ventilation and/or cardiac compressions in the presence of acute inadequate ventilation and/or cardiac output
   b. Continuous positive airway pressure without positive pressure ventilation
   c. Surfactant administration
   d. Endotracheal intubation
2. **True or false? Only 1 initial daily inpatient critical care code (99468, 99471, 99475) is reported per hospital stay for a given patient.**
   a. True
   b. False
3. **What code is reported for critical care of a neonate who becomes critically ill on a day when initial or subsequent intensive care services (99477–99480) has been provided by physician(s) or QHP(s) from the same group practice?**
   a. Codes for the intensive care and hourly critical care (99291–99292) services
   b. Either an initial or subsequent critical care code (99468 or 99469), as appropriate
   c. Codes for the intensive care and for subsequent daily critical care service (99469)
   d. Only the appropriate code for the intensive care service
4. **Which differentiates subsequent intensive care service codes 99478–99480?**
   a. The patient's age on the DOS
   b. The patient's current weight
   c. The type of unit to which the patient was admitted
   d. Whether or not the patient has previously received critical care services
5. **Which is true of ECMO initiation and management codes 33946–33949?**
   a. The service is time based and face-to-face time must be documented.
   b. The services include managing the ECMO or ECLS circuit and related patient issues.
   c. The services include managing the patient's overall medical condition and underlying disorders.
   d. Modifier 63 is appended to 33946–33949 when the patient weighs less than 4 kg.

CHAPTER 18

Common Surgical Procedures and Sedation in Facility Settings

Contents

Chapter Highlights

- Work that is included in the surgical package and global periods of surgery
- Reporting postoperative care
- Reporting special circumstances (eg, partial procedures, work of an assistant surgeon)
- Teaching physician guidelines for reporting surgical procedures
- Anesthesia and sedation

Surgical Package Rules

This chapter discusses coding for surgery and related services in a facility setting. *Current Procedural Terminology* (*CPT*®) surgical codes (**10004–69990**) are packaged or global codes including all the necessary services normally furnished by a surgeon before, during, and after a procedure. *CPT* defines only a surgical package, whereas the Centers for Medicare & Medicaid Services (CMS) defines the surgical package in terms of global periods based on the preoperative, intraoperative, and postoperative work values assigned to each procedure.

- Most Medicaid programs and private payers follow the CMS definition, but some plans apply different postoperative periods (eg, 30-day global period).

Both *CPT* and the CMS agree that

- Surgical codes include local infiltration, metacarpal/metatarsal/digital block, or topical anesthesia by the physician performing the procedure.
- Preoperative care
  - Includes evaluation and management (E/M) service(s) *subsequent to the decision for surgery* (eg, assessing the site and condition, explaining the procedure, obtaining informed consent) on the day before and/or on the date of the procedure, including history and physical examination.
  - When the initial decision to perform surgery is made on the day before or on the day of surgery, the appropriate-level E/M visit may be reported separately with modifier **57** (decision for surgery) appended. This modifier shows the payer that the E/M service was necessary to make the decision for surgery (ie, not the routine preoperative evaluation).
  - When an E/M service performed on the day of the procedure is unrelated to the decision to perform surgery and is significant and distinct from the usual preoperative care associated with the procedure, it may be reported with modifier **25** (significant, separately identifiable E/M service by the same physician on the same day of the procedure or other service) appended.
  - Medical record documentation must support that the service was significant, separately identifiable, and medically necessary. An E/M service performed before the decision to perform the procedure is separately reportable.
  - Different diagnoses are not required when reporting an E/M visit and procedure.

Medicare Policy Addresses Preoperative Care Differently for Minor and Major Procedures

When a payer adopts Medicare policy, the E/M visit on the date of a minor procedure (ie, procedure assigned a 0- or 10-day global period or endoscopy) is considered a routine part of the procedure regardless of whether it is prior or subsequent to the decision for surgery. In these cases, modifier 57 is not recognized.

An E/M code may be reported on the same day as a minor surgical procedure only when a significant, separately identifiable E/M service is performed; modifier 25 is appended to the E/M code.

When the initial decision to perform a major surgical procedure (ie, procedure assigned a 90-day global period) is made on the day before or on the day of a procedure, the E/M service may be reported with modifier 57 appended. Medical record documentation should support that the decision for surgery was made during the encounter and that time was spent in performing counseling of the risks, benefits, and outcomes.

- Postoperative care includes
  - All associated typical postoperative care (eg, dictating progress notes; counseling with the patient, family, and/or other physicians; writing orders; evaluating the patient in the postanesthesia recovery area)

Common Surgical Procedures and Sedation in Facility Settings

Chapter 18

- Only the care that is usually part of the surgical service for therapeutic surgical procedures (eg, suture and/or staple removal, care of incisions)
  - Only the care that is related to the recovery from the diagnostic procedure (eg, endoscopies, arthroscopies, injection procedures for radiography)

CPT allows separate reporting of postoperative management of complications, exacerbations, recurrence, treatment of unrelated diseases or injuries, or the presence of other diseases or injuries that require additional services in the postoperative care.

When Payers Adopt Medicare Policy for Reporting Postoperative Medical or Surgical Services

When a payer adopts Medicare's policy for care during the postoperative period, it is important to recognize one significant difference from *CPT*'s description of postoperative work, as follows:

- **All additional medical or surgical services required of the surgeon during the postoperative period of the surgery to address complications *that do not require additional trips to the operating/procedure room* (OR) are included in the global package (not separately reported).**

Like *CPT*, Medicare policy does not include treatment of the underlying condition or an added course of treatment that is not part of normal recovery from surgery. (Refer to discussion of related modifiers 24, 58, and 79 in the Global Periods and Modifiers for Reporting Postoperative Care section that follows.)

Global Periods and Modifiers for Reporting Postoperative Care

The CMS-designated global periods for each *CPT* procedure code can be found on the Resource-Based Relative Value Scale of the Medicare Physician Fee Schedule (MPFS) at www.cms.gov/medicare/payment/fee-schedules/physician/pfs-relative-value-files.

- It designates specific postoperative periods for certain procedure codes (ie, 0, 10, or 90 days). When determining the postoperative period, *the day after surgery* is day 1 of a 10- or 90-day period.
- Physicians append modifier 78 to the procedure code for return to the OR for a related procedure during a postoperative period. This includes return to the OR for treatment of complications of the first procedure.
- For return to the OR for staged or more extensive procedures and therapeutic procedures following a diagnostic procedure, append modifier 58.
- Report procedures during the postoperative period that are unrelated and not caused by complications of the original procedure with modifier 79 and unrelated E/M services with modifier 24 (documentation is typically required before payment).
- Other codes are designated YYY, which means the postoperative period is set by the carrier. There are no associated postoperative days included in the payment for codes assigned with status codes XXX (the global concept does not apply) or ZZZ (assigned to an add-on code [AOC] for a service that is always related to another service to which the global period is assigned).

Reporting Postoperative Care

- Report 99024 (postoperative follow-up visit) for follow-up care provided by the physician who performed a procedure (or the covering physician or other qualified health care professional [QHP]) during the global surgery period.
  - Reporting of inpatient or observation follow-up visits is typically not required.
  - Reporting 99024 allows a practice to track the number of visits performed by individuals during the postoperative period of specific procedures, calculate office overhead expenses (eg, supplies, staff, physician time) associated with the procedure, and potentially use the data to negotiate higher payment rates.

Payers track the postoperative care provided. If a physician is not providing or reporting the postoperative care (99024) typically performed for a procedure, payers may reduce payment for the surgical service because payment includes postoperative care as part of the procedure.

- When physicians from different practices perform part of a surgical package, the procedure should be reported with one of the following modifiers:
  - 54 (surgical care only)
  - 55 (postoperative management only)
  - 56 (preoperative management only)

Refer to Chapter 2 for a more detailed description of modifiers. For critical care following surgery, refer to the Patients Critically Ill After Surgery section in Chapter 17.

These situations require communication among the surgeon, the physician providing preoperative or postoperative care, and each physician's respective billing personnel to ensure accurate reporting and payment.

- No modifier is required when a physician (different specialty or group practice) other than the surgeon provides unrelated services to a patient during the postoperative period.

Despite the use of different National Provider Identifiers and diagnosis codes, some payers with assigned global surgical periods will deny unrelated services provided by any physician or QHP during a postoperative period. The claim should be appealed for payment with a letter advising the payer that the service was unrelated to any surgery.

Physicians and QHPs assuming postoperative management for a procedure performed by a physician in another group practice (eg, practicing in a different geographic area) should note payer policies for reporting these services.

Generally, the code for the procedure is appended with modifier 55 as described in this chapter. But Medicare has established an AOC, G0559, that is reported in addition to the first office or other outpatient E/M service for postoperative management when there is no formal transfer of care *and the physician who performed the procedure did not append modifier 54 to the procedure code.* The following components of service are required when reporting G0559:

- **Read available surgical note to understand the relative success of the procedure, the anatomy that was affected, and potential complications that could have arisen from the unique circumstances of the patient's operation.**
- **Research the procedure to determine expected postoperative course and potential complications (in the case of providing postoperative care for a procedure outside the specialty).**
- **Evaluate and physically examine the patient to determine whether the postoperative course is progressing appropriately.**
- **Communicate with the practitioner who performed the procedure if any questions or concerns arise.**

G0559 should not be billed by another physician or QHP in the same group practice as the individual who performed the surgical procedure. Report G0559 only once at the initial E/M service during the 90-day global period.

Removal of Sutures and/or Staples

15851 Removal of sutures or staples requiring anesthesia (ie, general anesthesia, moderate sedation)

Code 15851 is reported only when the patient requires general anesthesia or moderate sedation during suture or staple removal.

#+15853 Removal of sutures or staples not requiring anesthesia

#+15854 Removal of sutures and staples not requiring anesthesia

- Codes 15853 and 15854 are AOCs reported only in conjunction with a related E/M service in the office, emergency department (ED), or home/residence.

Do not report removal of sutures or staples

- In conjunction with hospital inpatient or observation E/M services
- Within the global period of the related procedure

Multiple Procedures on the Same Date

Multiple, separately reportable services are often provided in 1 session or on 1 date of service (DOS). But it is important to recognize which surgical services are considered a component of another procedure and which are separately reported.

- It is not appropriate to report multiple Healthcare Common Procedure Coding System (HCPCS)/*CPT* codes when a single, comprehensive HCPCS/*CPT* code describes the procedures performed.

Example

➤ **Code 42820 describes tonsillectomy and adenoidectomy in a patient younger than 12 years.** It would not be appropriate to separately report 42825 (tonsillectomy) and 42830 (adenoidectomy).

- Surgical access (eg, laparotomy) is integral to more comprehensive procedures (eg, appendectomy) and not separately reported.

Common Surgical Procedures and Sedation in Facility Settings

Chapter 18

• indicates a new code; ▲, revised; #, re-sequenced; +, add-on; ★, audiovisual technology; and ◀, synchronous interactive audio.

- When the surgical approach fails, report only the code for the approach that resulted in the completed procedure. For example, if laparoscopy fails and an open approach is used to complete the procedure, report only the open procedure.
- It is recommended to adopt a process for checking the National Correct Coding Initiative (NCCI) edits or payer-specific edit tools before submitting multiple procedure codes for services on the same date. Code edit tools may be provided through a provider portal.
- For Medicaid, the NCCI manual is informative regarding correct reporting and use of modifiers to override NCCI edits.
- When more than one procedure/service is performed on the same date, during the same session, or during a postoperative period, several *CPT* modifiers may apply. Documentation must support the reason for applying a modifier (eg, indicate a separate incision).
  - Modifier **59** (distinct procedural service) is often appended to surgical procedure codes to override payer edits that would otherwise not allow payment for services that may be components of other services.
  - It is important to carefully consider whether other modifiers are more appropriate (eg, **50**, bilateral service; an anatomical modifier such as **E4**, lower right eyelid) to indicate a distinct service.

Refer to Chapter 2 for more information on the NCCI.

Separate Procedure Designation

One designation in *CPT* helps identify procedures that are commonly performed as an integral component of another procedure. The parenthetical comment "(separate procedure)" follows the code descriptor for these services.

- Services designated as separate procedures should not be reported in addition to the code for the total procedure or service of which they are considered an integral component.
- A procedure or service that is designated as a separate procedure may be
  - Carried out independently and be the only code reported
  - Considered to be unrelated or distinct from other procedures/services provided at that time and reported in addition to other procedures/services by appending modifier **59** (distinct procedural service) or HCPCS modifiers **XE** (separate encounter), **XS** (separate structure), **XP** (separate practitioner), or **XU** (unusual non-overlapping service)

Modifiers Used in Reporting Procedural Services

Increased Procedural Service

Modifier **22** (increased procedural service) may be appended to the code for a surgical procedure when the work required to provide the service was *significantly greater* than typically required for that procedure. To substantiate modifier **22**, documentation must support that the procedure was more difficult because one or more of the following conditions were met:

- Increased intensity or time
- Technical difficulty
- The severity of the patient's condition
- Significantly increased physical and mental effort

Common Surgical Procedures and Sedation in Facility Settings

Chapter 18

Example

➤ **A child undergoes laparoscopic surgery for acute appendicitis with rupture.** The procedure takes 45 minutes longer than typical because of the subhepatic location and rupture of the appendix. The surgeon documents the increased work and time of the procedure and reports

44970 22 Laparoscopy, surgical, appendectomy

Teaching Point: The operative report should support the increased work of the procedure by detailing the increased work related to the subhepatic location and rupture of the appendix.

Reporting Terminated or Partial Procedures

- When a procedure is started but cannot be completed because of extenuating circumstances, physicians should consider the individual situation, including the reason for termination of the procedure and the amount of work that was performed, when determining how to report the service rendered.
- When a procedure is performed but not entirely successful (eg, portion of foreign body removed), it may be appropriate to report the procedure code that represents the work performed without modification.

- Report reduced services (modifier 52) or a discontinued procedure (modifier 53) only when the service was significantly reduced from the typical service and as instructed in *CPT.*

Examples

➤ ***CPT* instructs to append modifier 52 (reduced service) to 36572, 36573, or 36584 when insertion or replacement of a peripherally inserted central venous catheter (PICC) is performed without confirmation of catheter tip location (eg, via radiography or ultrasonography).**

➤ **A physician performs diagnostic flexible, transoral esophagogastroscopy on a patient without examination of the duodenum because it is not clinically indicated.** The physician reports 43235 52.

➤ **A physician performs diagnostic flexible, transoral esophagogastroscopy but cannot fully complete the examination because of concern for the patient's well-being if the procedure is continued.** The physician reports 43235 53.

- If the work performed before discontinuation is insignificant, it may be appropriate to not report the procedure.
- When not reporting the procedure, consider whether the level of a related E/M service was increased because of the level of medical decision-making (MDM) associated with the attempted procedure, any complicating factors, and the revised management or treatment plan.
- *CPT* includes specific instructions for reporting certain services when reduced or discontinued (eg, endoscopy). Be sure to verify *CPT* instructions before reporting reduced or terminated services.

Know Payer Policies for Modifiers 52 (Reduced Service) and 53 (Discontinued Procedure)

Individual payer policies may specify allowed uses and reporting requirements for reduced or discontinued services. Pediatricians should be aware that some payer policies automatically reduce payment to 25% to 50% of the fee schedule amount for the service reported with modifier 52 or 53.

Documentation should support the reason for reduced or discontinued service and the extent of the service performed. Payers may audit the patient's medical record or, for facility-based services, use electronic processes to compare a physician's claim to a facility claim for the same service that was reported with modifier 73 or 74 (outpatient hospital/ambulatory surgical center discontinued service). If modifier 52 or 53 is indicated but not reported, a payer may demand return of previous payments.

Anatomical or Laterality Modifiers

Use of modifiers for anatomical sites (eg, fingers and thumbs: FA, F1–F9; toes: TA, T1–T9; or eyelids: E1–E4) or laterality (RT, LT, or bilateral 50) may prevent denial of charges. Some payers have adopted payment policies that will deny charges submitted without the appropriate anatomical or laterality modifier(s) even when a single service is reported and the associated diagnosis code indicates site and laterality. For detailed discussions of modifiers, refer to **Chapter 2**.

Modifiers are also important when a payer's code edits bundle certain services that were provided on the same date or limit the allowable units of service per day (eg, Medicaid NCCI edits, published at www.cms.gov/medicare/coding-billing/ncci-medicaid).

Reporting by Assistant Surgeon

An assistant surgeon is a physician or other QHP who provides active assistance in the performance of a procedure when clinically indicated (eg, technically complex procedure).

- Refer to the Assistant Surgeon in a Teaching Facility section later in this chapter for guidance on reporting assistant surgeon services by a physician in a teaching facility.
- Global rules do not apply to services performed by an assistant surgeon. Payment is based on a percentage of the fee schedule amount allowed for the procedure performed (eg, Medicare allows 16%).
- Modifiers are appended to the code(s) for the procedure on the assistant's claim. Refer to **Box 18-1** for modifiers for reporting services by an assistant surgeon.
- Reductions for multiple procedures on the same date may apply.
- Refer to individual payer policies for an assistant at surgery, as many limit payment to only specific procedures and/or may require documentation substantiating the need for assistance.

- Follow payer policy for reporting assistant surgeon services by a QHP. Some payer policies specify that the assisting QHP must be qualified to take over the surgery should the surgeon become incapacitated. Modifier **AS** (physician assistant, nurse practitioner, or clinical nurse specialist services for assistant at surgery) may be required.

Box 18-1. Modifiers for Reporting Assistant Surgeon Services	
80	Assistant surgeon (Use for doctor of medicine or osteopathy.)
81	Minimum assistant surgeon
82	Assistant surgeon (when qualified resident surgeon not available; applicable only in teaching facility)

Procedures Performed With or Without Imaging Guidance

Some procedures include imaging guidance. When a code descriptor for a procedure or *CPT* instruction indicates that the procedure includes imaging guidance, do not separately report a code for supervision and interpretation of imaging (eg, radiography, fluoroscopy, ultrasonography, magnetic resonance imaging, computed tomography, nuclear medicine).

- ✖ Do not report imaging guidance when a non–imaging-guided tracking or localizing system (eg, radar, electromagnetic signals) is used.
- If you do not own or lease the equipment, append modifier **26** (professional component) to the procedure code to report only the professional service of interpreting the image and writing the report.
- Follow *CPT* instruction when reporting a procedure performed without imaging guidance when the code descriptor for the procedure includes imaging guidance.

Procedures Performed in Infants Less Than 4 kg

Modifier **63** is used to identify significantly increased complexity and physician or other QHP work commonly associated with procedures performed on neonates and infants with a present body weight of up to 4 kg.

- Append modifier **63** to codes for procedures performed in these infants only when there is no instruction prohibiting reporting.
- Services that cannot be reported with modifier **63** are those that have been valued according to the intensity of the service in patients weighing less than 4 kg. Refer to "Summary of *CPT* Codes Exempt from Modifier **63**" in your *CPT* appendixes for a list of codes exempt from modifier **63**.
- Unless otherwise designated, this modifier may be appended only to procedures or services listed in the **20100–69999** code series and **92920**, **92928**, **92953**, **92960**, **92986**, **92987**, **92990**, **92997**, **92998**, **93312–93318**, **93452**, **93505**, **93593–93598**, **93563**, **93564**, **93568**, **93569**, **93573–93575**, **93580–93582**, **93590–93592**, **93615**, and **93616**. Modifier **63** is not appended to codes from the E/M, anesthesia, radiology, or pathology/laboratory section of *CPT*.
- Use of modifier **63** may require submission of an operative note with the claim. The operative note should include the patient's weight. It is also beneficial to report the patient's weight on the claim.
- Payer acceptance of modifier **63** may be limited to specific procedures and increased payment allowance (above the payment for the same procedure in a patient weighing >4 kg) varies. Verify policies of individual health plans for reporting this modifier.

Examples

➤ **A 13-day-old weighing 2.4 kg requires peripheral cannulae insertion for extracorporeal membrane oxygenation.**
The physician reports

33951 63 Extracorporeal membrane oxygenation/extracorporeal life support provided by physician; insertion of peripheral (arterial and/or venous) cannula(e), percutaneous, birth through 5 years of age (includes fluoroscopic guidance, when performed)

Teaching Point: The patient weighed less than 4 kg, and the procedure is not listed as modifier-**63** exempt. Therefore, modifier **63** is appropriately appended to indicate the increased intensity and/or work of performing the procedure on the neonate. Note that modifier **63** cannot be appended to codes for initiation or daily management of extracorporeal membrane oxygenation/extracorporeal life support (**33646–33949**).

➤ **An infant weighing 3 kg undergoes diagnostic laryngoscopy.** The physician reports

31520 Laryngoscopy, direct, with or without tracheoscopy; diagnostic newborn

Teaching Point: The parenthetical instruction below 31520 ("Do not report modifier 63 in conjunction with 31520") prohibits reporting modifier 63, including when this procedure is performed on an infant weighing less than 4 kg.

Physicians at Teaching Hospitals Guidelines for Billing Procedures

The CMS established and maintains guidelines for documentation and billing by teaching physicians. Physicians at Teaching Hospitals guidelines for billing procedures are less complex than those for billing E/M services. Guidelines specify that

- When a procedure is performed by a resident, teaching physician attendance and participation are required and must be documented. For examples of appropriate documentation, refer to **Table 18-1**.

Table 18-1. Examples of Appropriate Documentation of Teaching Physician Presence

Presence	Documentation
Minor procedure	*"Dr Teaching Physician was present during the entire procedure."* —Nurse *"Dr Teaching Physician observed me as I performed this procedure."* —Dr Resident
Interpretation of diagnostic radiological findings and other diagnostic test results	*"I personally reviewed the MRI with Dr Resident and agree with their findings."* —Dr Teaching Physician *"I personally reviewed the EEG with Dr Resident. Findings indicate [cite specifics]."* —Dr Teaching Physician
Endoscopy	*"I was present during the entire viewing of this endoscopy."* —Dr Teaching Physician
Surgery other than minor procedure	*"Dr Teaching Physician was present during the entire surgery."* —Dr Resident *"I was present during and observed Dr Resident perform the key portion of this surgery."* —Dr Teaching Physician
Complex or high-risk surgery or procedure	*"I was physically present during this entire procedure except for the [opening and/or closing]."* —Dr Teaching Physician *"Dr Y was immediately available during the overlapping portions of this case, which included [cite specifics]."* —Dr Teaching Physician

Abbreviations: EEG, electroencephalogram; MRI, magnetic resonance image.

- The level of participation required by the teaching physician depends on the type of procedure being performed as described later in this section.
- A resident, nurse, or teaching physician may document the teaching physician's attendance.

To obtain the rules for supervising physicians in teaching settings, refer to Chapter 12 of the *Medicare Claims Processing Manual* at www.cms.gov/Regulations-and-Guidance/Guidance/Manuals/downloads/clm104c12.pdf.

Modifier GC must be appended to procedure codes for services performed by a resident under the direction of a teaching physician.

Minor Procedures

- The CMS defines a minor procedure as one taking *5 minutes or less* to complete with relatively little decision-making once the need for the procedure is determined. Minor procedures are usually assigned a 0- to 10-day global period.

Common Surgical Procedures and Sedation in Facility Settings

Chapter 18

- Teaching physicians may bill for a minor procedure when they personally perform the service or when a resident performs the service and they are present for the entire procedure.
- The resident may document the procedure but must attest to the teaching physician's presence.

Interpretation of Diagnostic Radiology and Other Diagnostic Tests

- The teaching physician may bill for interpretation of the diagnostic service if they interpret tests or review findings with the resident.
- Documentation must support a personal interpretation or a review of the resident's notes with indication of agreement with the resident's interpretation.
- Changes to the resident's interpretation must be documented.

Endoscopy

- The teaching physician must be physically present (ie, not remotely viewing the procedure) for the entire viewing starting at the time of insertion and ending at the time of removal of the endoscope.
- The presence of the teaching physician must be documented in the medical record. The teaching physician's presence must be stated.

Complex or High-Risk Surgery or Procedure

- A complex procedure or surgery (eg, cardiac catheterization) requires the direct or personal supervision of a physician as specified in Medicare or local policy or in the *CPT* description.
- A teaching physician must be present with a resident for the entire procedure when billing for a service identified by the CMS or local policy as complex and requiring personal supervision by a physician.
- Documentation must support that the teaching physician was present.

Surgery Other Than Minor, Complex, or High-Risk Procedure

- The teaching physician must assume the responsibility of preoperative, operative, and postoperative care of the patient. They must be present during all critical and key portions (as determined by the teaching physician) of the procedure. For example, if opening or closing is not considered key or critical, the teaching physician does not need to be present.
- The teaching physician must be immediately available to furnish services during the entire procedure.
- If circumstances prevent the physician from being immediately available, arrangements must be made with another qualified surgeon to be immediately available to assist with the procedure.
- The physician's presence for single surgical procedures may be demonstrated in notes made by the teaching physician, resident, or nurse.
- When the teaching physician is present for the entire procedure, only the written attestation of their presence is required.
- If the teaching physician is present during only the key or critical portions of the surgery, documentation must indicate their presence at those portions of the procedure (the resident may still document the operative report).
- When billing for 2 overlapping (concurrent) surgical procedures, the teaching physician must be present for the key or critical portions of both procedures and must personally document their presence. The surgeon cannot be involved in a second case until all key or critical portions in the first case have been completed.
- Arrangements may be made with another qualified surgeon to be present at one of the surgical procedures. The name of the other surgeon who was immediately available during overlapping surgical procedures must be documented.

Postoperative Care

- The teaching physician determines which postoperative visits are considered key or critical and require their presence.
- If the teaching physician is not providing postoperative care included in the global surgery package, they will report the procedure(s) with modifiers **54** (surgical care only) and **56** (preoperative management only).
- Postoperative care is reported by another physician with the same surgical procedure code with modifier **55** (postoperative management only).
- The surgeon and physician providing postoperative care must keep a copy of a written transfer agreement in the patient's medical record.

Assistant Surgeon in a Teaching Facility

Medicare will not pay for the services of assistants at surgery furnished in a teaching hospital that has a training program related to the medical specialty required for the surgical procedure and has a qualified resident available to perform the service. This policy may be applied by Medicaid and other payers.

- When the MPFS allows payment for an assistant surgeon and a physician assists a teaching physician because no qualified resident is available, modifier **82** (assistant surgeon [when qualified resident surgeon not available]) is appended to the code for the procedure performed on the assistant surgeon's claim.
- The unavailability of a qualified resident surgeon is a prerequisite for use of modifier **82**. Documentation must specify that no qualified resident was available.
- This modifier is used only in teaching hospitals and only if there is no approved training program related to the medical specialty required for the surgical procedure or no qualified resident was available.

Integumentary Procedures

Refer to Chapter 13 for discussions of laceration repairs and removal of foreign bodies from integumentary or musculoskeletal tissues.

Burn Care

CPT code **16000** (initial treatment, first-degree burn, where no more than local treatment is required) is reported when initial treatment is performed for the symptomatic relief of a first-degree burn that is characterized by erythema and tenderness.

Table 18-2 includes codes for dressings and/or debridement of partial-thickness burns.

Table 18-2. Dressings and/or Debridement of Partial-Thickness Burns

Includes initial or subsequent treatment of burns with dressings and/or debridement. The percentage of TBSA involved must be calculated and documented when reporting care of second- or third-degree burns.

16020	16025	16030
small or <5% TBSA (eg, finger)	medium or 5%–10% TBSA (eg, whole face or whole extremity)	large or >10% TBSA (eg, >1 extremity)

Abbreviation: TBSA, total body surface area.

Pediatric physicians often use the Lund-Browder classification method for estimating the total body surface area on the basis of the patient's age. (The Lund-Browder diagram and classification method table are in *CPT 2026 Professional Edition.*)

- An E/M visit (critical care, ED services, inpatient or outpatient E/M) may be provided for evaluation of the patient's injuries and management of complications such as dehydration, shock, infection, multiple organ dysfunction syndrome, electrolyte imbalance, cardiac arrhythmias, and respiratory distress.
  - Report the E/M code appropriate to the setting and care provided with modifier **25** appended to indicate that the significant, separately identifiable E/M service is medically indicated, performed, and documented in addition to the burn care.
- Codes **16000–16036** do not include other services such as pulmonary testing/therapy or procedures such as hyperbaric oxygenation, grafting, or tracheotomy. Separately report other services provided on the same date as burn care.
- It is advisable to use *International Classification of Diseases, 10th Revision, Clinical Modification* (*ICD-10-CM*) category **T31** (burns classified according to extent of body surface involved) as an additional code for reporting purposes when there is mention of a third-degree burn involving 20% or more of the body surface.
- Codes **16020–16030** include the application of materials (eg, dressings) not described in **15100–15278** (skin grafts and substitutes) or **15011–15018** (skin cell suspension autograft).

Category III code 0972T was implemented on July 1, 2025, to report assistive algorithmic classification of burn healing (ie, healing or nonhealing) by noninvasive multispectral imaging, including system setup and acquisition, selection, and transmission of images, with automated generation of report.

Category III temporary codes may have coverage limitations. See individual payer policies prior to providing these services.

Eschar Incision and Selective Enzymatic Debridement

16035 Escharotomy; initial incision
+16036 each additional incision

Codes **16035** and **16036**

- Are reported per incision of eschar (dead tissue cast off from the surface of the skin in full-thickness burns).
- Are not reported according to anatomical site; report with 1 unit of **16035** only for the first incision and 1 unit of **16036** for each additional incision regardless of body area.

Nonselective debridement of eschar is reported with **97602**.

97602 Removal of devitalized tissue from wound(s), non-selective debridement, without anesthesia (eg, wet-to-moist dressings, enzymatic, abrasion, larval therapy), including topical application(s), wound assessment, and instruction[s] for ongoing care, per session

Category III temporary codes **0973T–0976T** were implemented July 1, 2025, for reporting selective enzymatic debridement of partial-thickness and/or full-thickness burn eschar under separately reported general anesthesia or moderate sedation. For the full code descriptors and reporting instructions, refer to your *CPT* reference. As noted previously, it is important to verify payer policies for coverage of services reported with Category III codes.

Refer to "Skin Graft Codes" at www.aap.org/cfp2026.

Negative Pressure Wound Therapy

97605 Negative pressure wound therapy (eg, vacuum assisted drainage collection), utilizing durable medical equipment, including topical application(s), wound assessment, and instruction(s) for ongoing care, per session; total wound(s) surface area less than or equal to 50 square centimeters
97606 total wound(s) surface area greater than 50 square centimeters
97607 Negative pressure wound therapy (eg, vacuum assisted drainage collection), utilizing disposable, non-durable medical equipment including provision of exudate management collection system, topical application(s), wound assessment, and instructions for ongoing care, per session; total wound(s) surface area less than or equal to 50 square centimeters
97608 total wound(s) surface area greater than 50 square centimeters

Negative pressure wound therapy

- Requires direct (one-on-one) physician or QHP contact with the patient
- May be initiated in a hospital or surgical center setting and continued in the home setting after discharge
- Includes application of dressings
- Is separately reported when performed in conjunction with surgical debridement (**11042–11047**)
- Includes documentation of current wound assessment, including
  - Quantitative measurements of wound characteristics (eg, site, surface area, depth)
  - Any previous treatment regimens
  - Debridement (when performed)
  - Prescribed length of treatment
  - Dressing types and frequency of changes
  - Other concerns that affect healing
- Includes documentation of progress of healing and changes in the wound, including measurement, amount of exudate, and presence of granulation or necrotic tissue at encounters for ongoing negative pressure wound therapy

Codes **97605** and **97606** represent negative pressure wound therapy provided via a system that includes a *non-disposable* suction pump and drainage collection device. Supplies, including dressings, are reportable with HCPCS codes (eg, **A6550**, wound care set, for negative pressure wound therapy electrical pump, includes all supplies and accessories).

- Codes **97607** and **97608**
  - Report negative pressure wound therapy that uses a *disposable* suction pump and collection system
  - Are not reported in conjunction with **97605** and **97606**
  - Require verification of coverage by the patient's health plan before provision of services, as services may be subject to payer policies limiting to care of specific types of wounds that require negative pressure wound therapy to improve granulation tissue formation and to certain types of negative pressure wound therapy equipment

Supplies for a disposable system are reported with **A9272**, which also includes all dressings and accessories.

Musculoskeletal Procedures

Fracture and Dislocation Care Codes

Codes for fracture/dislocation care

- Are listed by anatomical location.
- Are provided (in most cases) for closed or open treatment, with or without manipulation and with or without internal fixation.
- Typically include a 90-day period of follow-up care under the Medicare global package.

An E/M service to determine the need for fracture or dislocation care may be separately reportable. Append modifier 57 (decision for surgery) to an E/M code when the decision for the procedure is made during a visit on the day before or day of the procedure.

Apply this guidance when reporting care of a fracture or dislocation.

- Fracture care services include the initial casting, splinting, or strapping, but do not include radiographs or subsequent cast changes.
- It is appropriate to append modifier 58 (staged or related procedure during the postoperative period) to a code reported for a cast change (29000–29799 58). However, payer guidance on use of modifier 58 may vary.
- Report routine follow-up visits during the global period with no charge with 99024 (post-op follow-up visit related to the original procedure).
- Append modifier 76 to the usual procedure code to indicate repeated procedure or service by the same physician or other QHP for re-reduction of a fracture and/or dislocation.

Fracture Care by Different Physicians or Other Qualified Health Care Professionals

Append modifier 54 to the usual procedure code if you provide initial fracture care (with or without manipulation) but transfer to another physician for follow-up care (applies to procedures with a 10- or 90-day global period). The transfer of care should be documented (eg, "Patient to see Dr X for continuing fracture care Monday morning").

Do not report a fracture care code when stabilization (eg, temporary cast/splint/strap) is performed to protect an injury and provide comfort to the patient until another physician performs initial fracture or dislocation care. Instead, report an E/M service and the application of a cast, splint, or strapping (29000–29584), as indicated.

The physician providing follow-up care will report the same DOS and procedure code appended with modifier 55. The claim will also denote the date of the transfer of care, which should be documented by both physicians.

Examples

➤ **An orthopedic surgeon is consulted to evaluate a child in the ED for an injury to the left elbow following a fall caused by overturning her bicycle on the sidewalk.** The orthopedic surgeon evaluates the child and diagnoses a displaced supracondylar humerus fracture. A decision is made to proceed with closed reduction and pinning. The surgeon's total time spent in provision and documentation of the E/M service is 40 minutes. The procedure takes place on the same date. The orthopedic surgeon provided consultation in the ED and a surgical procedure requiring an inpatient admission on the same date.

ICD-10-CM	*CPT*
S42.412A (displaced simple supracondylar fracture without intercondylar fracture of left humerus, initial encounter for closed fracture) V18.0XXA (pedal cycle driver injured in noncollision transport accident in nontraffic accident, initial encounter) Y92.480 (sidewalk as the place of occurrence of the external cause)	99244 57 (outpatient consultation with moderate MDM or ≥40 minutes) or, if the payer does not pay consultation codes, 99215 57 (office or other outpatient E/M service with high MDM or ≥40 minutes) 24538 (percutaneous skeletal fixation of supracondylar or transcondylar humeral fracture, with or without intercondylar extension)

Common Surgical Procedures and Sedation in Facility Settings

Chapter 18

Teaching Point: Because 24538 is assigned a 90-day global period in the MPFS, modifier 57 (decision for surgery) is appended to the E/M code reported for the same DOS. Individual payers may have different policies. The postoperative care in the hospital is not separately reported. Follow-up visits in the office should be reported with 99024 (postoperative follow-up visit).

➤ **An orthopedic surgeon sees a child for follow-up care after percutaneous skeletal fixation of a supracondylar fracture.** The surgeon replaces a splint that was applied at the time of the procedure with a long-arm cast.

ICD-10-CM	*CPT*
S42.412D (displaced simple supracondylar fracture without intercondylar fracture of left humerus, subsequent encounter for fracture with routine healing) V18.0XXD (pedal cycle driver injured in noncollision transport accident in nontraffic accident, subsequent encounter) Y92.480 (sidewalk as the place of occurrence of the external cause)	29065 58 (application cast; shoulder to hand)

Teaching Point: Because the cast is not part of the initial fracture care, it is separately reported. Cast removal on a later date will not be separately reported.

Vertebral Body Tethering

22836 Anterior thoracic vertebral body tethering, including thoracoscopy, when performed; up to 7 vertebral segments

22837 8 or more vertebral segments

22838 Revision (eg, augmentation, division of tether), replacement, or removal of thoracic vertebral body tethering, including thoracoscopy, when performed

0656T Anterior lumbar or thoracolumbar vertebral body tethering; up to 7 vertebral segments

0657T 8 or more vertebral segments

0790T Revision (eg, augmentation, division of tether), replacement, or removal of thoracolumbar or lumbar vertebral body tethering, including thoracoscopy, when performed

Vertebral body tethering is a means to correct scoliosis without fusion. The procedures involve use of a tether or cord to compress the convex vertebral growth plates to inhibit growth while allowing concave growth plates to grow.

When 2 surgeons perform distinct parts of the service, each acting as a primary surgeon, each surgeon reports their work using 22836–22838 appended with modifier 62 (2 surgeons).

Note that *CPT* Category III codes, including 0656T–0657T and 0790T, are not assigned relative value units or global periods in the MPFS. Individual payers will determine coverage and payment for these procedures. Verify benefits and requirements for prior authorization prior to these procedures.

- Do not report the following services in conjunction with 22836–22838:
  - ✖ Anterior instrumentation (22845–22847)
  - ✖ Diagnostic thoracoscopy (32601)
- Do not report the following services in conjunction with 0656T–0657T:
  - ✖ Arthrodesis procedures for spine deformity (22800–22819)
  - ✖ Anterior instrumentation (22845–22847)

Osteotomy With Insertion of Intramedullary Lengthening Device

New in 2026! Report 27458 or 27713 for a procedure to insert an externally controlled intramedullary lengthening device into the femur or tibia.

#●27458 Osteotomy(ies), femur, unilateral, with insertion of an externally controlled intramedullary lengthening device, including iliotibial band release when performed, imaging, alignment assessments, computations of adjustment schedules, and management of the intramedullary lengthening device

● indicates a new code; ▲, revised; #, re-sequenced; ✚, add-on; ★, audiovisual technology; and ◀, synchronous interactive audio.

#●27713 Osteotomy(ies), tibia, including fibula when performed, unilateral, with insertion of an externally controlled intramedullary lengthening device, including imaging, alignment assessments, computations of adjustment schedules, and management of the intramedullary lengthening device

Note that codes 27458 and 27713 report unilateral procedures that are performed to correct a limb length discrepancy (eg, Q72.812, congenital shortening of left lower limb).

- ✖ Do not report 27458 in conjunction with other osteotomy procedures (27450, 27466) or fracture treatment (27470, 27472, 27506).
- ✖ Do not report 27713 in conjunction with other osteotomy procedures (27705, 27709, 27712) osteoplasty (27715), or fracture treatment (27720, 27722, 27724, 27759).

Code 27468 (osteoplasty, femur; combined lengthening and shortening with femoral segment transfer) is deleted in 2026. This procedure is no longer commonly performed.

Removal of Musculoskeletal Hardware

An object intentionally placed by a physician or other QHP for any purpose (eg, diagnostic, therapeutic) is considered an implant. If an implant (or part thereof) has moved from its original position or is structurally broken and no longer serves its intended purpose or presents a hazard to the patient, it qualifies as a foreign body for coding purposes, unless *CPT* coding instructions direct otherwise or a specific *CPT* code exists to describe the removal of that broken/moved implant.

20665 Removal of tongs or halo applied by another individual
20670 Removal of implant; superficial (eg, buried wire, pin or rod) (separate procedure)
20680 deep (eg, buried wire, pin, screw, metal band, nail, rod or plate)

Removal of a halo or tongs is included in the placement procedure. Removal of a halo or tongs by another physician, however, is separately reported with 20665. (*Note:* Physicians of the same specialty and same group practice are typically considered the same physician for billing purposes.)

Codes 20670 and 20680 may be reported for removal of orthopedic hardware. If it is necessary to remove an implant within the global period (eg, to address breakage), report the appropriate removal code with modifier 78 (unplanned return to the OR by the same physician or other QHP following initial procedure for a related procedure during the postoperative period). Removal of an external fixation system under anesthesia (20694) requires more than local anesthesia.

Respiratory Procedures

Intubation and Airway Management

31500 Intubation, endotracheal, emergency

- Moderate sedation (99151–99157) may be reported in addition to the intubation if used to sedate the patient before and during the intubation procedure (eg, in rapid sequence intubation) and reporting criteria are met. Refer to the Sedation section later in this chapter for more on moderate sedation.
- Endotracheal intubation is included in the neonatal and pediatric critical care services reported with 99468–99476 and intensive care services reported with 99477–99480 and should not be billed separately. Code 31500 is separately reported for endotracheal intubation performed as part of neonatal resuscitation in the delivery room (ie, before admission).

31502 Tracheostomy tube change prior to establishment of fistula tract

Report 31502 only when an indwelling tracheostomy tube is replaced before establishment of a fistula tract.

Routine changing of a tracheostomy tube after a fistula tract has been established is included in a related E/M service. Code 31575 (laryngoscopy, flexible; diagnostic) may be reported when performed to check tracheostomy tube placement.

31505–31520 Indirect laryngoscopy

Report **31505** for indirect diagnostic laryngoscopy. If, while performing this procedure, a foreign body is removed, report **31511** (laryngoscopy with removal of foreign body).

31515 Direct laryngoscopy with or without tracheoscopy

Code **31515** is reported when laryngoscopy is performed for aspiration.

31520 Laryngoscopy direct, with or without tracheoscopy; diagnostic, newborn

Do not report modifier **63** (procedure performed on infant <4 kg) in conjunction with **31520**.

31525 Laryngoscopy, direct, with or without tracheoscopy; diagnostic except newborn

Thoracostomy, Thoracentesis, and Pleural Drainage

32551 Tube thoracostomy, includes connection to drainage system (eg, water seal), when performed, open (separate procedure)

32554 Thoracentesis, needle or catheter, aspiration of the pleural space; without imaging guidance

32555 with imaging guidance

32556 Pleural drainage, percutaneous, with insertion of indwelling catheter; without imaging guidance

32557 with imaging guidance

- Thoracostomy (**32551**) represents an open procedure involving incision into a rib interspace with dissection extending through the chest wall muscles and pleura. Thoracentesis and percutaneous pleural drainage may be more commonly performed in pediatrics except for neonatal and pediatric critical care.
  - ✖ Percutaneous image guidance cannot be reported in conjunction with **32551**, which represents an open procedure.
  - Diagnostic ultrasonography performed before thoracostomy to localize a collection in the pleural space is separately reportable only when the complete ultrasound study of the chest (**76604**) is performed with permanent recording of images.
- Thoracentesis codes **32554** and **32555** represent a procedure in which the surgical technique is puncture of the pleural space to remove fluid or air. Although a catheter (eg, pigtail catheter) may be used, it is not left in place at the end of the procedure.
- Percutaneous pleural drainage codes **32556** and **32557** represent procedures in which an indwelling catheter is inserted into the pleural space and remains at the end of the procedure. The catheter is secured in place and connected to a suction drainage system.
- Removal of chest tubes and non-tunneled indwelling pleural catheters is included in a related E/M service and not in a separately reportable procedure.
- For insertion of a tunneled pleural catheter with cuff, refer to **32550**. For removal of a tunneled pleural catheter with cuff, refer to **32552**.

Cardiovascular Procedures

Diagnostic Studies Performed in Conjunction With Interventional Procedures

CPT provides specific guidance regarding separate reporting of radiological supervision and interpretation performed as part of a vascular or cardiac procedure (eg, fluoroscopic guidance, contrast injections, angiography performed to accomplish the intervention). It is important that these guidelines are understood and used to distinguish studies included in interventional procedures from diagnostic studies that may be performed on the same date or at the same session.

Generally, diagnostic angiography, venography, and heart catheterization performed in conjunction with an interventional procedure may be separately reported (append modifier **59**) only when one of the following circumstances is true:

- No prior study is available and a full diagnostic study is performed.
- A prior study is available, but as documented in the medical record, one of the following circumstances applies:
  - There is inadequate visualization of the anatomy and/or pathology.
  - The patient's condition with respect to the clinical indication has changed since the prior study.
  - There is a clinical change during the procedure that requires new evaluation.
- ✖ Do not separately report diagnostic imaging that is specifically included in the code descriptor of an interventional procedure.

Prefatory instructions preceding codes for interventional services should be used to guide code selection.

Echocardiography

For discussion of limited transthoracic echocardiography (TTE) as part of the focused assessment with sonography for trauma examination, refer to Chapter 14.

Physicians and QHPs report codes for echocardiography with modifier 26 (professional component) when the facility bears the expense of the equipment and staff to perform the technical components of echocardiography. When applicable, and when all requirements for reporting are met, ultrasonography performed with physician-owned equipment is reported without a modifier (ie, modifiers 26 and TC are not applicable).

✖ Do not report echocardiography codes for a service without thorough evaluation of organ(s) or anatomical region, image documentation, and final, written report.

Multiple sets of codes describe echocardiography by type, purpose, and included components. Refer to "Echocardiography Code List" at www.aap.org/cfp2026 and your *CPT* reference for full code descriptors.

- The standard echocardiogram is TTE, 93303–93308, or TTE with stress, 93350–93352. But when necessary to obtain different views of the heart and blood flow, transesophageal echocardiography (TEE) (93312–93318) or TEE guidance of a transcatheter intervention (93355) is performed.

Codes 93319 (3D echocardiographic imaging and postprocessing during echocardiography) and 76987–76989 (intraoperative epicardial ultrasound) are discussed in the 3D Echocardiographic Imaging and Postprocessing section and the Diagnostic Intraoperative Epicardial Cardiac Ultrasound section that follow.

- Note that 93303–93304 and 93315–93317 are limited to the evaluation of congenital cardiac anomalies.
  - ✖ Congenital echocardiography should not be used when congenital heart disease is suspected but not found during echocardiographic evaluation. If so, noncongenital echocardiography codes should be reported.
  - — Codes for standard echocardiography are reported when congenital anomalies are limited to patent foramen ovale or bicuspid aortic valve.
- The work of complete echocardiography, in contrast to limited or follow-up study, is fully described in *CPT* prefatory instructions to echocardiography codes. Physicians and QHPs should document circumstances under which, despite significant effort, identification and measurement of some structures were not possible.

Where codes do not differentiate complete from limited/follow-up echocardiographic studies, modifier 52 (reduced service) or 53 (discontinued service) may be reported to indicate significantly reduced work.

- Administration of sedation or hypnotic agents for echocardiography is not separately reported except when services by an anesthesiologist or another provider of deep sedation are required.
- AOCs for spectral and color flow Doppler echocardiography and myocardial strain imaging provided in conjunction with echocardiography (93320, 93321, 93325, 93356) are reported in addition to certain echocardiography codes. Refer to *CPT* instructions below each AOC for a list of codes to which each is additionally reported.
- Codes for echocardiograms are not included in any of the critical care services. Separately report echocardiography when performed by the same physician or QHP providing critical care services on the same date.

3D Echocardiographic Imaging and Postprocessing

+93319	3D echocardiographic imaging and postprocessing during TEE, or during TTE for congenital cardiac anomalies, for the assessment of cardiac structure(s) (eg, cardiac chambers and valves, left atrial appendage, interatrial septum, interventricular septum) and function, when performed (List separately in addition to code for echocardiographic imaging)

When performed, report 93319 in conjunction with

- Transthoracic echocardiography for congenital cardiac anomalies (complete [93303] or follow-up/limited [93304] study)
- Transesophageal echocardiography, real time with image documentation (93312, 93314)
- Transesophageal echocardiography for congenital cardiac anomalies (93315, 93317).

● indicates a new code; ▲, revised; #, re-sequenced; +, add-on; ★, audiovisual technology; and ◀, synchronous interactive audio.

✖ Do not report 93319 in conjunction with 3D rendering with interpretation and reporting (76376, 76377), Doppler echocardiography color flow velocity mapping (93325), or echocardiography, transesophageal, for guidance of a transcatheter intracardiac or great vessel(s) structural intervention(s) (93355).

Diagnostic Intraoperative Epicardial Cardiac Ultrasound

76987 Intraoperative epicardial cardiac ultrasound (eg, echocardiography) for congenital heart disease, diagnostic; including placement and manipulation of transducer, image acquisition, interpretation and report

76988 placement, manipulation of transducer, and image acquisition only

76989 interpretation and report only

Intraoperative epicardial cardiac ultrasound for congenital heart disease is an alternative diagnostic imaging study to TEE (93312–93314).

Code 76987 is reported for the combined professional and technical components of intraoperative epicardial cardiac ultrasound for congenital heart disease service. Report 76989 when the physician provides only the professional components of interpretation and report. Code 76988 is reported for the technical components provided by an entity other than the physician performing interpretation and report.

✖ Do not report intraoperative ultrasound guidance (76998) in addition to 76987–76989.

Cardiac Catheterization for Congenital Heart Defects

Codes 93593–93598 are reported *only when cardiac catheterization is performed for evaluation of congenital cardiac defects.*

Diagnostic heart catheterization in a patient without congenital defect (eg, any acquired heart disease, such as dilated cardiomyopathy secondary to viral myocarditis, coronary artery diagnosis, or intervention in Kawasaki disease) is reported with 93451–93456, 93460, and 93461.

There is no age limit for services reported with 93593–93598. If there is evaluation of congenital cardiac defects, it is appropriate to report these codes. These codes take into account

- The added technical difficulty presented when structures may be in abnormal positions and locations and access is through abnormal native connections.
- Additional preservice time in both discussing the procedure with parents and reviewing noninvasive data, previous cardiac catheterizations, and previous surgical procedures.
- Procedures may be more time consuming because of small vessels, multiple measurements that must be made, hemodynamic instability of patients, frequency of multiple sites of arterial-venous admixture, and performance of other required interventions.

Heart catheterization includes ultrasound guidance of vascular access, generalized fluoroscopy to guide catheter manipulation, and any limited echocardiographic guidance when performed by the proceduralist. Echocardiography by another cardiologist during the same session is separately reported.

93593 Right heart catheterization for congenital heart defect(s) including imaging guidance by the proceduralist to advance the catheter to the target zone; normal native connections

93594 abnormal native connections

For reporting purposes, when the morphological left ventricle or left atrium is in a subpulmonic position as a result of congenital heart disease (eg, transposition of the great arteries), catheter placement in either of these structures is considered part of right-sided heart catheterization and does not constitute left-sided heart catheterization.

93595 Left heart catheterization for congenital heart defect(s) including imaging guidance by the proceduralist to advance the catheter to the target zone, normal or abnormal native connections

93596 Right and left heart catheterization for congenital heart defect(s) including imaging guidance by the proceduralist to advance the catheter to the target zone(s); normal native connections

93597 abnormal native connections

Report the appropriate code for right- and left-sided heart catheterization if catheter placement with hemodynamic assessment of the double outlet ventricle *is performed during the right-sided heart catheterization and separately from the arterial approach.* Catheter placement with hemodynamic assessment of the morphological left ventricle during right-sided heart catheterization alone (ie, not separately from the arterial approach) is considered part of that procedure.

- Codes for right-sided heart or right- and left-sided heart catheterization for congenital defects are determined depending on access through normal or abnormal native connections.
  - Normal native connections exist when blood flow follows the expected course (ie, superior vena cava/inferior vena cava to right atrium, then right ventricle, then pulmonary arteries, for the right side of the heart; left atrium to left ventricle, then aorta, for the left side of the heart). Examples of congenital heart defects with normal connections include acyanotic defects such as isolated atrial septal defect, ventricular septal defect, or patent ductus arteriosus.
  - Abnormal native connections exist when there are alternative connections for the pathway of blood flow through the heart and great vessels. Abnormal connections are typically present in patients with cyanotic congenital heart defects, any variation of single-ventricle anatomy (eg, hypoplastic right or left side of the heart, double outlet right ventricle), unbalanced atrioventricular canal (endocardial cushion) defect, transposition of the great arteries, valvular atresia, tetralogy of Fallot with or without major aortopulmonary collateral arteries, total anomalous pulmonary veins, truncus arteriosus, and any lesions with heterotaxia and/or dextrocardia.
- The work of imaging guidance, including fluoroscopy and ultrasound guidance for vascular access and catheter placement for hemodynamic evaluation, is included in the cardiac catheterization for congenital heart defects codes, when performed by the same operator.
- Procedures such as percutaneous transcatheter closure of patent ductus arteriosus (93582) include right- and left-sided heart catheterization for congenital cardiac anomalies. Be sure to read the *CPT* instructions for procedures performed in conjunction with congenital cardiac catheterization to determine if the catheterization is separately reportable.

Multiple AOCs may be reported for additional services performed in conjunction with codes for cardiac catheterizations for congenital heart defects. These include left-sided heart catheterization by transseptal or transapical puncture (93462), pharmacologic agent administration (93463), physiological exercise study (93464), cardiac output measurements (93598), injection procedures for angiography (93568, 93569, and 93573–93575), and venography (93584–93588).

Atrial Septostomy

33741 Transcatheter atrial septostomy for congenital cardiac anomalies to create effective atrial flow, including all imaging guidance by the proceduralist, when performed, any method (eg, Rashkind, Sang-Park, balloon, cutting balloon, blade)

33745 Transcatheter intracardiac shunt (TIS) creation by stent placement for congenital cardiac anomalies to establish effective intracardiac flow, all imaging guidance by the proceduralist when performed, left and right heart diagnostic cardiac catheterization for congenital cardiac anomalies, and target zone angioplasty, when performed (eg, atrial septum, Fontan fenestration, right ventricular outflow tract, Mustard/Senning/Warden baffles); initial intracardiac shunt

+33746 each additional intracardiac shunt location

Codes 33741–33746 are typically used to report creation of effective intracardiac blood flow in the setting of congenital heart defects. Report 93462 for transseptal puncture performed in conjunction with 33741.

Code 33741

- Involves the percutaneous creation of improved atrial blood flow (eg, balloon/blade method), typically in infants weighing 4 kg or less with congenital heart disease.
- ✖ Do not append modifier 63 (procedures performed on infants <4 kg) to 33741.
- Includes ultrasonographic guidance for vascular access and fluoroscopic guidance for the intervention, when performed. Intracardiac echocardiography including imaging supervision and interpretation is separately reported with 93662, when performed.
- Diagnostic cardiac catheterization is not typically performed at the same session as 33741; separately report each service when performed. Refer to *CPT* instructions addressing when it is appropriate to separately report cardiac catheterization.
- ✖ Do not separately report cardiac catheterization that is fluoroscopic guidance for the intervention or limited hemodynamic and angiographic data used solely for the purpose of accomplishing the intervention.

Codes 33745 and 33746

- Include intracardiac stent placement, target zone angioplasty preceding or following stent implantation, and *complete diagnostic right- and left-sided heart catheterization* (not separately reported), when performed.
  - Ultrasound guidance for vascular access and fluoroscopic guidance for the intervention is included, when performed. Intracardiac echocardiography including imaging supervision and interpretation is separately reported with 93662, when performed.
  - Includes all balloon angioplasties performed in the target lesion, including any pre-dilation or post-dilation following stent placement, or use of a larger/smaller balloon to achieve therapeutic result.
  - Angioplasty in a separate and distinct intracardiac lesion may be reported separately with modifier 59 (distinct procedural service) appended to the angioplasty code.
- Although diagnostic angiography (93563, 93565–93568, 93569, 93573–93575) is typically performed during 33745, target vessels and chambers are highly variable and, *when performed for an evaluation separate and distinct from the stent delivery,* may be reported separately with modifier 59.
- When additional, different intracardiac locations are treated in the same session, 33746 may be reported for each additional intracardiac shunt creation by stent placement at a separate location.

Report a single code, and not a first or additional unit of 33746, for placement of multiple stents in a single location.

Aortic Valvuloplasty

33390 Valvuloplasty, aortic valve, open, with cardiopulmonary bypass; simple (ie, valvotomy, debridement, debulking, and/or simple commissural resuspension)

33391 complex (eg, leaflet extension, leaflet resection, leaflet reconstruction, or annuloplasty)

✖ Do not report 33391 in conjunction with 33390.

Codes for open valvuloplasty of the aortic valve

- Are descriptive of currently performed valvuloplasty procedures
  - Code 33390 is specifically for reporting valvotomy, debridement, debulking, and/or simple commissural resuspension.
  - Code 33391 represents more complex procedures not limited to the examples in the code descriptor.
- May be reported in conjunction with the code for transmyocardial revascularization (33141), operative tissue ablation and reconstruction of atria (33255–33259), and reoperation, valve procedure, more than 1 month after original operation (33530), when appropriate

Open procedures for aortic valve replacement are reported with 33405, 33406, and 33410 according to the type of replacement valve (ie, prosthetic, homograft, or stentless).

Transcatheter Pulmonary Valve Implantation

33477 Transcatheter pulmonary valve implantation, percutaneous approach, including pre-stenting of the valve delivery site, when performed

The key instructions for reporting 33477 are that it

- Should be reported only once per session
- Includes, when performed,
  - Percutaneous access, placement of the access sheath, advancement of the repair device delivery system into position, repositioning of the device as needed and deployment of the device(s), angiography, all cardiac catheterization(s) for hemodynamic measurements, intraprocedural contrast injections, radiological supervision, and interpretation performed to guide transcatheter pulmonary valve implantation
  - Percutaneous balloon angioplasty of the conduit or treatment zone, valvuloplasty of the pulmonary valve conduit, and stent deployment within the pulmonary conduit or an existing bioprosthetic pulmonary valve

✖ Do not separately report diagnostic angiography (93563, 93566–93568, 93569, 93573) or right-sided heart catheterization (93451–93461; 93593, 93594; 93596–93598) that is intrinsic to the procedure.

Other cardiac catheterization services may be reported separately when performed for diagnostic purposes not intrinsic to transcatheter pulmonary valve implantation.

- **Does not include** (Report separately, when performed.)
  - ✖ Codes 92997 and 92998 when pulmonary artery angioplasty is performed at a site separate from the prosthetic valve delivery site

Common Surgical Procedures and Sedation in Facility Settings

Chapter 18

- ✖ Codes 37236 and 37237 when pulmonary artery stenting is performed at a site separate from the prosthetic valve delivery site
- ✖ Same-session/same-day *diagnostic* cardiac catheterization services (Refer to your *CPT* reference for further instruction, and append catheterization code with modifier 59.)
- ✖ Diagnostic coronary angiography performed at a separate session from an interventional procedure
- ✖ Percutaneous coronary interventional procedures
- ✖ Percutaneous pulmonary artery branch interventions
- ✖ Percutaneous ventricular assist device procedure codes (33990–33993), extracorporeal membrane oxygenation/extracorporeal life support procedure codes (33946–33989), or balloon pump insertion codes (33967, 33970, 33973)
- ✖ Percutaneous peripheral bypass (33367), open peripheral bypass (33368), or central bypass (33369)
- ✖ Ligation and takedown of a systemic to pulmonary artery shunt, performed in conjunction with a congenital heart procedure (33924)

Transcatheter Interventions for Revascularization/Repair for Coarctation of the Aorta

33894 Endovascular stent repair of coarctation of the ascending, transverse, or descending thoracic or abdominal aorta, involving stent placement; across major side branches

33895 not crossing major side branches

33897 Percutaneous transluminal angioplasty of native or recurrent coarctation of the aorta

Codes 33894, 33895, and 33897 include all fluoroscopic guidance of the intervention, diagnostic congenital left-sided heart catheterization, all catheter and wire introductions and manipulation, and angiography of the target lesion. For additional diagnostic right-sided heart catheterization in the same setting as 33894 and 33895, refer to 93593 and 93594.

Code 33897 may be reported in addition to 33894 or 33895 for balloon angioplasty of an additional coarctation of the aorta in a segment *separate from the treatment zone* for the coarctation stent. Balloon angioplasty *within the target treatment zone*, however, either before or after stent deployment, is not separately reportable in conjunction with 33894 or 33895. For angioplasty and other transcatheter revascularization interventions *of additional upper or lower extremity vessels* in the same setting as 33897, use the appropriate code from the Surgery/Cardiovascular System section of *CPT*.

- ✖ Do not report 33897 in conjunction with open or percutaneous transluminal angioplasty (37246) or with transcatheter stent placement for occlusive disease (37236).

Codes 33894 and 33895 include stent introduction, manipulation, positioning, and deployment, as well as any additional stent delivery in tandem with the initial stent for extension purposes.

- Codes 33894 and 33895 are differentiated by whether stent placement crosses major side branches of the aorta. Major side branches include
  - Thoracic aorta: brachiocephalic, carotid, and subclavian arteries
  - Abdominal aorta: celiac, superior mesenteric, inferior mesenteric, and renal arteries
- Do not separately report the following services when reporting 33894, 33895, and 33897:
  - ✖ Insertion of a temporary pacemaker (33210) to facilitate stent positioning, when performed
  - ✖ Introduction, positioning, and deployment of an endograft for treatment of abdominal aortic pathology (34701–34706)
  - ✖ Introduction of catheter, aorta (36200)
  - ✖ Thoracic or abdominal aortography (75600, 75605, 75625)
  - ✖ Left heart catheterization for congenital heart defect(s) (93595)
  - ✖ Right and left heart catheterization for congenital heart defect(s) for normal or abnormal native connections (93596, 93597)
- ✖ Do not separately report balloon angioplasty of the aorta *within the coarctation treatment zone* (transluminal angioplasty, 37246; open or percutaneous angioplasty with transcatheter stent placement for occlusive disease, 37236; or 33897) when reporting 33894 and 33895.
- The following services may be separately reported when performed before or after coarctation stent deployment during endovascular repair of coarctation of the aorta (33894, 33895):
  - Balloon angioplasty or stenting of the innominate, carotid, subclavian, visceral, iliac, or pulmonary artery
  - Arterial or venous embolization
  - Additional atrial, ventricular, pulmonary, or coronary or bypass graph angiography with injection procedure during cardiac catheterization (93563–93568)

For angiography of other vascular structures, use the appropriate code from the Radiology/Diagnostic Radiology section of *CPT*.

Percutaneous Pulmonary Artery Revascularization

33900 Percutaneous pulmonary artery revascularization by stent placement, initial; normal native connections, unilateral
33901 normal native connections, bilateral
33902 abnormal connections, unilateral
33903 abnormal connections, bilateral
+33904 Percutaneous pulmonary artery revascularization by stent placement, each additional vessel or separate lesion; normal or abnormal connections

Endovascular repair of pulmonary artery stenosis by stent placement is reported depending on normal native or abnormal connections and unilateral or bilateral procedures.

- Stent placement within the pulmonary arteries via normal native connections (33900, 33901) is reported when the pathway to stent placement is through the superior vena cava/inferior vena cava to right atrium, then right ventricle, then pulmonary arteries.
- Stent placement via abnormal connections with codes 33902 and 33903 includes placement within the pulmonary arteries, the ductus arteriosus, or a surgical shunt; via abnormal connections; or through postsurgical shunts (eg, Blalock-Taussig shunt, Sano shunt, or post Glenn operation or Fontan procedure).
- Code 33904 is an AOC that describes placement of stent(s) in additional vessels or lesions beyond the primary vessel or lesion treated regardless of whether access occurs via normal or abnormal connections.
- Codes 33900–33904 include vascular access and all catheter and guidewire manipulation; fluoroscopy to guide the intervention; any post-diagnostic angiography for the purpose of road mapping; post-implant evaluation; stent positioning and balloon inflation for stent delivery; and radiological supervision and interpretation of the intervention.
- Report 33904 only when also reporting 33900–33903.

Read the *CPT* instructions to determine whether diagnostic right- and left-sided heart catheterization, diagnostic coronary angiography, and diagnostic angiography performed in conjunction with 33900–33904 may be separately reported.

- Do not report diagnostic cardiac catheterization and diagnostic angiography codes (93451–93568, 93593–93598) in conjunction with 33900–33904 for any of the following procedures:
  - ✖ Contrast injections, angiography, road mapping, and/or fluoroscopic guidance for the stent placement
  - ✖ Pulmonary conduit angiography for guidance
  - ✖ Right-sided heart catheterization for hemodynamic measurements before, during, and after stent placement
- ✖ Do not report balloon angioplasty within the same target lesion as the stent implant, either before or after stent deployment. Balloon angioplasty for a distinct lesion or in a different artery may be separately reported with 92997 and 92998 when performed at the same session.

Percutaneous Transcatheter Closure of Patent Ductus Arteriosus

93582 Percutaneous transcatheter closure of patent ductus arteriosus

- Includes, when performed (do not separately report)
  - Introduction of catheter, right heart or main pulmonary artery (36013)
  - Selective catheter placement, left or right pulmonary artery (36014)
  - Introduction of catheter, aorta (36200)
  - Aortography, thoracic, without serialography, radiological supervision and interpretation (75600)
  - Aortography, thoracic, by serialography, radiological supervision and interpretation (75605)
  - Heart catheterization or catheter placement for coronary angiography (93451–94361)
  - Heart catheterization for congenital cardiac anomalies (93593–93598)
  - Injection procedure during cardiac catheterization including imaging supervision, interpretation, and report; for supravalvular aortography (93567)
- Separately report when performed at the time of transcatheter patent ductus arteriosus closure
  - Pharmacologic agent administration (93463)
  - Intracardiac echocardiography during therapeutic/diagnostic intervention, including imaging supervision and interpretation (93662)
  - AOCs for injection procedures during cardiac catheterization, including imaging supervision, with interpretation and report, for
    - Selective coronary angiography during congenital heart catheterization (93563)

- Selective opacification of aortocoronary venous or arterial bypass graft(s) to one or more coronary arteries and in situ arterial conduits, whether native or used for bypass to one or more coronary arteries during congenital heart catheterization, when performed (93564)
- Selective left ventricular or left atrial angiography (93565)
- Selective right ventricular or right atrial angiography (93566)
- Nonselective pulmonary arterial angiography (93568) or selective pulmonary angiography (93569, 93573–93575) performed during congenital heart catheterization

Modifier 63 may be appended to 93582 when the procedure is performed on an infant weighing less than 4 kg.

Vascular Access

Many vascular access procedures are included in the services reported with critical or intensive care codes. Refer to **Chapter 17** for a list of procedures not separately reported by a physician or QHP who is reporting critical care services on the same date.

Central Venous Access

There is no distinction between venous access achieved percutaneously or via cutdown. Report the venous access code appropriate to the

- Type of insertion (ie, centrally inserted or peripherally inserted)
- Type of catheter (eg, non-tunneled or tunneled)
- Device (eg, with or without port)
- Age of child

In non-facility settings, 96522 may be reported for refilling and maintenance of an implantable pump or reservoir for systemic (intravenous, intra-arterial) drug delivery.

Irrigation of an implanted venous access device for drug delivery (96523) is reported only in non-facility settings and when no other service is reported by the same individual on the same date.

✖ Do not report codes for refilling and maintenance and/or irrigation by physicians in facility settings.

If an existing central venous access device is removed and a new one *placed via a separate venous access site*, appropriate codes for both procedures (removal of old, if code exists, and insertion of new device) should be reported. Refer to replacement codes for removal with replacement *via the same venous access site*.

Insertion or Replacement of Centrally Inserted Central Venous Access Device

Refer to "Centrally Inserted Central Venous Catheter: Codes for Insertion and Replacement" at www.aap.org/cfp2026 for a comparison of codes by procedure and the patient's age.

- Codes 36555–36558 and 36560 and 36561 are selected according to the patient's age on the date of the procedure to insert the catheter.
- Codes for insertion of a tunneled centrally inserted central venous catheter (36563–36566) are not selected according to the patient's age.
- To qualify as a centrally inserted central venous access device, both the following circumstances must be true:
  - The entry site must be the *jugular, subclavian, or femoral vein or the inferior vena cava.*
  - The tip of the catheter must terminate in the *subclavian, brachiocephalic (innominate), or iliac veins; the superior or inferior vena cava; or the right atrium.*
- Moderate sedation services are separately reportable with 99151–99157. For more information on reporting moderate sedation, refer to the Moderate Sedation section in **Chapter 13**.
- Report imaging guidance for gaining access to venous entry site or manipulating the catheter into final central position (in addition to 36555–36558) with either of the following codes:
  - 76937 (ultrasound guidance for vascular access requiring ultrasound evaluation of potential access sites, documentation of selected vessel patency, concurrent real-time ultrasound visualization of vascular needle entry, with permanent recording and reporting)

  - 77001 (fluoroscopic guidance for central venous access device placement, replacement [catheter only or complete], or removal [includes fluoroscopic guidance for vascular access and catheter manipulation, any necessary contrast injections through access site or catheter with related venography radiologic supervision and interpretation, and radiographic documentation of final catheter position])
- ✖ *Do not separately report ultrasonography when performed only for vessel identification.*
- Report replacement of the catheter only with 36578, or report complete replacement with 36578–36583.

Insertion of Peripherally Inserted Central Venous Access Device

Refer to "Peripherally Inserted Central Venous Catheter: Codes" at www.aap.org/cfp2026 for comparison of codes for PICC insertion procedures and codes for PICC replacement procedures.

- To qualify as a PICC, both the following circumstances must be true:
  - The entry site must be a *peripheral vein (eg, axillary, basilic, or cephalic).*
  - The tip of the catheter *must terminate in the subclavian, brachiocephalic (innominate), or iliac veins; the superior or inferior vena cava; or the right atrium.*

Midline catheters terminate in the peripheral venous system. Midline catheter insertion is not reported as a PICC insertion. Refer to 36400, 36406, and 36410 for midline catheter insertion. Note that 36400, 36406, and 36410 are not separately reported when the same physician or QHP is reporting neonatal or pediatric critical or intensive care services.

- Codes 36568 and 36569 are reported for PICC insertion without a subcutaneous port *and without imaging guidance* according to the patient's age. This includes placement through magnetic guidance or any guidance modality that does not include imaging with image documentation.
- ✖ Do not report imaging guidance (76937, 77001) in conjunction with 36568 and 36569.
- If imaging guidance is used in PICC insertion, refer to 36572, 36573, and 36584. Imaging guidance is included in the placement (36572, 36573) or complete replacement (36584) of a PICC without subcutaneous port or pump.
- ✖ Do not report chest radiographs (71045–71048) for the purpose of documenting the final catheter position by the same physician on the same day of service as the PICC insertion (36572, 36573, or 36584). If PICC insertion is performed without confirmation of the catheter tip location, append modifier 52 (reduced service) to the code for catheter insertion (36572, 36573, or 36584).
- Documentation of services includes
  - Images from all modalities used (eg, ultrasonography, fluoroscopy) stored in the patient record
  - Associated supervision and interpretation
  - Venography performed through the same venous puncture
  - The final central position of the catheter with imaging
- Report PICC insertion *with a subcutaneous port* with 36570 and 36571.
  - Ultrasound (76937) or fluoroscopic guidance (77001) may be separately reported when performed and documented.
  - Documentation of ultrasound guidance for PICC placement should include evaluation of the potential puncture sites, patency of the entry vein, and real-time ultrasound visualization of needle entry into the vein.

Repair of Central Venous Catheters

36575	Repair of tunneled or non-tunneled central venous access catheter, without subcutaneous port or pump, central or peripheral insertion site
36576	Repair of central venous access device, with subcutaneous port or pump, central or peripheral insertion site
36593	Declotting by thrombolytic agent of implanted vascular access device or catheter
36595	Mechanical removal of pericatheter obstructive material (eg, fibrin sheath) from central venous device via separate venous access

For radiological supervision and interpretation of mechanical removal of pericatheter obstructive material from a central venous device via separate venous access, report 75901.

36596	Mechanical removal of intraluminal (intracatheter) obstructive material from central venous device through device lumen
36598	Contrast injection(s) for radiologic evaluation of existing central venous access device, including fluoroscopy, image documentation and report

Repair of a central venous catheter includes fixing the device without replacement of the catheter or port/pump.

- For the repair of a multi-catheter device, with or without subcutaneous ports or pumps, use the appropriate code describing the service with 2 units of service.
- Repair of any central venous access catheter *without a port or pump* is reported with **36575**.
- Repair of any central venous access catheter *with a port or pump* is reported with **36576**.
- Code **36593** is reported for declotting of an implanted vascular device or catheter *by thrombolysis.*
- Code **36593** *is not reported* for declotting of a pleural catheter. Use unlisted procedure code **32999** for declotting of a pleural catheter.
- Codes **36595** and **36596** are reported for a procedure with *mechanical removal* of pericatheter or intraluminal obstructive material.
  - Radiological supervision and interpretation are separately reported with **75901**.
- ✖ Do not report **36595** or **36596** in conjunction with **36593** or **36598**.
- When the patency of a central venous catheter is evaluated under fluoroscopy, **36598** is reported for the contrast injection, image documentation, and report.
  - Fluoroscopy (**76000**) is not separately reported.
  - Refer to **75820–75827** for complete venography studies.

Removal of Central Venous Catheters

36589	Removal of tunneled central venous catheter, without subcutaneous port or pump
36590	Removal of tunneled central venous access device, with subcutaneous port or pump, central or peripheral insertion

Removal codes are reported for removal of the entire device. Refer to replacement codes for partial replacement (catheter only) or complete exchange *in the same venous access site* of central venous access devices.

- For removal of both catheters (placed from separate venous access sites) of a multi-catheter device, with or without subcutaneous ports/pumps, use the appropriate code describing the procedure with 2 units of service.
- When removal of an existing central venous access device is performed in conjunction with placement of a new device *via a separate venous access site,* report both procedures.

Arterial Access

36600	Arterial puncture, withdrawal of blood for diagnosis
36620	Arterial catheterization or cannulation for sampling, monitoring or transfusion (separate procedure); percutaneous
36625	cutdown

- An arterial puncture for diagnosis is reported with **36600**.
- Codes **36620** and **36625** differentiate reporting for peripheral arterial catheterization by percutaneous insertion from when a cutdown is performed.

Transfusions

36430	Transfusion, blood or blood components
36440	Push transfusion; blood, 2 years or younger

Push transfusion (36440) is used only for patients younger than 3 years.

36450	Exchange transfusion, blood, newborn
36455	other than newborn
36456	Partial exchange transfusion, blood, plasma, or crystalloid necessitating the skill of a physician or other QHP; newborn

The placement of catheters to support exchange transfusions may be reported separately with the appropriate vascular access codes.

- Transfusion (36430) or push transfusion (36440) should be used only if the physician personally infuses the substance and not if the blood is administered by nursing personnel and allowed to enter the vessel via gravity or meter flow. Codes 36430 and 36440 are not separately reported when the same physician or physicians of the same specialty and same group practice are reporting neonatal or pediatric critical care (99468–99472, 99475, 99476).
- Complete exchange transfusions (double volume) performed during the neonatal period are reported with 36450; exchange transfusions for all other age-groups are reported with 36455.
  - The assumption is that the exchange for the neonate is performed via the umbilical vein, whereas an exchange for an older child or adult is performed via a peripheral vessel.
  - The actual placement of catheters to support the exchange transfusion may be reported separately with the appropriate vascular access codes.
- Partial exchange transfusions (eg, for hyperviscosity syndrome in the neonate) should be reported with 36456.
- ✖ Do not report other transfusion codes (36430, 36440, or 36450) with 36456.
- ✖ Do not append modifier 63 (procedure performed on infants <4 kg) when reporting 36450 or 36456.

Diagnosis codes Z67.A1–Z67.A4 are reported when a patient's Duffy phenotype influences MDM related to transfusions.

Ear, Nose, and Throat Procedures

69421	Myringotomy including aspiration and/or eustachian tube inflation requiring general anesthesia
69433	Tympanostomy (requiring insertion of ventilating tube), local or topical anesthesia
69436	Tympanostomy (requiring insertion of ventilating tube), general anesthesia

- For bilateral procedure, report code 69436 with modifier 50. Refer to **Chapter 2** for further discussion of modifier 50.
- Insertion of ventilation tube(s) is not separately reported when performed in conjunction with another middle ear procedure (eg, tympanoplasty) without significant increase in work.
- Cleaning debris from the lateral drum, including a pars flaccida retraction pocket, is inclusive to the tube placement code.
- Use of an operating microscope is included in the procedure described by 69436.

Code 69436 may be reported without a modifier (eg, 52, reduced service) when a ventilating tube is replaced under general anesthesia. Report 69433 (tympanostomy requiring insertion of a ventilation tube) for replacement under local or topical anesthesia.

Nasopharyngoscopy

92511	Nasopharyngoscopy with endoscope (separate procedure)

Code 92511 is designated as a "separate procedure" and should not be reported in addition to the code for the total procedure or service of which it is considered an integral component.

- When carried out independently, report 92511.
- When considered to be unrelated or distinct from other procedures or services provided at that time, report 92511 59 in addition to other procedures or services.

Laryngoplasty

#31551	Laryngoplasty; for laryngeal stenosis, with graft, without indwelling stent placement, younger than 12 years of age
#31552	age 12 years or older
#31553	Laryngoplasty; for laryngeal stenosis, with graft, with indwelling stent placement, younger than 12 years of age
#31554	age 12 years or older
31580	Laryngoplasty; for laryngeal web, with indwelling keel or stent insertion
31584	Laryngoplasty; with open reduction and fixation of (eg, plating) fracture, includes tracheostomy, if performed

- ✖ Do not report the graft separately if harvested through the laryngoplasty incision (eg, thyroid cartilage graft).
- Report only 1 of the following codes for a single operative session: 31551–31554 or 31580.
- Codes for treatment of laryngeal stenosis by laryngoplasty with the graft are selected depending on whether the procedure includes indwelling stent placement and on the age of the patient (<12 years or ≥12 years).

- Open treatment of a hyoid fracture is reported with 31584 (repair procedure on the larynx).
- To report tracheostomy, refer to 31600, 31601, 31603, 31605, or 31610.
- Report laryngoplasty, not otherwise specified or for removal of a keel or stent, with 31599.

Adenoidectomy and Tonsillectomy

42820 Tonsillectomy and adenoidectomy; younger than age 12
42821 age 12 or over
42825 Tonsillectomy, primary or secondary; younger than age 12
42826 age 12 or over
42830 Adenoidectomy, primary; younger than age 12
42831 age 12 or over
42835 Adenoidectomy, secondary; younger than age 12
42836 age 12 or over

Report only the code for the combined tonsillectomy and adenoidectomy (42820–42821) when both are provided.

For partial ablation of the tonsils with a laser, report the appropriate code from 42820 or 42821, or 42825 or 42826, with modifier 52 (reduced service).

For control of hemorrhage following tonsillectomy or adenoidectomy, refer to 42960–42972. Modifier 22 (increased service) may be reported in conjunction with tonsillectomy codes when significant bleeding *during the procedure* requires extensive dissection.

- ✖ Do not append modifier 52 (reduced service) when intracapsular tonsillectomy is performed. Report the procedure (tonsillectomy or tonsillectomy with adenoidectomy) with the appropriate code without a modifier, as the work of the procedure and outcome are unchanged.
- ✖ Do not separately report incision and drainage of a peritonsillar abscess (42700) when performed in conjunction with tonsillectomy.

Digestive System Procedures

Gastric Intubation and Aspiration

43752 Naso- or orogastric tube placement, requiring physician's skill and fluoroscopic guidance (includes fluoroscopy, image documentation and report)
43753 Gastric intubation and aspiration(s), therapeutic (eg, for ingested poisons), including lavage if performed

Do not report 43752 or 43753 in conjunction with critical or intensive care services (99291, 99292; 99466–99469; 99471–99476; or 99477–99480). Append modifier 25 to codes for other significant, separately identifiable E/M services (eg, hospital care, consultation).

Note that 43752 is reported when a physician's skill and fluoroscopic guidance are required for placement of a nasogastric or orogastric tube. Use of fluoroscopic guidance must be documented (ie, image documentation and report).

- ✖ Do not separately report 43752 for tube placement to insufflate the stomach before percutaneous gastrointestinal tube placement.
- ✖ Do not report 43752 when a physician's skill is not required or placement is performed without fluoroscopic guidance.

Examples

➤ **A patient requires placement of a nasogastric tube.** Attempts by nursing staff are unsuccessful, so placement by the physician is required. The physician places the tube using fluoroscopic guidance.

➤ **A child is brought to the ED after having ingested drugs.** Gastric intubation and lavage are performed.

Code 43753 is reported in addition to the appropriate E/M service (eg, ED services [99281–99285]).

Appendectomy

44950 Appendectomy
+44955 when done for indicated purpose at time of other major procedure

• indicates a new code; ▲, revised; #, re-sequenced; +, add-on; ★, audiovisual technology; and ◀, synchronous interactive audio.

44960 for ruptured appendix with abscess or generalized peritonitis
44970 Laparoscopy, surgical, appendectomy
44979 Unlisted laparoscopy procedure, appendix

As a sole procedure, appendectomy coding is fairly straightforward, with 3 code choices: 44950, 44960, and 44970.

CPT instructs that incidental appendectomy (ie, not caused by disease or symptom) during intra-abdominal surgery does not usually warrant reporting a code for the appendectomy procedure.

- If it is necessary to report an incidental appendectomy performed during another intra-abdominal procedure, append modifier 52 (reduced service).
- The Medicaid NCCI manual also instructs that incidental removal of a normal appendix during another abdominal surgery is not separately reportable. This instruction is likely followed by other payers.

Appendectomy performed for an indicated purpose (ie, problem with the appendix) in conjunction with another procedure is separately reported.

- Report AOC 44955 in addition to the code for the primary procedure when open appendectomy is performed (because clinically indicated) in conjunction with another procedure.
- For a laparoscopic appendectomy when done for an indicated purpose at the time of another major procedure, report 44979.
- A separate diagnosis code (distinct from the diagnoses for which other intra-abdominal procedures were performed) should be linked to the appendectomy procedure code to indicate the medical necessity of the procedure.

Inguinal Hernia Repair

Diagnosis codes for reporting an inguinal hernia are shown in **Table 18-3**. Report additional codes that specify preterm birth/gestational age (P07.3-, additional character required to designate completed weeks of gestation) and/or comorbidities that affect patient management in addition to codes for inguinal hernia.

Table 18-3. Inguinal Hernia Diagnosis Codes

Laterality	Without Obstruction or Gangrene	With Obstruction	With Gangrene
Unilateral	K40.90	K40.30	K40.40
Unilateral, recurrent	K40.91	K40.31	K40.41
Bilateral	K40.20	K40.00	K40.10
Bilateral, recurrent	K40.21	K40.01	K40.11

Laparoscopic Inguinal Hernia Repair

For laparoscopic inguinal hernia repair, report either 49650 or 49651. Append modifier 50 (bilateral procedure) to the code for inguinal hernia repair performed bilaterally. Modifier 63 (procedure performed in infants less than 4 kg) may be appended to codes 49650–49651 when the procedures are performed in neonates and infants up to a present body weight of 4 kg.

49650 Laparoscopy, surgical; repair initial inguinal hernia
49651 repair recurrent inguinal hernia

Open Inguinal Hernia Repair

For open hernia repair, refer to the procedure codes in **Table 18-4**.

- For the purpose of reporting inguinal hernia repair codes 49491–49492 and 49495–49496, selection is based, in part, on preterm or full-term birth and age at the time of the procedure. For preterm neonates and infants, postconception age equals gestational age at birth plus age of newborn/infant in weeks at the time of the hernia repair.

Table 18-4. Codes for Open Repair of Inguinal Hernia in Infants and Children

Infant's Birth Status (preterm/term) and Age at Time of Surgery	Reducible Hernia	Incarcerated or Strangulated Hernia
Preterm (up to 50 wk PC age)—initial repair	49491[a]	49492[a,b]
Term <6 mo old, or preterm >50 wk PC age and <6 mo old—initial repair	49495[a]	49496[a,b]
Any infant 6 mo to <5 y old—initial repair	49500[a]	49501[a,b]
Child ≥5 y—initial repair	49505[c]	49507[b,c]
Any age, recurrent hernia	49520	49521[b]
Any age, sliding	49525	

Abbreviation: PC, postconception.

[a] Procedures reported with codes 49491–49501 include hydrocelectomy, when performed.

[b] Excision or repair of strangulated organs or structures (eg, 44120) is reported in addition to the repair of a strangulated hernia.

[c] Separately report simple orchiectomy (54520) or excision of hydrocele (54840 or 55040), when performed, in conjunction with 49505 or 49507.

Examples of Calculating Postconception Age

➤ **Postconception age up to 50 weeks (eg, 35-weeks'-gestational age infant now 6 weeks old = 41 weeks' postconception age)**

➤ **Postconception age greater than 50 weeks (eg, 35-weeks'-gestational age infant now 16 weeks old = 51 weeks' postconception age)**

- ✖ Do not append modifier 63 (procedure performed on infants <4 kg) to 49491, 49492, 49495, or 49496.
- Separately report inguinal hernia repair (49495–49525) performed in conjunction with inguinal orchiopexy (54640).
- Append modifier 50 when procedures are performed bilaterally.

Refer to 49591–49618 for reporting anterior abdominal hernia(s) (ie, epigastric, incisional, ventral, umbilical, spigelian) and 49621 or 49622 for reporting repair of parastomal hernia.

Genitourinary System Procedures

Anogenital Examination

99170 Anogenital examination, magnified, in childhood for suspected trauma including image recording when performed

Example

➤ **A child is brought to the ED for concern of sexual abuse after blood was found in the child's underpants.** The physician performs a comprehensive history and physical examination. Because of the findings on general examination, the physician elects to further examine the child's genitalia with magnification to document findings.

Common Surgical Procedures and Sedation in Facility Settings

Chapter 18

ICD-10-CM	*CPT*
Report confirmed abuse with all the following codes: T74.22XA (child sexual abuse, confirmed, initial encounter) An appropriate injury code (eg, S39.848A, other specified injuries of external genitals, initial encounter) A code from categories X92–Y06 or Y08 for assault A code from category Y07 to identify the perpetrator of assault If abuse is suspected but not confirmed, report T76.22XA (child sexual abuse, suspected, initial encounter) and a code for injury. If there are no findings, report Z04.42 (encounter for examination and observation following alleged child rape or sexual abuse).	99285 (comprehensive ED examination) 99170 (anogenital examination) If the same physician performs moderate (conscious) sedation, also report 99152.

Refer to the Moderate Sedation section in **Chapter 13** for a detailed discussion of the codes for reporting this service.

Correction of Chordee and Hypospadias

54300 Plastic operation of penis for straightening of chordee (eg, hypospadias), with or without mobilization of urethra

54304 Plastic operation on penis for correction of chordee or for first stage hypospadias repair with or without transplantation of prepuce and/or skin flaps

54340 Repair of hypospadias complication(s) (ie, fistula, stricture, diverticula); by closure, incision, or excision, simple

54344 requiring mobilization of skin flaps and urethroplasty with flap or patch graft

54348 requiring extensive dissection, and urethroplasty with flap, patch or tubed graft (including urinary diversion, when performed)

54352 Revision of prior hypospadias repair requiring extensive dissection and excision of previously constructed structures including re-release of chordee and reconstruction of urethra and penis by use of local skin as grafts and island flaps and skin brought in as flaps or grafts

Code 54300 is appropriately reported for *straightening* of the chordee to correct congenital concealed penis (Q55.64). This procedure may also be performed to correct an entrapped penis after newborn circumcision (eg, release of concealed penis with coverage of deficient penile ventral skin by penile skin-raised Byars flaps and re-circumcision).

Codes 54304–54336 describe procedures performed to *correct* hypospadias in either single- or multiple-stage procedures.

- ✖ Do not separately report 54300, 54304, or 54360 (plastic operation on penis to correct angulation) when reporting single-stage repair of hypospadias.

Correction of penile chordee or penile curvature is included in all single-stage repairs of hypospadias.

- ● Repair or revision of hypospadias complication is reported with 54340–54352.
- ✖ Do not separately report the following procedures when reporting 54352: application of skin substitute graft (15275); formation of direct or tubed pedicle (15574); island pedicle flap (15740); excision of urethral diverticulum (53235); one-stage urethroplasty of anterior urethra (53410); repair of hypospadias or hypospadias correction described by codes 54300, 54336, 54340, 54344, and 54348; or plastic operation to correct penile angulation (54360).

Sedation

Moderate Sedation

Moderate sedation is reported with 99151–99153 (provided by the same physician or QHP performing the diagnostic or therapeutic service) and 99155–99157 (provided by a different physician or QHP who is not performing the diagnostic or therapeutic service). Refer to **Table 13-3** for full code descriptors and time requirements.

Moderate sedation codes are not used to report administration of medications for pain control, minimal sedation (anxiolysis), deep sedation, or monitored anesthesia care (00100–01999).

For more detailed discussion of moderate sedation, refer to **Chapter 13**.

Deep Sedation/Anesthesia Services

Deep sedation/analgesia is a drug-induced depression of consciousness during which patients cannot be easily aroused but respond purposefully after repeat verbal or painful stimulation (eg, purposefully pushing away the noxious stimuli). A state of deep sedation may be accompanied by partial or complete loss of protective airway reflexes. Cardiovascular function is usually maintained.

CPT codes for reporting anesthesia services, including deep sedation, monitored anesthesia care, or general anesthesia, are **00100–01999**. These codes are not as specific as codes for other services and generally identify a body area or type of procedure.

00102 Anesthesia for procedures involving plastic repair of cleft lip

01820 Anesthesia for all closed procedures on radius, ulna, wrist, or hand bones

Anesthesia services include

- Preoperative evaluation of the patient
- Administration of anesthetic, other medications, blood, and fluids
- Monitoring of physiologic parameters
- Other supportive services
- Postoperative E/M related to the surgery (Ongoing critical care services by an anesthesiologist may be separately reportable.)

Pediatricians who provide deep sedation services for procedures performed outside the operating suite should follow the same anesthesia policies and coding instructions as other providers of anesthesia services.

If surgery is canceled subsequent to the preoperative evaluation, payment may be allowed to the anesthesiologist for an E/M service and the appropriate E/M code (eg, consultation) may be reported. Refer to Chapter 16 for information on reporting these services.

AOCs may be reported to identify special circumstances that increase the complexity of providing anesthesia care, including

+99100 Patient under 1 year or older than 70 years (not reported in conjunction with codes **00326**, **00561**, **00834**, or **00836**)

+99116 Anesthesia complicated by total body hypothermia

+99135 Anesthesia complicated by controlled hypotension

+99140 Emergency conditions

Emergency is defined by *CPT* as a situation in which delay in treatment of the patient would lead to a significant increase in the threat to life or body part.

Modifiers are reported in addition to anesthesia codes to indicate the physical status of the patient. The American Society of Anesthesiologists classification of the patient's physical status is represented by the following HCPCS modifiers:

P1 Normal healthy patient

P2 Patient with mild systemic disease

P3 Patient with severe systemic disease

P4 Patient with severe systemic disease that is a constant threat to life

P5 Moribund patient who is not expected to survive without the operation

P6 Declared brain-dead patient whose organs are being removed for donor purposes

Base units for anesthesia services are published in the American Society of Anesthesiologists *Relative Value Guide* and by the CMS for each anesthesia procedure code. Payers do not typically require reporting of base units on the claim for services.

- Many private payers will allow additional base units for physical status modifiers **P3** (1 unit), **P4** (2 units), and **P5** (3 units).
- Anesthesia time is reported in minutes unless a payer directs to report units (eg, 1 unit per 15 minutes). Start and stop times must be documented, including multiple start and stop times when anesthesia services are discontinuous.

Other modifiers that may be required by payers for anesthesia services by pediatric physicians are those identifying the type of anesthesia or anesthesia provider.

AA Anesthesia services performed personally by anesthesiologist

Payers may also require this modifier for services personally rendered by physicians other than anesthesiologists. This signifies that services were not rendered by a nonphysician provider, such as a certified registered nurse anesthetist.

GC	This service has been performed in part by a resident under the direction of a teaching physician
G8	Monitored anesthesia care for deep complex, complicated, or markedly invasive surgical procedure
G9	Monitored anesthesia care for patient who has history of severe cardiopulmonary condition
QS	Monitored anesthesia care service

Medicare considers deep sedation equivalent to monitored anesthesia care. Private payers may vary.

Postoperative Pain Management

Generally, the surgeon is responsible for postoperative pain management. However, a surgeon may request assistance with postoperative pain management (eg, epidural or peripheral nerve block).

- Payers may require a written request by the surgeon for postoperative pain management by the anesthesia provider.
- When a catheter is placed as the mode of anesthesia (eg, epidural catheter) and retained for use in postoperative pain management, this is not separately reported.
- When separately reporting postoperative pain management, append modifier 59 (distinct procedural service) to indicate the separate service and document this service distinctly (and preferably separately) from the anesthesia record.
- When an epidural catheter is used for postoperative pain management, 01996 (daily management of epidural) may be reported on days subsequent to the day of surgery. Daily management of other postoperative pain management devices may be reported with subsequent hospital care codes (99231–99233).

Example

➤ **An orthopedic surgeon requests preanesthetic insertion of a catheter to provide a continuous infusion of the femoral nerve for postoperative pain relief for a patient undergoing an arthroscopy of the knee with lateral meniscectomy.** The anesthesiologist uses ultrasound guidance to insert a catheter for continuous infusion before inducing general anesthesia for the surgical procedure.

ICD-10-CM	*CPT*
Appropriate diagnosis code	01400 (anesthesia for open or surgical arthroscopic procedures on knee joint; not otherwise specified) 64448 59 (injection, anesthetic agent[s] and/or steroid; femoral nerve, continuous infusion by catheter [including catheter placement])

Teaching Point: Because the anesthetist provided a distinct service separate from the anesthesia for the procedure, the catheter insertion is separately reported with modifier 59. Had the procedure been performed under an epidural block and the epidural catheter left in place for postoperative pain management, no additional code would have been reported.

To test your knowledge of the information presented in this chapter, complete the quiz found at the end of it, after the resources. Answers to each quiz are found in **Appendix II**.

Chapter Takeaways

This chapter addressed many aspects of coding for surgical care in a facility setting. Following are some takeaways from this chapter:

- Surgical services are packaged to include all the necessary services normally furnished by a surgeon before, during, and after a procedure.
- Payers may assign a global period (eg, 0, 10, or 90 days) according to the periods published in the MPFS or assign other global periods. It is important to identify the global periods when contracting with payers.
- Report **99024** (postoperative follow-up visit) for follow-up care during the global surgery period.
- Report other modifiers as needed to indicate circumstances such as distinct procedures performed by the same physician or QHP on the same date (**59**), increased (**22**) or decreased (**52**) procedural services, assistant surgeon (**80**, **81**, or **82**), or procedures performed in infants less than 4 kg (**63**).
- Teaching physicians should follow policies for physical presence during all or key portions of a procedure and be sure that the required presence is documented in the surgical record.
- *CPT* instructions preceding codes for surgical procedures provide important details on what services are or are not separately reported. These instructions should be reviewed when reporting multiple services on the same date or within a global period.

Resources

AAP Pediatric Coding Newsletter™

"*CPT 2024:* Reporting Unlisted Procedure Codes," December 2023 (https://doi.org/10.1542/pcco_book236_document004)

"Procedural Services: Modifiers to Report Site and Laterality," January 2025 (https://doi.org/10.1542/pcco_book249_document005)

"Q&A: Coding for Pediatric Echocardiography," August 2023 (https://doi.org/10.1542/pcco_book232_document003)

"What Stories Do the Modifiers on Your Claims Tell?" July 2023 (https://doi.org/10.1542/pcco_book231_document003)

Online-Exclusive Content at www.aap.org/cfp2026

"Centrally Inserted Central Venous Catheter: Codes for Insertion and Replacement"

"Codes and Instructions for Reporting Preparation for and Skin Grafting"

"Echocardiography Code List"

"Peripherally Inserted Central Venous Catheter: Codes"

Surgery

American Urological Association policy and advocacy brief, "Pediatric Hypospadias Repair: A New Consensus Document on Coding" (www.auanet.org/Documents/practices-resources/coding-tips/Pediatric-Hypospadias-Repair.pdf)

CMS-designated global periods, Medicare Resource-Based Relative Value Scale Physician Fee Schedule (www.cms.gov/medicare/payment/fee-schedules/physician/pfs-relative-value-files; refer to Column O in the PPRRVU Excel file included in the file for the most recent version of the fee schedule)

Teaching Physician

Medicare Claims Processing Manual, Chapter 12 (www.cms.gov/Regulations-and-Guidance/Guidance/Manuals/downloads/clm104c12.pdf)

Test Your Knowledge!

1. **Which of the following is a difference between the *CPT* surgical package and Medicare policy for postoperative care provided within the global period?**
   a. *CPT* does not describe any postoperative care in the surgical package.
   b. Medicare does not recognize global periods and pays separately for preoperative and postoperative care.
   c. Medicare policy includes services to address complications that do not include a return to the operating room in the surgical package during the global period.
   d. Medicare policy includes all services to address complications in the surgical package during the global period.
2. **What codes are reported when stabilization (eg, temporary cast/splint/strap) is performed to protect an injury and provide comfort to the patient until another physician performs initial fracture or dislocation care?**
   a. Only an E/M service (eg, emergency department E/M service)
   b. An E/M service and any application of a cast/splint/strap
   c. An appropriate fracture care code appended with modifier **54**
   d. An appropriate fracture care code appended with modifier **52**
3. **True or false? Codes for cardiac catheterization for congenital heart defect are reported only when the procedure is performed in a neonate or infant.**
   a. True
   b. False
4. **What type of code(s) is reported when an existing central venous access device is removed and a new one placed via a separate venous access site?**
   a. A code for removal of central venous access device
   b. A code for insertion
   c. Separate codes for removal and insertion
   d. A code for replacement
5. **Which is true when selecting codes for open repair of a strangulated inguinal hernia?**
   a. Codes do not differentiate strangulated hernia from a reducible hernia.
   b. Codes for excision/repair of strangulated organs or structures are not separately reported.
   c. Repair of a strangulated inguinal hernia is included in the procedure reported for excision or repair of the strangulated organs or structures.
   d. Excision or repair of strangulated organs or structures is reported in addition to the repair of a strangulated hernia.

Part 4

Digital Medicine Services

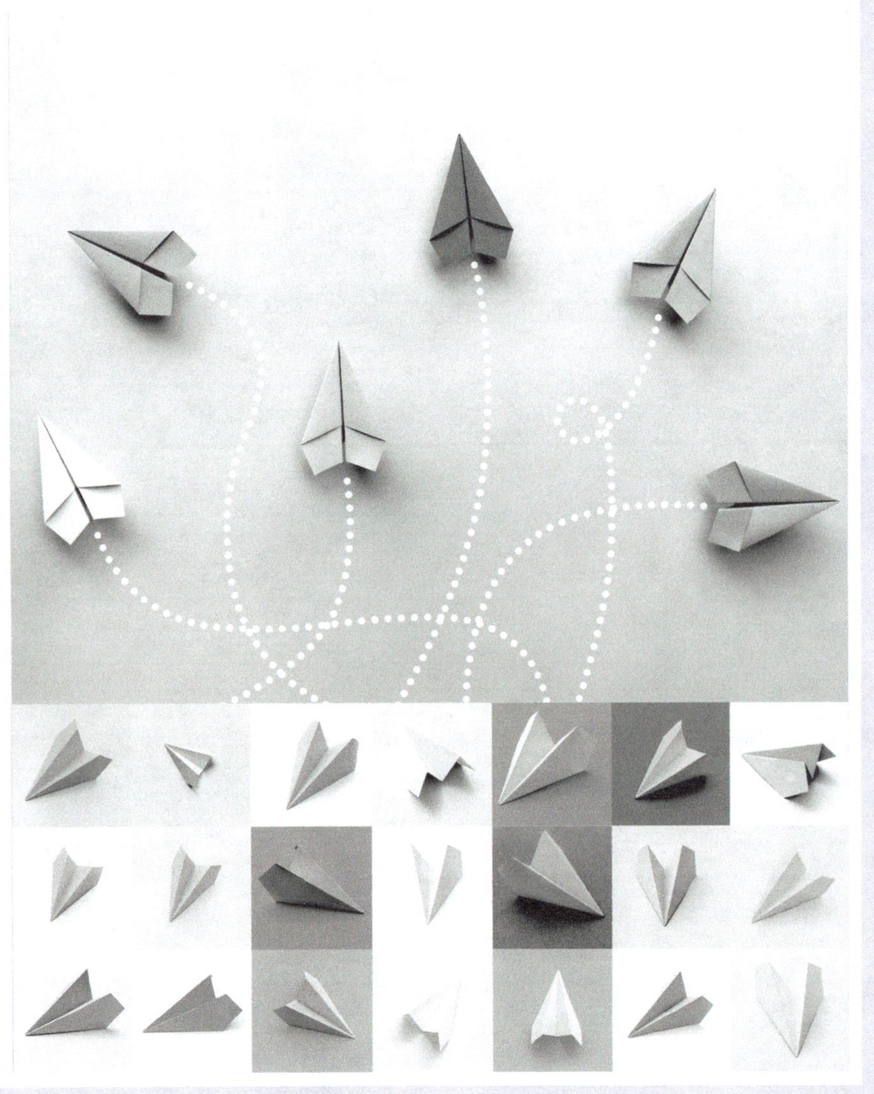

Part 4. Digital Medicine Services

CHAPTER 19

General Telemedicine Coding and Documentation Concepts

Contents

Chapter Highlights

- Definitions of telemedicine services
- Compliance with regulations for privacy and accessibility to services
- Identification of codes, modifiers, and place of service (POS) for telemedicine services in settings other than an office or other outpatient setting
- Differentiation of telemedicine services from telephone or online digital evaluation and management (E/M) services

This chapter addresses current definitions of telemedicine services and compliant provision, documentation, and coding. The general guidelines and regulatory compliance discussed in this chapter apply to all telemedicine services. However, codes and modifiers discussed here are not applicable when the service is reported with codes specific to synchronous audio-video or audio-only telemedicine services in office and outpatient settings or E/M services provided via asynchronous technology such as secure email or messaging (discussed in **Chapter 20**).

Defining Telemedicine Services

Put simply, telemedicine allows a physician or other qualified health care professional (QHP) and, for some services, a nonphysician qualified health care professional (NQHCP) (eg, psychologist, medical nutritionist) in a distant location to provide medical services to a patient without the need for either party to physically travel. Telemedicine is part of a larger category of digital medicine services that includes other services such as remote physiologic monitoring and digital diagnostic services such as multianalyte assays with algorithmic analysis. Provision of and payment for telemedicine services expanded greatly during the COVID-19 public health emergency. Demand for telemedicine continues to grow in both primary and subspecialty care.

Telemedicine Terminology

Key terms in differentiating telemedicine services from other digital services are *synchronous* and *asynchronous*. Telemedicine services (other than a special Medicare demonstration project) always include synchronous communication.

- **Synchronous telemedicine services include simultaneous (real-time) interaction between a physician/QHP/NQHCP and a patient who is located at a distant site.**
- **Asynchronous communication does not require simultaneous interaction from both parties. Examples of asynchronous communication are email correspondence and data and/or images transferred for review and subsequent response.**

The Centers for Medicare & Medicaid Services and some payers may use the term *telehealth* rather than *telemedicine* in payment policies. However, *telehealth* generally refers to a broader scope of remote health care services than telemedicine per the Assistant Secretary of Technology Policy and Office of the National Coordinator for Health Information Technology. Whereas *telemedicine* refers specifically to remote clinical services, *telehealth* can refer to remote nonclinical services, such as provider training, administrative meetings, and continuing medical education, in addition to clinical services.

Current Procedural Terminology (*CPT*) does not limit telemedicine services to services reported only by physicians and QHPs whose scope of practice includes E/M services. Many of the services that may be reported as telemedicine are reported by NQHCPs such as psychologists, licensed clinical social workers, dietitians, and speech pathologists.

Compliant Provision of Digital Medicine Services

This section addresses general compliance in delivery and documentation of telemedicine and other digital medicine services. Practice compliance includes proper documentation to support the services rendered, correct code assignment, and adherence to regulations for privacy and security of personal health information (PHI). Practice policies may vary depending on differences in state regulations or local and regional payer policies. Compliant provision and reporting of telemedicine services involves addressing many of the same concerns addressed for face-to-face services but with considerations of the type of technology used, state and federal regulations that are specific to telemedicine, and certain documentation requirements. Requirements may vary by state or payer.

Changes to state regulations and payer policies for telemedicine services are ongoing. These changes may limit the locations where a patient may receive care via telemedicine (eg, excluding home or a non-rural locale), coverage of services to new and/or established patients, and payment parity with in-person services.

- Practices must be aware of state regulations and local or regional payment policies.
- Physicians, QHPs, and NQHCPs must be aware of licensure requirements when providing telemedicine services to patients located in other states. States require licensure to practice in the patient's location at the time of service. Some states allow professionals from another state to provide telehealth services if they share a common border or have interstate medical licensure compacts that provide an expedited pathway to licensure in multiple states and territories for physicians who qualify.

Learn more about the Interstate Medical Licensure Compact at https://imlcc.com/a-faster-pathway-to-physician-licensure.

When providing telemedicine to any patients, a practice must make accommodations for access and effective delivery to a patient and/or parent or caregiver with disabilities or with limited English proficiency. Telemedicine services must be provided in a nondiscriminatory manner.

Protecting Privacy and Securing Protected Health Information

Before providing telemedicine or any digital medicine service, understand local and state laws, in addition to federal regulations such as the Health Insurance Portability and Accountability Act (HIPAA) of 1996 Privacy, Security, and Breach Notification Rules. Typically, where state and federal regulations differ, the stricter rule applies.

- Effort must be made to protect the privacy of communications that include PHI. Examples include
  - Providing services in a private setting and/or implementing reasonable safeguards to limit disclosure of PHI (eg, using a headset for telephone or computer audio rather than speakers)
  - Verifying the identity of individuals not known to the physician or QHP
- Electronic communication technologies, including cellular and Wi-Fi technology and computer or mobile device applications, are subject to the HIPAA security rule. The security rule requires risk analysis and risk management, which may include adoption of user authentication, encryption of data, and locking or termination of an application session after a period of inactivity. (Traditional or landline phones are not subject to the security rule.)
- HIPAA requires business associate agreements with any developer/provider of an electronic application that creates and/or receives and stores PHI (eg, application that includes transcription or recording and storage of PHI; language translation application). A business associate agreement with the telephone service provider (landline or cellular) is not required when the service is limited to connecting the call without routine access to or maintenance of the PHI transmitted on a call.

Choice of Service Delivery Method

Patients and/or caregivers must be given the options to receive or transition to audiovisual telemedicine or in-person visits when necessary or preferred.

State regulation or Medicaid plan policy may be more stringent. Some plans require documentation that the patient and/or caregiver is aware of the potential advantages and disadvantages of telemedicine, was given the option of not participating in telemedicine services, and was informed of their right to request a change in service delivery mode at any time.

Documentation of Services

Some plans require documentation of the patient's and/or caregiver's oral or written consent to receive services via telemedicine and, as discussed in the previous sections, may require documentation that the patient and/or caregiver made an informed choice to receive services via telemedicine.

In general, documentation of telemedicine services should be similar to that of services provided in traditional patient care settings, such as the following documentation of an E/M service:

- The reason for the visit and the requesting party (eg, patient, another physician or QHP)
- Relevant history and physical examination, if there is one
- Assessment and plan of care and/or recommendations
- The reporting individual's time, when code selection is based on time

Documentation must support the service reported. For instance, the time requirements for codes selected on the basis of total time or time of medical discussion must be met and supported in the documentation for the service. When codes are selected based on medical decision-making (MDM), the elements of MDM must be distinguishable in the documentation (eg, number and complexity of problems addressed, tests ordered).

Refer to Chapter 6 for more information on documentation of E/M services and instructions for reporting based on time.

Other documentation elements include

- Patient or family consent to receive a service via telemedicine
- Platform or modality by which the service is occurring (must be HIPAA compliant)
- Patient and physician location (Specificity may be necessary for locations other than the patient's home address, such as a school, group home, or out-of-state location.)
- Any other individuals present with the patient, including, when offered, identification of and contributions from a telepresenter (ie, a health care professional who is present with the patient to facilitate the service)
- Start and end times, when required, for the telemedicine encounter

Document any technology (eg, digital examination camera, digital stethoscope) used during a telemedicine encounter.

Payer Coverage

Payment for telemedicine services may be affected by state and federal regulations in addition to payer policy. Review the payment policies of health plans and payers such as Medicaid before initiating telemedicine services, as coverage and payment policies may vary.

Although state regulations may require that health plans originating in the state cover and pay equitably for telemedicine services, plans subject to other regulations (eg, self-funded health plans governed by the Employee Retirement Income Security Act of 1974) may be exempt from state regulations.

When contracting with payers, be aware of plans that include virtual-first or other restrictions of patient access to telemedicine services by community physicians. Virtual-first plans require or encourage patients to use one select telemedicine agency for initial health care services and receive a referral before receiving services from a physician or QHP in the patient's community. (This process does not typically apply to services such as recommended preventive services that require in-person examination.) The patient may have access to the plan's virtual care network without out-of-pocket costs versus application of a co-payment and/or deductible to services by other physicians and QHPs. A plan may also limit patient access by covering telemedicine services only when received from the plan's telemedicine vendor.

Medicare has published a list of codes covered when provided via telemedicine (www.cms.gov/medicare/coverage/telehealth/list-services; see the link on this page to "Medicare List of Telehealth Services for Calendar Year 2026 [ZIP]"), but this list may be more or less restrictive than the lists used by Medicaid plans and other payers. Private payers may limit telemedicine services to those described by specific codes and create benefit policy that allows only services for which state regulations mandate coverage. It is important to verify the services and sites of service that are covered by each patient's health plan.

Many health plans develop policies that designate covered and noncovered telemedicine services and reporting instructions for each. Health plan policies may be presented under various names (eg, telemedicine, telehealth/virtual health, virtual visits).

Services that are most often *not reportable* as a telemedicine service include

- A service provided on the same day as an in-person visit, when performed by the same provider and for the same condition
- A service that is incidental to an E/M service and limited to clinical staff communication of test results, scheduling additional services, or providing educational resources
- Any service that is not a covered benefit, such as travel counseling

Though not separately paid, a routine postoperative visit (**99024**) via telemedicine may be reportable based on payer policy. Code **99024** is not designated as a telemedicine service in *CPT*.

Individual plans vary in their payment policies for telemedicine and the Healthcare Common Procedure Coding System (HCPCS), *CPT* codes, and modifiers used to report telemedicine services. Managers and billing staff must maintain an awareness of these policies to receive appropriate payment.

A service that would not be separately reportable when provided in person is typically not separately reportable when provided via telemedicine. Follow *CPT* and payer instructions when reporting telemedicine services that are provided on the same date or that may be included another reported service.

Medicaid and Children's Health Insurance Plan Payment

For Medicaid and CHIP purposes, telemedicine (telehealth is the term used in Medicaid and CHIP guidelines) is a service that includes 2-way, real-time interactive communication between the patient at an originating site (eg, clinical facility or home) and the physician/QHP/NQHCP at a distant site (eg, physician practice location).

States have broad flexibility in designing the parameters of telemedicine delivery methods to furnish services. State regulations may restrict or allow use of audio-only interactive communication. However, states must observe telehealth delivery requirements set forth by Medicaid regulations for specific benefits (eg, coverage of specific telemedicine services). States that pay for covered telemedicine services at a rate equal to in-person provision of the same services do not need approval from the Centers for Medicare and Medicaid Services to cover the telemedicine services.

Policies may also vary between Medicaid managed care plans (eg, a specific plan may allow more than is required by standard Medicaid policy or regulation).

Medicaid plans may pay the physician or other QHP at the distant site for each service rendered via telemedicine and also pay **T1014** (telehealth transmission, per minute) to originating sites (other than patient's home) or **Q3014** (telehealth originating site facility fee).

States may also choose to pay for services delivered with technology that does not meet the definition of telemedicine services (eg, text messaging applications, facsimile machines, email systems, remote patient monitoring).

Refer to Chapter 21 for information on remote patient monitoring services.

States may cover telemedicine services reported with a variety of *CPT* and HCPCS codes. Because state regulations and coverage criteria are frequently changing, state- and plan-level guidance for provision and billing for telemedicine services must be monitored. Some states provide a list of *CPT* and HCPCS codes that are eligible for payment when provided via telemedicine. Modifiers are often required to designate a telemedicine service. For further discussion, refer to the Telemedicine Modifiers section later in this chapter.

Reporting Telemedicine Services

Place of Service Codes

Use of the correct POS code on claims for telemedicine services is important for appropriate payment. There are 2 POS codes that identify that a service was provided either to a patient in a place other than their home (ie, clinical setting) or to a patient in their home (eg, private residence or residential facility).

02 Telehealth provided other than in patient's home
10 Telehealth provided in patient's home

Payment may be affected by the POS code, as some services include payment for a physician's or QHP's practice expense for services provided in a non-facility setting (eg, office) versus a facility setting (eg, hospital or hospital-based clinic). POS code **02** typically triggers payment at a lower facility-based rate, when applicable.

Some payers accept the POS code for the location at which the physician or QHP would provide the service if performed in person (eg, **11**, office) in addition to appending a modifier (eg, **93** or **95**, discussed later in this chapter) to the procedure code to indicate that the service was delivered via telemedicine. However, POS codes **02** and **10** are more commonly required.

Billing staff should be aware of policies that affect how telemedicine services are reported to individual payers. Refer to Chapter 4 for more information on POS codes. Physicians and QHPs practicing in a hospital outpatient department (including a hospital-based practice) should verify the required POS (eg, 19, off-campus—outpatient hospital versus 02, telehealth provided in other than patient's home).

Refer to an individual payer's telemedicine policy to determine if there are reporting requirements for the specific site of service (eg, physical location from which services were rendered or received).

Field 32 of the 1500 paper professional claim form and its electronic equivalent is used to report the site of service (eg, hospital name, address, National Provider Identifier). This is typically the physical location of the physician or other provider of service at the time of service when payment is influenced by geographic location. The Medicare program currently allows a physician or other provider to use their currently enrolled practice location instead of their home address when providing telemedicine services from their home. Other payers may also allow listing the address where in-person care is typically rendered.

Telemedicine Modifiers

Modifiers are used to indicate that a service was somehow modified from what is typical (eg, reduced or increased service). *CPT* and HCPCS include modifiers for indicating that a service was provided by telemedicine. It is important to append an indicated modifier as directed by *CPT* or, when applicable, in compliance with an individual health plan's payment policy. Some health plans now accept telemedicine modifiers as informational only (ie, not affecting payment) and instead rely on the POS code to identify services provided via telemedicine and determine appropriate payment.

✖ Do not report telemedicine codes **98000–98015** with a telemedicine modifier.

Individual payers, especially those adopting Medicare policy to use office and other outpatient E/M service codes in lieu of telemedicine codes **98000–98015**, may require use of telemedicine modifiers in conjunction with codes that are not included in Appendixes P and T of the American Medical Association *CPT* manual.

Telemedicine modifiers include

93—Synchronous Telemedicine Service Rendered via Telephone or Other Real-Time Interactive Audio-Only Telecommunications System

Modifier **93** has limited utility for physicians and QHPs. It is appended to services preceded by an audio symbol (◀) and included in *CPT* Appendix T. Some services included in *CPT* Appendix T are

- Individual behavior change interventions (**99406–99409**)
- Advance care planning (**99497**, **99498**)
- Psychiatric services (**90791**, **90792**; **90832–90840**; **90845**; **90846**, **90847**; and **90785**)
- Health risk assessment (**96160**, **96161**)
- Developmental screening (**96110**)

✖ Do not report modifier **93** in conjunction with codes not included in *CPT* Appendix T (eg, E/M services other than those listed previously) unless directed by payer policy.

Refer to modifier **FQ**, discussed later in this chapter, when payer policy requires use of modifier **FQ** (eg, when reporting follow-up behavioral health and substance use disorder treatment services provided via audio-only technology).

95—Synchronous Telemedicine Service Rendered via a Real-Time Interactive Audio and Video Telecommunications System

Modifier **95** may be appended to the codes preceded by a star (★) and included in *CPT* Appendix P. Appending modifier **95** to the appropriate procedure code identifies to the payer that telemedicine services were rendered via real-time interactive audio and video telecommunications.

CPT Appendix P codes that may be of particular interest to pediatricians include

- Subsequent hospital inpatient or observation care (**99231–99233**, **99418**)
- Inpatient or observation (**99252–99255**, **99418**) and outpatient (**99242–99245**, **99417**) consultations
- Administration of patient-focused health risk assessment instrument (eg, health hazard appraisal) with scoring and documentation, per standardized instrument (**96160**)
- Administration of caregiver-focused health risk assessment instrument (eg, depression inventory) for the benefit of the patient, with scoring and documentation, per standardized instrument (**96161**)
- Individual behavior change interventions (**99406–99409**)
- Transitional care management services (**99495**, **99496**)

Notably, the following codes are not included in Appendix P:

✖ Initial hospital inpatient or observation care codes (**99221–99223**)
✖ Hospital inpatient or observation care with same date admission and discharge services (**99234–99236**)
✖ Hospital inpatient or observation discharge day management (**99238–99239**)
✖ Emergency department services (**99281–99285**)

General Telemedicine Coding and Documentation Concepts

Chapter 19

CPT Appendix P also includes codes for services such as psychotherapy, health and behavior assessment and intervention, medical nutrition therapy, and education and training for patient self-management, allowing for telemedicine services provided by certain nonphysician qualified health care professionals in addition to physicians and QHPs.

When providing services via telemedicine, it is important to note whether each service may be reported with a telemedicine modifier. For instance, use of a structured screening instrument to assess mental or behavioral health (96127) is not included in *CPT* Appendixes P or T. Individual payers may provide unique lists of codes that may be reported when provided via telemedicine with either *CPT* or HCPCS modifiers.

Healthcare Common Procedure Coding System Modifiers

FQ—The Service Was Furnished Using Audio-Only Communication Technology

Modifier FQ is used specifically for reporting *telehealth for behavioral health and substance use disorder treatment services* furnished to a patient in their home through audio-only communications technology. This modifier is not reported in conjunction with codes for other services unless specified as such in payer policy. Refer to **Chapter 2** for additional information.

Modifier FQ may apply to either E/M services or psychiatric services when the reason for the service is continuing management of a diagnosed behavioral health or substance use disorder.

GQ—Via Asynchronous Telecommunications System

The application of GQ is limited to services provided via asynchronous technology (eg, store-and-forward of digital images for interpretation and report).

GT—Via Interactive Audio and Video Telecommunication Systems

Some payers accept modifier GT in lieu of modifier 95. Critical access hospitals billing under Method II report modifier GT (via interactive audio and video telecommunication systems) because no POS code is reported on Method II claims to identify telemedicine services. Some health plans may also require modifier GT, although this modifier is no longer accepted by Medicare on claims for physician services.

Medicaid plans may also use modifiers U1–UD (as defined by the state) to identify, track, and pay for telemedicine services.

Telemedicine in *Current Procedural Terminology*

As defined by *CPT*, synchronous telemedicine services include real-time interaction between a physician or QHP and a patient who is located at a separate site. The total communication between the physician or QHP and the patient during the course of the synchronous telemedicine service must be of an amount and nature that would be sufficient to meet the requirements of the same service when rendered in person.

CPT provides 2 reporting methods for synchronous telemedicine services provided via a real-time interactive audio-only or audio-video telecommunications system.

1. Codes that specifically describe services delivered via telemedicine (ie, 98000–98015)
2. Codes that are typically reported for an in-person service to which a modifier is appended to identify that the service was provided via either synchronous real-time interactive audio-video or audio-only telecommunications.

Symbols preceding certain *CPT* codes indicate the applicability of telemedicine modifiers 93 and 95.

- *CPT* codes for services that are typically performed in person but may be rendered via a synchronous interactive audio-video telecommunications system are preceded by a star (★) and listed in *CPT* Appendix P.
- *CPT* codes for telemedicine services that may be delivered by technology including at least synchronous interactive audio communication, in lieu of audiovisual technology, are preceded by an audio symbol (◀) and listed in *CPT* Appendix T.

Refer to the Telemedicine Modifiers section earlier in this chapter for examples of codes included in Appendix P or T.

Refer to Chapter 20 for information on coding for E/M services provided via online digital communication technology (eg, secure email, patient portal). *CPT* does not include these services in the listing of telemedicine services for the purpose of code assignment.

HCPCS Telemedicine Codes

Although *CPT* codes are accepted by most plans covering telemedicine services, payers may require HCPCS codes that are used in the Medicare/Medicaid programs for consultations and other services with specific coverage policies (eg, telemedicine critical care consultation).

- HCPCS codes are used for telemedicine consultations with Medicare beneficiaries because *CPT* consultation codes are not payable under the Medicare Physician Fee Schedule.
- Verify the individual payer's policies for the following HCPCS codes, including required documentation of time (eg, face-to-face time with patient versus total time on the date of the visit) and medical decision-making. For Medicare purposes, these time-based codes may also be selected on the basis of 2 of 3 of documented history, physical examination, and medical decision-making. Individual payer policies may vary.
- Also, verify the place of service code required on claims (typically **02**).

G0406 Follow-up inpatient consultation, limited, physicians typically spend 15 minutes communicating with the patient via telehealth

G0407 intermediate, physicians typically spend 25 minutes communicating with the patient via telehealth

G0408 complex, physicians typically spend 35 minutes communicating with the patient via telehealth

G0425 Telehealth consultation, emergency department or initial inpatient, typically 30 minutes communicating with the patient via telehealth

G0426 typically 50 minutes communicating with the patient via telehealth

G0427 typically 70 minutes or more communicating with the patient via telehealth

G0459 Inpatient telehealth pharmacologic management, including prescription, use, and review of medication with no more than minimal medical psychotherapy

G0508 Telehealth consultation, critical care, physicians typically spend 60 minutes communicating with the patient via telehealth (initial)

G0509 Telehealth consultation, critical care, physicians typically spend 50 minutes communicating with the patient via telehealth (subsequent)

Refer to the Critical Care via telemedicine section that follows for more information on this topic.

When payer policies include payment for the cost of telemedicine transmission and/or a site facility fee, report **T1014** (telehealth transmission, per minute to originating sites [other than the patient's home]) and/or **Q3014** (telehealth originating site facility fee).

Critical Care via Telemedicine

CPT codes for critical and intensive care services are not included in *CPT* Appendix P. *CPT* instructs to report unlisted E/M service code **99499** for critical care provided via telemedicine. (Payers may instruct to append modifier **95** when reporting **99499**.) Alternatively, payers may include either HCPCS codes **G0508** and **G0509** as covered critical care consultation services when provided via telemedicine or the less specific *CPT* inpatient or observation consultation codes appended with modifier **95** (ie, **99252–99255 95**).

For an example of codes for reporting critical care via telemedicine, refer to the Example: Critical Care Consultation section later in this chapter.

Examples of Coding for Telemedicine Services (*CPT*®, HCPCS)

The following examples are solely for the purpose of demonstrating coding and are not clinical guidelines. Additionally, code assignment depends on the nature of the service provided as documented in the patient record.

For each example, assume that health plan benefits for telemedicine services have been verified before the encounter.

Example: Hospital Consultation

➤ **A consultation is requested of a physician at a children's hospital for an inpatient in a rural hospital, 75 miles away.** Through real-time interactive technology, the physician performs a consultation, including moderate MDM. The total time of the interactive communication with the patient and/or parents/caregivers is 30 minutes. A written report to the requesting physician is transmitted via secure electronic health information exchange. The physician's total time, including pre-consultation review of records, documentation, and report to the requesting physician, is 50 minutes.

	CPT
MDM: Moderate *History:* Comprehensive *Physical examination:* Comprehensive	99254 95 (initial inpatient consultation, which requires moderate MDM or total time of ≥60 minutes) or, if payer does not accept consultation codes or requires HCPCS codes, G0425 (telehealth consultation, emergency department or initial inpatient, typically 30 minutes communicating with the patient via telehealth)

Teaching Point: Although the physician's total time was less than 60 minutes, the moderate level of MDM supports 99254. The physician's total time may include time interacting with the facility's clinical staff, who act as telepresenter to assist with the examination.

Note that *CPT* does not include initial hospital care codes 99221–99223 in *CPT* Appendix P, so these codes are used to report telemedicine services only as specifically instructed by a payer.

If payer policy allows payment for overhead expenses related to telemedicine services, also report T1014 (telehealth transmission, per minute, professional services bill separately). Because this is billed per minute, 30 units are reported. The rural hospital, as the originating facility, may also report Q3014 (telehealth originating site facility fee).

Example: Telemedicine With Prolonged Service

➤ **A physician provides an initial consultation to a 9-year-old who was admitted with symptoms of fatigue and decreased appetite for about 3 days.** The admitting physician provides examination findings, including stage 2 hypertension with urgency, oliguria, weight gain of 1.8 kg (4 lbs) since a primary care visit 3 months ago, periorbital edema without conjunctival injection or discharge, mild pitting edema of bilateral extremities, and scrotal edema. History obtained from parents includes a febrile illness with sore throat that resolved about 2 weeks ago. The consultant spends 97 minutes on this date determining diagnoses of acute poststreptococcal glomerular nephritis with acute kidney injury, hypertensive urgency, and hypervolemia; developing a plan for treatment; and monitoring/adjusting treatment intermittently throughout the day.

ICD-10-CM	*CPT*
N00.9 (acute nephritic syndrome with unspecified morphologic changes) N17.9 (acute kidney failure, unspecified) I16.0 (hypertensive urgency) I15.1 (hypertension secondary to other renal disorders) E87.70 (fluid overload, unspecified) B94.8 (sequelae of other specified infectious and parasitic diseases)	99255 95 (inpatient or observation consultation for a new or established patient, which requires high level of MDM or ≥80 minutes) 99418 95 × 1 unit (prolonged hospital E/M service[s] time with or without direct patient contact beyond the required time of the primary service when the primary service level has been selected using total time, each 15 minutes)

Teaching Point: The physician's total time of 97 minutes supports 99255 (first 80 minutes) and one 15-minute period of prolonged outpatient service, 99418 (first 15-minute period [80–95 minutes]). The final 2 minutes of total time are not reported because prolonged service requires at least 15 minutes beyond the time of the prior period. Had the service been reported with 99223 95 (initial hospital care, ≥75 minutes) owing to payer policy, 1 unit of 99418 would also be reported for the 15-minute period beyond the first 75 minutes.

Both E/M codes are reported with modifier 95 because the service was provided via synchronous audiovisual telemedicine. The first 4 diagnosis codes listed on the claim are linked to the procedure codes. (See **Chapter 1, Figure 1-1** for an example of how codes are linked.)

Example: Audio-Only Telemedicine

➤ **A 16-year-old is scheduled for a telemedicine consultation for reevaluation of generalized anxiety disorder.** The patient was scheduled to receive a synchronous audiovisual service, but the parent's internet service has been discontinued because they are unable to afford increased rates. The patient's health plan covers audio-only health follow-up services for behavioral health conditions when provided to patients in their homes. At the appointment, the physician spends 30 minutes communicating with the patient and his mother by telephone and recommends a medication change and an in-person follow-up visit in 4 weeks. After the telephone service, the physician spends another 10 minutes ordering a different medication that requires prior authorization by the patient's health plan and documenting the service.

ICD-10-CM	*CPT*
F41.1 (generalized anxiety disorder) **Z59.868** (other specified financial insecurity)	**99244 FQ** (outpatient consultation, moderate level MDM or total time of ≥40 minutes) or, if the payer does not accept consultation codes, **99215 FQ** (office or other outpatient visit for an established patient, high level MDM or total time of ≥40 minutes)

Teaching Point: The physician's total time on the date of the encounter (40 minutes) supports **99244** or **99215**. Clinical staff time is not included in the time of the E/M service. Modifier **FQ** is reported in lieu of modifier **93** because a behavioral health service was provided via audio-only communication.

If the patient completed a standardized instrument for assessing anxiety and this was scored and documented in the visit note, it could be possible to report **96127** for the practice expense of the provision, scoring, and documentation of the instrument. This code is not, however, included in the *CPT* appendixes of codes for telemedicine services, and payment will depend on individual payer policy.

When an audiovisual connection cannot be achieved or maintained, some payers advise that the service be reported according to the method by which most of the service was provided. For instance, if a real-time audiovisual encounter is scheduled but the service must be changed to an audio-only (eg, telephone) service because of lack of connectivity, an audio-only E/M service should be reported rather than a service provided via real-time audiovisual communication. Payer instructions on these circumstances may vary.

Example: Critical Care Consultation

➤ **A pediatric intensivist is contacted via live audiovisual telecommunications to provide remote critical care to an infant who presented with fever, lethargy, and suspected sepsis.** The intensivist views radiographs and other data from monitoring devices in addition to performing visual and audio examination of the infant. The attending physician at the hospital where the infant is an inpatient performs necessary procedures as advised by the intensivist (eg, lumbar puncture). The infant remains at the same hospital under the care of the pediatrician. A total of 65 minutes of remote critical care service is provided.

The consulting physician reports	The attending physician reports
G0508 (telehealth consultation, critical care, physicians typically spend 60 minutes communicating with the patient via telehealth [initial]) or, if a payer does not accept this code, **99499 95** (unlisted E/M service) (Enter description of service on claim or attachment.)	*CPT* codes for services personally performed (eg, initial hospital care or hourly critical care, intubation, lumbar puncture)

Teaching Point: Code **G0508** is reported only once per date of service per patient. Alternatively, the pediatric intensivist may report an inpatient consultation (**99252–99255 95**) as allowed under the specific payer's policy for telemedicine.

A payer may require modifier **GT** (via interactive audio and video telecommunication systems) appended to **G0508**.

Continuing Changes in Telemedicine Services

Payer policies and legislation (state and Federal) that affect provision of and payment for telemedicine services continue to evolve. It is important that physician practices monitor local and regional payer policies for opportunities to provide medical care via telemedicine, when appropriate, and are paid for the physician work and practice expense of providing these services.

To test your knowledge of the information presented in this chapter, complete the quiz found at the end of it, after the resources. Answers to each quiz are found in **Appendix II**.

Chapter Takeaways

Telemedicine is an evolving practice resulting in frequent changes to codes, modifiers, guidelines, and payer policies. Following are some takeaways from this chapter:

- From a coding perspective, telemedicine describes synchronous (real-time) provision of medical services via telecommunications.
- Telemedicine services provided using real-time audio-video telecommunications technology are typically reported with a code for the service provided appended with modifier **95**. *CPT* includes telemedicine codes for certain outpatient E/M services.
- Telemedicine services have traditionally required real-time audio-video communication, but certain services may be reported with modifier **93** or **FQ** (telehealth for behavioral health and substance use disorder treatment services) when provided via audio-only communication technology.
- State regulations and payer policies for coverage of and payment for telemedicine services vary. Practices must monitor and adapt to these changes to support provision and payment for telemedicine services.

Resources

AAP Coding Resources

Pediatric Telehealth Coding: Expert Guidance for Your Practice. American Academy of Pediatrics; 2025

AAP Telemedicine Resources

AAP policy statement, "Telehealth: Improving Access to and Quality of Pediatric Health Care" (https://doi.org/10.1542/peds.2021-053129)

AAP technical report, "Telehealth: Opportunities to Improve Access, Quality, and Cost in Pediatric Care" (https://doi.org/10.1542/peds.2021-056035)

AAP practice management telehealth resource page (www.aap.org/en/practice-management/care-delivery-approaches/telehealth)

Pediatric Telehealth Best Practices paperback and eBook package (www.aap.org/Pediatric-Telehealth-Best-Practices-Paperback-and-eBook-Package)

AAP Section on Telehealth Care (SOTC) (www.aap.org/en/community/aap-sections/telehealth-care)

CPT Telemedicine Code List

CPT list of codes that may be reported with modifier **93** and **95** (Refer to *CPT* Appendixes P and T.)

Interstate Licensure

Interstate Medical Licensure Compact (https://imlcc.com/a-faster-pathway-to-physician-licensure/)

Licensing Across State Lines (https://telehealth.hhs.gov/licensure/licensing-across-state-lines)

Licensure compacts (https://telehealth.hhs.gov/licensure/licensure-compacts)

Medicare Telehealth Policies and Service List

Medicare list of codes covered when provided via telehealth (www.cms.gov/medicare/coverage/telehealth/list-services)

Telehealth Compliance Guidance

"Guidance on Nondiscrimination in Telehealth: Federal Protections to Ensure Accessibility to People with Disabilities and Limited English Proficient Persons," US Department of Health and Human Services (HHS) (www.hhs.gov/sites/default/files/guidance-on-nondiscrimination-in-telehealth.pdf)

"Resource for Health Care Providers on Educating Patients about Privacy and Security Risks to Protected Health Information when Using Remote Communication Technologies for Telehealth," HHS (www.hhs.gov/hipaa/for-professionals/privacy/guidance/resource-health-care-providers-educating-patients/index.html)

"Telehealth," Americans with Disabilities Act, US Department of Justice Civil Rights Division (www.ada.gov/topics/telehealth)

Telehealth Privacy Tips for Providers, Health Resources and Services Administration (HRSA) (https://telehealth.hhs.gov/documents/Telehealth+Privacy+Tips+for+Providers.pdf)

"Your Mobile Device and Health Information Privacy and Security," HealthIT.gov (www.healthit.gov/topic/privacy-security-and-hipaa/your-mobile-device-and-health-information-privacy-and-security)

Telemedicine Originating Site Eligibility Analyzer

HRSA Medicare Telehealth Payment Eligibility Analyzer for originating site payment (https://data.hrsa.gov/tools/medicare/telehealth)

Test Your Knowledge!

1. **True or false? Synchronous communication includes correspondence via email.**
   a. True
   b. False
2. **Which of the following should be documented for all telemedicine services?**
   a. The reason for the visit and the requesting party (eg, patient, another physician or QHP)
   b. Platform or modality by which the service is occurring
   c. Patient and physician location
   d. All of the above
3. **Which of the following is a telemedicine modifier?**
   a. 02, telehealth provided other than in patient's home
   b. 10, telehealth provided in patient's home
   c. 95, synchronous telemedicine service rendered via a real-time interactive audio and video telecommunications system
   d. Either a or b
4. **Which telemedicine services are most specifically described by HCPCS codes when provided via telemedicine?**
   a. Critical care services
   b. Office and other outpatient visits
   c. Telephone E/M services
   d. Prolonged hospital services
5. **Which is appropriate when a service began as an audio-video telemedicine service but was completed with audio-only owing to a drop in connectivity?**
   a. The service is reported as audio-video because that was the intended method of communication.
   b. The service is reported using the code for the type of telemedicine service by which most of the service was provided.
   c. Modifiers 95 and 52 (reduced service) are reported with the code for the service to indicate that audio-video communication was reduced during the service.
   d. Audio-only modifier 93 is reported when the service is not delivered completely via audio-video communication.

CHAPTER 20

Outpatient Telemedicine and Online Digital Services

Contents

● indicates a new code; ▲, revised; #, re-sequenced; ✚, add-on; ★, audiovisual technology; and ◀, synchronous interactive audio.

Chapter Highlights

- Codes for synchronous audio-video telemedicine evaluation and management (E/M) services
- Codes for synchronous audio-only telemedicine E/M services
- Brief virtual check-in services – brief communications to determine if a more extensive visit is indicated
- Codes and instructions for reporting online digital E/M services
- Reporting evaluation of recorded video and/or images (eg, rash)

This chapter discusses codes that are specific to reporting telemedicine E/M and online digital health services.

Refer to **Chapter 19** for the following topics:

- A general overview of how to appropriately provide telemedicine services in compliance with state and federal regulations
- Discussion of appropriate documentation of telemedicine services, including compliance with potential regulatory requirements (eg, patient or parent/caregiver consent to services)
- Reporting telemedicine services using Healthcare Common Procedure Coding System codes
- Reporting telemedicine services with codes that are typically reported for face-to-face services and appended with modifiers to designate delivery via telemedicine

Related topics discussed in other chapters include interprofessional telephone/internet/electronic health record consultation services (refer to **Chapter 9**) and remote monitoring services (refer to **Chapter 21**).

Examples included in this chapter are solely for the purpose of demonstrating coding and are not clinical guidelines. Additionally, code assignment depends on the nature of the service provided as documented in the patient record. For each example, assume that the patient's and/or parent's or caregiver's consent for telemedicine or online digital E/M services is documented and the health plan benefits for telemedicine services have been verified before the encounter.

Payer policies for telemedicine services change frequently because of changes in state regulations, changes in code sets, and availability of communications technology. It is important that practice and billing managers maintain an awareness of state regulations for telemedicine and individual payer policies that may specify allowable codes and required modifiers.

Office and Outpatient Synchronous Telemedicine Services

Current Procedural Terminology (*CPT*®) includes 3 categories of E/M codes that describe synchronous telemedicine services. Unlike other telemedicine services that may be reported with the same codes reported for in-person services (but appended with a telemedicine modifier), these codes always describe telemedicine services. No modifiers are required.

The first 2 categories differentiate telemedicine visits by type of synchronous communication (audio-video or audio-only) with code descriptors that define the levels of physician work through levels of medical decision-making (MDM) or total time on the date of the encounter.

- Synchronous audio-video communication, new patient (98000–98003) and established patient (98004–98007)
- Synchronous telephone/audio-only communication, new patient (98008–98011) and established patient (98012–98015)

Report new patient codes only when the patient has not received a professional face-to-face service (including any prior telemedicine services) from the same physician or qualified health care professional (QHP) or another physician or QHP of the same exact specialty and subspecialty within 3 years prior to the current service.

The third category includes a single code (98016) to report a brief patient-initiated service provided via synchronous communication technology for the purpose of determining whether a more extensive service (eg, in-person office visit) is needed.

- Code 98016 represents an established patient service and is not reported for a service provided to a new patient.

Modifiers 93 and 95 are not appended to codes 98000–98016.

Modifiers 93 and 95 are appended to other codes for services provided in conjunction with telemedicine E/M services (ie, services described by codes included in Appendixes P [*CPT* Codes That May Be Used for Synchronous Real-Time Interactive Audio-Video Telemedicine Services] and T [*CPT* Codes That May Be Used for Synchronous Real-Time Interactive Audio-Only Telemedicine Services]) of the American Medical Association *CPT* manual.

Example

➤ **A patient receives an established patient audio-video telemedicine E/M service meeting the requirements of code 98006 and also 30 minutes of psychotherapy provided by the same physician. The physician reports**
98006 (synchronous audio-video E/M visit, established patient, with moderate MDM or total time meeting or exceeding 30 minutes)
★✚◀90833 95 Psychotherapy, 30 minutes with patient when performed with an evaluation and management service
Teaching Point: Although no modifier is indicated with code 98006, the psychotherapy code is appended with modifier 95 to indicate the service was provided via synchronous audio-video communications technology.

Place of Service Codes

Payers may also require specific place of service (POS) codes to identify where the patient received a telemedicine service. Telemedicine POS codes are

02 Telehealth provided other than in the patient's home
10 Telehealth provided in the patient's home

Practices should verify POS requirements in payment policies, as these may vary by payer and type of practice. For instance, a practice that operates as an outpatient department of a hospital may be instructed to report POS codes for outpatient hospital locations because this indicates the reporting physician's or QHP's service does not include the practice expense portions of the service (eg, clinic space, supplies, and staff employed by a facility).

Refer to **Chapter 4** for further discussion of POS codes and how practice expense is included in values assigned to codes.

Synchronous Telemedicine Service Codes

As discussed in detail in **Chapter 19**, telemedicine service codes are not reported for routine communications related to a previous visit (eg, communication of test results without additional E/M work) or when included in another reported service (eg, post-procedural care within a global period).

- As with all services, the telemedicine service should be clinically appropriate to address the health care needs of the patient.

Synchronous telemedicine visit codes 98000–98016 are reported only for services provided via communication technology that allows real-time interactive audio-video or audio-only communication between the physician or QHP providing the service and the patient and/or parents/caregivers located at a distant site.

A synchronous telemedicine visit provided to an established patient by clinical staff working under a physician's or QHP's direct supervision (ie, without a physician's or QHP's presence) may be reported with established patient code 99211 appended with the appropriate telemedicine modifier, 93 or 95. Payer policies for incident-to services may apply. Learn more about 99211 and incident-to services in Chapter 7.

✖ Do not report 98000–98016 for services provided by asynchronous communication (eg, secure email).

Refer to the Online Digital Evaluation and Management Services (99421–99423) section later in this chapter for guidance on reporting E/M services provided via asynchronous communication technology.

When audio-video connections are lost during an encounter *and only audio is restored,* report the service that accounted for the majority of the time of the interactive portion of the service. Documentation should include the time spent to support the code selection.

Table 20-1 provides a quick reference to codes for synchronous telemedicine services. Refer also to **Table 6-4** to review the elements that are used in selecting a level of MDM.

Table 20-1. Synchronous Telemedicine Evaluation and Management Service Codes

Services described by codes 98000–98015 require a medically appropriate history and/or examination. Communication via a telecommunication technology device for deaf patients is synchronous communication.

Type of Service by Communication Technology	Codes and Level of MDM/Total Minutes Met or Exceeded per Calendar Date
Synchronous audio-video visit, new patient	98000 Straightforward or 15 min
	98001 Low or 30 min
	98002 Moderate or 45 min
	98003 High or 60 min; add 99417 for ≥75 min[a]
Synchronous audio-video visit, established patient	98004 Straightforward or 10 min
	98005 Low or 20 min
	98006 Moderate or 30 min
	98007 High or 40 min; add 99417 for ≥55 min[a]
Synchronous audio-only (verbal communication) visit *including* >*10 minutes of medical discussion,*[b] new patient	98008 Straightforward or 15 min
	98009 Low or 30 min
	98010 Moderate or 45 min
	98011 High or 60 min; add 99417 for ≥75 min[a]
Synchronous audio-only (verbal communication) visit *including* >*10 minutes of medical discussion,*[b] established patient	98012 Straightforward or >10 min
	98013 Low or 20 min
	98014 Moderate or 30 min
	98015 High or 40 min; add 99417 for ≥55 min[a]

Virtual Check-in

Service Description	Patient Description	Code and Required Minutes of Medical Discussion	
Brief communication technology-based service (eg, virtual check-in) by a physician or other QHP who can report E/M services	Established patient initiates to evaluate whether a more extensive type of service is required.	98016	≥5–10 min of medical discussion[c] Discussion is unrelated to E/M service in prior 7 days and does not lead to an E/M service in the next 24 hours.

Abbreviations: E/M, evaluation and management; MDM, medical decision-making; QHP, qualified health care professional.

[a] Add prolonged service outpatient E/M code 99417 only when the code is selected based on total time and the total time of 98003, 98007, 98011, or 98015 has been exceeded by ≥15 minutes. Report 1 unit of 99417 for each full 15-minute period beyond the total time required for the primary service. Telemedicine modifiers (eg, 93 or 95) are appended to 99417 when prolonged service is provided via telemedicine.

[b] Codes 98008–98015 require >10 minutes (ie, ≥11 minutes) of medical discussion. Do not report 98008–98015 for service of ≤10 minutes. Report 98016 (established patient only) when applicable.

[c] >10 minutes of medical discussion may be reported with 98000–98015.

Synchronous Audio-Video Services (98000–98007)

#98000 Synchronous audio-video visit for the E/M of a new patient, which requires a medically appropriate history and/or examination and straightforward medical decision making.

When using total time on the date of the encounter for code selection, 15 minutes must be met or exceeded.

#98001 Synchronous audio-video visit for the E/M of a new patient, which requires a medically appropriate history and/or examination and low medical decision making.

When using total time on the date of the encounter for code selection, 30 minutes must be met or exceeded.

#98002 Synchronous audio-video visit for the E/M of a new patient, which requires a medically appropriate history and/or examination and moderate medical decision making.
When using total time on the date of the encounter for code selection, 45 minutes must be met or exceeded.

#98003 Synchronous audio-video visit for the E/M of a new patient, which requires a medically appropriate history and/or examination and high medical decision making.
When using total time on the date of the encounter for code selection, 60 minutes must be met or exceeded.

#98004 Synchronous audio-video visit for the E/M of an established patient, which requires a medically appropriate history and/or examination and straightforward medical decision making.
When using total time on the date of the encounter for code selection, 10 minutes must be met or exceeded.

#98005 Synchronous audio-video visit for the E/M of an established patient, which requires a medically appropriate history and/or examination and low medical decision making.
When using total time on the date of the encounter for code selection, 20 minutes must be met or exceeded.

#98006 Synchronous audio-video visit for the E/M of an established patient, which requires a medically appropriate history and/or examination and moderate medical decision making.
When using total time on the date of the encounter for code selection, 30 minutes must be met or exceeded.

#98007 Synchronous audio-video visit for the E/M of an established patient, which requires a medically appropriate history and/or examination and high medical decision making.
When using total time on the date of the encounter for code selection, 40 minutes must be met or exceeded.

Codes **98000–98007** are specific for reporting services that are provided via telecommunications technology that includes both audio and video components with interactive communication in real time (ie, synchronous).

Code selection is based on either MDM or the physician's or QHP's total time directed to care of the individual patient as discussed in **Chapter 6** and as used in code selection for other services such as office and other outpatient E/M services (**99202–99205** and **99212–99215**).

Codes **98000–98007**

- Are initiated by either the physician or QHP (eg, scheduled follow-up visit) or the patient and/or parent or caregiver.
- Are reported for new or established patients as defined in *CPT*.
- ✖ Do not require a specific time interval from the last in-person or telemedicine visit.
- Require a medically appropriate history and/or examination.
- Are selected according to MDM or total time.
- May be reported in addition to **99417** (prolonged outpatient E/M service) when the code for the highest level of synchronous audio-video service (**98003** or **98007**) is selected according to total time and the required total time is exceeded by 15 minutes or more. Report 1 unit of **99417** appended with the appropriate telemedicine modifier for each full 15-minute period beyond the total time of the primary service.

Time establishing the connection or arranging the appointment is not included in the physician's or QHP's total time, even when performed by the physician or other QHP (ie, count time spent in activities that require a physician's or QHP's skills).

Do not report **98000–98007**

- ✖ When another E/M visit is reported on the same date
- ✖ For time spent by clinical staff even when performed with a physician's or QHP's oversight
- ✖ For any time counted toward chronic or principal care management services (**99437**, **99491**, or **99424–99425**)
- ✖ For services provided by asynchronous communication (eg, secure messaging)
- ✖ During the global period of a procedure

When the video component of an audio-video E/M service is lost and the service is continued with audio-only communication, the service is reported according to the service that accounted for the majority of the time spent in interactive medical discussion and/or patient observation. *In this event, the service is reported only when the time of medical discussion and/or patient observation exceeds 10 minutes.*

Refer to **Table 20-1** as you review the following examples to identify the levels of MDM and/or required total time for the services described:

● indicates a new code; ▲, revised; #, re-sequenced; ✚, add-on; ★, audiovisual technology; and ◀, synchronous interactive audio.

Examples

➤ **A parent of a 3-year-old established patient requests an audio-video telemedicine service for possible pinkeye.** The physician providing the service uses a preconfigured template to document the service.

Date: January 7, 2026

Parent's consent obtained at log-on to telemedicine application.

Patient location: Home **Service provided from:** Care for Kids Pediatrics

Individuals present: Parents and child

History: Per parents, recent symptoms of an upper respiratory infection (URI) followed by development of symptoms of redness, itching, and clear discharge of first the left eye and then the right eye over the past 24 hours. Matting of eyelashes was cleaned with a warm cloth this morning.

Examination: Child is resting comfortably in a parent's lap. Temperature is 98.4 °F per digital thermometer. Eyes are red and watery in appearance, consistent with viral conjunctivitis.

Assessment and plan: Viral conjunctivitis. Parents instructed to use cold compresses and lubricants, such as artificial tears, for comfort. Parents also instructed that symptoms may worsen over 24 to 48 hours but that they can contact the office for further evaluation if the condition worsens or is not improving within 72 hours. Antibiotics are requested and parents are counseled regarding lack of indication or benefit. Next scheduled appointment in 2 months for routine health examination and immunization.

Total time on this date: 15 minutes

Electronic signature applied

Problem(s) addressed ➡ ***Low*** (an acute uncomplicated illness)
Data reviewed and analyzed ➡ ***Limited*** (independent historian required)
Risk of patient management ➡ ***Moderate*** (decision regarding antibiotic prescription)

ICD-10-CM	*CPT*
B30.9 (Viral conjunctivitis, unspecified) **J06.9** (acute URI, unspecified)	**98005** (synchronous audio-video visit for E/M of an established patient, which requires a medically appropriate history and/or examination and low MDM or total time of 20 minutes met or exceeded)

Teaching Point: The MDM is low, given the low number and complexity of problems addressed and limited data to be reviewed and analyzed. Although the risk of patient management is moderate, this alone does not support a moderate level of MDM. Although the 15-minute total time would support **98004**, *CPT* instructs to select the code based on MDM or total time, and the physician or QHP may use the most favorable method.

➤ **Same as previous example except the physician's total time on the date of the encounter is 30 minutes because of prolonged discussion of the contraindications to prescription of antibiotics.**

Problem(s) addressed ➡ ***Low*** (an acute uncomplicated illness)
Data reviewed and analyzed ➡ ***Limited*** (independent historian)
Risk of patient management ➡ ***Moderate*** (decision against prescription drug management)

ICD-10-CM	*CPT*
J06.9 (acute URI, unspecified)	**98006** (synchronous audio-video visit for E/M of an established patient, which requires a medically appropriate history and/or examination and moderate MDM or total time of 30 minutes met or exceeded)

Teaching Point: Total time on the date of the established patient encounter supports **98006** (≥30 minutes), although a low level of MDM is supported by the low number and complexity of problems addressed and the limited data. Either total time or MDM must support the level of service reported.

➤ **An adolescent established patient is seen via audio-video telemedicine for increasingly symptomatic mental health problems.** The physician reviews the patient's current medications and results of psychological tests and speaks to the patient's psychologist. After extensive discussion with the patient and a parent, new medication is prescribed and a follow-up visit is scheduled in 1 week. The physician sends the psychologist a secure message about changes in treatment. The physician's total time spent in medical management (not psychotherapy, which would be reported separately, when provided) is 55 minutes.

Teaching Point: The physician reports **98007** (synchronous audio-video visit for the E/M of an established patient with either high MDM or ≥40 minutes total time) and **99417 95** (prolonged outpatient E/M service time beyond the required time of the primary service, each 15 minutes) with 1 unit for the 15 minutes beyond the 40 minutes required to report **98007**. The scheduled follow-up visit in 1 week does not limit reporting this service.

➤ **A synchronous audio-video telemedicine visit is being provided to an established patient.** After 10 minutes of audio-video communication, the patient loses internet service. The service is completed via a 5-minute telephone call. The combined interactive time of medical discussion and observation is 15 minutes. The physician's total time of service is 20 minutes, not including time to establish or reestablish connections.

Teaching Point: The physician reports **98005** (synchronous audio-video E/M visit to an established patient with low MDM or total time of ≥20 minutes) because the greater portion of the interactive communication time was conducted via audio-video telecommunication. Had the greater portion (>10 minutes) of the interactive communication been via telephone or other audio-only communication technology, **98013** (synchronous audio-only E/M visit to an established patient with more than 10 minutes of medical discussion and low MDM or total time of ≥20 minutes) would have been reported.

When services are provided in part by audio-video and in part by audio-only telecommunication, more than 10 minutes must be spent in medical discussion or patient observation.

Synchronous Audio-Only Services (98008–98015)

#●98008 Synchronous audio-only visit for the E/M of a new patient, which requires a medically appropriate history and/or examination, straightforward medical decision making, and more than 10 minutes of medical discussion.

When using total time on the date of the encounter for code selection, 15 minutes must be met or exceeded.

#●98009 Synchronous audio-only visit for the E/M of a new patient, which requires a medically appropriate history and/or examination, low medical decision making, and more than 10 minutes of medical discussion.

When using total time on the date of the encounter for code selection, 30 minutes must be met or exceeded.

#●98010 Synchronous audio-only visit for the E/M of a new patient, which requires a medically appropriate history and/or examination, moderate medical decision making, and more than 10 minutes of medical discussion.

When using total time on the date of the encounter for code selection, 45 minutes must be met or exceeded.

#●98011 Synchronous audio-only visit for the E/M of a new patient, which requires a medically appropriate history and/or examination, high medical decision making, and more than 10 minutes of medical discussion.

When using total time on the date of the encounter for code selection, 60 minutes must be met or exceeded.

#●98012 Synchronous audio-only visit for the E/M of an established patient, which requires a medically appropriate history and/or examination, straightforward medical decision making, and more than 10 minutes of medical discussion.

When using total time on the date of the encounter for code selection, 10 minutes must be exceeded.

#●98013 Synchronous audio-only visit for the E/M of an established patient, which requires a medically appropriate history and/or examination, low medical decision making, and more than 10 minutes of medical discussion.

When using total time on the date of the encounter for code selection, 20 minutes must be met or exceeded.

#●98014 Synchronous audio-only visit for the E/M of an established patient, which requires a medically appropriate history and/or examination, moderate medical decision making, and more than 10 minutes of medical discussion.

When using total time on the date of the encounter for code selection, 30 minutes must be met or exceeded.

#●98015 Synchronous audio-only visit for the E/M of an established patient, which requires a medically appropriate history and/or examination, high medical decision making, and more than 10 minutes of medical discussion.

When using total time on the date of the encounter for code selection, 40 minutes must be met or exceeded.

Codes **98008–98015**

- May be initiated by either the physician or QHP (eg, scheduled follow-up visit) or the patient and/or parent or caregiver.
- Are reported for new or established patients as defined in *CPT.*

Although not a face-to-face service, synchronous audio-only services are comparable with a face-to-face E/M service. It is advisable to report E/M services provided to patients who have previously received an E/M service via synchronous audio-only services by using codes for an established patient visit.

- Require a medically appropriate history and/or (probably rarely) examination.
- ✖ Do not require a specific time interval from the last in-person or telemedicine visit.
- *Must include documentation of more than 10 minutes (ie, ≥11 minutes) of medical discussion.*
  - For established patient services with more than 5 and less than 10 minutes of medical discussion, consider whether a brief virtual check-in code (**98016**) may be reported. Refer to the Brief Synchronous Communication Technology Service (Virtual Check-In [**98016**]) section later in this chapter.
  - The time of medical discussion must be documented in addition to total time when a code is selected on the basis of total time.
- Are selected according to either MDM or total time but must always include more than 10 minutes of medical discussion.
- May be reported in addition to **99417** (prolonged outpatient E/M service) when the code for the highest level of synchronous audio-video service (**98003** or **98007**) is selected according to total time and the total time is exceeded by 15 minutes or more. Report 1 unit of **99417** appended with an appropriate telemedicine modifier for each full 15-minute period beyond the total time of the primary service.

Do not report **98008–98015**

- ✖ When 10 minutes or less is spent in medical discussion with the patient and/or parent or caregiver even when the required total time has been met or exceeded.
- ✖ When another E/M visit is reported on the same date
- ✖ For time spent by clinical staff even when performed with a physician's or QHP's oversight
- ✖ For any time counted toward chronic or principal care management services (**99437**, **99491**, or **99424–99425**)
- ✖ For services provided by asynchronous communication (eg, secure messaging)
- ✖ During the global period of a procedure provided by the same physician or QHP or individuals of the same specialty and same group practice

Do not report **98012–98015**

- ✖ When provided in the same month as complex chronic care management (**99487**, **99489**)

Refer to **Table 20-1** as you review the following examples to identify the levels of MDM and/or required total time for the services described:

Examples

➤ **A parent requests a telephone call to learn their child's test results.** A physician speaks with the parent and advises that the test results were within reference limits and no further testing or evaluation is indicated. The patient is to return for the next well-child visit or as needed. The physician documents total time of 10 minutes.

Teaching Point: The physician's documentation of total time does not support that more than 10 minutes was spent in medical discussion. Additionally, the purpose of the call—to communicate test results in the absence of an indication for additional E/M—does not support a billable service.

When a patient- or parent-initiated call addresses abnormal results and/or need for additional testing or management, documentation of the clinical indications and time spent may support a reportable audio-only E/M service.

All communications with patient and/or parents or caregivers should be documented, even when the communication is not a separately reportable service.

➤ **A 17-year-old new patient requests a telephone E/M service after a positive COVID-19 test result.** The patient provides history of mild symptoms for 2 days prior to testing. Although not very ill, they are especially concerned about what precautions they should take to prevent spreading the condition to their mother, who has multiple chronic conditions. A nurse practitioner (NP) spends 12 minutes obtaining the patient's history, discussing indications for an in-person visit, answering questions about long COVID, and advising the patient on precautionary measures aimed at preventing spread of the infection. The NP documents 12 minutes of interactive medical discussion, low-complexity MDM, and a total time of 20 minutes.

Teaching Point: The NP, whose scope of practice includes E/M services, selects the code on the basis of the low-level MDM and reports **98009** (synchronous audio-only E/M for a new patient with >10 minutes of medical discussion and either low MDM or total time of ≥30 minutes). The NP's total time would support **98008**, which requires at least 15 minutes of total time.

➤ **A 16-year-old established patient is scheduled for a telephone appointment for reevaluation of anxiety.** The physician spends 30 minutes in medical discussion with the patient during the call. After the telephone service, the physician spends another 10 minutes ordering a new medication that requires prior authorization by the patient's health plan and documenting the service. *The physician documents the 30 minutes spent in medical discussion and the total time of 40 minutes.*

ICD-10-CM	*CPT*
F41.9 (anxiety)	**98015** (audio-only E/M service to an established patient, including >10 minutes in medical discussion, and either high-level MDM or total time of ≥40 minutes)

Teaching Point: The physician's documented times of medical discussion (30 minutes) and total time on the date of the encounter (40 minutes) support **98015**.

Brief Synchronous Communication Technology Service (Virtual Check-In [98016])

Code **98016** represents an established patient E/M service that is specifically for the purpose of determining whether a more extensive E/M service is indicated.

#●98016 Brief communication technology-based service (eg, virtual check-in) by a physician or other QHP who can report E/M services, provided to an established patient, not originating from a related E/M service provided within the previous 7 days nor leading to an E/M service or procedure within the next 24 hours or soonest available appointment, 5–10 minutes of medical discussion

Code **98016**

- Is reported only for a service that is initiated by the established patient and/or parent or caregiver
- Is reported according to the time of medical discussion, not total time or MDM
- Requires documentation of at least 5 and up to 10 minutes of medical discussion
- Must take place via synchronous telecommunication (ie, not asynchronous communication [eg, messaging]) but does not require video technology

Do not report **98016**

- ✖ For a service provided to a new patient or for a visit that was not initiated by an established patient and/or parent or caregiver
- ✖ For a service with less than 5 minutes of medical discussion
- ✖ When the service originates from a related E/M service within the previous 7 days
- ✖ When the service leads to an E/M service or procedure within the next 24 hours or at the soonest available appointment
- ✖ During the postoperative period of a procedure

When the virtual check-in leads to an E/M service provided by the same physician or QHP or an individual of the same group practice and same specialty on the same date, the time of the **98016** service may be added to the total time on the date of the encounter.

● indicates a new code; ▲, revised; #, re-sequenced; ✚, add-on; ★, audiovisual technology; and ◀, synchronous interactive audio.

Examples

➤ **A parent requests a telephone E/M service to discuss whether an appointment is indicated for their child's refill of medication.** The patient was most recently seen by the physician 4 months ago. The physician speaks with the parent and explains that a follow-up visit is required to verify that the medication is still appropriate for the child. The total time of medical discussion is 6 minutes. The patient is scheduled for the next available in-person appointment.

Teaching Point: The service is not reported. Code 98016 is not reported when the patient is scheduled for the next available in-person appointment. The physician's time of medical discussion (6 minutes) may be added to the total time of the in-person visit when the code for the in-person visit is selected based on total time.

➤ **A parent requests a telephone E/M service to discuss whether an appointment is indicated for their 5-year-old's symptoms, which began with nasal congestion 3 days ago and have progressed to nasal drainage with a cough.** The physician speaks with the parent and explains that the symptoms are consistent with a viral URI. The parent is advised regarding appropriate home care. The total time of medical discussion is 6 minutes. The visit is not related to a prior visit and does not lead to scheduling a visit.

Teaching Point: The physician's time of medical discussion (6 minutes) does not support a synchronous audio-only E/M service (which would require >10 minutes of medical discussion) but does support 98016.

Online Digital Evaluation and Management Services (99421–99423)

#99421	Online digital E/M service, for an established patient, for up to 7 days, cumulative time during the 7 days; 5–10 minutes
#99422	11–20 minutes
#99423	21 or more minutes

Digital communication technology (eg, patient portal messaging, secure email) that supports only asynchronous communication is increasingly used to provide online digital E/M services.

Online digital E/M services differ from telemedicine services. The required delivery mechanism for telemedicine (ie, synchronous [real-time] audiovisual or audio-only communication) is not required for online digital E/M services. Communication for online digital E/M services may be an exchange of messages through technology such as secure email, secure text messaging, or a patient portal.

Verify individual health plan policies for payment for digital E/M services.

Codes 99421–99423 are reported by physicians and other QHPs whose scope of practice includes E/M services as described by 98000–98016, 99202–99499. Online assessment and management codes 98970–98972 are reported by health care professionals (eg, speech or physical therapists) whose scope of practice does not include E/M services as described by 98000–98016, 99202–99499.

Online digital E/M services must be patient or caregiver initiated. Online digital E/M services include

- *Cumulative physician or other QHP time* devoted to the patient's care over 7 days whether the time is spent addressing *single or multiple different problems* within the 7-day period
- Cumulative service time beginning at the physician's personal review of the patient's initial inquiry, including
  - Review of patient records or data pertinent to assessment of the patient's problem
  - Physician's or QHP's personal interaction with clinical staff focused on the patient's problem
  - Development of management plans, including physician or QHP generation of prescriptions or ordering of tests
  - Subsequent communication with the patient through online, telephone, email, or other digitally supported communication that does not otherwise represent a separately reported E/M service
- The cumulative time of multiple physicians and/or QHPs in the same group practice and same specialty and subspecialty over the course of a service period (up to 7 days from the initiating physician's initial review of the patient's inquiry)

A physician or QHP may instruct clinical staff to relay a response to a patient and/or caregiver, but only the physician's or QHP's time is included in the service time used to select a code for the online digital E/M service.

- Permanent documentation storage (electronic or hard copy) of the encounter

Document but do not report online digital services

- ✖ Of less than 5 minutes' total time
- ✖ Based on any time spent by clinical staff
- ✖ During the global period of a procedure
- ✖ If another E/M service (in person or via telemedicine) for the same or related problem occurred within 7 days before the online digital service
- ✖ When a separately reported E/M visit occurs within 7 days of initiation of an online digital E/M service

If a patient generates the initial online digital inquiry for a new problem within 7 days of a previous E/M visit that addressed a different problem, the online digital E/M service may be reported separately. Table 20-2 illustrates reporting instructions for 99421–99423 with or without additional services within a 7-day period.

Table 20-2. Decision-Making Guide for Reporting Online Digital Evaluation and Management Services

Use the questions and directions following each question in this table to guide reporting of online digital E/M codes 99421–99423 when using the *CPT* guidelines.[a]

Question	Direction
1. Is this service related to and within the global period of a procedure provided by the same physician or other QHP or an individual in the exact same specialty and same group practice?	No: Go to question 2. Yes: Stop and do not bill the online digital E/M service.
2. Has the 7-day period for the online digital E/M service concluded?	No: Hold the claim to determine if another E/M service within the 7-day period of the online digital E/M service will affect reporting.[b] Yes: Go to question 3.
3. Was the cumulative time of service over the 7-day period at least 5 minutes?	No: Stop and do not report the online digital E/M service. Yes: Continue to question 4.
4. Did the patient receive a face-to-face E/M service (in person or via telemedicine) within the 7 days *following receipt of the online digital E/M service* by a physician or QHP of the exact same specialty and same group practice?	No: Continue to question 5. Yes: Stop and report only the in-person or telemedicine E/M service.
5. Did the patient receive the online digital E/M service *within 7 days following receipt of a face-to-face E/M service* (in person or via telemedicine) by a physician or QHP of the same specialty and same group practice?	No: Continue to row 7. Yes: Continue to question 6.
6. Did the patient receive the online digital E/M service *for the same or a related problem* within the 7 days following receipt of a face-to-face E/M service (in person or via telemedicine) by a physician or QHP of the same specialty and same group practice?	No: Continue to row 7. Yes: Stop and report only the prior E/M service.
7. Report the online digital E/M service based on the cumulative time of service by all physicians and other QHPs in the exact same specialty and same group practice over the 7-day period.[c]	99421 5–10 minutes 99422 11–20 minutes 99423 21 minutes or more (no upper limit)

Abbreviations: *CPT, Current Procedural Terminology;* E/M, evaluation and management; QHP, qualified health care professional.

[a] Refer to your *CPT* reference for full reporting guidelines.

[b] *CPT* does not require that billing for online digital E/M services be held until completion of the 7-day service period. However, billing prior to completion of the 7-day period may result in the need to cancel a claim for an online digital E/M service and file a separate claim for another E/M service within the 7-day period.

[c] When indicated, append a modifier to indicate that an unrelated problem was addressed within 7 days following receipt of another E/M service (eg, XU, unusual non-overlapping service) or during a postoperative period (24, unrelated E/M service by the same physician or QHP during a postoperative period).

Examples

➤ **On July 1, a pediatrician provides an online digital E/M service to a patient with a rash, which includes obtaining history, reviewing digital photographs of the rash, and advising the parent/caregiver on home treatment.** The time of service is 10 minutes and is reportable with 99421. The service is reported when the 7-day service period is complete and no face-to-face E/M service has been rendered during that period. In addition to the documented request for service and images received through the patient portal, the physician uses a template to document the service.

Date: July 1, 2026

Service initiated and consent by: Ms Smith (mother) **Provided via:** Electronic health record portal

History: Per mother, rash began 2 days ago and she thinks it may be impetigo. No known allergies or exposures. Mother has washed it with soap and water and applied neomycin.

Examination: Reviewed digital images of rash. Appears to be nonbullous impetigo of the skin above the mouth and right cheek.

Response: Advised to keep area clean with soap and water with removal of crusts and to stop neomycin and start a prescription of mupirocin ointment at 3 times a day for 7 days. Instructed to return to office in 1 to 2 days if rash not improving because patient may need oral antibiotics. Advised that this is contagious and can spread, so may wash patient's face 2 to 3 times a day and change towels frequently.

Total time: 8 minutes

Electronic signature applied

Teaching Point: The time of any *subsequent* online E/M service within the 7-day service period is added to the time of the first service and 1 code is reported (eg, 99422) for the combined services.

➤ **For the same patient as in the previous example, the parent/caregiver sends a new photograph on July 3 because they are concerned that the rash is not responding to treatment.** The pediatrician sees the patient in the office later that day.

Teaching Point: Code 99421 is not reported for the prior online digital E/M services. Only the appropriate code for the office visit (eg, 99213) is reported.

➤ **A patient is seen in the office by a pediatrician for a URI on January 9.** On January 14, the same patient receives an online digital E/M service for advice on managing fear of sleeping in their own bed. Because the problem addressed by the online service is unrelated to the problem addressed at the office encounter, the online service is separately reported (eg, 99422).

Teaching Point: Follow payer instructions for reporting an unrelated online service within 7 days of an office E/M service (eg, append modifier XU [unusual non-overlapping service]). Append modifier 24 (unrelated E/M service by the same physician or QHP during a postoperative period) when an online service occurs during a postoperative period of an unrelated procedure (eg, within a 10- or 90-day global period).

➤ **A 10-year-old patient is seen in the office by a pediatrician for concern of serous otitis media on January 9.** On January 11, a parent/caregiver contacts the pediatrician via secure email with concern that the patient's symptoms have worsened, so the pediatrician prescribes an antibiotic.

Teaching Point: Only the office encounter (eg, 99213) is reported because the online digital E/M service is provided within 7 days for the same problem addressed at the in-person visit.

➤ **A patient receives an online digital E/M service on January 9.** The physician's total time spent providing the service is 10 minutes. On January 15, the same patient receives an online digital E/M service for an unrelated problem with a total physician time of 15 minutes.

Teaching Point: The 2 services occurring within 7 days are combined, even though each service addressed different problems, and reported with 99423. A practice may choose to delay billing of online services until the 7-day period of service is completed. Alternatively, if the initial service has been reported and another service is provided within 7 days

Outpatient Telemedicine and Online Digital Services

Chapter 20

such that the combined time supports a higher level of service, the initial claim may be canceled and a new claim submitted for the combined services with the code that accounts for additional time. Follow payer guidelines for the date of service, typically the date that the service was completed, although the range of dates from the first to last service may be included in the notes field on the claim.

Do not include the time of separately reported online digital E/M services in the time attributed to other services (eg, care plan oversight [99374, 99375, 99377–99380] or chronic or principal care management services [99487, 99489, 99490, #99439, 99491, 99424–99427]).

Remote Evaluation of Recorded Video and/or Images

G2010 Remote evaluation of recorded video and/or images submitted by an established patient (eg, store and forward), including interpretation with follow-up with the patient within 24 business hours, not originating from a related E/M service provided within the previous 7 days nor leading to an E/M service or procedure within the next 24 hours or soonest available appointment

The Centers for Medicare & Medicaid Services created G2010 as a virtual check-in service allowing payment for evaluation of patient images and/or recorded video sent via digital technology (eg, secure email or text messaging, patient portal) to a physician or QHP by an established patient or their caregiver and the physician's or QHP's response regarding recommended management.

G2010 represents a service that includes review of the patient-submitted images and/or video and communications with the patient/caregiver in response to the findings *but is not a time-based service.*

Report G2010 when the service

- Is initiated and agreed to by an established patient (although the practice may inform the patient of the option to access care via submission of recorded video or images)
- Includes interpretation and follow-up communication with the patient within *24 business hours*
- Is unrelated to a medical visit within the previous 7 days and does not lead to a medical visit within the next 24 hours (or soonest appointment available)
- Is a physician or QHP service in response to receipt of images and/or video from an established patient and/or caregiver
- Is reported for work personally performed by a physician or QHP, not clinical staff, in review of images and/or video and preparation of a response to the patient and/or caregiver

Example

➤ **A physician receives and reviews images of a rash on a 9-month-old's trunk.** The patient's mother sent the images in a secure email that included history of the patient's being feverish earlier in the week but not acting or appearing ill and not showing any signs of itching or discomfort. The mother also notes suspicion that the rash is caused by roseola. The physician agrees that the rash is likely caused by roseola and advises clinical staff to relay this information with instruction to follow up if any new symptoms develop. The service is reported to a payer that allows payment when reported with G2010.

Teaching Point: The physician's review of the images and provision of medical advice to the caregiver via clinical staff supports G2010. When the patient requires an in-person or telemedicine E/M service on the same date or at the next available appointment in response to the review of images/video, G2010 is not separately reported. There is no requirement for time spent providing this service.

To test your knowledge of the information presented in this chapter, complete the quiz found at the end of it, after the resources. Answers to each quiz are found in **Appendix II**.

Chapter Takeaways

Telemedicine is an evolving practice, which results in frequent changes to codes, guidelines, and payer policies. Following are some takeaways from this chapter:

- Codes **98000–98007** are reported for synchronous audio-visual visits according to either MDM or total time.
- Codes **98008–98015** are reported for synchronous audio-only visits based on either MDM or total time but with an additional requirement of more than 10 minutes spent in medical discussion.
- Code **99417 95** (prolonged outpatient E/M service) may be reported in addition to **98003**, **98007**, **98011**, and **98015** when code selection is based on total time and the required total time is exceeded by 15 minutes or more.
- When the video component of an audio-video E/M service is lost and the service is continued with audio-only communication, the service is reported according to the service that accounted for the majority of the time spent in interactive medical discussion and/or patient observation. A requirement of more than 10 minutes of medical discussion applies.
- Code **98016** is reported for a brief (5- to 10-minute) synchronous communication technology visit for the purposes of determining whether a more extensive service is required.
- Modifiers **93** and **95** are not appended to codes **98000–98016**.
- Payers may require specific POS code **02** or **10** to identify where the patient received a telemedicine service.
- Codes **99421–99423** are reported for E/M services provided via asynchronous communication technology. Limitations apply regarding services within 7 days of a previous E/M service or resulting in an appointment for another E/M service within 24 hours or at the soonest available appointment.
- Codes discussed in this chapter are not reported when another E/M service is provided by the same physician or QHP or individuals of the same group practice and same exact specialty on the same date.

Resources

AAP Coding Assistance and Education

AAP Section on Telehealth Care (www.aap.org/en/community/aap-sections/telehealth-care)

Pediatric Telehealth Best Practices Paperback and eBook Package (www.aap.org/Pediatric-Telehealth-Best-Practices-Paperback-and-eBook-Package)

Pediatric Telehealth Coding: Expert Guidance for Your Practice (www.aap.org/Pediatric-Telehealth-Coding-Paperback)

AAP Pediatric Coding Newsletter™

"*CPT 2025:* An Overview of Telemedicine Code Changes," November 2024 (https://doi.org/10.1542/pcco_book247_document002)

"*CPT 2025:* Audio-Only Telemedicine Services," December 2024 (https://doi.org/10.1542/pcco_book248_document004)

"*CPT 2025:* Audio-Video Telemedicine Visits," December 2024 (https://doi.org/10.1542/pcco_book248_document003)

"*CPT 2025:* Reporting a Brief Communication Technology-Based Service," December 2024 (https://doi.org/10.1542/pcco_book248_document002)

"Q&A: Coding for Telemedicine Services in 2025," January 2025 (https://doi.org/10.1542/pcco_book249_document004)

"Telemedicine in 2025: Beyond the New Codes," January 2025 (https://doi.org/10.1542/pcco_book249_document002)

Test Your Knowledge!

1. **True or false? Telemedicine codes 98000–98015 may be selected on the basis of either level of MDM or total time on the date of the encounter.**
   a. True
   b. False
2. **Which service may be reported with synchronous audio-video telemedicine visit codes 98004–98007?**
   a. A telemedicine service provided within 7 days of an in-person visit
   b. A service that includes only communication between the patient and clinical staff who relay a physician's or QHP's instructions to the patient
   c. A synchronous audio-video telemedicine service provided to a new patient
   d. A telemedicine service that was provided via audio-only communication because the patient's video technology failed
3. **Which of the following is reported with audio-only telemedicine service codes 98012?**
   a. An audio-only E/M service to answer questions relating a procedure performed by the same physician or QHP during a 10-day post-operative period.
   b. An E/M service provided to an established patient by clinical staff under a physician's direct supervision and in continuation of the physician's plan of care.
   c. An audio-only E/M service with 11 minutes spent in medical discussion and total time of 16 minutes.
   d. An audio-only E/M service with 8 minutes of medical discussion and total time of 15 minutes.
4. **Which is correct when reporting a synchronous audio-video E/M service with prolonged service of 20 minutes beyond the 40 minutes total time used to select code 98007?**
   a. *CPT* does not allow reporting of prolonged services when a service is provided via telemedicine so only **98007** is reported.
   b. Report **98007** and **99417 95** × 1 unit.
   c. Report only **99417 95** with 4 units.
   d. Report **98007** and **99417 95** × 2 units.
5. **Which of the following may be reported with code 98016?**
   a. A telephone call by a physician to advise a patient/parent that their health plan has denied prior authorization of a test and an alternative test has been ordered and scheduled
   b. An audio-only E/M service provided at the request of and to an established patient with 8 minutes of medical discussion
   c. An exchange of secure emails with a patient or parent that required 9 minutes of a physician's time
   d. A 3-minute E/M service provided via synchronous communication technology

CHAPTER 21

Remote Data Collection and Monitoring Services

Contents

Chapter Highlights

- General documentation elements for remote data collection and monitoring services
- Identification and differentiation of codes for condition-specific types of remote data collection and monitoring or management services
- Codes for collection and interpretation of digitally stored physiologic data
- Updates to remote physiologic monitoring treatment management services
- Updates to remote therapeutic monitoring with or without therapeutic intervention

This chapter reviews codes for reporting services that include collection of data over time with submission/transmission of data for review and report at the conclusion of the service period and for reporting remote monitoring of patient data with concurrent treatment management services.

Codes included describe the following related services:

- Device supply and data capture/transfer services
- Patient education/training and device calibration

Note: All relative value units (RVUs) included in this chapter are 2025 Medicare Physician Fee Schedule (MPFS) values that are unadjusted for geographic locality. The RVUs for 2026 were not available at the time of this publication. Individual payers may utilize different fee schedule methodologies or the MPFS from a different year (eg, 2023).

Getting Paid for Remote Data Monitoring

Although some remote data collection and monitoring services have been available for decades, increased access to and advances in technology have expanded the types of data that may be collected, monitored, and used in patient management.

According to the Center for Connected Health Policy, as of 2024, Medicaid plans in 42 states offer some form of payment for remote patient (ie, patient data) monitoring services (www.cchpca.org/resources/state-telehealth-laws-and-reimbursement-policies-report-fall-2024). Medicaid payment policies often include restrictions on the clinical indications for monitoring, types of monitoring devices used, and health care professionals paid for monitoring services (eg, only home health agencies).

Commercial health plans may or may not provide clear payment policy for remote data collection and/or monitoring services. Physicians and other qualified health care professionals (QHPs) should review local and regional payment policies (which may be included in policies for telehealth or virtual health care) prior to providing remote monitoring or remote treatment management services.

State regulations and payer policies for all types of digitally enhanced health services continue to evolve. It is important for physicians and other QHPs to research and understand local and regional payment policies for remote data collection and monitoring services before offering these services.

Refer also to the discussion of care management services in Chapter 9, as care management services may be an alternative or addition to remote data monitoring services.

General Documentation Guidance

Documentation of all remote monitoring services should include

- Patient name and other identifying information (eg, patient ID number)
- Documented order, including clinical indications for the services provided

Payment policies published by commercial, exchange, or Medicaid plans may include required clinical indications for remote data collection or monitoring services. Verify your contractual terms regarding direct billing to patients including use of advance notice of noncoverage or waiver of liability prior to billing patients for noncovered services.

- Patient/caregiver agreement to receive services (Documented notification of potential financial responsibility may also be required.)

Remote Data Collection and Monitoring Services

Chapter 21

- Any accommodations used to facilitate the service (eg, language assistance services)
- Dates of each episode of service (eg, start and stop dates of equipment use; dates of physician, QHP, or clinical staff communication with patients and caregivers)
- Description of services provided on each date of service (DOS) (eg, patient education, review of data transmission), including type of technology used
- Time, when applicable (eg, time spent in patient/caregiver communication)
- Identification and authentication by each author entering documentation into the patient's health record

Types of Remote Data Collection and/or Monitoring Services

Current Procedural Terminology (*CPT*®) describes multiple services that may include utilization of data acquired remotely by

- Patient self-collection and data transmission/submission to a physician for review and interpretation outside a face-to-face visit
- Remote physiologic monitoring with treatment management services
- Remote therapeutic monitoring of non-physiologic data (eg, level of function, adherence to treatment plan) with treatment management services

Appendix R of the AMA *CPT* manual is a digital medicine taxonomy table for quickly identifying and differentiating digital medicine services, including clinical data monitoring services. (The taxonomy table does not include all services that may be considered digital medicine services and does not supersede specific coding guidance found elsewhere in *CPT*.)

Devices used for digitally storing data and/or remote physiologic or therapeutic monitoring must be medical devices as defined by the US Food and Drug Administration (FDA). Medical devices may be listed as *FDA approved* or *FDA cleared*. Storage, transfer, and access of personal health information must also comply with federal and state regulations for protection of personal health information (eg, privacy provisions of the Health Insurance Portability and Accountability Act).

Collection and Interpretation of Digitally Stored Physiologic Data

Certain codes describe specific physiological data collection/monitoring (eg, apnea monitoring), whereas other codes describe more generalized services (eg, remote monitoring of physiologic parameter[s] [eg, weight, blood pressure, pulse oximetry, respiratory flow rate]). The code that most specifically describes a service should be reported.

Self-Measured Blood Pressure Monitoring

#99473 Self-measured blood pressure using a device validated for clinical accuracy; patient education/training and device calibration (RVUs: work, 0.00; total in a facility or non-facility setting, 0.43)

#99474 separate self-measurements of two readings one minute apart, twice daily over a 30-day period (minimum of 12 readings), collection of data reported by the patient and/or caregiver to the physician or other QHP, with report of average systolic and diastolic pressures and subsequent communication of a treatment plan to the patient (RVUs: work, 0.18; total non-facility, 0.51; total facility, 0.26).

Self-measured blood pressure monitoring is a non–face-to-face service in which the patient or caregiver uses a home blood pressure measurement device to measure and record readings that are then provided to the ordering physician on paper, digitally (eg, email), or by electronic transmission from the device to an application that allows the patient to directly share data with the ordering physician or other QHP.

The work of managing or treating the patient's blood pressure is not included in **99474**. But when provided on the same date as a patient visit, **99474** is considered part of the visit and not separately reported. The review and analysis of the patient's readings would contribute to the data to be reviewed and analyzed at the visit.

Self-measured blood pressure monitoring is used for

- Ruling out white-coat hypertension, which can prevent unnecessary treatment, adverse medication effects, and laboratory or diagnostic costs
- Identifying masked hypertension, which, if left untreated, carries a higher risk of cardiovascular disease and stroke
- Assessing control of hypertension and ensuring appropriate treatment is being ordered

Table 21-1 provides an overview of work included in each code.

Table 21-1. Self-Measured Blood Pressure Monitoring by the Patient	
#99473	Clinical staff or physician work • Patient education/training on self-measurement and reading collection • Calibration of home blood pressure monitoring device Report once per device.
#99474	Physician work • Review the report of individual and average systolic/diastolic blood pressure readings (it must include ≥12 readings; the patient performs/documents 2 readings 1 minute apart at each measurement). • Communicate the treatment plan to clinical staff or the patient/caregiver. Report once per calendar month.

- ✖ Codes 99473 and 99474 are not reported for automated ambulatory blood pressure monitoring using report-generating software worn continuously for 24 hours or longer; refer to 93784–93790.

Do not report 99473 or 99474 when reporting the following services in the same calendar month:

- ✖ Ambulatory blood pressure monitoring (93784, 93786, 93788, 93790)
- ✖ Collection and interpretation of physiologic data (99091)
- ✖ Remote physiologic monitoring and treatment management (99453, 99454, 99457)
- ✖ Remote therapeutic monitoring treatment management services (98980, 98981)
- ✖ Chronic care management (CCM) (99487, 99489, 99490, 99439, 99491, 99437)
- ✖ Principal care management (PCM) (99424–99427)

Example

➤ **A 16-year-old patient with moderate obesity presents with primary hypertension that is not responsive to lifestyle management.** The patient is struggling with dietary guidelines and exercises only during physical education at school. A low-dose medication is prescribed with instruction to adhere to an agreed-on diet and exercise regimen. The patient has previously been intolerant of ambulatory blood pressure monitoring but agrees to monitoring by self-measurement. The patient's parents have a home blood pressure monitor. The physician's documented evaluation and management (E/M) service supports moderate medical decision-making.

On the next day, the patient returns with the device. Clinical staff calibrate the device and provide training for measurement and download and transmission of readings via the practice patient portal.

At the end of the 30-day period, the clinical staff review the patient's transmitted readings and average the systolic and diastolic pressures. The readings and calculated averages are reviewed by the physician, who communicates an ongoing treatment plan to the patient and/or caregivers.

ICD-10-CM	*CPT*
I10 (hypertension) for all dates of service	*Initial DOS* 99214 (office or other outpatient E/M service with moderate medical decision-making) *Return visit for device setup after receipt of blood pressure device* 99473 (patient education/training and device calibration) *Data analysis and patient communication after 30-day period* 99474 (collection and averaging of blood pressure readings with communication of plan of care)

Teaching Point: At least 12 blood pressure readings must be obtained and averaged to create a treatment plan for the patient. Code 99474 includes collection, analysis, and communication of treatment plan(s) within a 30-day period.

If the patient returned for an office or other outpatient E/M service to review the readings and obtain the physician's recommended care plan, an E/M service (eg, 99214) would be reported in lieu of 99474.

Nonspecific Physiologic Data Collection and Interpretation

#99091 Collection and interpretation of physiologic data (eg, electrocardiography, blood pressure, glucose monitoring) digitally stored and/or transmitted by the patient and/or caregiver to the physician or other QHP, qualified by education, training, licensure/regulation (when applicable) requiring a minimum of 30 minutes of time, each 30 days (1.10 work RVUs, 1.60 total RVUs in a facility or non-facility setting)

Code **99091** *does not require active monitoring of physiologic data* or live interactive communication with the patient during the service period as required for remote physiologic monitoring treatment management service codes **99470**, **99457**, and **99458**, discussed in the Remote Physiologic Monitoring Treatment Management Services section later in this chapter.

Code **99091** represents a 30-day episode of care. Time spent by a physician or QHP in the following activities is included in the time supporting **99091**:

- Accessing, reviewing, and interpreting data
- Modifying the care plan as necessary and communicating to the patient/caregiver
- Completing associated documentation
- Report **99091** for a minimum of 30 minutes (cumulative time), each 30 days.

If the services described by 99091 are provided on the same day that the patient presents for an E/M service, these services should be considered part of the E/M service and not separately reported.

Do not report **99091**

- ✖ If other, more specific *CPT* codes exist (eg, **93227**, **93272** for electrocardiographic services; **95251** for continuous glucose monitoring)
- ✖ For time spent by clinical staff
- ✖ For transfer and interpretation of data from hospital or clinical laboratory computers
- ✖ For time used to meet the criteria for care plan oversight services (**99374–99380**), personally performed CCM (**99437**, **99491**) or PCM (**99424–99427**), or remote physiologic monitoring treatment management services (**99457**, **99458**)

***CPT* does not require use of a medical device as defined by the FDA for services reported with 99091. Live interactive contact during the reporting period is also not a required element of service for 99091.**

Example

➤ **An adolescent with cystic fibrosis transmits physiologic data (self-reported and data from a combination of FDA-approved and non–FDA-approved medical devices) to their physician.** The data includes results from a handheld spirometry device and a Bluetooth oximeter, wellness and cough scores, temperature, weight, and smartwatch measurements of heart rate, exercise, and sleep. A care coordinator in the physician's practice receives the patient's data and notifies the physician of symptoms/trends that are outside the acceptable range designated by the physician. Over a 30-day period, the physician documents 30 minutes spent in review of the patient's data, updating the patient's plan of care, and providing instructions to the patient and patient's parents (as indicated). The physician reports **99091** linked to a diagnosis code for the current state of the child's cystic fibrosis (eg, **E84.0**, cystic fibrosis with pulmonary manifestations).

Circadian Respiratory Pattern Recording

94772 Circadian respiratory pattern recording (pediatric pneumogram), 12–24-hour continuous recording, infant

- This code is not assigned RVUs in the MPFS (used by many payers). Allowable fees are determined by the payer.
- Report **94772** when circadian respiratory pattern recording (pediatric pneumogram), at least 12- to 24-hour continuous recording, is performed on an infant (generally defined as a child younger than 12 months old).
- Physicians may be required to append modifier **26** to indicate that only the professional component of this service was provided.
- Report 1 unit per recording period unless otherwise instructed by a payer.

Pediatric Home Apnea Monitoring Event Recording

94774 Pediatric home apnea monitoring event recording including respiratory rate, pattern and heart rate per 30-day period of time; includes monitor attachment, download of data, review, interpretation, and preparation of a report by a physician or other QHP

94775 monitor attachment only (includes hook-up, initiation of recording and disconnection)

94776 monitoring, download of information, receipt of transmission(s) and analyses by computer only

94777 review, interpretation and preparation of report only by a physician or other QHP

- Codes 94774–94777 are not assigned RVUs in the MPFS (used by many payers). Allowable fees are determined by the payer.
- Codes 94775 and 94776 are reported by the home health agency because there is no physician work involved.
- Report either 94774 or 94777 once per 30-day period.
  - Report 94774 when the physician or QHP orders home monitoring, chooses the monitor limits, arranges for a home health care provider to teach the parents, and, after receiving downloaded information, also provides an interpretation and report of the findings and recommendations for continuation or discontinuation of monitoring.
  - Report 94777 when the physician or QHP receives the downloaded information and provides an interpretation and report of the findings and recommendations for continuation or discontinuation of monitoring. This information is provided to the primary care physician and/or the family.
- ✖ Codes 94774–94777 are not reported in conjunction with 93224–93272 (electrocardiographic monitoring).
- ✖ The apnea recording device cannot be reported separately.
- ✖ When oxygen saturation monitoring is used in addition to heart rate and respiratory monitoring, it is not reported separately.

Example

➤ **An infant born at 23 weeks' gestation, corrected age now 38 weeks old, has chronic lung disease due to bronchopulmonary dysplasia and requires prolonged low-flow oxygen.** The infant continues to have occasional episodes of self-stimulated apnea lasting less than 15 seconds and goes home with heart rate and respiratory monitoring during unattended periods and sleep. The physician orders the monitor, contacts the home health agency for its provision, and instructs the home health agency to teach the parents about cardiopulmonary resuscitation, proper attachment of the monitor leads, and resetting of the monitor. The home health agency provides the physician with the downloaded recordings. The first month's data are interpreted by the physician and a written report is generated. The physician counsels the parents about the need to continue monitoring.

Teaching Point: Report 94774 and the appropriate *International Classification of Diseases, 10th Revision, Clinical Modification* codes (eg, P27.1, bronchopulmonary dysplasia originating in the perinatal period; P28.49, other apnea of newborn [apnea of prematurity]; P07.18, other low birth weight newborn, 2000-2499 grams; and Z99.81, dependence on supplemental oxygen).

In subsequent months, the physician receives the downloaded recordings, interprets them, and generates reports with recommendations for continued or discontinued monitoring. These services are reported with 94777.

Ambulatory Continuous Glucose Monitoring

95250 Ambulatory continuous glucose monitoring of interstitial tissue fluid via a subcutaneous sensor for a minimum of 72 hours; physician or other QHP (office) provided equipment, sensor placement, hook-up, calibration of monitor, patient training, removal of sensor, and printout of record (4.31 total facility or non-facility RVUs)

#95249 patient-provided equipment, sensor placement, hook-up, calibration of monitor, patient training, and printout of recording (1.98 total facility or non-facility RVUs)

95251 Ambulatory continuous glucose monitoring of interstitial tissue fluid via a subcutaneous sensor for a minimum of 72 hours; analysis, interpretation and report (0.70 work RVUs and 1.03 total facility or non-facility RVUs)

- The supplier of the equipment (patient or physician office) determines code selection for the sensor placement, hookup, calibration of the monitor, patient training, and printout of record 95250 and 95249.
- Report 95249 or 95250 only when use of an ambulatory glucose monitor is initiated and data are captured for a minimum of 72 hours.

- Physicians report 95249 only if the patient brings the data receiver into the physician's or other QHP's office and the entire initial data collection procedure is conducted in the office.
- Report 95249 only once for the entire duration that a patient has a receiver, even if the patient receives a new sensor and/or transmitter. If a patient receives a new or different model of receiver, 95249 may be reported again when the entire initial data collection procedure is conducted in the office.
  - Report 95249 on the date the continuous glucose monitoring recording is printed in the office.
  - Removal of a sensor is not a required component of 95249.
- Analysis, interpretation, and report (95251) may be performed with or without a face-to-face encounter on the same DOS. This service is reported only once per month when at least 72 hours of monitoring is analyzed with interpretation and report.
- Codes 95249 and 95250 do not include physician work (ie, valued only for practice expense and liability). **Table 21-2** lists the physician and clinical staff work components of 95249–95251.

Table 21-2. Ambulatory Continuous Glucose Monitoring of Interstitial Tissue Fluid via a Subcutaneous Sensor

A minimum of 72 hours of monitoring is required for each code.	
95251	Physician work includes correlation of individual data points with the patient's daily log and interpretation and report. Do not report more than once per month.
#95249 (patient-provided equipment only)	Clinical staff work includes sensor placement, hookup, calibration of the monitor, patient training, and printout of the record. Report only once during the time a patient owns a given data receiver.
95250 (physician office–provided equipment only)	Clinical staff work includes sensor placement, hookup, calibration of the monitor, patient training, removal of the sensor, and printout of the record. Do not report more than once per month.

Refer to discussion of 99091 and 99457 for collection and interpretation of glucose monitoring data other than continuous ambulatory glucose monitoring of interstitial fluid (eg, review of data transmitted from a patient's blood glucose monitor).

Remote Physiologic Monitoring Services

New in 2026! Report device supply with daily recordings or programmed alert transmission for 2 to 15 days within a 30-day period (99445) or 16 to 30 days in a 30-day period (99454). Remote physiologic treatment management services may now be reported for 10 to 19 minutes of time in a calendar month using 99470. Continue reporting codes 99457–99458 for 20 minutes or more of remote physiologic treatment management services in a calendar month.

Remote physiologic monitoring services include use of a medical device approved by the FDA to record and transmit daily recordings or programmed alerts. Codes distinguish equipment setup and patient education, device supply with transmission of data, and use of results to treat a patient under a specific treatment plan.

- ✖ Do not report 99453, 99445, 99454, 99470, 99457, and 99458 for remote physiologic monitoring services when the parameters monitored are more specifically identified by other codes.
- A physician practice may provide all components (eg, equipment supply, initial setup, calibration, training, monitoring, treatment management services) or, perhaps more frequently, only the remote physiologic monitoring treatment management component (ie, 99470, 99457 and 99458).

Remote Monitoring Setup and Device Supply

#▲99453 Remote monitoring of physiologic parameter(s) (eg, weight, blood pressure, pulse oximetry, respiratory flow rate); initial set-up and patient education on use of equipment (0.61 RVUs in a facility or non-facility setting)

#●99445 device(s) supply with daily recording(s) or programmed alert(s) transmission, 2–15 days in a 30-day period (RVUs not available at time of publication)

#▲99454 device(s) supply with daily recording(s) or programmed alert(s) transmission, 16–30 days in a 30-day period (1.33 RVUs in a facility or non-facility setting)

To report **99453**, **99445**, and **99454**, the device used must be a medical device as defined by the FDA (eg, spirometer) and the service must be ordered by a physician or QHP.

Codes 99453 describes setup and patient education provided to an individual patient. When setup and education are provided in a group setting, report an unlisted E/M service (99499).

- Codes **99453**, **99445**, and **99454** represent only practice expense; no physician work is valued in these codes.
- Initial setup and patient education on use of equipment (**99453**) is reported only once for each episode of care (begins when the remote monitoring physiological service is initiated and ends with attainment of targeted treatment goals).

Do not report

- ✖ **99453**, **99445**, and **99454** in conjunction with codes for more specific physiologic parameters (eg, **94762**, home apnea monitoring) or when these services are included in other *CPT* codes for the duration of the physiologic monitoring service (eg, **95250**, ambulatory continuous glucose monitoring sensor placement and removal and data download).
- ✖ **99453** in conjunction with **0811T** (setup and patient education for remote multi-day complex uroflowmetry) or **0812T** (remote multi-day complex uroflowmetry device supply with automated report generation, up to 10 days).
- ✖ **99454** in conjunction with **0812T**.
- ✖ **99454** in the same 30-day period as **99445**.
- ✖ **99453** and **99445** when cumulative monitoring is less than 2 days in a 30-day period.

Examples

➤ **A child with epilepsy is prescribed an FDA-approved wearable device that detects seizures and notifies caregivers in addition to transmitting data to the prescribing physician.** The patient is provided with setup and education for use of the device and the program's monitoring application by clinical staff in the prescribing physician's practice. The practice directly receives and monitors daily recordings and/or programmed alerts for at least a 2-day period. Education on equipment use is provided as needed. Codes **99453** and **99454** are reported.

Teaching Point: The device must be used for monitoring for at least 2 days to report device training and supply with **99453** and/or **99445**. For cumulative monitoring of at least 16 days in a 30-day period, report device supply with **99454** in lieu of **99445**.

The patient and caregivers are provided separately reported treatment management services (**99470**, **99457**, **99458**) of at least 10 minutes in the month, as discussed later in this chapter.

➤ **A child with poorly controlled asthma is enrolled in a remote monitoring program.** A Bluetooth-enabled device that promotes and monitors effective inhaler use and measures forced expiratory volume in 1 second and peak expiratory flow is provided to the patient by a remote monitoring technology provider. The patient's physician and/or clinical staff provide education to the patient and caregivers on device use. The physician reports **99453**.

Teaching Point: Because the physician practice furnishes only the initial setup and patient education, only **99453** is reported for setup and education encounter. This service is reported only at the time of the initial 2 to 30 days of monitoring. Either **99445** or **99454** would be reported by the equipment supplier and monitoring service for cumulative monitoring of at least 2 days.

The patient and caregivers are provided separately reported treatment management services (**99470**, **99457**, **99458**) of at least 10 minutes in the month, as indicated.

Remote Physiologic Monitoring Treatment Management Services

#●99470 Remote physiologic monitoring treatment management services, clinical staff/physician/other QHP time in a calendar month requiring 1 real-time interactive communication with the patient/caregiver during the calendar month; first 10 minutes (RVUs not yet published)

#▲99457 first 20 minutes (0.61 work RVUs; 1.48 total RVUs in a non-facility setting and 0.89 total RVUs in a facility setting)

#✚▲99458 each additional 20 minutes (0.61 work RVUs; 1.19 total RVUs in a non-facility setting and 0.89 total RVUs in a facility setting)

● indicates a new code; ▲, revised; #, re-sequenced; ✚, add-on; ★, audiovisual technology; and ◀, synchronous interactive audio.

Remote physiologic monitoring treatment management services include time spent in a calendar month monitoring, analyzing, and using the results of transmitted physiologic data to treat a patient under a specific treatment plan. These services may be rendered by physicians, QHPs, and/or clinical staff working under supervision of a physician or QHP.

The reporting period for 99470, 99457, and 99458 is a calendar month. At least 10 minutes must be spent in treatment management services in a calendar month to report 99470.

The time spent in activities listed in **Table 21-3** is included in the time supporting **99470**, **99457**, and **99458**.

Table 21-3. Remote Physiologic Monitoring Treatment Management Services	
#●99470	Physician work, performed personally or by clinical staff under physician or QHP supervision Access, review, and interpret data. Modify the treatment plan as necessary and communicate to the patient/caregiver. Complete associated documentation. Report for a total time of 10–19 minutes each calendar month. Do not report **99470** for <10 minutes or in addition to **99457** and **99458**.
#99457	Physician work, performed personally or by clinical staff under physician or QHP supervision as described for **99470**, except report **99457** for the initial time of 20–39 minutes each calendar month.
#+99458	Physician work, performed personally or by clinical staff under physician or QHP supervision, as described for **99470** with 1 unit for each additional period of no less than 20 minutes beyond the first 20 minutes reported with **99457**
Abbreviation: QHP, qualified health care professional.	

Documentation of remote physiologic monitoring treatment management must include

- An order by a physician or QHP
- Data access, review, and interpretation, as indicated by daily transmittals and/or alerts
- *Live interactive communication* (eg, 2-way conversation via telephone or secure messaging) with the patient and/or caregiver at least once in a calendar month
- Time of service of 10 or more minutes in a calendar month, including time in live interactive communication, data access, review and interpretation, and documentation

Reporting instructions

- Report **99470** once with 1 unit of service for total time of 10–19 minutes of service in a calendar month, or
- Report **99457** once with 1 unit of service for the initial 20–39 minutes of service regardless of the number of physiologic monitoring modalities performed in a calendar month. When the time of service extends a full 20 minutes beyond the first 20 minutes, report **99458** in addition to **99457**.

Do not report **99470**, **99457** or **99458**

- ✖ For any time on a day when the physician or QHP reports an E/M service (office or other outpatient services [**99202–99205**, **99211–99215**], home or residence services [**99341–99345**, **99347–99350**], initial or subsequent hospital inpatient or observation services [**99221–99223**, **99231–99233**], or inpatient or observation consultations [**99252–99255**]).
- ✖ For any time related to other reported services (eg, **93290**, interrogation of implantable cardiovascular physiologic monitor system).
- ✖ In conjunction with collection and interpretation of physiologic data (**99091**).
- Codes **99470**, **99457** and **99458** may be reported during the same service period as CCM (**99437**, **99439**, **99487–99491**), PCM (**99424–99427**), transitional care management (**99495**, **99496**), and behavioral health integration services (**99484**, **99492–99494**). But the time for each service must be distinct and not overlapping and must be separately documented.

Remote Data Collection and Monitoring Services

Chapter 21

Example

➤ **Data are received for a child with poorly controlled asthma who is enrolled in a remote physiologic monitoring program.** Clinical staff of the ordering physician review the data and note that the patient's plan of care calls for patient contact because forced expiratory volume in 1 second and/or peak expiratory flow measurements are outside a specific range. A care coordinator contacts the patient's parent to inquire about medication use and signs and symptoms. The child's physician is consulted by the care coordinator, and advice or orders for a change in management are relayed to the parent. At the end of the calendar month, documentation supports 25 minutes spent in remote physiologic monitoring treatment management services with at least 1 episode of live interactive communication with the patient's caregiver. Code **99457** is reported.

Had the time of service in the calendar month been 10–19 minutes, **99470** would be reported in lieu of **99457**. Had the time in the calendar month totaled 40 minutes or more, code **99458** would be reported in addition to **99457** with one unit of **99458** for each full 20 minutes beyond the initial 20 minutes of service reported with **99457**.

Remote Therapeutic Monitoring Services

Remote therapeutic monitoring services (eg, musculoskeletal function, therapy adherence, therapy response) represent the review and monitoring of transmitted data related to signs, symptoms, and functions of a therapeutic response as opposed to physiologic data such as heart rate and rhythm. In addition to its monitoring functionality, the device may also provide a therapeutic intervention. The data may represent objective device-generated integrated data or subjective inputs reported by a patient (eg, the patient's reported outcome of therapeutic exercise). These data are reflective of therapeutic responses that provide a functionally integrative representation of patient status.

Remote therapeutic monitoring services are included in the Non-face-to-face Nonphysician Services category of the Medicine section of *CPT*. The services require an order by a physician or other QHP. However, nonphysician qualified healthcare professionals (NQHCP) who may provide and independently report therapeutic services (eg, physical therapist) may report the codes in this category.

Remote Therapeutic Monitoring Setup and Device Supply

New in 2026! Codes 98984, 98985, and 98986 are added to allow reporting of device supply and data transmissions for remote therapeutic monitoring of 2 to 15 days during a 30-day period. The requirement for at least 16 days of monitoring during a 30-day period still applies to codes 98976–98978.

98975 Remote therapeutic monitoring (eg, therapy adherence, therapy response, digital therapeutic intervention); initial set-up and patient education on use of equipment

#●98984 device(s) supply for data access or data transmissions to support monitoring of respiratory system, 2–15 days in a 30-day period

▲98976 device(s) supply for data access or data transmissions to support monitoring of respiratory system, 16–30 days in a 30-day period

#●98985 device(s) supply for data access or data transmissions to support monitoring of musculoskeletal system, 2–15 days in a 30-day period

▲98977 device(s) supply for data access or data transmissions to support monitoring of musculoskeletal system, 16–30 days in a 30-day period

#●98986 device(s) supply for data access or data transmissions to support monitoring of cognitive behavioral therapy, 2–15 days in a 30-day period

▲98978 device(s) supply for data access or data transmissions to support monitoring of cognitive behavioral therapy, 16–30 days in a 30-day period

Report **98975**, **98984**, **98976**, **98985**, **98977**, **98986**, and **98978** only when supplying devices used by the patient to capture and transmit data used in remote therapeutic monitoring treatment management services, **98979**, **98980**, and **98981**. These codes may be more frequently reported by a device vendor.

Code **98975** is reported once per episode of care for the initial setup and patient education on use of the equipment. An *episode of care* is defined as beginning when the remote therapeutic monitoring service is initiated and as ending with attainment of targeted treatment goals.

- ✖ Codes **98975**, **98984**, **98985**, and **98986** are not reported for less than 2 days of cumulative monitoring during the 30-day period.
- ✖ Codes **98976**, **98977**, and **98978** are not reported for less than 16 days of cumulative monitoring during the 30-day period.

Codes **98984**, **98985**, **98986** and **98975–98978** are specific to remote therapeutic monitoring services and are not used in conjunction with physiologic monitoring services (eg, **95250**, ambulatory continuous glucose monitoring or **99453**, **99445**, or **99454**).

Remote Data Collection and Monitoring Services

Chapter 21

Example

➤ **An adolescent patient with moderate persistent asthma is learning to take responsibility for following a QHP's guidance for use of the control medication, identification and avoidance of triggers, and response to symptoms.** The QHP has prescribed remote therapeutic monitoring using an FDA-cleared medical device that automatically transmits data regarding the patient's use of an inhaler.

Initial setup of the medical device and education on its use are provided and reported with 98975. A device(s) is supplied and used for therapeutic monitoring for at least 16 days in a 30-day period. Code 98976 is reported.

When device supply for data access or data transmissions is limited to 2–15 days, 98984 is reported in lieu of 98976. Initial set-up and device supply with monitoring for less than 2 days are not reported. (Codes 98975, 98984, and 98976 may be reported by a device vendor rather than a physician or QHP, when applicable.)

Remote Therapeutic Monitoring Treatment Management Services

●98979 Remote therapeutic monitoring treatment management services, physician/other QHP time in a calendar month requiring at least 1 real-time interactive communication with the patient/caregiver during the calendar month; first 10 minutes

▲98980 first 20 minutes

+▲98981 each additional 20 minutes

Remote therapeutic monitoring treatment management service codes 98979, 98980, and 98981 are reported for a physician's, QHP's, or NQHCP's cumulative time in a calendar month spent in remote therapeutic monitoring to treat a patient under a specific treatment plan. *At least 1 real-time (synchronous) interactive communication with the patient/caregiver is required* in the calendar month. Time of interactive communication with the patient/caregiver contributes to the cumulative time of remote therapeutic monitoring treatment management services.

Codes 98979, 98980, and 98981 are found in the medicine section of *CPT* to indicate that these services may be provided by any physician, other QHP, or NQHCP (eg, physical or occupational therapist, psychologist). In contrast, codes for remote physiologic monitoring are E/M services reported only by professionals whose scope of practice includes independent provision and reporting of E/M services.

- Either code 98979 or 98980 is reported once per calendar month regardless of the number of therapeutic parameters monitored.
- Code 98979 is reported for a service of 10–19 minutes in a calendar month.
- ✖ Do not report 98979 when time spent in remote therapeutic monitoring treatment management services during a calendar month is less than 10 minutes or in conjunction with 98980 and 98981.
- Report 98980 for 20–39 minutes in a calendar month. Report add-on code 98981 in addition to 98980 with 1 unit for each additional full 20-minute period beyond the first 20 minutes reported with 98980.
- ✖ Do not report 98981 for a period of less than 20 minutes.

Do not report 98979, 98980, and 98981

- ✖ According to time spent by clinical staff (ie, only include time spent by a physician, QHP, or NQHCP)
- ✖ In conjunction with remote monitoring of a wireless pulmonary artery pressure sensor (93264), collection and interpretation of physiologic data (99091), or remote physiologic data monitoring treatment management (99470, 99457, 99458)
- ✖ In the same calendar month as self-measured blood pressure (99473, 99474)
- ✖ For any time spent on the date of an E/M service, including home, office or other outpatient, domiciliary, rest home, or inpatient services
- ✖ For time counted toward separately reported CCM services (99437, 99439, 99487–99491), PCM services (99424–99427), transitional care management services (99495, 99496), behavioral health integration services (99484, 99492–99494), psychotherapy services (90832–90853), health behavior assessment and intervention services (96156–96161, 96164–96171), or psychiatric collaborative care services (99492–99494) (When provided in the same time period, each service must be separately documented and no time should be counted toward the required time for both services.)

Documentation of remote physiologic monitoring treatment management must include

- An order by a physician or QHP
- *Live interactive communication* (eg, 2-way conversation via telephone or audio-video technology) with the patient and/or caregiver
- Time of service of 10 or more minutes in a calendar month

● indicates a new code; ▲, revised; #, re-sequenced; ✚, add-on; ★, audiovisual technology; and ◀, synchronous interactive audio.

Although a live, interactive communication with the patient/caregiver is required within the calendar month, there is no requirement for 10 minutes of interactive communication. The total time includes time spent in interactive communication in addition to time in data analysis and interpretation and overseeing, coordinating, and/or modifying the patient's care.

Example

➤ **An adolescent patient with moderate persistent asthma is learning to take responsibility for following a QHP's guidance for use of a control medication, identification and avoidance of triggers, and response to symptoms.** The QHP has prescribed remote therapeutic monitoring using an FDA-cleared medical device that automatically transmits data regarding the patient's use of an inhaler.

The QHP reviews the transmissions and, at least once during the calendar month, telephones the patient to discuss medication adherence. The QHP's total time spent in remote therapeutic monitoring treatment management during the calendar month is 35 minutes. Code **98980** is reported. Had time during the calendar month exceeded 39 minutes, **98981** would have also been reported (ie, for 20 minutes beyond the first 20-minute service period).

Time of less than 10 minutes in the calendar month would not be reported. Time of 10–19 minutes would be reported with **98979**.

To learn more about remote data monitoring services, refer to the February 2022 *Pediatrics*® article "Remote Monitoring of Patient- and Family-Generated Health Data in Pediatrics" (https://doi.org/10.1542/peds.2021-054137).

To test your knowledge of the information presented in this chapter, complete the quiz found at the end of it, after the resources. Answers to each quiz are found in **Appendix II**.

Chapter Takeaways

This chapter discussed multiple types of remote data collection and/or monitoring services. Following are some takeaways from this chapter:

- Documentation of remote data collection or remote monitoring services should include details such as the clinical indication for ordering the services, dates of service, activities such as communicating findings and recommendations to the patient/caregiver, and, for time-based code selection, total time spent during the service period.
- Report the most specific *CPT* code, when applicable, for remote physiologic data monitoring services. For example, codes **95249–95251** are reported for ambulatory continuous blood glucose monitoring of interstitial fluid, rather than **99091**, which is less specific regarding the type of physiologic data monitored.
- Remote therapeutic monitoring treatment management services are differentiated from remote physiologic monitoring treatment management by the type of data monitored and by the type of service (ie, management of a patient's response to a specific treatment plan vs E/M of a condition based on physiologic data).

Resources

AAP Coding Assistance and Education

"Remote Monitoring of Patient- and Family-Generated Health Data in Pediatrics," *Pediatrics* (https://doi.org/10.1542/peds.2021-054137)

AAP Pediatric Coding Newsletter™

"Report the Right Codes: Remote Monitoring Treatment Management Services," June 2025 (https://doi.org/10.1542/pcco_book254_document001)

Coverage of Digital Medicine Services

"AMA Future of Health issue brief: Commercial Payer Coverage for Digital Medicine Codes" (www.ama-assn.org/practice-management/digital/ama-future-health-issue-brief-commercial-payer-coverage-digital)

Center for Connected Health Policy (www.cchpca.org)

Digital Medical Taxonomy

Digital Medicine Taxonomy: *CPT* Appendix R

Test Your Knowledge!

1. **Where can physicians find a resource for identifying and differentiating digital medicine services?**
   a. *CPT* Alphabetic Index
   b. *CPT* telemedicine appendixes P and T
   c. *CPT* digital medicine taxonomy table (Appendix R)
   d. *CPT* telemedicine section
2. **What is the episode of care (reporting period) for collection and interpretation of physiologic data reported with 99091?**
   a. A calendar month
   b. A 30-day period
   c. A 14-day period
   d. A 10-day period
3. **Which of the following differentiates the services reported with 95250 and 95249?**
   a. The supplier of the equipment
   b. The time of service during a 30-day period
   c. The number of days the equipment is used for monitoring
   d. The time of service during a calendar month
4. **Which service requires active monitoring of physiologic data and live interactive communication with the patient during the service period?**
   a. 99091, collection and interpretation of physiologic data
   b. 99474, self-measured blood pressure
   c. 94774, pediatric home apnea monitoring
   d. 99470 or 99457, remote physiologic monitoring treatment management services
5. **Which of the following is true of remote therapeutic monitoring treatment management services?**
   a. Remote therapeutic treatment management services are reported for a physician's, QHP's, or NQHCP's cumulative time in a calendar month.
   b. At least 1 real-time (synchronous) interactive communication with the patient/caregiver is required in the calendar month.
   c. Either code 98979 or 98980 is reported once per calendar month regardless of the number of therapeutic parameters monitored.
   d. All of the above.

Appendixes

Additional coding resources are available at www.aap.org/cfp2026.

I. Quick Reference to 2026 *ICD-10-CM* Pediatric Code Changes

This list does not include all changes made to *International Classification of Diseases, 10th Revision, Clinical Modification* (*ICD-10-CM*). Every effort has been made to include the diagnosis code changes that most apply to pediatric practices. Revisions and/or additional codes may have been published after the date of this printing. Always begin in the *ICD-10-CM* Alphabetic Index to locate the code most specific to the condition or other reason for encounter. Codes are valid as of October 1, 2025, unless otherwise noted.

Quick Reference to 2026 *ICD-10-CM* Pediatric Code Changes	
Abdominal Pain of Multiple Sites	
●R10.85	Abdominal pain of multiple sites
Abnormal Rheumatoid Factor and Anti-citrullinated Protein Antibody	
●R76.81 ●R76.89	Abnormal rheumatoid factor and anti-citrullinated protein antibody without rheumatoid arthritis Other specified abnormal immunological findings in serum
Acute Disseminated Demyelination, Other	
●G37.3	Acute transverse myelitis in demyelinating disease of central nervous system
Adverse Food Reaction, Not Elsewhere Classified	
●Z91.0110 ●Z91.0110X-	Allergy to milk products, unspecified Other adverse food reactions, not elsewhere classified
Adverse Food Reaction, Specified, Not Elsewhere Classified	
●T78.19-	Other adverse food reactions, not elsewhere classified
Allergy Status to Milk Products or Eggs	
●Z91.0110 ●Z91.0111 ●Z91.0112 ●Z91.0120 ●Z91.0121 ●Z91.0122	Allergy to milk products, unspecified Allergy to milk products with tolerance to baked milk Allergy to milk products with reactivity to baked milk Allergy to eggs, unspecified Allergy to eggs with tolerance to baked egg Allergy to eggs with reactivity to baked egg
Anaphylactic or Other Adverse Reaction to Egg	
●T78.080- ●T78.081- ●T78.089- ● T78.12 ●T78.120- ●T78.121- ●T78.129-	Anaphylactic reaction due to egg with tolerance to baked egg Anaphylactic reaction due to egg with reactivity to baked egg Anaphylactic reaction due to eggs, unspecified Other adverse food reaction due to eggs Other adverse food reaction due to egg with tolerance to baked egg Other adverse food reaction due to egg with reactivity to baked egg Other adverse food reaction due to egg with baked egg tolerance/reactivity, unspecified
Anaphylactic or Other Adverse Reaction to Milk and Dairy Products	
●T78.070- ●T78.071- ●T78.079- ●T78.11X- ●T78.110- ●T78.111- ●T78.119-	Anaphylactic reaction due to milk and dairy products with tolerance to baked milk Anaphylactic reaction due to milk and dairy products with reactivity to baked milk Anaphylactic reaction due to milk and dairy products, unspecified Other adverse food reactions due to milk and dairy products Other adverse food reactions due to milk and dairy products with tolerance to baked milk Other adverse food reaction due to milk and dairy products with reactivity to baked milk Other adverse food reaction due to milk and dairy products with baked milk tolerance/reactivity, unspecified

Continued on next page

Appendixes

● indicates a new code; ▲, revised; #, re-sequenced; ✚, add-on; ★, audiovisual technology; and ◀, synchronous interactive audio.

Quick Reference to 2026 *ICD-10-CM* Pediatric Code Changes (*continued*)	
Bite, Open, Flank with Penetration into Peritoneal Cavity	
●S31.656-	Open bite of abdominal wall, right flank with penetration into peritoneal cavity
●S31.657-	Open bite of abdominal wall, left flank with penetration into peritoneal cavity
●S31.65A-	Open bite of abdominal wall, unspecified flank with penetration into peritoneal cavity
Bite, Open, Flank, without Penetration into Peritoneal Cavity	
●S31.156-	Open bite of abdominal wall, right flank without penetration into peritoneal cavity
●S31.157-	Open bite of abdominal wall, left flank without penetration into peritoneal cavity
●S31.15A-	Open bite of abdominal wall, unspecified flank without penetration into peritoneal cavity
Cannabis Hyperemesis Syndrome	
●R11.16	Cannabis hyperemesis syndrome
Craniosynostosis of Unspecified Type	
▲Q75.001	Craniosynostosis, unspecified type, unilateral
▲Q75.002	Craniosynostosis, unspecified type, bilateral
Degenerative Diseases of Nervous System, Not Elsewhere Classified, Other	
●G31.87	Primary progressive apraxia of speech
Diabetes Mellitus, Type 2, In Remission	
●E11.A	Type 2 diabetes mellitus without complications in remission
Diethylstilbestrol, Personal Risk Factor of Exposure To	
● Z91.B	Personal risk factor of exposure to diethylstilbestrol
Disorders of Adrenal Gland, Other	
●E27.5	Adrenomedullary hyperfunction
Disorders of Pyrophosphate Metabolism	
●E83.82	Disorders of pyrophosphate metabolism
●E83.820	Generalized arterial calcification of infancy with unspecified genetic causality
●E83.821	ENPP1 deficiency causing generalized arterial calcification of infancy
●E83.822	ENPP1 deficiency causing autosomal recessive hypophosphatemic rickets type 2
●E83.823	ABCC6 deficiency causing generalized arterial calcification of infancy
●E83.824	ABCC6 deficiency causing pseudoxanthoma elasticum
●E83.825	CD73 deficiency causing arterial calcification
Eyelid Inflammation, Other Specified	
●H01.81	Other specified inflammation of right upper eyelid
●H01.82	Other specified inflammation of right lower eyelid
●H01.83	Other specified inflammation of right eye, unspecified eyelid
●H01.84	Other specified inflammation of left upper eyelid
●H01.85	Other specified inflammation of left lower eyelid
●H01.86	Other specified inflammation of left eye, unspecified eyelid
●H01.89	Other specified inflammation of unspecified eye, unspecified eyelid
●H01.8A	Other specified inflammation of right eye, upper and lower eyelids
●H01.8B	Other specified inflammation of left eye, upper and lower eyelids
Familial Hypercholesterolemia	
●E78.010	Homozygous familial hypercholesterolemia [HoFH]
●E78.011	Heterozygous familial hypercholesterolemia [HeFH]
●E78.019	Familial hypercholesterolemia, unspecified
Family History of Colon Polyps	
▲Z83.718	Family history of other colon polyps

Quick Reference to 2026 *ICD-10-CM* Pediatric Code Changes (*continued*)	
Family History of Diethylstilbestrol Exposure	
●Z84.A	Family history of exposure to diethylstilbestrol
Family History of Primary Malignant Neoplasm	
●Z80.44	Family history of malignant neoplasm of fallopian tube(s)
Financial Insecurity	
●□Z59.861	Financial insecurity, difficulty paying for utilities
●□Z59.868	Other specified financial insecurity
●□Z59.869	Financial insecurity, unspecified
Fishing Hook Injury to Skin	
●W45.3XX-	Fishing hook entering through skin
Flank Infections	
▲L02.212	Cutaneous abscess of back [any part, except buttock and flank]
●L02.217	Cutaneous abscess of flank
▲L02.222	Furuncle of back [any part, except buttock and flank]
●L02.227	Furuncle of flank
●L03.31A	Cellulitis of flank
●L03.32A	Acute lymphangitis of flank
Flank and Suprapubic Tenderness	
●R10.8A	Flank tenderness
●R10.8A1	Right flank tenderness
●R10.8A2	Left flank tenderness
●R10.8A3	Suprapubic tenderness
●R10.8A9	Flank tenderness, unspecified
Flank Pain (localized)	
●R10.A	Pain localized to flank
●R10.A0	Flank pain, unspecified side
●R10.A1	Flank pain, right side
●R10.A2	Flank pain, left side
●R10.A3	Flank pain, bilateral
Fluoroquinolone Antibiotics Poisoning, Adverse Effect, Underdosing	
●T36.A	Poisoning by, adverse effect of and underdosing of fluoroquinolone antibiotics
●T36.AX	Poisoning by, adverse effect of and underdosing of fluoroquinolone antibiotics
●T36.AX1-	Poisoning by fluoroquinolone antibiotics, accidental (unintentional)
●T36.AX2-	Poisoning by fluoroquinolone antibiotics, intentional self-harm
●T36.AX3-	Poisoning by fluoroquinolone antibiotics, assault
●T36.AX4-	Poisoning by fluoroquinolone antibiotics, undetermined
●T36.AX5-	Adverse effect of fluoroquinolone antibiotics
●T36.AX6-	Underdosing of fluoroquinolone antibiotics
Fontan-Related Circulation	
●I27.84	Fontan-related circulation
●I27.840	Fontan-associated liver disease [FALD]
●I27.841	Fontan-associated lymphatic dysfunction
●I27.848	Other Fontan-associated condition
●I27.849	Fontan-related circulation, unspecified

Continued on next page

• indicates a new code; ▲, revised; #, re-sequenced; ✚, add-on; ★, audiovisual technology; and ◀, synchronous interactive audio.

Quick Reference to 2026 *ICD-10-CM* Pediatric Code Changes (*continued*)

Functional Disorders of Polymorphonuclear Neutrophils	
●**D71.1**	Leukocyte adhesion deficiency
●**D71.8**	Other functional disorders of polymorphonuclear neutrophils
●**D71.9**	Functional disorders of polymorphonuclear neutrophils, unspecified
Genetic Susceptibility to Malignancy	
●**Z15.05**	Genetic susceptibility to malignant neoplasm of fallopian tube(s)
●**Z15.06**	Genetic susceptibility to malignant neoplasm of digestive system
●**Z15.060**	Genetic susceptibility to colorectal cancer
●**Z15.068**	Genetic susceptibility to other malignant neoplasm of digestive system
●**Z15.07**	Genetic susceptibility to malignant neoplasm of urinary tract
Genitourinary System, Other Signs and Symptoms Involving The	
●**R39.85**	Costovertebral (angle) tenderness
●**R39.851**	Costovertebral (angle) tenderness, right side
●**R39.852**	Costovertebral (angle) tenderness, left side
●**R39.853**	Costovertebral (angle) tenderness, bilateral
●**R39.859**	Costovertebral (angle) tenderness, unspecified side
Hereditary Nephropathy	
●**N07.B**	Hereditary nephropathy, not elsewhere classified with APOL1-mediated kidney disease [AMKD]
●**Z15.3**	Genetic susceptibility to kidney disease
●**Z84.11**	Family history of APOL1-mediated kidney disease [AMKD]
●**Z84.19**	Family history of other disorders of kidney and ureter
Hyperoxaluria	
●**E72.530**	Primary hyperoxaluria, type 1
●**E72.538**	Other specified primary hyperoxaluria
●**E72.539**	Primary hyperoxaluria, unspecified
●**E72.54**	Secondary hyperoxaluria
●**E72.540**	Dietary hyperoxaluria
●**E72.541**	Enteric hyperoxaluria
●**E72.548**	Other secondary hyperoxaluria
●**E72.549**	Secondary hyperoxaluria, unspecified
Immune Complex-mediated Membranoproliferative Glomerulonephritis	
●**N00.B**	Acute nephritic syndrome with immune complex membranoproliferative glomerulonephritis (IC-MPGN)
●**N00.B1**	Acute nephritic syndrome with idiopathic immune membranoproliferative glomerulonephritis (IC-MPGN)
●**N00.B2**	Acute nephritic syndrome with secondary immune complex membranoproliferative glomerulonephritis (IC-MPGN)
●**N04.B1**	Nephrotic syndrome with idiopathic immune complex membranoproliferative glomerulonephritis (IC-MPGN)
●**N04.B2**	Nephrotic syndrome with secondary immune complex membranoproliferative glomerulonephritis (IC-MPGN)
Infestation by Demodex Mites and Other Acariasis	
●**B88.01**	Infestation by Demodex mites
●**B88.09**	Other acariasis

Quick Reference to 2026 *ICD-10-CM* Pediatric Code Changes (*continued*)	
Injury, Superficial, Abdominal Wall, Groin, or Flank	
●S30.11X-	Contusion of abdominal wall
●S30.12X-	Contusion of groin
●S30.13X-	Contusion of flank (latus) region
●S30.81A-	Abrasion of flank
●S30.82A-	Blister (nonthermal) of flank
●S30.84A-	External constriction of flank
●S30.85A-	Superficial foreign body of flank
●S30.86A-	Insect bite (nonvenomous) of flank
●S30.87A-	Other superficial bite of flank
●S30.9AX-	Unspecified superficial injury of flank
Kabuki Syndrome	
●Q89.81	Kabuki syndrome
●Q89.89	Other specified congenital malformations
Laceration, Flank, With Foreign Body, With Penetration Into Peritoneal Cavity	
●S31.626-	Laceration with foreign body of abdominal wall, right flank with penetration into peritoneal cavity
●S31.627-	Laceration with foreign body of abdominal wall, left flank with penetration into peritoneal cavity
●S31.62A-	Laceration with foreign body of abdominal wall, unspecified flank with penetration into peritoneal cavity
Laceration, Flank, With Foreign Body, Without Penetration Into Peritoneal Cavity	
●S31.126-	Laceration with foreign body of abdominal wall, right flank without penetration into peritoneal cavity
●S31.127-	Laceration with foreign body of abdominal wall, left flank without penetration into peritoneal cavity
●S31.12A-	Laceration with foreign body of abdominal wall unspecified flank without penetration into peritoneal cavity
Laceration, Flank, Without Foreign Body, With Penetration Into Peritoneal Cavity	
●S31.616-	Laceration without foreign body of abdominal wall, right flank with penetration into peritoneal cavity
●S31.617-	Laceration without foreign body of abdominal wall, left flank with penetration into peritoneal cavity
●S31.61A-	Laceration without foreign body of abdominal wall, unspecified flank with penetration into peritoneal cavity
Laceration, Flank, Without Foreign Body, Without Penetration Into Peritoneal Cavity	
●S31.116-	Laceration without foreign body of abdominal wall, right flank without penetration into peritoneal cavity
●S31.117-	Laceration without foreign body of abdominal wall, left flank without penetration into peritoneal cavity
●S31.11A-	Laceration without foreign body of abdominal wall, unspecified flank without penetration into peritoneal cavity
Lipodystrophy	
●E88.10	Lipodystrophy, unspecified
●E88.11	Partial lipodystrophy
●E88.12	Generalized lipodystrophy
●E88.13	Localized lipodystrophy
●E88.14	HIV-associated lipodystrophy
●E88.19	Other lipodystrophy, not elsewhere classified
Liver Diseases, Inflammatory, Other	
●K75.8	Other specified inflammatory liver diseases
●K75.81	Nonalcoholic steatohepatitis (NASH)

Continued on next page

● indicates a new code; ▲, revised; #, re-sequenced; ✚, add-on; ★, audiovisual technology; and ◀, synchronous interactive audio.

Quick Reference to 2026 *ICD-10-CM* Pediatric Code Changes (*continued*)	
Multiple Sclerosis	
●G35.A	Relapsing-remitting multiple sclerosis
●G35.B	Primary progressive multiple sclerosis
●G35.B0	Primary progressive multiple sclerosis, unspecified
●G35.B1	Active primary progressive multiple sclerosis
●G35.B2	Non-active primary progressive multiple sclerosis
●G35.C	Secondary progressive multiple sclerosis
●G35.C0	Secondary progressive multiple sclerosis, unspecified
●G35.C1	Active secondary progressive multiple sclerosis
●G35.C2	Non-active secondary progressive multiple sclerosis
●G35.D	Multiple sclerosis, unspecified
Muscular Dystrophy	
●G71.036	Limb girdle muscular dystrophy due to fukutin related protein dysfunction
Neonatal Hearing Screening	
▲P09.6	Abnormal findings on neonatal hearing screening
Nutritional Anemias, Other	
●D53.8	Other specified nutritional anemias
Open Wound, Flank, With Penetration Into Peritoneal Cavity	
●S31.606-	Unspecified open wound of abdominal wall, right flank with penetration into peritoneal cavity
●S31.607-	Unspecified open wound of abdominal wall, left flank with penetration into peritoneal cavity
●S31.60A-	Unspecified open wound of abdominal wall, unspecified flank with penetration into peritoneal cavity
Open Wound, Flank, Without Penetration Into Peritoneal Cavity	
●S31.106-	Unspecified open wound of abdominal wall, right flank without penetration into peritoneal cavity
●S31.107-	Unspecified open wound of abdominal wall, left flank without penetration into peritoneal cavity
●S31.10A-	Unspecified open wound of abdominal wall, unspecified flank without penetration into peritoneal cavity
Pelvic and Perineal Pain	
●R10.20	Pelvic and perineal pain unspecified side
●R10.21	Pelvic and perineal pain right side
●R10.22	Pelvic and perineal pain left side
●R10.23	Pelvic and perineal pain bilateral
●R10.24	Suprapubic pain
Pulmonary Heart Diseases, Other Specified	
●I27.89	Other specified pulmonary heart diseases
Puncture Wound, Flank, With Foreign Body, With Penetration Into Peritoneal Cavity	
●S31.646-	Puncture wound of abdominal wall with foreign body, right flank with penetration into peritoneal cavity
●S31.647-	Puncture wound of abdominal wall with foreign body, left flank with penetration into peritoneal cavity
●S31.64A-	Puncture wound of abdominal wall with foreign body, unspecified flank with penetration into peritoneal cavity
Puncture Wound, Flank, With Foreign Body, Without Penetration Into Peritoneal Cavity	
●S31.146-	Puncture wound of abdominal wall with foreign body, right flank without penetration into peritoneal cavity
●S31.147-	Puncture wound of abdominal wall with foreign body, left flank without penetration into peritoneal cavity
●S31.14A-	Puncture wound of abdominal wall with foreign body, unspecified flank without penetration into peritoneal cavity

• indicates a new code; ▲, revised; #, re-sequenced; ✚, add-on; ★, audiovisual technology; and ◀, synchronous interactive audio.

Quick Reference to 2026 *ICD-10-CM* Pediatric Code Changes (*continued*)	
Puncture Wound, Flank, Without Foreign Body, With Penetration Into Peritoneal Cavity	
●**S31.636-**	Puncture wound of abdominal wall without foreign body, right flank with penetration into peritoneal cavity
●**S31.637-**	Puncture wound of abdominal wall without foreign body, left flank with penetration into peritoneal cavity
●**S31.63A-**	Puncture wound of abdominal wall without foreign body, unspecified flank with penetration into peritoneal cavity
Puncture Wound, Flank, Without Foreign Body, Without Penetration Into Peritoneal Cavity	
●**S31.136-**	Puncture wound of abdominal wall without foreign body, right flank without penetration into peritoneal cavity
●**S31.137-**	Puncture wound of abdominal wall without foreign body, left flank without penetration into peritoneal cavity
●**S31.13A-**	Puncture wound of abdominal wall without foreign body, unspecified flank without penetration into peritoneal cavity

● indicates a new code; ▲, revised; #, re-sequenced; ✚, add-on; ★, audiovisual technology; and ◀, synchronous interactive audio.

II. Test Your Knowledge! Answer Key

Chapter 1

1. ***a.*** *CPT* is used for reporting most professional services, immunizations, and performance measurement tracking.
2. ***b.*** An *Excludes1* note indicates codes for conditions that would not occur in conjunction with the code category in which the note is found.
3. ***d.*** Unspecified codes are valid *ICD-10-CM* codes used to report conditions for which a more specific diagnosis has not yet been determined and/or when testing to determine a more specific diagnosis would not be medically necessary.
4. ***b.*** To differentiate discussion of *CPT* and HCPCS Level II codes, the abbreviation HCPCS is typically used in reference to Level II codes unless otherwise stated. HCPCS Level I codes are more commonly called *CPT* codes.
5. ***c.*** Up to 4 diagnosis fields may be linked to a service line. A diagnosis pointer in field 24E indicates which diagnosis codes relate to each service line by indicating the letter(s) of the related diagnosis field. The diagnosis code may be the same or different for each service performed.

Chapter 2

1. ***b.*** The 1 indicator is assigned to a code pair for which an appropriate modifier may be used to override the edit.
2. ***d.*** Modifier **22** is appended only to anesthesia, surgery, radiology, laboratory, pathology, and medicine codes.
3. ***c.*** The units of service provided were clinically indicated and exceed the MUE for the procedure. Modifier **59** is not applicable when procedures are performed bilaterally, in conjunction with an E/M service, or when another modifier better describes the reason for separately reporting a service (eg, anatomical modifier).
4. ***c.*** Modifier **63** is appropriately reported only when procedures or services described by codes listed in the *CPT* description of modifier **63** are provided to a neonate or infant with a present body weight of 4 kg or less. Codes in *CPT* Appendix F are not reported with modifier **63**.
5. ***b.*** Payer policies may require use of anatomical modifiers even when reporting a single procedure and despite site identification that may be included in a reported *ICD-10-CM* code. The anatomical modifiers are designated as appropriate modifiers under NCCI edits and may be reported as alternatives to or in conjunction with modifier **59** (distinct procedure).

Chapter 3

1. ***b.*** Category II codes were developed and are used by physicians and hospitals to report performance measures and certain aspects of care not yet included in performance measures. Category II codes are intended for reporting purposes only and are reported in addition to and not in place of Category I *CPT* codes.
2. ***a.*** Payers may use physician- or practice-level data to determine qualifications for incentive programs that pay greater than FFS revenue (eg, pay-for-performance or a quality bonus) when care that aligns with quality measures is performed, documented, and appropriately reported. Employed physicians may also earn bonuses based on meeting the organization's quality measurement goals.
3. ***c.*** Health plans may provide more specific documentation and coding guidance for reporting quality and performance measures.
4. ***c.*** Eight visits are included in the well-child visits in the first 30 months of life: 6 prior to turning 15 months old and 2 prior to turning 30 months old.
5. ***b.*** False. Codes for patient or caregiver immunization refusal do not exclude a patient from the population for immunization measures.

Chapter 4

1. ***d.*** Pediatricians can recommend values for services to the CMS by participation in AAP surveys conducted through the AMA/RUC. AAP staff sends out requests for participation to AAP section members to allow completion by physicians who most typically perform the service being surveyed.
2. ***a.*** Physician payments in value-based care arrangements may be based on a combination of FFS and alternative payment methodologies. Physicians and QHPs in smaller practices may enter into a contract to participate in a network or an organization with other physician practices, and sometimes hospitals or health care systems, that offer support for demonstrating lower cost and higher value.
3. ***b.*** Physicians should not sign contracts without reading and considering the impact of entering into the contractual agreement. Fee schedules, tiering, and allowances for billing patients for non-covered services will vary across payers and plans.
4. ***a.*** The physician must have the ability to fully describe patient diagnoses for each encounter (ie, not to merely select a diagnosis code). Code descriptors may be generalized and do not capture the physician's differential diagnoses, and many codes do not indicate when a condition is worsening or poorly controlled.

Continued on next page

5. ***d.*** All of the above are true. Physicians can reject contract terms requiring payment by credit card that may result in processing fees. Health plans must provide payment in compliance with HIPAA's electronic fund transfer standards rather than virtual card or wire transfer when requested by a physician.

Chapter 5

1. ***d.*** Both A and B. The Civil Monetary Penalties law authorizes the HHS to impose civil money penalties on and/or exclude from the Medicare and Medicaid programs physicians who commit various forms of fraud and abuse involving Medicare and Medicaid.
2. ***a.*** A key aspect is that the organization exercises due diligence to prevent and detect criminal conduct and promotes a culture that encourages ethical conduct and a commitment to compliance with the law.
3. ***b.*** Do not allow cut-and-paste functionality in the EHR. Any use of copy and paste, copy forward, macros, or auto-population should be regulated by office policies that address maintenance of record integrity and supplementation via free text, where indicated.
4. ***c.*** Use of internal audits to identify and correct errors shows a good-faith effort to be compliant.
5. ***d.*** Reply in writing to inform the carrier that you are willing to work with it and to ask that it identify each of the claims in question as well as the specific criteria or standards it is applying to the audit.

Chapter 6

1. ***c.*** The categorization of new and established patients influences coding for office or other outpatient E/M services (new patient, **99202–99205**; established patient, **99211–99215**). No distinction is made between new and established patients for ED services, for consultations, or for observation, inpatient, or nursing facility care.
2. ***b.*** False. When an E/M service is caused or prompted by the symptoms or condition for which another diagnostic or therapeutic service (eg, ECG, injection of medication, surgery) is provided on the same date, different diagnoses are not required for reporting the 2 services on the same date.
3. ***d.*** Time is the physician's and/or QHP's total time on the date of service, not their time in a 24-hour period.
4. ***d.*** When a test with multiple components can be reported with a single code (eg, **80047**, basic metabolic panel or a test with a specific number of images), count the test once for the purpose of data to be reviewed and analyzed.
5. ***a.*** To select a code for E/M services based on MDM, you must determine which code is supported by 2 of 3 elements of MDM.

Chapter 7

1. ***d.*** **G2211** is reported in addition to an office E/M code appended with modifier **25** only when reporting certain preventive services (eg, immunization administration, **90460–90461**) on the same date. Do not report **G2211** in addition to an office E/M code appended with modifier **25** when reporting other diagnostic or therapeutic services (eg, medication administration) on the same date.
2. ***a.*** True. Under Medicare's incident-to policy, code **99211** may be reported for services provided by clinical staff to established patients under the direct supervision of a physician or QHP who is either in the office suite or immediately available via real-time audio-video technology at the time of service.
3. ***b.*** The total time included in the code descriptor must be met or exceeded and includes only the physician's or QHP's total time devoted the patient's care on the date of the visit.
4. ***a.*** The straightforward MDM supports a new patient service reported with **99202**. It is not necessary to also meet or exceed the total time included in the code descriptor.
5. ***c.*** The office E/M code selected by the physician or QHP, based on MDM or total time, and the total face-to-face clinical staff time are necessary to determine if the time requirement for **99415** has been met. The starting point for **99415** is 30 minutes beyond the typical clinical staff time that is included in the value assigned to the office or other outpatient E/M code reported.

Chapter 8

1. ***b.*** Codes **90460–90461** and **96380** require counseling by a physician or other QHP. Counseling is not required to support codes **90471–90474** or **90480**, although counseling is included in code **90480**, when provided.
2. ***d.*** Report code **90482** for *at least 3 minutes* of counseling for one or more immunizations that are not administered in the physician's or QHP's practice on the date of counseling. Code **90482** includes up to 10 minutes of counseling. For more than 10 minutes of counseling, see **90483** or **90484**.
3. ***b.*** False. Codes **90482–90484** may be reported when immunization counseling is provided for multiple immunizations and some, but not all, immunizations are administered. Do not include the time spent counseling for administered immunizations (reported with any IA code) in the time reported with codes **90482–90484**.

4. ***a.*** The appropriate *ICD-10-CM* code for the infant's routine child health examination (eg, **Z00.129**) is reported in conjunction with **96161**. Depression screening codes (**Z13.31** or **Z13.32**) are not appropriate for maternal screening for the benefit of the infant.
5. ***a.*** Behavior change interventions involve validated interventions provided to either a new or an established patient who has a behavior that is often considered an illness itself. Specific time requirements are included in the code descriptors, so the midpoint rule is not applicable to **99406–99408**.

Chapter 9

1. ***b.*** CCM is reported by a physician or QHP who provides or oversees the management and/or coordination of services, as needed, for all the patient's health care needs.
2. ***d.*** PCM services require development, monitoring, or revision of disease-specific care plan for a patient.
3. ***a.*** Complex CCM requires at least 60 minutes of clinical staff time and moderate or high MDM.
4. ***b.*** On a date when no other E/M service is furnished to the patient, the treating/requesting physician or QHP who spends 16 to 30 minutes preparing for the referral and/or communicating with the consultant may report the service with **99452**.
5. ***b.*** False. Indirect prolonged services may be reported in relation to any level or category of E/M service that was or will be provided on another date of service regardless of whether time was used to select the level of the face-to-face service.

Chapter 10

1. ***b.*** *Nonphysician qualified health care professional* is used to describe professionals (eg, licensed clinical psychologists and licensed clinical social workers) who may provide and independently report non-E/M services as allowed by state regulations and payer policy.
2. ***d.*** Psychiatric collaborative care management (**99492–99494**) represent services provided by a team that includes 3 distinct roles: a treating physician or QHP, BHCM, and psychiatric consultant.
3. ***c.*** Report testing evaluation services according to the face-to-face time with the patient and the time spent integrating and interpreting data. A minimum of 31 minutes must be provided to report a 1-hour unit of service. Time spent by technicians (eg, in test administration and scoring) is not included.
4. ***b.*** Health and behavior assessment and intervention procedures (**96156**, **96158**, **96159**, and **96164–96171**) are provided by NQHCPs who cannot report E/M services but can independently provide and report assessment and intervention procedures. Physicians and QHPs who can provide and report E/M services do not report these codes.
5. ***d.*** Although family members may act as informants during individual psychotherapy, psychotherapy using family psychotherapy techniques is reported with **90846** or **90847** depending on whether the patient is present for the service. When multiple families participate in family psychotherapy at the same session, **90849** is reported once for each family.

Chapter 11

1. ***c.*** None. Modifiers **26** and **TC** are not appended because **93010** designate that only the professional component (interpretation and report) was provided. Codes **93000** and **93005** are used to report the global service or technical component, respectively. A reduced service modifier **52** is not indicated because the full service was completed.
2. ***d.*** Report collection of blood samples for testing (eg, venipuncture) in a physician practice regardless of whether the laboratory test is performed in the office or at an outside facility. Other specimen collection (eg, nasal or oral swab, urine collection) is typically not separately reported. Code **51701** is reported when a non-indwelling bladder catheter (straight catheterization) is inserted for a urine culture collection.
3. ***d.*** Laboratories and physician offices performing waived tests should append modifier **QW** to the *CPT* code for CLIA-waived procedures. Only a small number of CLIA-waived tests are exempt from use of modifier **QW** (eg, **81002**, non-automated urinalysis without microscopy; **81025**, urine pregnancy test; **82272**, occult blood by peroxidase for other than colorectal neoplasm screening).
4. ***c.*** Codes for proprietary laboratory analyses or multianalyte assays with algorithmic analyses are selected on the basis of the analysis performed and the proprietary name of the test.
5. ***d.*** All of the above. The physician's or QHP's analysis of test results that do not require interpretation and report is part of an E/M service. Time spent providing a separately reported testing service does not contribute to the total time of an E/M service. Modifier **25** may be required on the E/M service to indicate the service was significant and is separately identifiable in the documentation.

Chapter 12

1. *a.* Scope of practice is used to define the procedures, actions, and processes that are permitted for a licensed individual. Scope of practice may also address the delegation of health care activities to unlicensed individuals who the delegating physician or other QHP/NQHCP has ascertained have the education, training, and/or certification necessary to safely perform the activity.
2. *b.* Online medical assessment and management (**98970–98972**) are independently provided and reported by NQHCPs. NQHCPs typically have a scope of practice that does not include independent provision and reporting of evaluation and management services.
3. *d.* The cumulative time is used in code selection for the online assessment and management services. One code and 1 unit of service are reported for the sum of communications pertaining to the online encounter during a 7-day period.
4. *a.* True. Lactation consultation services do not have a specific *CPT* code. HCPCS code **S9443** is the code most specific to lactation services.
5. *a.* A standardized curriculum is used, and the time-based services are prescribed by a physician or QHP.

Chapter 13

1. *a.* For minor procedures, separate payment for a significant, separately identifiable E/M service may be allowed when modifier **25** is appended to the E/M code.
2. *d.* Codes **15853** and **15854** are add-on codes reported when sutures and/or staples are removed without anesthesia at a follow-up E/M service to a procedure with a 0-day global period.
3. *d.* Removal of an umbilical clamp is one of several services that are included in an E/M service and not separately reported.
4. *a.* If multiple wounds belong to the same category of difficulty and location, add the lengths and report with a single code. If multiple wounds do not belong in the same category, report each repair separately.
5. *c.* Intravenous infusion for hydration, **96360**, may be reported for hydration infusion lasting longer than 31 minutes and up to 1 hour. But subsequent code **96361** is reported if an IV hydration infusion is provided secondary or subsequent to a therapeutic, prophylactic, or diagnostic infusion.

Chapter 14

1. *a.* When multiple symptoms are listed as chief complaints during the ED triage process, the physician needs to designate only 1 sign, symptom, disease, or injury as the chief complaint (principal reason for the visit). This diagnosis is used to help support the urgency of the ED visit under prudent layperson guidelines as well as support resource utilization.
2. *d.* Report one of the following codes from category **Z04** for an encounter at which neglect, abuse, or exploitation is suspected but ruled out. However, report codes for the problems addressed in lieu of a category **Z04** code when maltreatment is ruled out but problems are addressed.
3. *c.* The physician's dated and timed order for observation status is the starting point of the observation service.
4. *d.* All of the above. A physician or QHP providing ED care does not report a procedure that is performed by hospital personnel under general supervision or the global or technical component code for services that include use of hospital equipment. However, the professional component, such as interpretation and report of radiographic findings, may be reported by appending modifier **26** [professional component] to the procedure code.
5. *c.* *CPT* instructs that **99292** be reported in conjunction with **99291** when critical care time extends *up to 30 minutes* beyond the first 74 minutes and for each additional period of up to 30 minutes. Report 1 unit of **99292** for critical care time of 75 to 104 minutes and then an additional unit for each additional period of up to 30 minutes.

Chapter 15

1. *a.* True. For *ICD-10-CM* and *CPT* coding purposes, the day of birth is day zero (0) of life and the next day is day 1. Monday is day 1 of life for the newborn delivered on Sunday.
2. *d.* Perinatal conditions are considered clinically significant if the condition has implications for future health care needs or any of the clinical indications for reporting codes from other chapters (ie, requires clinical evaluation, therapeutic treatment, diagnostic procedures, extended hospital stay, or increased nursing care or monitoring).
3. *b.* A single normal newborn care code is reported. Codes **99460–99463** are reported once per date of service regardless of the number of visits or time spent.
4. *d.* **99026** (hospital-mandated on-call service; in hospital, each hour) is reported in addition to the initial hospital care of the normal newborn (**99460**). Attendance at delivery (**99464**) is not reported when hospital-mandated attendance is the only basis for providing the service.

5. *c.* If the circumcision with a clamp or other device is performed without dorsal penile or ring block, append modifier **52** (reduced services) to **54150**.

Chapter 16

1. *b.* False. Admission orders should distinctly designate the patient's admission status, including transitions from observation to inpatient status, as this may be important for payer coverage and payment rates.
2. *c.* The service is a subsequent service because the patient has received professional service(s) from another physician or QHP of the exact same specialty and subspecialty who belongs to the same group practice on a prior date during the current admission and stay.
3. *b.* Only initial hospital inpatient or observation service codes **99221–99223** are reported for initial hospital care and discharge services provided at a single visit.
4. *a.* *CPT* defines consultations as *initial encounters* provided by a physician or QHP at the request of another physician, QHP, or appropriate source *to recommend care for a specific condition or problem.* Subsequent visits are reported with codes for subsequent hospital care (**99231–99233**).
5. *c.* Code **99418** is used to report prolonged total time that exceeds the minimum total time of the highest level of service in the code category (eg, **99223**) *by no less than 15 minutes.* The code for the primary E/M service must be selected on the basis of time, and only time spent on the date of the encounter is included in the total time.

Chapter 17

1. *a.* Positive pressure ventilation, delivered by any means (resuscitation bag or T-piece resuscitator), and/or cardiac compressions are required for **99465**.
2. *a.* True. Only 1 initial daily inpatient critical care code (**99468**, **99471**, **99475**) is reported per calendar day and *per hospital stay* for a given patient.
3. *b.* Report only initial or subsequent critical care (**99468–99469**), according to whether this is the first or subsequent episode of neonatal critical care during the same hospital stay when the neonate becomes critically ill on a day when initial or subsequent intensive care services (**99477–99480**) have been provided by the same physician(s) or QHP(s) from the same group practice.
4. *b.* Subsequent intensive care services (**99478–99480**) are differentiated by the infant's weight in grams on the date of service.
5. *b.* Codes **33946–33949** include managing the ECMO or ECLS circuit and related patient issues.

Chapter 18

1. *c.* All additional medical or surgical services required of the surgeon during the postoperative period of the surgery to address complications *that do not require additional trips to the OR* are included in the global package (not separately reported) under Medicare policy.
2. *b.* Stabilization (eg, temporary cast/splint/strap) that is performed to protect an injury and provide comfort to the patient until another physician performs initial fracture or dislocation care is reported with the appropriate E/M and casting/splinting/strapping codes.
3. *b.* False. There is no age limit for cardiac catheterization for congenital heart defect (**93593–93598**). If there is evaluation of congenital cardiac defects, it is appropriate to report these codes.
4. *c.* When an existing central venous access device is removed and a new one placed via a separate venous access site, appropriate codes for both procedures (removal of old, if code exists, and insertion of new device) should be reported. Refer to replacement codes for removal with replacement via the same venous access site.
5. *d.* Excision or repair of strangulated organs or structures (eg, **44120**, enterectomy, resection of small intestine; single resection and anastomosis) is reported in addition to the repair of a strangulated hernia.

Chapter 19

1. *b.* False. Synchronous communication occurs in real-time. Email correspondence is an example of asynchronous communication.
2. *d.* All of the above. Documentation elements specific to telemedicine services include consent to receive the service via telemedicine, platform or modality used, and patient and physician locations. Additional documentation may include individuals present with the patient, time of service, and any digital technology used (eg, digital otoscope).
3. *c.* Modifier **95** is 1 of 2 telemedicine modifiers found in *CPT.* Answers a and b (**02** and **10**) are POS codes.
4. *a.* HCPCS codes **G0508** and **G0509** most specifically describe critical care services when provided via telemedicine. *CPT* instructs to report unlisted E/M service code **99499** for critical care provided via telemedicine.
5. *b.* The service is reported using the code for the type of telemedicine service by which most of the service was provided.

Chapter 20

1. *a.* True. Telemedicine codes **98000–98015** may be selected according to either level of MDM or total time on the date of the encounter.
2. *a.* Codes **98000–98007** do not require a specific time interval from the last in-person or telemedicine visit. Codes **98004–98007** are reported for established patient synchronous audio-video visits.
3. *c.* Code **98012** is supported by greater than 10 minutes of medical discussion in combination with total time exceeding 10 minutes.
4. *b.* Report **99417** (prolonged outpatient E/M service) appended with modifier **95** × 1 unit for 20 minutes of prolonged service. Report 1 unit of **99417 95** for each full 15-minute period beyond the total time of the primary service (ie, **98003** or **98007** selected on the basis of total time).
5. *b.* Code **98016** is reported for a service that is initiated by the established patient and/or parent or caregiver and that includes at least 5 and up to 10 minutes of medical discussion.

Chapter 21

1. *c.* *CPT* Appendix R is a digital medicine taxonomy table for quickly identifying and differentiating digital medicine services, including clinical data monitoring services.
2. *b.* Code **99091** represents a 30-day episode of care.
3. *a.* The supplier of the equipment (patient or physician office) determines code selection for the sensor placement, hook-up, calibration of monitor, patient training, and printout of recording **95250** and **95249**.
4. *d.* **99470** and **99457** include time spent in a calendar month monitoring, analyzing, and using the results of transmitted physiologic data to treat a patient under a specific treatment plan. At least 1 interactive communication with the patient/caregiver is required in the calendar month of service.
5. *d.* All of the above are correct. The remote therapeutic monitoring treatment management services require a minimum of 10 minutes of a physician's, QHP's, or NQHCP's time in a calendar month and 1 real-time interactive communication, and only 1 initial service is reported per calendar month.

Subject Index

A

B

C

Q

R

S

Subject Index

Code Index

References are to pages. **Boldface** page numbers indicate the pages on which the primary code descriptions reside. *Current Procedural Terminology* (*CPT®*) codes begin on this page; *International Classification of Diseases, 10th Revision, Clinical Modification (ICD-10-CM)* codes begin on page 576; Healthcare Common Procedure Coding System (HCPCS) codes begin on page 579; and modifiers begin on page 580.

CPT Codes

ICD-10-CM Codes

HCPCS Codes

Modifiers

American Academy of Pediatrics
DEDICATED TO THE HEALTH OF ALL CHILDREN®

Recommendations for Preventive Pediatric Health Care

Bright Futures/American Academy of Pediatrics

Bright Futures. prevention and health promotion for infants, children, adolescents, and their families™

Each child and family is unique; therefore, these Recommendations for Preventive Pediatric Health Care are designed for the care of children who are receiving nurturing parenting, have no manifestations of any important health problems, and are growing and developing in a satisfactory fashion. Developmental, psychosocial, and chronic disease issues for children and adolescents may require more frequent counseling and treatment visits separate from preventive care visits. Additional visits also may become necessary if circumstances suggest concerns.

These recommendations represent a consensus by the American Academy of Pediatrics (AAP) and Bright Futures. The AAP continues to emphasize the great importance of continuity of care in comprehensive health supervision and the need to avoid fragmentation of care.

Refer to the specific guidance by age as listed in the *Bright Futures Guidelines* (Hagan JF, Shaw JS, Duncan PM, eds. *Bright Futures: Guidelines for Health Supervision of Infants, Children, and Adolescents.* 4th ed. American Academy of Pediatrics; 2017).

The recommendations in this statement do not indicate an exclusive course of treatment or serve as a standard of medical care. Variations, taking into account individual circumstances, may be appropriate.

The Bright Futures/American Academy of Pediatrics Recommendations for Preventive Pediatric Health Care are updated annually.

	INFANCY								EARLY CHILDHOOD							MIDDLE CHILDHOOD						ADOLESCENCE										
AGE[1]	Prenatal[2]	Newborn[3]	3-5 d[4]	By 1 mo	2 mo	4 mo	6 mo	9 mo	12 mo	15 mo	18 mo	24 mo	30 mo	3 y	4 y	5 y	6 y	7 y	8 y	9 y	10 y	11 y	12 y	13 y	14 y	15 y	16 y	17 y	18 y	19 y	20 y	21 y
HISTORY Initial/Interval	●	●	●	●	●	●	●	●	●	●	●	●	●	●	●	●	●	●	●	●	●	●	●	●	●	●	●	●	●	●	●	●
MEASUREMENTS																																
Length/Height and Weight		●	●	●	●	●	●	●	●	●	●	●	●	●	●	●	●	●	●	●	●	●	●	●	●	●	●	●	●	●	●	●
Head Circumference		●	●	●	●	●	●	●	●	●	●	●																				
Weight for Length		●	●	●	●	●	●	●	●	●	●																					
Body Mass Index[5]												●	●	●	●	●	●	●	●	●	●	●	●	●	●	●	●	●	●	●	●	●
Blood Pressure[6]		★	★	★	★	★	★	★	★	★	★	★	★	●	●	●	●	●	●	●	●	●	●	●	●	●	●	●	●	●	●	●
SENSORY SCREENING																																
Vision[7]		★	★	★	★	★	★	★	★	★	★	★	★	●	●	●	●	★	●	★	●	★	●	★	★	●	★	★	★	★	★	★
Hearing		●[8]	●[9]	—	→	★	★	★	★	★	★	★	★	★	●	●	●	★	●	★	●	←	—	●[10]	→	←	●	→	←	—	●	→
DEVELOPMENTAL/SOCIAL/BEHAVIORAL/MENTAL HEALTH																																
Maternal Depression Screening[11]				●	●	●	●																									
Developmental Screening[12]								●			●		●																			
Autism Spectrum Disorder Screening[13]											●	●																				
Developmental Surveillance		●	●	●	●	●	●		●	●		●		●	●	●	●	●	●	●	●	●	●	●	●	●	●	●	●	●	●	●
Behavioral/Social/Emotional Screening[14]		●	●	●	●	●	●	●	●	●	●	●	●	●	●	●	●	●	●	●	●	●	●	●	●	●	●	●	●	●	●	●
Tobacco, Alcohol, or Drug Use Assessment[15]																						★	★	★	★	★	★	★	★	★	★	★
Depression and Suicide Risk Screening[16]																							●	●	●	●	●	●	●	●	●	●
PHYSICAL EXAMINATION[17]		●	●	●	●	●	●	●	●	●	●	●	●	●	●	●	●	●	●	●	●	●	●	●	●	●	●	●	●	●	●	●
PROCEDURES[18]																																
Newborn Blood		●[19]	●[20]	—	→																											
Newborn Bilirubin[21]		●																														
Critical Congenital Heart Defect[22]		●																														
Immunization[23]		●	●	●	●	●	●	●	●	●	●	●	●	●	●	●	●	●	●	●	●	●	●	●	●	●	●	●	●	●	●	●
Anemia[24]						★			●	★	★	★	★	★	★	★	★	★	★	★	★	★	★	★	★	★	★	★	★	★	★	★
Lead[25]							★	★	● or ★[26]		★	● or ★[26]		★	★	★	★															
Tuberculosis[27]				★			★		★			★		★	★	★	★	★	★	★	★	★	★	★	★	★	★	★	★	★	★	★
Dyslipidemia[28]												★			★		★		★	←	●	→	★	★	★	★	★	←	—	—	●	→
Sexually Transmitted Infections[29]																						★	★	★	★	★	★	★	★	★	★	★
HIV[30]																						★	★	★	★	●	—	—	—	—	—	→
Hepatitis B Virus Infection[31]		★	—	—	—	—	—	—	—	—	—	—	—	—	—	—	—	—	—	—	—	—	—	—	—	—	—	—	—	—	—	→
Hepatitis C Virus Infection[32]																													●	—	—	→
Sudden Cardiac Arrest/Death[33]																						★	—	—	—	—	—	—	—	—	—	→
Cervical Dysplasia[34]																																●
ORAL HEALTH[35]							●[36]	●[36]	★		★	★	★	★	★	★	★															
Fluoride Varnish[37]							←	—	—	—	●	—	—	—	—	→																
Fluoride Supplementation[38]							★	★	★		★	★	★	★	★	★	★	★	★	★	★	★	★	★	★	★	★					
ANTICIPATORY GUIDANCE	●	●	●	●	●	●	●	●	●	●	●	●	●	●	●	●	●	●	●	●	●	●	●	●	●	●	●	●	●	●	●	●

1. If a child comes under care for the first time at any point on the schedule, or if any items are not accomplished at the suggested age, the schedule should be brought up to date at the earliest possible time.
2. A prenatal visit is recommended for parents who are at high risk, for first-time parents, and for those who request a conference. The prenatal visit should include anticipatory guidance, pertinent medical history, and a discussion of benefits of breastfeeding and planned method of feeding, per "The Prenatal Visit" (https://doi.org/10.1542/peds.2018-1218).
3. Newborns should have an evaluation after birth, and breastfeeding should be encouraged (and instruction and support should be offered).
4. Newborns should have an evaluation within 3 to 5 days of birth and within 48 to 72 hours after discharge from the hospital to include evaluation for feeding and jaundice. Breastfeeding newborns should receive formal breastfeeding evaluation, and their mothers should receive encouragement and instruction, as recommended in "Policy Statement: Breastfeeding and the Use of Human Milk" (https://doi.org/10.1542/peds.2022-057988). Newborns discharged less than 48 hours after delivery must be examined within 48 hours of discharge, per "Hospital Stay for Healthy Term Newborn Infants" (https://doi.org/10.1542/peds.2015-0699).
5. Screen, per "Clinical Practice Guideline for the Evaluation and Treatment of Children and Adolescents with Obesity" (https://doi.org/10.1542/peds.2022-060640).
6. Screening should occur per "Clinical Practice Guideline for Screening and Management of High Blood Pressure in Children and Adolescents" (https://doi.org/10.1542/peds.2017-1904). Blood pressure measurement in infants and children with specific risk conditions should be performed at visits before age 3 years.
7. A visual acuity screen is recommended at ages 4 and 5 years, as well as in cooperative 3-year-olds. Instrument-based screening may be used to assess risk at ages 12 and 24 months, in addition to the well visits at 3 through 5 years of age. See "Visual System Assessment in Infants, Children, and Young Adults by Pediatricians" (https://doi.org/10.1542/peds.2015-3596) and "Procedures for the Evaluation of the Visual System by Pediatricians" (https://doi.org/10.1542/peds.2015-3597).
8. Confirm initial screen was completed, verify results, and follow up, as appropriate. Newborns should be screened, per "Year 2007 Position Statement: Principles and Guidelines for Early Hearing Detection and Intervention Programs" (https://doi.org/10.1542/peds.2007-2333).
9. Verify results as soon as possible, and follow up, as appropriate.
10. Screen with audiometry including 6,000 and 8,000 Hz high frequencies once between 11 and 14 years, once between 15 and 17 years, and once between 18 and 21 years. See "The Sensitivity of Adolescent Hearing Screens Significantly Improves by Adding High Frequencies" (https://www.sciencedirect.com/science/article/abs/pii/S1054139X16000483).
11. Screening should occur per "Incorporating Recognition and Management of Perinatal Depression Into Pediatric Practice" (https://doi.org/10.1542/peds.2018-3259).
12. Screening should occur per "Promoting Optimal Development: Identifying Infants and Young Children With Developmental Disorders Through Developmental Surveillance and Screening" (https://doi.org/10.1542/peds.2019-3449).
13. Screening should occur per "Identification, Evaluation, and Management of Children With Autism Spectrum Disorder" (https://doi.org/10.1542/peds.2019-3447).

(continued)

KEY: ● = to be performed ★ = risk assessment to be performed with appropriate action to follow, if positive ←—— ★ or ● ——→ = range during which a service may be provided

BFNC.2025.PSMAR
3-372/0325

(continued)

14. Screen for behavioral and social-emotional problems per "Promoting Optimal Development: Screening for Behavioral and Emotional Problems" (https://doi.org/10.1542/peds.2014-3716), "Mental Health Competencies for Pediatric Practice" (https://doi.org/10.1542/peds.2019-2757), "Clinical Practice Guideline for the Assessment and Treatment of Children and Adolescents With Anxiety Disorders" (https://pubmed.ncbi.nlm.nih.gov/32439401), "Screening for Anxiety in Adolescent and Adult Women: A Recommendation From the Women's Preventive Services Initiative" (https://pubmed.ncbi.nlm.nih.gov/32510990), and "Anxiety in Children and Adolescents: Screening" (https://www.uspreventiveservicestaskforce.org/uspstf/recommendation/screening-anxiety-children-adolescents). The screening should be family centered and may include asking about caregiver emotional and mental health concerns and social determinants of health, racism, poverty, and relational health. See "Poverty and Child Health in the United States" (https://doi.org/10.1542/peds.2016-0339), "The Impact of Racism on Child and Adolescent Health" (https://doi.org/10.1542/peds.2019-1765), and "Preventing Childhood Toxic Stress: Partnering With Families and Communities to Promote Relational Health" (https://doi.org/10.1542/peds.2021-052582).
15. A recommended tool to assess use of alcohol, tobacco and nicotine, marijuana, and other substances, including opioids is available at http://crafft.org. If there is a concern for substance or opioid use, providers should consider recommending or prescribing Naloxone (see https://www.cdc.gov/ore/search/pages/2018-evidence-based-strategies.html and https://nida.nih.gov/publications/drugfacts/naloxone).
16. Screen adolescents for depression and suicide risk, making every effort to preserve confidentiality of the adolescent. See "Guidelines for Adolescent Depression in Primary Care (GLAD-PC): Part I. Practice Preparation, Identification, Assessment, and Initial Management" (https://doi.org/10.1542/peds.2017-4081), "Mental Health Competencies for Pediatric Practice" (https://doi.org/10.1542/peds.2019-2757), "Suicide and Suicide Attempts in Adolescents" (https://doi.org/10.1542/peds.2016-1420), and "The 21st Century Cures Act & Adolescent Confidentiality" (https://adolescenthealth.org/press_release/naspag-sahm-statement-the-21st-century-cures-act-adolescent-confidentiality/).
17. At each visit, age-appropriate physical examination is essential, with infant totally unclothed and older children undressed and suitably draped. See "Use of Chaperones During the Physical Examination of the Pediatric Patient" (https://doi.org/10.1542/peds.2011-0322).
18. These may be modified, depending on entry point into schedule and individual need.
19. Confirm initial screen was accomplished, verify results, and follow up, as appropriate. The Recommended Uniform Screening Panel (https://www.hrsa.gov/advisory-committees/heritable-disorders/rusp/index.html), as determined by The Secretary's Advisory Committee on Heritable Disorders in Newborns and Children, and state newborn screening laws/regulations (https://www.babysfirsttest.org/) establish the criteria for and coverage of newborn screening procedures and programs.
20. Verify results as soon as possible, and follow up, as appropriate.
21. Confirm initial screening was accomplished, verify results, and follow up, as appropriate. See "Clinical Practice Guideline Revision: Management of Hyperbilirubinemia in the Newborn Infant 35 or More Weeks of Gestation" (https://doi.org/10.1542/peds.2022-058859).
22. Screening for critical congenital heart disease using pulse oximetry should be performed in newborns, after 24 hours of age, before discharge from the hospital, per "Endorsement of Health and Human Services Recommendation for Pulse Oximetry Screening for Critical Congenital Heart Disease" (https://doi.org/10.1542/peds.2011-3211).
23. Schedules, per the AAP Committee on Infectious Diseases, are available at https://publications.aap.org/redbook/pages/immunization-schedules. Every visit should be an opportunity to update and complete a child's immunizations.
24. Perform risk assessment or screening, as appropriate, per recommendations in the current edition of the AAP *Pediatric Nutrition: Policy of the American Academy of Pediatrics* (Iron chapter).
25. For children at risk of lead exposure, see "Prevention of Childhood Lead Toxicity" (https://doi.org/10.1542/peds.2016-1493) and "Low Level Lead Exposure Harms Children: A Renewed Call for Primary Prevention" (https://stacks.cdc.gov/view/cdc/11859).
26. Perform risk assessments or screenings as appropriate, based on universal screening requirements for patients with Medicaid or in high prevalence areas.
27. Tuberculosis testing per recommendations of the AAP Committee on Infectious Diseases, published in the current edition of the AAP *Red Book: Report of the Committee on Infectious Diseases*. Testing should be performed on recognition of high-risk factors.
28. See "Integrated Guidelines for Cardiovascular Health and Risk Reduction in Children and Adolescents" (http://www.nhlbi.nih.gov/guidelines/cvd_ped/index.htm).
29. Adolescents should be screened for sexually transmitted infections (STIs) per recommendations in the current edition of the AAP *Red Book: Report of the Committee on Infectious Diseases*.
30. Screen adolescents for HIV at least once between the ages of 15 and 21, making every effort to preserve confidentiality of the adolescent, as per "Human Immunodeficiency Virus (HIV) Infection: Screening" (https://www.uspreventiveservicestaskforce.org/uspstf/recommendation/human-immunodeficiency-virus-hiv-infection-screening); after initial screening, youth at increased risk of HIV infection should be retested annually or more frequently, as per "Adolescents and Young Adults: The Pediatrician's Role in HIV Testing and Pre- and Postexposure HIV Prophylaxis" (https://doi.org/10.1542/peds.2021-055207).
31. Perform a risk assessment for hepatitis B virus (HBV) infection according to recommendations per the USPSTF (https://www.uspreventiveservicestaskforce.org/uspstf/recommendation/hepatitis-b-virus-infection-screening) and in the 2021–2024 edition of the AAP *Red Book: Report of the Committee on Infectious Diseases*, making every effort to preserve confidentiality of the patient.
32. All individuals should be screened for hepatitis C virus (HCV) infection according to the USPSTF (https://www.uspreventiveservicestaskforce.org/uspstf/recommendation/hepatitis-c-screening) and Centers for Disease Control and Prevention (CDC) recommendations (https://www.cdc.gov/mmwr/volumes/69/rr/rr6902a1.htm) at least once between the ages of 18 and 79. Those at increased risk of HCV infection, including those who are persons with past or current injection drug use, should be tested for HCV infection and reassessed annually.
33. Perform a risk assessment, as appropriate, per "Sudden Death in the Young: Information for the Primary Care Provider" (https://doi.org/10.1542/peds.2021-052044).
34. See USPSTF recommendations (https://www.uspreventiveservicestaskforce.org/uspstf/recommendation/cervical-cancer-screening). Indications for pelvic examinations prior to age 21 are noted in "Gynecologic Examination for Adolescents in the Pediatric Office Setting" (https://doi.org/10.1542/peds.2010-1564).
35. Assess whether the child has a dental home. If no dental home is identified, perform a risk assessment (https://www.aap.org/en/patient-care/oral-health/oral-health-practice-tools/) and refer to a dental home. Recommend brushing with fluoride toothpaste in the proper dosage for age. See "Maintaining and Improving the Oral Health of Young Children" (https://doi.org/10.1542/peds.2022-060417).
36. Perform a risk assessment (https://www.aap.org/en/patient-care/oral-health/oral-health-practice-tools/). See "Maintaining and Improving the Oral Health of Young Children" (https://doi.org/10.1542/peds.2022-060417).
37. The USPSTF recommends that primary care clinicians apply fluoride varnish to the primary teeth of all infants and children starting at the age of primary tooth eruption (https://www.uspreventiveservicestaskforce.org/uspstf/recommendation/prevention-of-dental-caries-in-children-younger-than-age-5-years-screening-and-interventions1). Once teeth are present, apply fluoride varnish to all children every 3 to 6 months in the primary care or dental office based on caries risk. Indications for fluoride use are noted in "Fluoride Use in Caries Prevention in the Primary Care Setting" (https://doi.org/10.1542/peds.2020-034637).
38. If primary water source is deficient in fluoride, consider oral fluoride supplementation. See "Fluoride Use in Caries Prevention in the Primary Care Setting" (https://doi.org/10.1542/peds.2020-034637).

Summary of Changes Made to the Bright Futures/AAP Recommendations for Preventive Pediatric Health Care (Periodicity Schedule)

This schedule reflects recommendations approved in December 2024 and published in February 2025. For updates and a list of previous changes made, visit www.aap.org/periodicityschedule.

RECOMMENDATIONS APPROVED IN DECEMBER 2024

No changes have been made to clinical guidance or footnotes in the recommendations published in 2025.

HRSA
Health Resources & Services Administration
This program is supported by the Health Resources and Services Administration (HRSA) of the U.S. Department of Health and Human Services (HHS) as part of an award totaling $1,566,000 with 0% financed with non-governmental sources. The contents of this document are those of the author(s) and do not necessarily represent the official views of, nor an endorsement, by HRSA, HHS, or the U.S. Government. For more information, please visit HRSA.gov.